39

Springer Series in Chemical Physics

Edited by Fritz Peter Schäfer

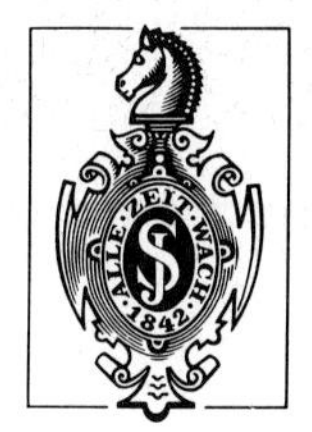

# Springer Series in Chemical Physics

Editors: V. I. Goldanskii R. Gomer F. P. Schäfer J. P. Toennies

1 **Atomic Spectra and Radiative Transitions** By I. I. Sobelman
2 **Surface Crystallography by LEED** Theory, Computation and Structural Results. By M. A. Van Hove, S. Y. Tong
3 **Advances in Laser Chemistry** Editor: A. H. Zewail
4 **Picosecond Phenomena** Editors: C. V. Shank, E. P. Ippen, S. L. Shapiro
5 **Laser Spectroscopy** Basic Concepts and Instrumentation By W. Demtröder 2nd Printing
6 **Laser-Induced Processes in Molecules** Physics and Chemistry Editors: K. L. Kompa, S. D. Smith
7 **Excitation of Atoms and Broadening of Spectral Lines** By I. I. Sobelman, L. A. Vainshtein, E. A. Yukov
8 **Spin Exchange** Principles and Applications in Chemistry and Biology By Yu. N. Molin, K. M. Salikhov, K. I. Zamaraev
9 **Secondary Ion Mass Spectrometry SIMS II** Editors: A. Benninghoven, C. A. Evans, Jr., R. A. Powell, R. Shimizu, H. A. Storms
10 **Lasers and Chemical Change** By A. Ben-Shaul, Y. Haas, K. L. Kompa, R. D. Levine
11 **Liquid Crystals of One- and Two-Dimensional Order** Editors: W. Helfrich, G. Heppke
12 **Gasdynamic Laser** By S. A. Losev
13 **Atomic Many-Body Theory** By I. Lindgren, J. Morrison
14 **Picosecond Phenomena II** Editors: R. M. Hochstrasser, W. Kaiser, C. V. Shank
15 **Vibrational Spectroscopy of Adsorbates** Editor: R. F. Willis
16 **Spectroscopy of Molecular Excitions** By V. L. Broude, E. I. Rashba, E. F. Sheka
17 **Inelastic Particle-Surface Collisions** Editors: E. Taglauer, W. Heiland
18 **Modelling of Chemical Reaction Systems** Editors: K. H. Ebert, P. Deuflhard, W. Jäger
19 **Secondary Ion Mass Spectrometry SIMS III** Editors: A. Benninghoven, J. Giber, J. László, M. Riedel, H. W. Werner
20 **Chemistry and Physics of Solid Surfaces IV** Editors: R. Vanselow, R. Howe
21 **Dynamics of Gas-Surface Interaction** Editors: G. Benedek, U. Valbusa
22 **Nonlinear Laser Chemistry** Multiple-Photon Excitation By V. S. Letokhov
23 **Picosecond Phenomena III** Editors: K. B. Eisenthal, R. M. Hochstrasser, W. Kaiser, A. Laubereau
24 **Desorption Induced by Electronic Transitions DIET I** Editors: N. H. Tolk, M. M. Traum, J. C. Tully, T. E. Madey
25 **Ion Formation from Organic Solids** Editor: A. Benninghoven
26 **Semiclassical Theories of Molecular Scattering** By B. C. Eu
27 **EXAFS and Near Edge Structures** Editors: A. Bianconi, L. Incoccia, S. Stipcich
28 **Atoms in Strong Light Fields** By N. B. Delone, V. P. Krainov
29 **Gas Flow in Nozzles** By U. Pirumov, G. Roslyakov
30 **Theory of Slow Atomic Collisions** By E. E. Nikitin, S. Ya. Umanskii
31 **Reference Data on Atoms, Molecules, and Ions** By A. A. Radzig, B. M. Smirnov
32 **Adsorption Processes on Semiconductor and Dielectric Surfaces I** By V. F. Kiselev, O. V. Krylov
33 **Surface Studies with Lasers** Editors: F.R. Aussenegg, A. Leitner, M.E. Lippitsch
34 **Inert Gases** Potentials, Dynamics, and Energy Transfer in Doped Crystals. Editor: M. L. Klein
35 **Chemistry and Physics of Solid Surfaces V** Editors: R. Vanselow, R. Howe
36 **Secondary Ion Mass Spectrometry, SIMS IV** Editors: A. Benninghoven, J. Okano, R. Shimizu, H. W. Werner
37 **X-Ray Spectra and Chemical Binding** By A. Meisel, G. Leonhardt, R. Szargan
38 **Ultrafast Phenomena IV** By D. H. Auston, K. B. Eisenthal
39 **Laser Processing and Diagnostics** Editor: D. Bäuerle

# Laser Processing and Diagnostics

Proceedings of an International Conference,
University of Linz, Austria, July 15–19, 1984

Editor: D. Bäuerle

With 399 Figures

Springer-Verlag
Berlin Heidelberg New York Tokyo 1984

Professor Dr. Dieter Bäuerle

Institut für Angewandte Physik, Johannes-Kepler-Universität
A-4040 Linz, Austria

*Series Editors*

Professor Vitalii I. Goldanskii

Institute of Chemical Physics
Academy of Sciences
Kosygin Street 3
Moscow V-334, USSR

Professor Robert Gomer

The James Franck Institute
The University of Chicago
5640 Ellis Avenue
Chicago, IL 60637, USA

Professor Dr. Fritz Peter Schäfer

Max-Planck-Institut für
Biophysikalische Chemie
D-3400 Göttingen-Nikolausberg
Fed. Rep. of Germany

Professor Dr. J. Peter Toennies

Max-Planck-Institut für Strömungsforschung
Böttingerstraße 6–8
D-3400 Göttingen
Fed. Rep. of Germany

ISBN 3-540-13843-9 Springer-Verlag Berlin Heidelberg New York Tokyo
ISBN 0-387-13843-9 Springer-Verlag New York Heidelberg Berlin Tokyo

Library of Congress Cataloging in Publication Data. Main entry under title: Laser processing and diagnostics. (Springer series in chemical physics ; 39). Includes bibliographies and indexes. 1. Lasers – Industrial applications – Congresses. I. Bäuerle, D. (Dieter), 1940– . II. Series: Springer series in chemical physics ; v. 39. TA1673.L365 1984 621.36'6 84-22144



Offset printing: Beltz Offsetdruck, 6944 Hemsbach/Bergstr. Bookbinding: J. Schäffer OHG, 6718 Grünstadt
2153/3130-543210

# Preface

Laser processing is now a rapidly increasing field with many real and potential applications in different areas of technology such as micromechanics, metallurgy, integrated optics, and semiconductor device fabrication. The necessity for such sophisticated light sources as lasers is based on the spatial coherence and the monochromaticity of laser light. The spatial coherence permits extreme focussing of the laser light resulting in the availability of high energy densities which can be used for strongly localized heat- and chemical-treatment of materials, with a resolution down to less than 1 µm. When using pulsed or scanned cw-lasers, localization in time is also possible. Additionally, the monochromaticity of laser light allows for control of the depth of heat treatment and/or selective, nonthermal bond breaking - within the surface of the material or within the molecules of the surrounding reactive atmosphere - simply by tuning the laser wavelength.

These inherent advantages of laser light permit micromachining of materials (drilling, cutting, welding etc.) and also allow single-step controlled area processing of thin films and surfaces. Processes include structural transformation (removal of residual damage, grain growth in polycrystalline material, amorphization, surface hardening etc.), etching, doping, alloying, or deposition. In addition, laser processing is *not* limited to planar substrates.

While other sources of energy such as electron or ion beams, or even incoherent lamps, have shown particular desirability in some processing techniques, there are presently many cases where, because of the abovementioned properties, lasers offer a unique application.

The aim of this book is to give an overview of the present understanding of the possibilities and of the limitations of laser processing, with special emphasis on electronic materials.

The book is composed of invited reviews and contributed papers, presented during an international conference on "Laser Processing and Diagnostics - Applications in Electronic Materials", held at the Johannes-Kepler-Universittt in Linz, Austria, July 15-19, 1984. This meeting constituted, in essence, the first international conference intended to cover all aspects of laser applications in electronic materials technology, ranging from the fundamentals of the physics and chemistry of laser surface interactions to semiconductor processing and the diagnostics of electronic materials, device properties and semiconductor fabrication processes.

The book is divided into five parts. The first part is devoted to the basic interaction mechanisms between laser radiation and solid surfaces and to applications which are essentially based on rapid thermal heating and quenching of surfaces (in vacuum or in a non-reactive atmosphere). The second part deals with laser photochemistry of adsorbates and basic molecule-surface interaction mechanisms. Part three gives an overview of both direct writing and large area laser *chemical* processing including deposition, doping, oxide formation and etching of materials as well as compound formation by mainly pyrolytic or mainly photolytic processes, incorporating laser fabrication and repair of devices. The fourth part summarizes the equally important area of the diagnostics of laser processing and of electronic materials and devices. Finally, the fifth part is devoted to laser diagnostic techniques which allow *in situ* measurement of temperature and molecular concentration fields in reactive gaseous systems, with special emphasis on those which are relevant to semiconductor fabrication processes.

Inevitably, several papers could be equally well fitted into two or more subject categories, and this made classification by chapter very difficult. Therefore, the reader is urged to make use of the comprehensive subject index at the end of the book. Furthermore, although some contributions may appear to overlap with others in broad content, the finer details of each will alert the reader to the various perspectives taken by different groups following similar paths.

I would like to thank all contributors to the book and especially the invited speakers. All papers in this volume were reviewed by the editor and reviewers, mainly from the international advisory committee, which included M. Balkanski, H. Beneking, I.W. Boyd, T.J. Chuang, T.F. Deutsch, D.J. Ehrlich, R.J. v. Gutfeld, M. Hanabusa, A.W. Johnson, K.L. Kompa, V.S. Letokhov, R.L. Melcher, R.M. Osgood, J.M. Poate, R. Salathé, and T. Tokuyama. I would like to thank all of them for their help and advice in organizing this conference.

The conference was attended by more than 200 scientists representing Australia, Austria, Belgium, Brazil, Bulgaria, China, Czechoslovakia, Egypt, Hungary, France, Germany, Great Britain, Israel, Italy, Japan, The Netherlands, Poland, Romania, Spain, Switzerland, USA, and USSR.

The essential financial support provided by the Austrian Bundesministerium für Wissenschaft und Forschung, the Linzer Hochschulfonds, IBM Austria, the USAF European Office of Aerospace Research and Development (EOARD) and European Research Office (USARDSG), and the European Research Office of the United States Navy (ORNL) is gratefully acknowledged.

Last but not least, I would like to thank all my co-workers and especially the conference secretary, Maria Rauch, for their superb support and help. I am indebted to my wife, Barbara, for her encouragement and continuous assistance, before, during and after the conference.

Linz, Austria, July 1984 *Dieter Bäuerle*

# Contents

*Part 5* Laser Diagnostics in Reactive Gaseous Systems

# Part 1

# Laser – Solid Interactions: Fundamentals and Applications

# Fundamentals of Laser Annealing

M. Balkanski

Laboratoire de Physique des Solides, Associé au C.N.R.S.,
Université Pierre et Marie Curie, 4, Place Jussieu
F-75230 Paris Cédex 05, France

## 1. INTRODUCTION

One of the most fascinating debates in the field of semiconductor physics in recent years centers on the fundamental interpretation of laser annealing. The question of the energy transfer from an intense laser beam to a disordered material, such as amorphous silicon, resulting in the crystallization of the amorphous substance has been approached from two different points of view, both referring to a set of fairly clear experimental results. On one hand, a large number of publications concludes that the laser beam simply heats the sample up to melting the amorphous material which on cooling crystallizes from melt. On the other hand, one has considered that amorphous to crystalline phase transitions can occur at low temperatures without passing through the molten state. Many arguments have been developed in support of these interpretations. A large number of publications have appeared in the literature.

In addition to the fundamental interest, laser annealing has been considered to have a strong potential in the technology of semiconductor doping by ion implantation. For all these reasons, the attention of a large audience has been focussed on this problem. It seems appropriate to-day to attempt to analyse the different arguments and to strike the balance on the present status of a field which will probably take a new dimension as subpicosecond spectroscopy develops.

After a short historical survey, we shall describe the crucial experiments and then discuss different theoretical approaches.

In the concluding part, we shall address two main questions : today, what is the extent of understanding of the physical mechanism of laser annealing and what is its applicability to industrial processes. For both aspects, we have to recognize the significant progress achieved in recent years. We have also to admit that the actual status is not completely up to the initial expectations.

The first investigation on the effect of an intense laser beam on a solid were motivated by the damaging of mirrors and windows of the lasers themselves [1]. At this time, the effect produced on the material was attributed to the local heating due to energy transfer from the intense laser beam to the crystal lattice mediated by "out of equilibrium free carriers" created by the laser beam [2].

The first experiments aiming directly at laser annealing of ion implanted semiconductors seems to be those of Khaibullin et al.[3] who claim to have discovered the photostimulated recrystallization of disordered implanted semiconductor layers. These authors describe the effect as an extremely quick recrystallization of the disordered ion-implanted material under the action of short, nanosecond, powerful pulse of laser radiation, the wavelength of which is chosen in the fundamental absorption band of the semiconductor. This effect was then called "laser annealing" and it was admitted that in the nanosecond regimes, one cannot reduce it to the ordinary thermal effect [3]. The authors have considered that different factors such as photoionization, impact wave, powerful light fields play a significant role. They do not give a complete description of the laser annealing mechanism but they clearly do not satisfy themselves with the thermal mechanism. Yet, in many other publications dealing with the annealing of amorphous silicon by pulsed lasers, the thermal melting and recrystallization mechanism has been taken as perfectly satisfactory to explain the observations. It has been generally considered that the energy of the incident laser beams is converted into heat in the lattice by means of non-radiative recombination. Then the recrystallization process which occurs as the material cools is liquid phase epitaxial growth [4]. The thermal melting - recrystallization mechanism remained generally accepted until 1979 when Van Vechten, R. Tsu and F.W. Saris [5] sharply criticised the thermal hypothesis and proposed that the description of pulsed laser annealing must take account of the dense plasma produced by the absorption of light.

For a long time, the controversy has persisted, kept up by experiments some of which have been one sidedly interpreted using theoretical arguments which have not always been convincing.

The general tendency to-day is to admit that within a delay of the order of few ps after the laser impact the irradiated material melts and then recrystallizes.

The question which remains to be considered is, is it necessary to reach thermal melting in order to achieve the amorphous to crystalline transition and what is the time ordering of the processes which would be monitoring this transition.

## 2. STRUCTURAL ANALYSIS AFTER LASER ANNEALING

### 2.1. Amorphous - Crystalline transformation

The aim of laser annealing is to achieve the transformation of the amorphous material obtained by ion implantation into a perfect crystal. Therefore, we shall first discuss the results of the structural analysis after annealing.

One of the methods which seems to be most appropriate to define the degree of crystallinity of the material is light scattering. The light scattering spectrum of amorphous silicon, for example, is very different from that of the perfect crystal.

Laser annealing performed with a Q-switched ruby laser delivering pulses of about one hundred nanoseconds duration with an energy density of the order of one $J/cm^2$ is described by Morhange [6]. At this energy density, the diameter of the laser beam was of the order of one mm. The annealed region was explored with an argon laser probe beam focussed to a diameter of 80 μm. The probe beam was used for Raman spectroscopy. With this arrangement, it was possible to explore the annealed region in the xy plane by moving the sample with regard to the probe beam and in the z direction by varying the frequency of the probe beam which causes changes in the penetration depth in the a-Si sample.

Two parameters characterize the annealed Si : the frequency position of the Raman line and its half width. For monocrystalline Si, the Raman active normal mode is observed at 520,5 $cm^{-1}$ with a half width of 3 $cm^{-1}$. When ion-implanted samples having a thickness of the amorphous layer of 5000 Å are investigated, the annealed region does not show a uniform single crystal structure. At the center of the irradiated region, the Raman peak frequency is 519 $cm^{-1}$, shifted by 1,5 $cm^{-1}$ towards lower frequencies. The width of the peak is 6 $cm^{-1}$ significantly broader than the single crystal peak. When the probe beam is moved towards the periphery of the laser irradiated region, the frequency shift increases and reaches 5,5 $cm^{-1}$ at the edge of the annealed area. The band is also broader and has a width of 10 $cm^{-1}$ near the edge. These results are displayed in Figure 1, where the circles represent the extent of the primary laser beam and the dots indicate the position of the probe beam for the spectrum represented on the left side of the figure.

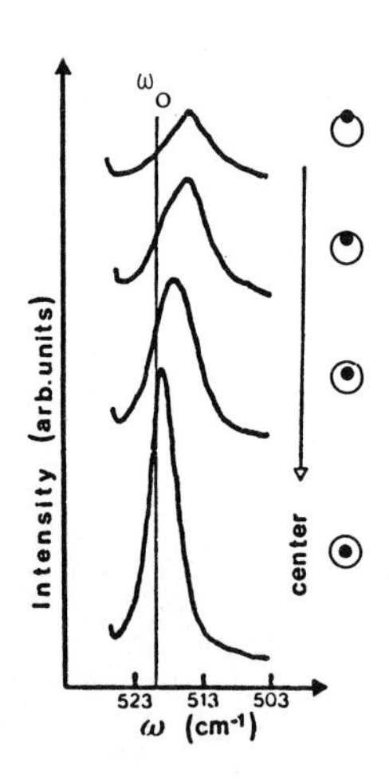


Figure 1. Raman spectra originating from various points along the diameter of a laser annealed region. From J.F. MORHANGE et al. Proceedings of the Material Research Society Annual Meeting, Boston, 1978 (American Institute of Physics, New-York 1979) p. 429.

These results could be viewed as follows. Even at the center of the annealed region, laser annealing does not lead to a large single crystal in the way it would be obtained in equilibrium epitaxial regrowth. Instead, the annealed material consists of large polycrystallites whose dimensions decrease as one approaches the interface between annealed and amorphous material. The recrystallization occurs as a result of random nucleation in the amorphous layer. The dimensions of the crystallites depend on the energy distribution in the incident power laser beam. The crystallite dimensions determine the frequency shift of the Raman active normal mode band. An account of the normal mode frequency shift as a function of the dimension of the crystallite is given by a simple lattice dynamics calculation developed by Kanellis [7] . The model used in this calculation is that of a thin slab limited in one direction and infinite in the plane perpendicular to that direction. In the case of Si, the results obtained are shown in Figure 2.

In this figure the frequency shift of the two high frequency modes are represented. These are the surface modes which in the limit of infinite crystal tends toward the Raman active mode at the center of the Brillouin Zone. These calculations show that for crystallites having dimensions smaller than 80 Å, a noticeable frequency shift should occur. Indeed, the experimental observations show that in the region near the crystalline-amorphous interface a significant frequency shift is measured. From this theoretical model and the experimental results, we draw the conclusion that in laser annealing, the crystallization occurs randomly.

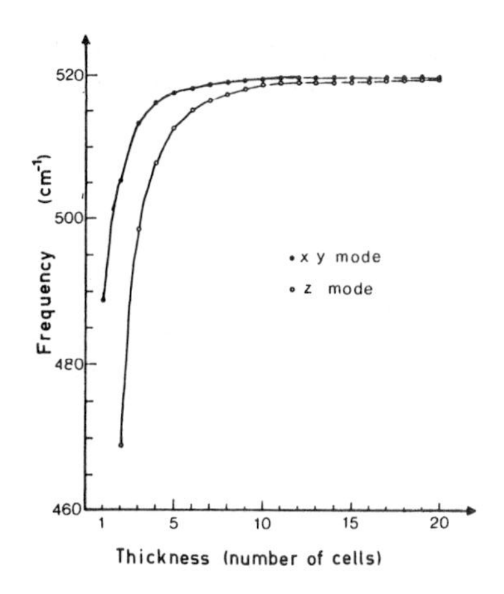


Figure 2. Frequency variation of the higher-frequency optical modes as a function of the number of cells.
From G. KANELLIS et al., Phys. Rev. B21, 1543 (1980)

An amorphous network is not a perfectly regular structure. The energy supplied by the laser beam at threshold is sufficient to soften bonds in the less favourable topological situation and allow nucleation. Crystallographic ordering develops around the randomly distributed nucleus embedded in the amorphous background creating microcrystalline clusters whose size depends on the energy density distribution.

First-order phase transitions such as melting or crystallization take place, in general, via nucleation and growth of microphases. Unstable phases of Si have also been prepared in high-pressure experiments [8]. Phillips [9] has given evidence of metastable phases in laser-induced and thermally reversible microcrystallization in chalcogenide glass formers such as $GeSe_2$. Recent light scattering experiments [10] show the existence of microcrystallites embedded in the glass ($GeSe_2$) during laser annealing. The microcrystalline clusters initially formed are free to rotate and form larger clusters, a fact which is deduced from the observations of Raman line narrowing; this demonstrates a precursor effect in the laser induced glass to crystal transition. These experiments although achieved in different materials and on a very different time scale might be suggestive of the processes occurring in silicon.

## 2.2. Picosecond laser-induced patterns on silicon single crystal surface

It is generally believed that monocrystalline silicon being a well-defined target would yield unambiguous indication about the mechanism of the transformations produced by a laser beam on a semiconductor.

The surface of a silicon single crystal may be transformed into an amorphous layer by a single picosecond pulse [11]. Optical observation show the formation of an amorphous ring pattern on a (111) crystal surface after exposure to a laser pulse at 532 nm with an average duration of 30 ps and with a spot having a size of the order of $5.10^{-4}$ cm$^2$. At lower intensities, the ring diameter becomes smaller, the amorphous region coalesces to a spot at the center and disappears below a critical intensity threshold. At 532 nm, the threshold is reported to be 0,18 J/cm$^2$ for (100) and 0,08 J/cm$^2$ for (111) surfaces. Amorphous rings rather than central spots are formed for intensity levels exceeding 0,24 J/cm$^2$ for (100) and 0,12 J/cm$^2$ for (111) surfaces. The center in this case is a single crystal with the same orientation as the substrate. The amorphous nature of the rings was deduced from an increase of the reflectivity compared to crystalline silicon and was confirmed by electron diffraction with a transmission electron microscope.

The annular pattern of the amorphous phase is interpreted in terms of cooling rate and crystal-growth speed. It is first assumed that above threshold the laser pulse induces melting of the silicon target.

Following laser pulse melting, two limiting cases are then proposed : just above the threshold intensity, a layer of depth somewhat smaller than $5.10^{-6}$ cm is cooled in $t_p = 3.10^{-11}$ s and the condition, $d/U_M > t_p$, for nucleation of an amorphous solid phase, is fulfilled. Well above the threshold intensity, the temperature of the molten layer rises far above $T_m$ and the cooling rate in the critical region below 0.8 $T_m$ becomes longer. This gives a description of the annular pattern of the amorphous phase.

## 2.3. Picosecond laser annealing of implanted silicon

Experiments analogous to that described in the previous section for silicon single crystal surface have been performed by Liu et al.[12] on ion implanted amorphous silicon.

With a laser beam of 1.06 μm, beside the annular amorphous region and recrystallized center, one also observes a recrystallized ring. Both the ring and the center are polycrystals. The energy fluence level to form the ring is 0.22 J/cm$^2$. It is 0.35 J/cm$^2$ for the a-Si region and 0.85 J/cm$^2$ or the recrystallized region.

Rozgonyi et al.[13] have re-examined the structural modification of amorphized silicon surfaces following picosecond laser irradiation using cross-section transmission electron microscopy and showed that the center is always a dislocation free single crystal encircled by poly-silicon ring. This observation is consistent with the results of Morhange et al. [14] obtained by Raman spectroscopy.

More recently, Nissim et al.[15] have performed light scattering measurements analogous to that reported by Morhange et al. [14]. The irradiated area was scanned with a probe laser beam focussed to a 1 μm diameter spot. When a single 30ps pulse at 1.06 and 0.532 μm wavelengths from a mode-locked Nd:YAG laser is used, a multi annular recrystallization pattern is observed on implanted silicon. At high incident energies, single crystal silicon is observed in the central spot and in the first recrystallized ring of the annealed area. With an irradiation at 1.06 μm, the threshold of laser induced damage was found to be above 2 J/cm$^2$. The multi annular pattern has been ascribed to a multiple melting resolidification process during the pulse duration leading to the superposition of basic structures of different sizes.

For the understanding of this complex structure , it should also be remembered that periodic surface structures on solids may result from inhomogeneous energy deposition associated with the interference of the incident beam with a surface scattered field as discussed by Van Driel et al.[16].

## 3. TIME RESOLVED ANALYSIS OF PULSED LASER IRRADIATION OF SEMICONDUCTORS

For the discussion of the data obtained by short laser irradiation pulses one could distinguish three different time ranges : i) very short time scale, $t << 10^{-12}$ s, where the system is in a stage far from equilibrium, the region of highly non linear processes, ii) intermediate time scale, $t \sim 10^{-12}$ s when different elementary relaxation processes take place and iii) long time range $t > 10^{-9}$ s when thermalization occurs and the system tends toward equilibrium.

## 3.1. Investigations in the very short time range

A radiation beam of energy density of 1 J/cm$^2$ is bound to produce a strong perturbation on the material at the instant of interaction. The photon density is such that a hot electron plasma might be produced.

The experiments in the shortest time scale are those of optical pulse induced phase transitions in silicon described by Shank, Yen and Hirlimann [17]. They reported the first observations of optically induced reflectivity changes in silicon with 90 fs optical pulses.

The results of reflectivity measurements are shown in Figure 3. The energy $E_{th}$ is defined as the excitation energy density where visual evidence of amorphous layer formation is observed. This energy corresponds to 0.1 J/cm$^2$.

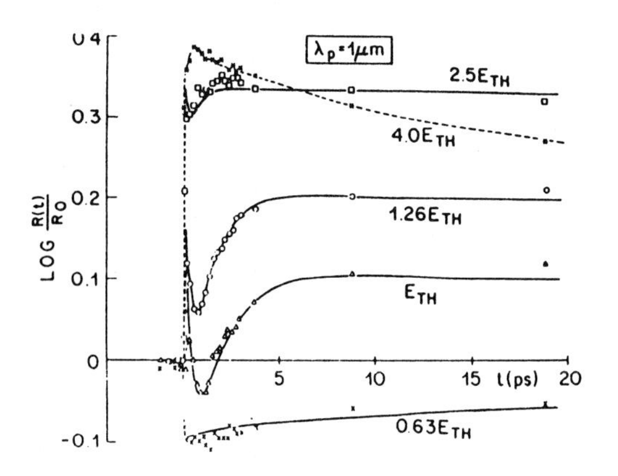


Figure 3. Transient reflectivity data in silicon at probe wavelength 1 μm and pump wavelength 620 nm at various incident energies. From C.V. SHANK et al., Phys. Rev. Letters 50, 454 (1983).

Shank et al. [17] discuss the results shown in Figure 3 in the following way. Optical excitation of Si with a 2.0 eV optical pulse results in the generation of a dense electron-hole plasma within the optical absorption depth : $\alpha^{-1} = 3$ μm. They suppose that during the earlier time following excitation, the reflectivity is dominated by the electron-hole plasma. As the pulse intensity is increased, the energy is transferred to the crystal lattice and the crystal melts. It is also supposed that melting begins at the surface and moves inward into the bulk.

Probably, the most important contribution of this investigation is the demonstration that when the crystal is excited with a short optical pulse of 90 fs a form of unstable highly excited silicon is created which persists for a fraction of a picosecond. A challenging problem now is to determine the properties of this material with at least 10 % of the available electrons excited.

### 3.2. Intermediate time range. Picosecond irradiation

Most of the work on time resolved spectroscopy is in the picosecond range for the simple reason that this is the time scale for which short pulse laser sources are readily available.

Experiments in the picosecond range on transmission and reflectivity were performed by Liu et al. [18] at the fundamental and doubled frequency of a mode-locked Nd : YAG laser producing a 30 ps single pulse. In this work are presented measurements on self-reflectivity and self-transmission at $\lambda$ = 532 nm for increasing energy fluence with 20 ps pulses. The self-reflectivity of bulk silicon with (111) surface starts to increase when the energy fluence of the pump beam reaches 0.2 J/cm$^2$. The initial rise of the reflectivity from the crystalline value of 0.37 to a maximum value of 0.48 is in agreement with changes in the index of refraction due to melting of a thin surface layer. In this case, it is supposed that the hot e-h plasma transfers sufficient energy for melting within the duration of the pulse itself. Below the critical fluence level of 0.2 J/cm$^2$, the photoexcited e-h plasma causes a decrease in the real part n of the complex refractive index.

A pump and probe technique was also used where a picosecond excitation pulse is followed by a slightly focussed weak probe with a variable time delay.

At 100 ps delay, the probe pulse is temporarily completely separated from the pump pulse and an abrupt rise in reflectivity at the threshold fluence of 0.2 J/cm$^2$ is observed [18] . This discontinuity in the carrier density should be associated with local structural changes. The reflectivity rises to 0.75 $\pm$ 0.03 which is characteristic of molten silicon at the probe wavelength of 1.064 μm. This behaviour is observed even at zero delay indicating that melting occurs within the pulse duration of 20 ps.

### 3.3. Long time phenomena

At long times, the energy is transferred to the lattice which eventually melts. For the long time phenomena, we are faced with three major problems :

i) what is the mechanism of melting,
ii) do intermediate, metastable phase exist during thermalization,
iii) what is the microscopic mechanism of resolidification?

There are two experimental approaches to these questions :

a) determination of the temperature of the system,
b) direct observation of the structural phase transformation during the evolution of the system towards thermalization.

We have discussed structural observations in section 2 and the insight they provide for understanding the dynamical evolution of the system. We shall now focuss on considerations regarding the determination of the temperature of the system : the electron gas temperature and the lattice temperature.

### 3.4. Energy transfer and carrier density

Of particular interest for understanding the effects of laser action on a solid is the analysis of the initial events following the irradiation by an intense optical pulse. Femtosecond spectroscopy has already shown to be a valuable method for such an analysis [17, 19, 20] . Measurements of the time dependent reflectivity leads to estimation of the electron hole density initially created as well as its evolution with time. Such measurements are also suggestive for models for the energy transfer during and after the irradiation.

The questions to be considered are the following :

i) what is the electron-hole (e-h) density resulting from the excitation,

ii) what are the interaction processes behind the excitation,

iii) how is the energy stored in the excited carriers and transferred to the rest of the system?

i) electron-hole density produced by femtosecond pulse

The high density electron-hole plasma in silicon created by a 90 femtosecond pulse has been investigated [17] by measuring the time dependent reflectivity over a 20 picoseconds time scale, at various laser energies. Such short pulses lead to the possibility to break so many covalent bonds that the crystal becomes fluid even at T = 0 K. The carrier density created at this time scale was estimated to be of the order of $5.10^{21}$ $cm^{-3}$ under an incident energy density of 0.063 $J/cm^2$. The phenomena produced in such very short pulses can be viewed in the following way [20]. The part of the initial laser beam absorbed over a penetration depth of d = 3 μm creates an electron hole plasma with a decreasing density profile. After the surface density reaches a fraction of $N_p$, the plasma density, the reflectivity and the penetration depth fall, because of the decrease of the real part of the dielectric constant as well as of the increase of the induced free carrier absorption. For high enough power, the surface density goes beyond $N_p$ within the pulse, yielding an instantaneous reflectivity larger than $R_o$, the initially reflected beam. At that high surface density the laser beam becomes a vanishing wave which can create e-h pairs only very close to the surface.

The reflectivity during the pulse R(t) is obtained through a general resolution of the Maxwell equations, taking into account the variation of the dielectric constant via the modification of the e-h density profile.

The experimental data [20] are fitted with a relaxation time $\tau = 3.10^{-16}$ s. For $\lambda = 0,31$ μm the plasma frequency density can be as high as $2.10^{22} < N_p < 8.10^{22}$ $cm^{-3}$ which is indeed very high in view of the total number of valence band electrons ($2.10^{23}$ $cm^{-3}$).

ii) electron-gas temperature

An interesting investigation of the photoexcited electron distribution is performed by non-linear photoemission from silicon by Bensoussan and Moison [21]. They show that in Si, at moderate fluences an equilibrium distribution coexists with the electrons at very high energies in the conduction band, generated by two and three quantum processes. The equilibrium distribution is described by a well-defined temperature which differs significantly from the lattice temperature. Because of the fast photogeneration of the carriers, and of the two photon absorption and biparticle Auger recombination processes in which carriers are sent continuously high in the bands, the electron gas can reach an internal equilibrium characterized by a temperature $T_e$ higher than the lattice temperature $T_e$. The experimentally measured thermal emission is interpreted by the Richardson equation. The temperatures deduced for different fluences are shown in Figure 4.

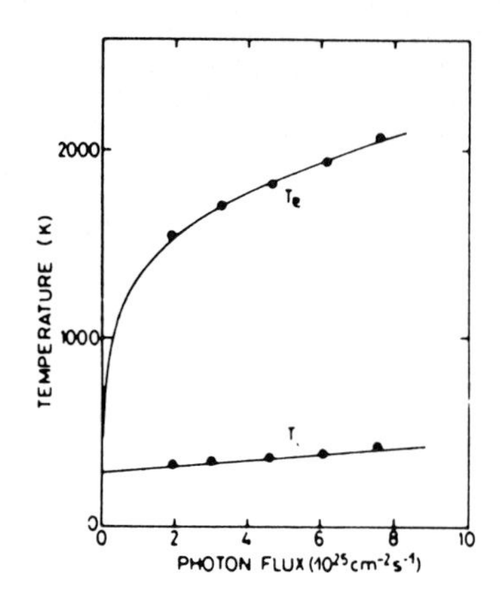


Figure 4. Electron and lattice temperatures vs. photon flux.
From M. BENSOUSSAN. Proceedings of the 16th International Conference on the Physics of Semiconductors. North-Holland, Editor M. Averous (1982) p. 405.

iii) lattice temperature

Lattice temperature at equilibrium can be inferred from light scattering measurements of the frequency shift and line width of the LO mode 22 and Stokes to anti-Stokes ratio [23] . The Stokes to anti-Stokes ratio indicates a lattice temperature of 1400 K for a delay of 150 ns after excitation with a beam of 0.8 J/cm$^2$ at 532 nm. Raman measurements are evidently taken after the high reflectivity falls off.

## 4. DISCUSSION AND CONCLUSIONS

Laser annealing has now a long history and an abundant literature. The interesting question, which still remains to be answered, is what are the elementary processes in the interaction of a strong radiation field with matter.

The process of laser annealing consists of two sets of phenomena. The first concerns the effect of a dense radiation field on matter creating elementary excitation far from equilibrium. The initial hot plasma redistributes through interactions between carriers and ultimately thermalizes giving up energy to heavier particles which are the lattice constituents. The second set of phenomena, of a completely different nature, concerns the modifications induced to the solid as a result of the creation of the dense hot plasma. If the laser pulse is short enough, the e-h density reached corresponds to an amount of broken covalent bonds which is a significant portion of the total number of bonds, the crystal could become fluid even at T = 0 K. Ultimately, the solid sets in a new phase whose structure depends on the elementary mechanisms of interaction and organization of the lattice constituents. We shall examine successively these two states as : i) direct laser effect and ii) consequences of the laser action.

### 4.1. Direct laser effect

The incident laser energy is absorbed by electron-hole pair creation and by free carrier excitation. In indirect gap semiconductors, electron-hole pairs are created via indirect absorption processes involving the emission and absorption of phonons. Because phonon energies are much smaller than photon energy, the amount of energy transferred to the lattice during absorption is negligible in comparison to the total amount absorbed. The rise of carrier density leads, in turn, to increased free carrier absorption. The net result is the production of hot electrons and holes far from equilibrium which subsequently thermalize with the set of the carriers and eventually with the lattice. The observations by Shank et al. [17] demonstrate that with a short (90 femtosecond) optical pulse an unstable, highly excited state is created near the surface which persists for a fraction of picosecond.

For very short pulses of radiation one perceives clear indications from the experiments [17,20] that there are two steps of the laser action on a crystal well separated in time. In the first step, the electromagnetic energy transferred from the laser beam to the solid is retained in the highly excited non-equilibrium electronic state. In a second step, this energy is transferred to the lattice.

Recently, a theoretical model [20] is proposed which takes into account the space time evolution of the plasma during the pulse in order to explain the processes for densities higher than $10^{22}$ $cm^{-3}$ reached in 100 fs pulses. The novelty of this model is the argument that free carrier absorption is dominated by e-h collisions with a characteristic relaxation time $\tau = 3.10^{-16}$ s.

A different situation is reached with much longer pulses : $\tau_L = 10$ ns and a photon absorption rate $g \sim 10^{31}$ $cm^{-3}$ $s^{-1}$ : Auger recombination becomes the dominant recombination mechanism at these densities.

Most of the laser energy is absorbed by the carriers within the absorption depth. Eventually these carriers lose their energy to the lattice, the rise of the lattice temperature then depends on the distance they have diffused before substantial phonon emission occurs. At moderate density, the phonon scattering time is $\tau \sim 10^{-13}$ s. Screening does not affect the rate of intervalley phonon emission until $N_e \sim 10^{21}$ $cm^{-3}$. Because screening increases the electron-phonon scattering time, it not only decreases the rate of phonon emission but also enhances diffusion. This increases the volume of the region in which the energy of the excited carriers is transferred to the lattice. Owing to the extreme non-linearity of the hot carrier effects, it is impossible to make an accurate estimate of the precise temperature to which the lattice is heated or to determine the laser power threshold above which melting will occur.

### 4.2. Consequences of the laser action

The equilibrium observations are clear : an amorphous or glass solid is transformed into crystal under laser action and a crystal submitted to very short laser irradiation is transformed into amorphous material. An implication of both of these transformations is that melting precedes the transition. Another alternative is that the phase transition is directly induced in the highly excited state.

The effect of a dense plasma on the melting temperature is itself an interesting problem of solid state theory. This question has been recently addressed by Bok and Combescot [24]. It is shown that in the presence of a dense plasma, the melting temperature of a solid changes. The melting temperature decreases with increasing plasma density. For a laser pulse of 1 $J/cm^2$ during 10 ns, it is considered that an e-h plasma reaches a steady state in a time shorter than the laser pulse. Considering the plasma expansion due to its high pressure, its collision with phonons and Auger recombination, the highest plasma density is of the order $10^{21}$ $cm^{-3}$. This density is nevertheless considered to be sufficient to considerably reduce the melting temperature so that a metallic layer of liquid silicon is formed at the surface.

The role of a high plasma density in laser annealing has been discussed by Van Vechten et al. [5] in a quite different way but still involving electron-phonon coupling and lattice instability induced by this interaction. Above a critical carrier density estimated at $8.10^{21}$ $cm^{-3}$, a second-order phase transition occurs. At this plasma density, the bond charges will be so depleted that they will no longer be able to stabilize the TA phonon modes [25] . The crystal will no longer resist shearing stresses and will become fluid. This fluid is distinct from the normal molten phase of Si, the latter being the result of a strictly first-order phase transition driven by the atomic motion at high temperatures. The assumption of Van Vechten is that the plasma is supposed to directly induce the structural transformation. The energy is retained in the electronic system instead of being entirely associated with atomic motion. As the plasma becomes less dense due to expansion and to transfer of energy to the lattice, the material will pass back through the second-order phase transition at $8.10^{21}$ $cm^{-3}$ and covalent bonding will gradually appear. The material will finally recrystallize if this process is relatively slow or will solidify in the amorphous phase if the process is very fast.

This dense plasma phase could be compared to the highly excited silicon which persists for a fraction of a picosecond [17, 20] . The interpretation of the laser action differs nevertheless with regard to the following step ; it is generally considered that the solid melts after the initial interaction stage.

In conclusion, few points appear clear today. The laser interaction with solids results first in the creation of a dense plasma which persists for a fraction of a picosecond. Melting seems to occur after the excitation pulse. The mechanism of melting is not clear and consequently the mechanism of solidification is not clear either. Further investigations in the very short impulse regime are certainly desirable to clarify the physical processes in laser annealing.

ACKNOWLEDGMENT

The research reported here in has been sponsored in part by the United States Army through its European Research Office.

REFERENCES

1. Y.M. Fairfield and G.H. Schwuttke : Sol. Stat. Electronics 11, 1175 (1968)
   A.A. Grynberg, R.F. Mekhtiev, S.M. Ryvkin, V.A. Salamanov and I.D. Yaroshetskii : Sov. Phys. Sol. Stat. 9, 1085 (1967)
2. S.M. Ryukin, V.M. Salamanov and I.D. Yaroshetskii : Sov. Phys. Sol. Stat. 10, 807 (1968)
3. I.B. Khaibullin, E.I. Shtyrkov, M.M. Zaripov, R.M. Bayazitov and M.F. Galjavtdinov : Rad. Eff. 36, 225 (1978)
4. J.C. Wang, R.F. Wood and P.P. Pronko : Appl. Phys. Lett. 33, 455 (1978)
   P. Baeri, S.U. Campisano, G. Foti and E. Rimini : J. Appl. Phys. 50, 788 (1979)

C.M. Surko, A.L. Simons, D.H. Auston, J.A. Golovchenko and R.E. Sluster : Appl. Phys. Lett. 34, 635 (1979)
J.C. Schultz and R.J. Collins : Appl. Phys. Lett. 34, 363 (1979)
5. J.A. Van Vechten, R. Tsu and F.W. Saris : Phys. Lett. 74A, 417 (1979) and 74A, 422 (1979)
6. J-F. Morhange : Thesis, Paris (1982)
7. G. Kanellis, J-F. Morhange and M. Balkanski : Phys. Rev. B21, 1543 (1980)
8. J.S. Kasper and S.M. Richards : Acta Cryst. 17, 752 (1964)
9. J.C. Phillips : Comments Solid State Phys. 10, 165 (1982)
10. M. Balkanski, E. Haro, G.P. Espinosa and J.C. Phillips : Sol. Stat. Commun. 51, 639 (1984)
11. P.L. Liu, R. Yen, N. Bloembergen and R.T. Hodgson : Mat. Res. Proc. Ed. White and Peercy (Academic Press), 1980 p. 156
12. J.M. Liu, R. Yen, H. Kurz and N. Bloembergen : Appl. Phys. Lett. 39, 755 (1981)
13. G.A. Rozgonyi, H. Baugart, F. Phillipp, R. Uebbing and H. Oppolzer : Mat. Res. Soc. Proc. Ed. B.R. Appleton and B.K. Celler, (North Holland), 1982 p. 177
14. J-F. Morhange, G. Kanellis and M. Balkanski : Solid State Commun. 31, 805 (1979)
15. Y.I. Nissim, J. Sapriel and J-L. Oudar : Appl. Phys. Lett. 42, 504 (1983)
16. H.M. Van Driel, J.S. Preston and M.I. Galant : Appl. Phys. Lett. 40, 385 (1982)
17. C.V. Shank, R. Yen and C. Hirlimann : Phys. Rev. Lett. 50, 454 (1983)
18. J.M. Liu, H. Kurz and N. Bloembergen : Appl. Phys. Lett. 41, 643 (1982)
19. C.V. Shank, R. Yen and C. Hirlimann : Phys. Rev. Lett. 51, 900 (1983)
D. Von der Linde and G. Wartmann : Appl. Phys. Lett. 41, 700 (1982)
20 D. Hulin, M. Combescot, J. Bok, A. Migus, J.Y. Vinet and A. Antonetti : Phys. Rev. Lett. 52, 1998 (1984)
21. M. Bensoussan and J. de Moison : Proceedings of the Intern. Conf. on the Physics of Semiconductors. Part I (Ed. by M. Averous, North Holland, Amsterdam) p. 404 (1982)
22. M. Balkanski, R.F. Wallis and E. Haro : Phys. Rev. B28, 1928 (1983)
23. A. Compaan : High Excitation and Short Pulse Phenomena, Trieste (1984)
24. J. Bok : Phys. Lett. 84A, 488 (1981)
M. Combescot : Phys. Lett. 85A, 308 (1981)
M. Combescot and J. Bok : Phys. Rev. Lett. 48, 1413 (1982)
25. R.M. Martin : Phys. Rev. 186, 871 (1969)

# Inhomogeneous Energy Deposition in Crystalline Silicon with Picosecond Pulses of One Micron Radiation

Ian W. Boyd, Steven C. Moss, Thomas F. Boggess, and Arthur L. Smirl

Center for Applied Quantum Electronics, Department of Physics, North Texas State University, Denton, TX 76203, USA

In recent years, the extensive use of ultrashort laser pulses to time resolve the transmission and reflectivity of Si has led to a much improved understanding of the kinetics of energy deposition and redistribution immediately preceding and following optically induced phase transitions [1]. With few exceptions, visible sources of radiation with photon energies well above the indirect bandgap have been used for excitation in these studies. By contrast, because the interaction of near-bandgap picosecond 1 μm radiation with Si is more complicated, it has received little attention. We have recently presented preliminary results of the first studies of the pulsewidth dependence of the nonlinear absorption [2] and the various phase transitions and changes in surface morphology [3] for 1 μm excitation pulses in the 4-260 ps range. These measurements demonstrate that the absorption of 1 μm picosecond radiation below the melting point is strictly fluence dependent, with no observable intensity-dependent contributions. Moreover, the nonlinear behavior of the absorption in this regime can be completely accounted for by indirect and free-carrier absorption, when lattice-heating effects are included. In addition, the fluence required for single-shot melting of the Si at 1 μm is found to decrease significantly with decreasing pulsewidth. This decrease goes roughly as the square root of the pulsewidth, suggesting that significant energy diffusion occurs during the pulse duration. Not only is the melting threshold highly pulsewidth dependent, but the observed morphology and solid state following irradiation depend dramatically on the irradiation time. For pulses of more than 30 ps in duration, the silicon is found to have recrystallized to a state of relative order. By contrast, for pulses of less than roughly 12 ps duration, the liquid silicon cools so rapidly that it freezes in an amorphous layer before it can reorganize in the crystalline state. This observation is in contrast to predictions that picosecond pulses of 1 micron radiation would not be capable of producing amorphous material from crystalline Si [4] because of relatively long absorption depth at this wavelength. It is our intent to emphasize in this paper the short pulse regime (<20 ps) where amorphization occurs. We first describe the resulting morphology and then demonstrate that the observed features have well-defined thresholds. We also report the formation of alternate regions of amorphous and crystalline stripes, and suggest that these stripes are evidence for inhomogeneous and localized melting of the surface.

In these studies, a well-characterized mode-locked Nd:glass laser that produced pulses of ~7 ps duration at 1.054 μm was used. Single pulses were selected from the mode-locked trains by means of an electro-optic shutter and were then amplified. A small fraction of the pulses was delivered to calibrated pulsewidth and energy monitors so that the absolute energy and pulse duration could be determined on a shot-to-shot basis. The major portion was then directed through a polarizer-half-waveplate-polarizer combination that provided a variable attenuation of a factor of up to 300

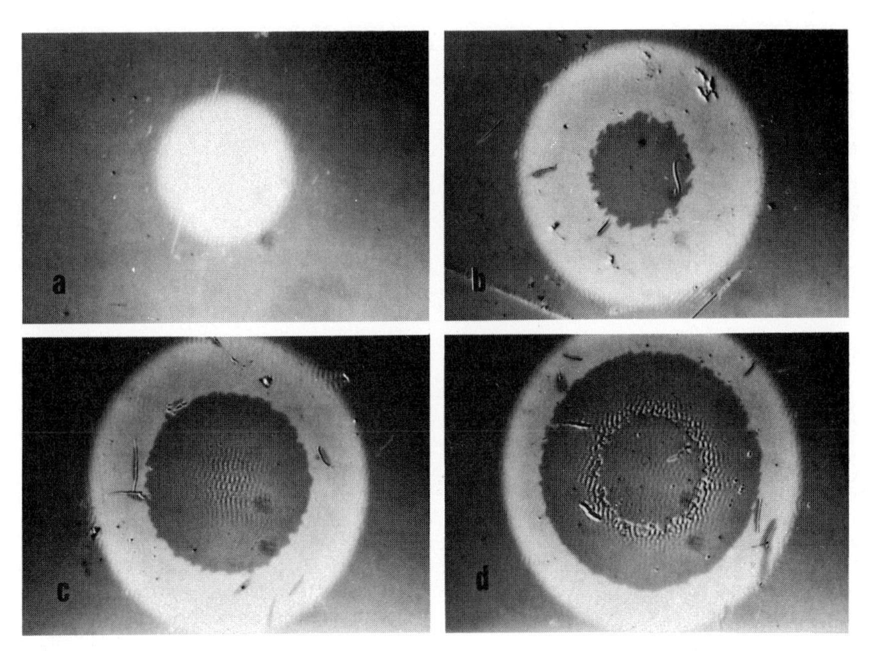


Fig.1 Morphological changes induced in c-Si by 7 ps pulses at 1 micron, for increasing fluence (a)-(d)

and was focused by a "best form" lens on to the sample. Pinhole scans of the spatial beam profile at various positions from the output coupler and near focus indicated that the beam was Gaussian and obeyed the usual propagation laws. The sample was a 1-mm-thick, optically polished, single-crystal (<111>-orientation) Si wafer. The back surface was anti-reflection coated to eliminate Fabry-Perot effects. Irradiation was performed in a 1-on-1 fashion in order to eliminate the occurrence of multi-shot damage resulting from N-on-1 exposure at fluences below the single shot melting threshold [3]. The surface morphology of the irradiated c-Si was studied using Nomarski interference high contrast optical microscopy.

Figure 1 shows the fluence dependence of the morphological changes induced by these pulses. At threshold, $E_a$, amorphization is restricted to a small disc in the center of the irradiated zone. At higher fluences the conditions for amorphization are satisfied only at the perimeter of the melted region, and as the energy density is increased, the amorphous band becomes wider and thinner. For fluences above the upper limit for amorphization, recrystallization occurs. This has been confirmed qualitatively by scanning a tightly focused HeNe beam across a structure similar to that shown in Fig.1b. The reflectivity of the lighter amorphous region was some 17% higher than the value found for the outlying unmelted region and also ~17% higher than the recrystallized inner region. Inside the recrystallized region, another very narrow ring of structure always appears at a well defined fluence ($E_c$), above the amorphization ($E_a$) and recrystallization ($E_b$) thresholds. Figure 2 shows the relationship of incident fluence to the size of these features. As can be seen, the square of the radius of these characteristic rings is linearly proportional to the logarithm of the incident fluence:

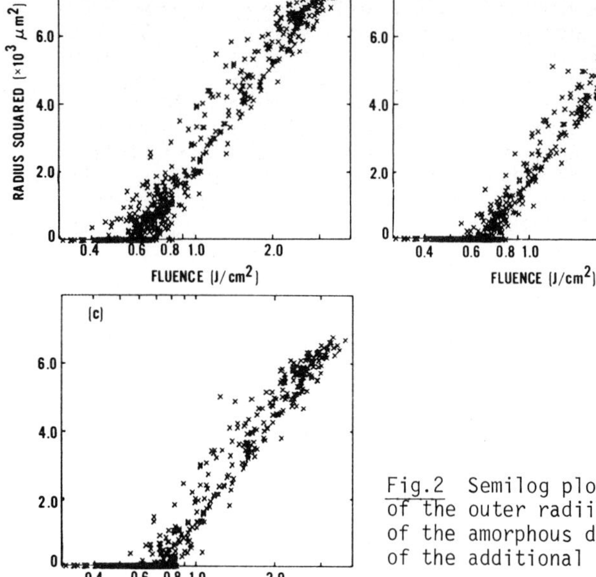


Fig.2 Semilog plot of the energy dependence of the outer radii (a) and inner radii (b) of the amorphous disc, and the outer radii of the additional ring of structure (c)

$$r_x^2 = R^2(\ln E_0 - \ln E_x) \quad , \tag{1}$$

where $r_x$ is the radius of feature x, $E_x$ is the fluence at which this feature is initiated, $E_0$ is peak incident fluence, and R is the incident beam radius (1/e of the intensity). This relationship is identical to the one used previously by Liu [5] to fit the radii of the amorphous and recrystallized rings in c-Si following irradiation with 30 ps pulses at 0.53 μm. We also observe that the difference in the squares of the radii of any two features is a constant:

$$r_a^2 - r_c^2 = R^2(\ln E_c - \ln E_a) = C_1 \tag{2a}$$

$$r_a^2 - r_b^2 = R^2(\ln E_b - \ln E_a) = C_2 \tag{2b}$$

$$r_b^2 - r_c^2 = R^2(\ln E_c - \ln E_b) = C_3 \quad , \tag{2c}$$

where $r_a$, $r_b$, $r_c$ are the radii of the three features described above, and $C_1$, $C_2$ $C_3$ are constants where $C_1 = C_2 + C_3$. Although the scatter of points on Fig. 2 is larger than similar fluctuations observed for an excitation wavelength of 0.53 μm, we emphasize that amorphization always occurs at lower fluence levels than recrystallization for these pulsewidths.

Another feature often observed within the morphology described above is the appearance of permanent periodic ripple patterns aligned perpendicularly to the incident electric field of the laser beam. These structures have previously been observed on the surface of many semiconductors as well as various metals and insulators [6-11]. Attempts to explain these characteristics in terms of properties of the incident laser beam [6], interference of the beam with a surface-scattered wave originating at a scratch [7], nonradiative short-range fields associated with surface defects [9], and surface plasmons or polaritons [8,10] have been published over the years. Although each of these models invokes inhomogeneous energy deposition resulting from interference with some surface scattered field, the nature of this field is different in each case. More recently, van Driel et al. [11] have proposed a more universal model. This model predicts inhomogeneous melting, in contrast to other models [10] which require uniform surface melting.

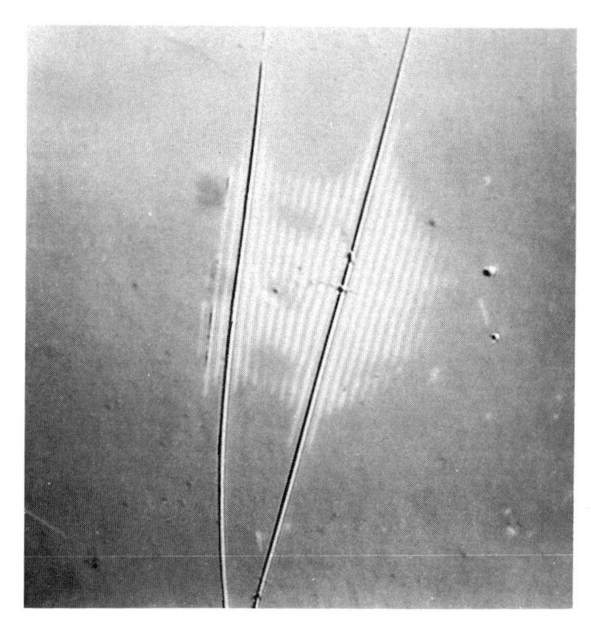

Fig.3 Periodic ripple pattern consisting of alternate regions of amorphous and crystalline silicon. The period is approximately 1 micron

In our case, the formation of ripple patterns within the recrystallized material could be adequately explained by either of the models. However, we have observed features evident of inhomogeneous and localized melting. In Fig.3 we show one particular case where the scattering has been enhanced by a surface scratch and has resulted in the formation of alternate regions of crystalline and amorphous material. Although such patterns are often seen outside but near the perimeter of the amorphous ring, they are most evident near defects. Suppose that during irradiation the silicon melted uniformly over the irradiated region and that a scattered surface wave propagated across the molten material to interfere with the incident radiation to result in differential energy deposition and inhomogeneous solidification. Keeping in mind then that recrystallization occurs for higher fluences than amorphization,such a set of events would require that the material at either end of the vertical crystalline lines be amorphous or that an amorphous ring surround the rippled region. Clearly there is no indication of any amorphous interface with the surrounding unmelted c-Si, suggesting that the crystalline material has remained in the solid phase throughout the entire interaction.

In conclusion, we have discussed the nature of the absorption of 1 micron picosecond pulses in c-Si and described a pulsewidth dependence of the single shot melting threshold. We have shown changes in surface morphology associated with irradiation by 1 μm pulses shorter than 12 ps and have presented indirect evidence for inhomogeneous energy deposition. Specifically, we have observed the presence of alternating regions of amorphous and crystalline silicon that we have tentatively taken to be the result of localized melting.

References


1. H. Kurz, in "Festkoerperprobleme XXIII", 1983, p. 115.
2. A. L. Smirl, T. F. Boggess, I. W. Boyd, S. C. Moss, 17th International Conference on the Physics of Semiconductors, San Francisco, California, 6-10 August 1984 (to be published).
3. I. W. Boyd, S. C. Moss, T. F. Boggess, A. L. Smirl, Appl. Phys. Lett., (1984).
4. P. L. Liu, R. Yen, N. Bloembergen R. T. Hodgson, in "Laser and Electron Beam Processing of Materials," edited by C. W. White and P. S. Peercy (Academic, New York, 1980).
5. J. M. Liu, Rev. Sci. Inst., Optics Letters, 7, 196 (1982).
6. M. Birnbaum, J. Appl. Phys. 36, 3688 (1965).
7. D. C. Emmony, R. P. Howson, K. J. Willis, Appl. Phys. Lett., 23, 598 (1977).
8. N. R. Isenor, Appl. Phys. Lett., 31, 148 (1977).
9. P. A. Temple, M. J. Soileau, IEEE J. Quantum Electron., 17, 2067 (1981).
10. S. R. J. Brueck, D. J. Ehrlich, Phys. Rev. Lett., 48, 1678 (1982).
11. H. M. van Driel, J. E. Sipe, J. F. Young, Phys. Rev. Lett., 49, 1955 (1982).

# Instabilities of Crystallization in Amorphous Germanium Under Pulsed Laser Irradiation

P. Fontaine, J. Marfaing, W. Marine, F. Salvan

Faculté des Sciences de Luminy, ERA 373, Département de Physique, Case 901, F-13288 Marseille Cedex 9, France

B. Mutaftschiev

Campus de Luminy, CRMC, Case 913, F-13288 Marseille Cedex 9, France

Several crystallization mechanisms of amorphous solids under laser irradiation have been proposed in the last few years. In previous work, an explosive crystallization mechanism of thin amorphous germanium films under pulsed laser irradiation in a transmission electron microscope has been reported [1,2]. It was shown that a solid phase crystallization mechanism occurs at the crystallization threshold. Different results strongly depending on the crystallization conditions have been obtained on a-Ge by several workers. For example, pulsed laser and pulsed electron beam crystallizations may give similar [3,4] results or may not [5,6]; thermal crystallization [7,8] is different from laser recrystallization. We have also noted in our series of experiments that the morphological features of the crystallized pattern are very dependent on the thermal "prehistory" of the film. In order to gain further insight on the structural properties and the growth kinetics, we undertook a systematically controlled study where we examined the crystallization mechanism as a function of controlled parameters. We investigated the influence of the thickness of the films, the evaporation rate, repetitive laser pulses, as well as thermal preannealing of the film. We also calculated the maximal temperature reached in the film in the different regimes of crystallization observed.

## 1 Experimental Conditions and Results

Crystallization of unsupported Ge films (220-1000 Å thick) has been performed in situ in a TEM microscope with a Nd:YAG laser ($\lambda$ = 0.53 µm, 14 ns FWHM). When irradiations with one single pulse of increasing incident energy density were made, no crystallization occurred below a minimum energy density defined as the crystallization threshold. Three regimes were observed:

i) Just above the crystallization threshold, typical features consist of spherulites with dendritic crystals inside 2-3 µm long and 1 µm wide with a number of quasi periodic rings 0.6-0.7 µm large on their periphery.

ii) Increasing the energy density, a second regime appears : fine polycrystallites of about 0.1-0.2 µm large are formed in the center of the irradiated zone. At the periphery of this zone long dendrites and rings exist as in the first regime.

iii) When the energy density is about twice the threshold value, a third regime -coalescence- is characterized by four zones with different structures. In the center, spherical, separated grains ($\sim$ 1 µm diameter) are formed, held by a very thin film of oxide (in diffraction the diagrams present large rings like amorphous material). Polycrystalline, then dendritic zones, and finally annular rings appear.

Let us look now at the influence of different parameters on the first regime described above. We first of all verify that in the range of evaporation

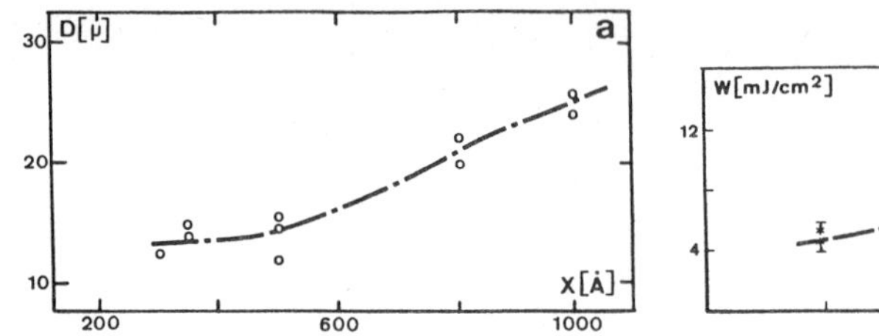


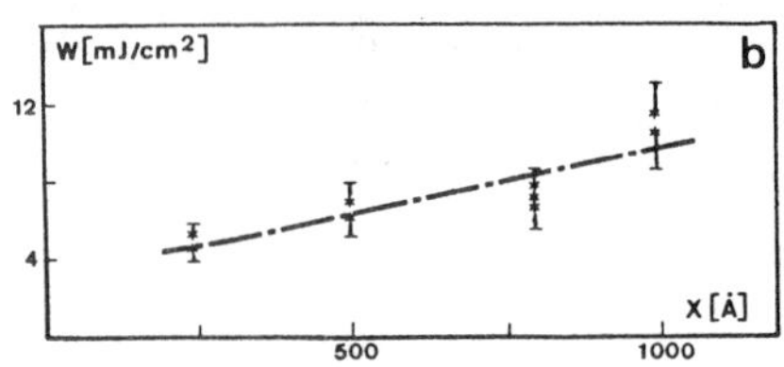


Fig. 1 -
(a) Diameter of the dendritic zone versus thickness of the Ge film
(b) Threshold energy density (TED) versus thickness of the germanium film under one single laser irradiation

rate used (0.5 to 2 Å $s^{-1}$) no significant difference in the threshold energy density of crystallization (TED) is visible. Also, controls by diffraction patterns of the different amorphous films give identical results. The second parameter tested was the thickness X of the film. Fig. 1a shows that the diameter of the dendritic zone increases with the thickness of the film in the ranges studied. Likewise the (TED) increases when the film becomes thicker as seen in Fig. 1b. It was also noticed that the number of rings varied from one for the thinner specimens to 6 or 7 for the thickest ones. This is due to a change of the internal stress energy ($\gamma$). The stresses are associated with defects in the random structure which give an $x^2$ dependence in the bending forces per unit width [9]. This causes a change in the barrier height of the activation energy $W_0$ for the amorphous to crystalline phase transformation. We can show that the energy condition for self-sustaining crystallization is

$$\Delta H_{a-c} + 2\gamma > W_0 \qquad (1)$$

where $\Delta H_{a-c}$ is the heat of crystallization released. The energy balance between the $\Delta H_{a-c}$ and $W_0$ which depends on the internal stress energy allows propagation of the crystallization up to a certain distance from the spot centre and gives the dependence of the crystallized zone dimensions and the number of rings versus the film thickness.

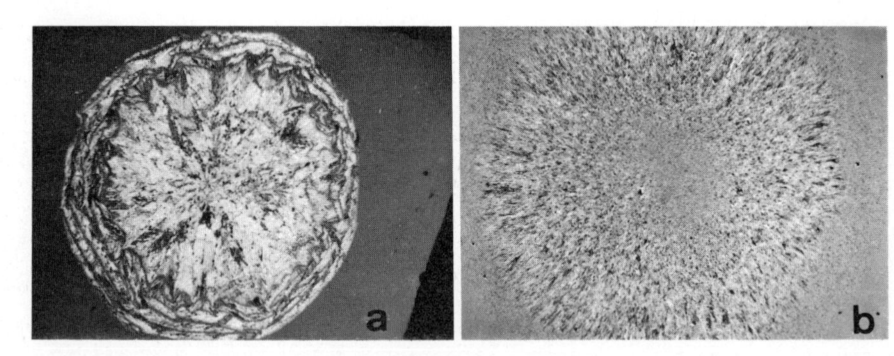


Fig. 2 - Morphologies of amorphous germanium films crystallized by a single laser pulse of threshold energy density (TED) :
- without preannealing of the film (a)
- with 1 hour thermal preannealing at 100°C in a furnace (b)

Let us consider now the influence of different preannealings.

Furnace preannealing - Thermal annealing in a furnace at a temperature T < 250°C for one hour causes a decrease of about 20 % of the TED. Figure 2 also shows that the crystallization pattern is different. Fine polycrystalline grains are preferentially formed with thermal preannealing followed by laser irradiation; the large dendrites become very fine in comparison to those observed without pretreatment. Generally no final ring is formed and if one exists, it is separated from the preceding grains by a very fine polycrystalline zone.

Laser preannealing - Then we tested the influence of preannealing with laser irradiation on the TED. Successive irradiations (from 20 to 1000) at one second interval with an energy density 25 % smaller than the TED were made and no crystallization occurs after such a treatment. Then, by continuously increasing the irradiation energy density of one single pulse, crystallization was observed with an increase of the threshold (TED) of 25-30 %. The changes in the morphology of the crystallization are i) a decrease in the size of the spot, ii)the dendrites become more fine, iii) a decrease of the polycrystallite dimensions with a larger density, iv) we observe a displacement of the final ring which is separated by a very fine polycrystalline zone from the central dendrites.

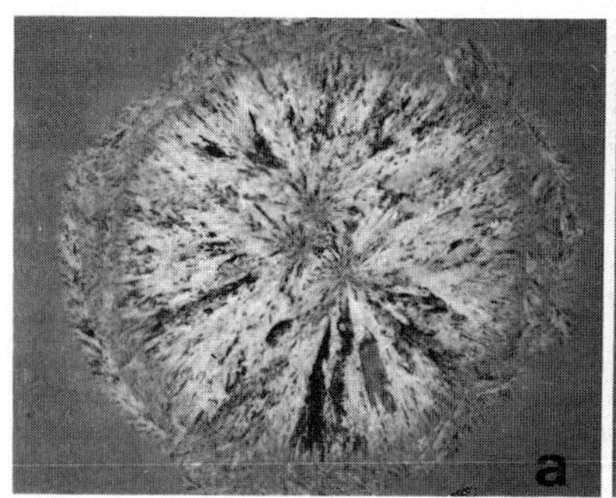


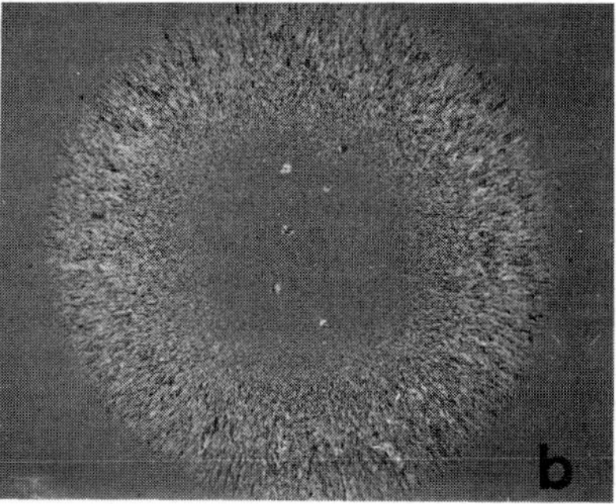


Fig. 3 - Influence of laser preannealing (successive laser irradiation 25 % energy density smaller than TED):
- without thermal preannealing of the film (a)
- with 1 hour thermal preannealing at 250°C in a furnace (b)

If prior to the successive laser irradiations, specimens are heated in a furnace, only 10 % energy higher than TED is needed to cause crystallization. Thermal and laser annealing morphologies of crystallization are shown in Fig. 3. The crystallization features, after laser preannealing, give evidence of a decrease of the $\gamma$ value (eq. 1), which governs explosive crystallization. When thermal annealing is applied to the a-film, the TED decreases and at the same time the explosive crystallization seems inhibited. During the thermal annealing time, for the a-film several zones with short range order can be rearranged but the critical dimension of the nucleus is not reached, and under laser irradiation these preoriented zones are more easily crystallized with a lower value of energy than TED.

## 2 Discussion

The morphology of the different crystallized zones can be discussed in terms of the temperature at the centre and along a radius of the crystallized spot. In our laser annealing experiments, the temperature distribution is governed by the Gaussian spatial laser beam profile (thermal diffusion plays a minor role during the excitation because the thermal diffusion length $\sim 1$ µm is much smaller than the excitation beam dimension $\sim 50$ µm and greater than the film thickness).

Our dynamical studies [10] show that nucleation and crystallization under TED conditions starts during excitation. From classical nucleation theories, the nucleation rate is given by :

$$V \propto \frac{kT}{h} e^{-W_0/kT} e^{-A/kT(\Delta T)^2} \qquad (2)$$

where $W_0$ is the activation energy of migration, kT/h the Debye frequency, A is a constant depending on the form of nuclei and $\Delta T = T - T_f$ (with $T_f$ denoting the fusion temperature) the surfusion.

Such a function, schematically represented in Fig. 4, shows a maximum for the temperature value $T_m$.

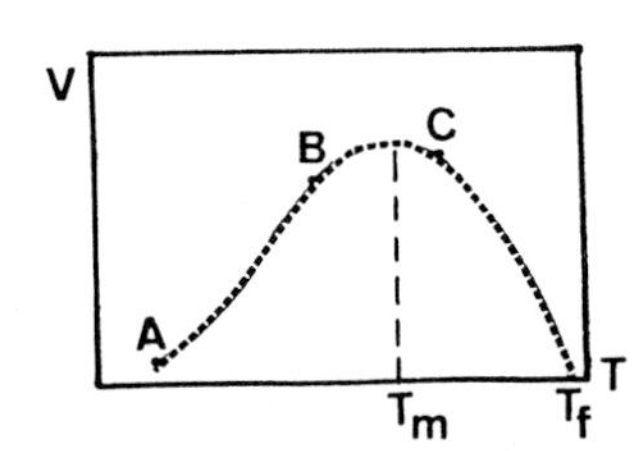


Fig. 4 - Schematic diagram of the nucleation rate versus temperature

The number of critical nuclei increases with the surfusion and the nucleation rate is maximal at $T_m$. Then the atomic diffusion phenomena are important and the nucleation rate decreases for temperatures less than $T_m$. It causes an auto-regulation of the phenomenon. Such a case corresponds to the decreasing part of the curve in Fig. 4 where $T > T_m$. If the surfusion is important -as in amorphous materials- the phenomena can be explained in a nonclassical nucleation model where transport phenomena are predominant. At ambient temperature, the atomic diffusion is quasi-zero and the term $e^{-Wo/kT}$ is negligible. When the temperature is increased, this term increases as well as the atomic diffusion(which then is sufficient and so allows atoms to move from equilibrium positions) and the amorphous matrix crystallizes. Such a behaviour exists when $T < T_m$ (corresponding to the positive slope of the curve in Fig. 4). Nuclei appear through an amorphous-crystalline transformation. The exothermic crystallization heat gives additional heating in the neighbourhood of the preexistent nuclei. Two phenomena can then exist depending on the ratio between the crystal growth rate and the crystallization heat dissipation :

i) if the heat generation rate caused by crystallization is slow, the exothermic heat diffuses in the material to such a distance that the additional temperature near the nuclei is not important : the isolated nuclei formation rate follows the shape given in Fig. 4 at the beginning of the curve (point A). It corresponds to thermal crystallization;

ii) if the heat generation rate is fast, the crystallization heat cannot diffuse far away from the crystallized zone. At neighbouring regions, the amorphous matrix undergoes an incrase in temperature that creates an increase of the nucleation and crystal growth rates. The phenomenon is auto-induced and is characteristic of the explosive crystallization, often observed in amorphous materials. In this case, the crystal growth rate is very far from the equilibrium rate.

In our experiments, using nanosecond laser pulses, we can reach and instantaneously go beyond the crystallization threshold temperature (point B in Fig. 4) on a well-localized zone of the amorphous film. As the heat diffusion through the film is negligible during the irradiation time, the crystallization heat easily increases the temperature of the amorphous crystalline interface. Thus the explosive phenomenon can start, and a crystallized zone of significant diameter ($\sim$ 10 μm) is created.

Our temperature estimations from the measurements of TED give a value of 660 K in the thicker films under laser irradiation. From the centre of the crystallized spot along a radius r, this temperature decreases because of the spatial Gaussian distribution of the irradiation. In the centre, one or more nuclei appear and the process is as explained in ii). Explosive crystallization propagates with a high rate : 10-40 m/s [5]. The ring formation is produced by thermal diffusion as stated above (Eq. 1).

Analogous considerations are made in the polycrystalline regime. The temperature in the centre (point C, Fig. 4) is higher than in the preceding case and a high nucleus density exists. The growth of the nuclei is obstructed because of their density, and their growth rate is low $\sim$ 0.05 m/s [5]. After crystallization, the temperature in the spot centre increases and the nucleation rate decreases. Simultaneously along a radius and at a certain distance from the centre depending on the temperature, explosive crystallization has been induced as in the preceding regime.

Our estimations show that the nucleation rate ,V, under laser irradiations is more than $10^{18}$ $cm^{-3}$ $s^{-1}$, well above the V = $10^{7}$ $cm^{-3}$ $s^{-1}$ [7] measured under furnace conditions at the same temperature. This difference, due to the presence of the strong concentration (N $\sim$ $10^{20}$ $cm^{-3}$) involves a decrease in the activation energy ($W_0$) for nucleation.

In conclusion, we show that explosive crystallization of thin unsupported germanium films under laser irradiation can occur in a solid phase and is propagated further when the films contain additional internal stresses. Thermal preannealing has an influence on the morphology of the crystallized zones and promotes the formation of polycrystallites.

The observed phenomena can be explained by classical theories if we assume that the activation energy for nucleation is dependent on the free carrier density.

References


1 J. Marfaing, P. Pierrard, W. Marine, B. Mutaftschiev and F. Salvan : Microscopy of Semiconducting Materials, edited by A.G. Cullis, S.M. Davidson and G.R. Booker, 1983.
2 P. Pierrard, B. Mutaftschiev, W. Marine, J. Marfaing and F. Salvan : Thin Solid Films 111, 141 (1984).
3 R. Andrew, M. Lovato : J. Appl. Phys. 50, 1142 (1979).
4 R.K. Sharma, S.K. Bansal, R. Nath and R.M. Mehra : J. Appl. Phys. 55, 387 (1984).
5 O. Bostanjoglo : Phys. Stat. Sol.(a) 70, 473 (1982).

6 G. Andrä, H.D. Geiler, G. Götz, K.H. Heinig and H. Woittennek : Phys. Stat. Sol.(a) 74, 511 (1982).
7 P. Germain, K. Zellama, S. Squelard, J.C. Bourgoin and A. Gheorghiu : J. Appl. Phys. 50, 6988 (1979).
8 A. Barna, P.B. Barna, Z. Bodo, J.F. Pocza, I. Pozsgai and G. Radnoczi : Thin Solid Films 23, 49 (1974).
9 M.A. Paesler: Amorphous and Liquid Semiconductors, edited by J. Stuke and W. Brenig, Taylor and Francis, London (1974).
10 W. Marine, J. Marfaing, P. Mathiez and F. Salvan: J. Phys. C (1984), to be published.

# Time Resolved Calorimetry of 30 nm Te-Films During Laser Annealing

H. Coufal and W. Lee
IBM Research Laboratory 5600 Cottle Road, K34/281
San Jose, California 95193 U.S.A.

The temperature of 30 nm thick Te films has been studied during annealing with a XeCl Excimer laser. Using a pyroelectric thin film calorimeter melting, boiling and recrystallization were observed. Boiling was identified as the prevalent mechanism for the loss of material.

## 1. Introduction

The laser annealing of 30 nm thick Te films has been studied using a pyroelectric thin film calorimeter [1]. Pyroelectric calorimeters are particularly suitable for the study of transient heating phenomena of thin films because of their sensitivity and time resolution. If the sample can be directly deposited onto the calorimeter it can be used as an ultrafast thermometer with a response time in the order of few picoseconds: Assuming a temperature-independent pyroelectric coefficient the charge generated in a pyroelectric element is proportional to the heat content of this element and independent of the temperature distribution. For a thin film deposited onto such a calorimeter the heat flow from the film into the calorimeter is, however, proportional to the average temperature at the interface. To be able to probe the generated charge,electrodes have to be deposited on both sides of the calorimeter, *i.e.*, also between the pyroelectric detector material and the heat source, the sample. Assuming the validity of classical heat conduction processes an electrode with a thickness of 30 nm introduces due to its finite thermal diffusivity a time delay of several picoseconds. The same is true also for the heat diffusion from the sample surface to the interface between sample and electrode. With an electronic bandwidth of 100 MHz for the existing experimental set up,time delay and dispersion due to thermal diffusion from the sample into the calorimeter are, therefore, negligible. The observed signal is thus within the above limits a true representation of the temperature of the sample.

## 2. Experimental

In this study, 9 $\mu$m thick ferroelectric $PVF_2$ foils (Pennwalt KYNAR®) were used as the active pyroelectric element. The $PVF_2$ foils were coated on both sides with a 0.3 nm Ni electrode. The coated foil was stretched over a 8 mm diameter stainless steel supporting ring and held in place by a retaining ring. These rings served as heat sinks, electrical contacts and for mechanical support. The complete assembly was housed in a standard microbalance housing for RF shielding.

The tellurium films in this work were thermally evaporated onto the assembled calorimeters from Knudsen cells charged with pure Te (99.9995%) source material. During the deposition the substrate was at room temperature, and the pressure in the vacuum chamber was in the order of $1 \times 10^{-7}$ Torr. The Te film thickness and deposition rate (30 nm/min) was controlled by a quartz microbalance. Films deposited under similar conditions have been found to be polycrystalline with a grain size of 100- 250 nm [2]. Upon exposure to air a 2 nm thick surface layer of these films was found to be oxidized according to ESCA data [2].

Samples were excited at ambient conditions with a XeCl Excimer laser (Lambdaphysik EMG 201) at a wave length of 308 nm. At the sample position fluences between 100 $\mu J/cm^2$ and 70 $mJ/cm^2$ were achieved by suitably attenuating the raw beam. The half-width of the laser pulses was determined to be 12 ns. A custom designed preamplifier (Comlinear CLC-B-600) with a 450 ps risetime and a 100 MHz transient digitizer (Dataprecision D6000) were used to record and analyze the time-dependent signals.

Depending on the laser fluence typical signal shapes as shown in Fig. 1 are observed. The temperature rises almost instantaneously and depending on the initial temperature either falls continuously (Fig. 1a) or shows a plateau (Figs. 1b,c). If the plateau temperature is tentatively assigned to the recrystallization temperature of Te at 449°C the peak temperature in Fig. 1c would correspond to the boiling point of Te at 989°C.

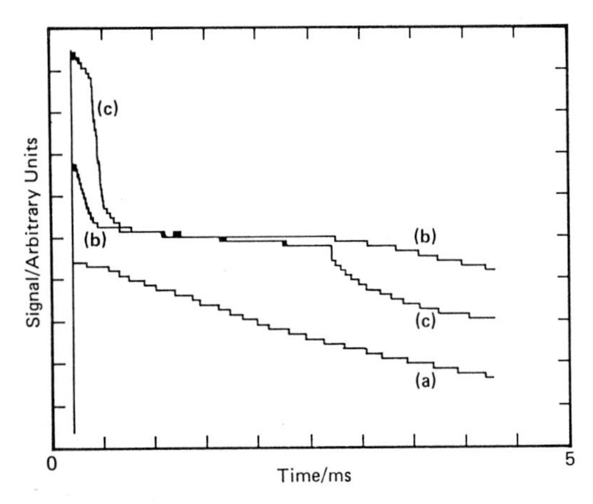


Fig. 1: Temperature during annealing of 30 nm thick Te films with a XeCl Excimer laser for 3 different laser fluences: (a) 0.7 $mJ/cm^2$, (b) 7 $mJ/cm^2$ and (c) 70 $mJ/cm^2$.

This assignment of temperatures is supported by experiments at higher time resolution. With increasing laser fluence (Figs. 2a-2e) the sample temperature does not increase proportionally. Despite a substantial increase in laser power from 2d to 2e the same final temperature is reached. These observations are consistent with the latent heat of the assigned first-order phase transitions. Tellurium being a semiconductor has of course two different relaxation mechanisms, a fast vibrational relaxation with a ps life time and a subsequent electronic relaxation with a life time of the order of tens of nanoseconds. Figure 2d then would be consistent with instantaneous melting during the laser pulse by vibrational relaxation and subsequent heating of the molten Te to the boiling point by electronic deexcitation. To a lesser degree these two relaxation mechanisms are visible also at other fluences. To test this interpretation of the data an experiment at a wavelength of 3.7 $\mu m$ is under preparation which should show the effect of electronic relaxation only.

Independent of the incident laser power all molten samples cool to the same crystallization temperature (Fig. 3). The latent heat for crystallization depends of course on the amount of material lost due to evaporation. As shown in Fig. 4 the transition from

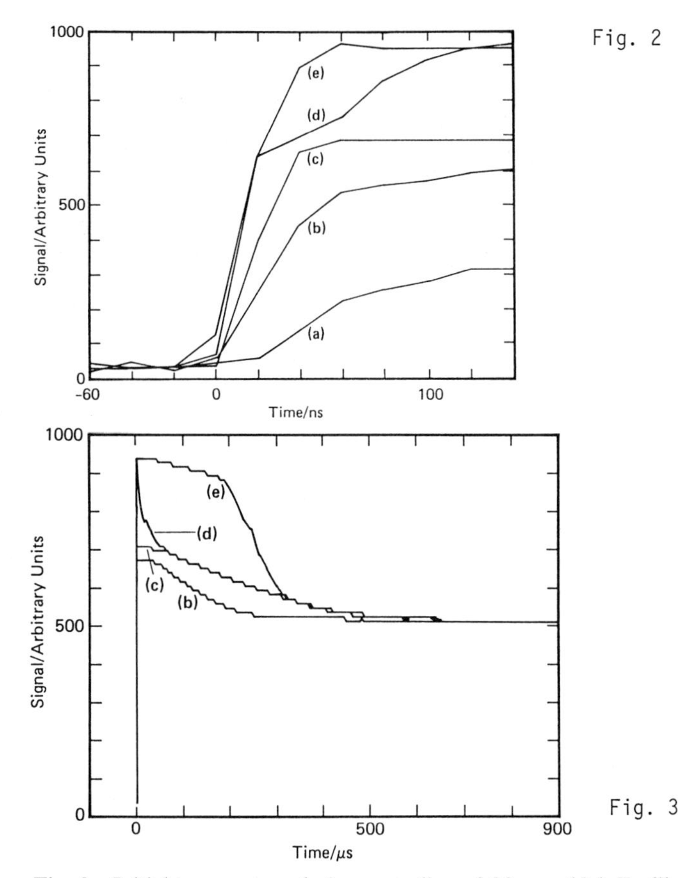


Fig. 2: Initial temperature during annealing of 30 nm thick Te films with a XeCl Excimer laser with 5 different fluences: (a) 0.7 mJ/cm$^2$, (b) 2 mJ/cm$^2$, (c) 7 mJ/cm$^2$, (d) 24 mJ/cm$^2$ and (e) 70 mJ/cm$^2$.

Fig. 3: Temperature during the liquid phase observed when annealing 30 nm thick Te films with a XeCl Excimer laser with different laser fluences (b)-(e) as in Fig. 2.

crystallization to cooling by heat conduction in solidified material occurs earlier for increasing laser fluences. The largest increase in material loss is observed for Fig. 4e, the exposure with the longest boiling time (Fig. 3e). In the molten phase several time constants are observed. Before the onset of crystallization one time constant which is attributed to heat conduction in liquid tellurium is observed for all samples. The initial plateau and the subsequent rapid cooling at the highest laser fluences might be due to heating of part of the calorimeter above its Curie temperature and subsequent evaporation of the sample.

Computer simulations of the heating and cooling processes using a *finite differences* method for the solution of the heat diffusion equation are under way. Preliminary results are in agreement with the general pulse shape observed and the peak temperatures reached. These calculations also indicate that a thin layer of the $PVF_2$ material should be for a short time above its melting point and, therefore, no longer pyroelectric. Measurements of the capacitance of the calorimeters before and after laser annealing did,

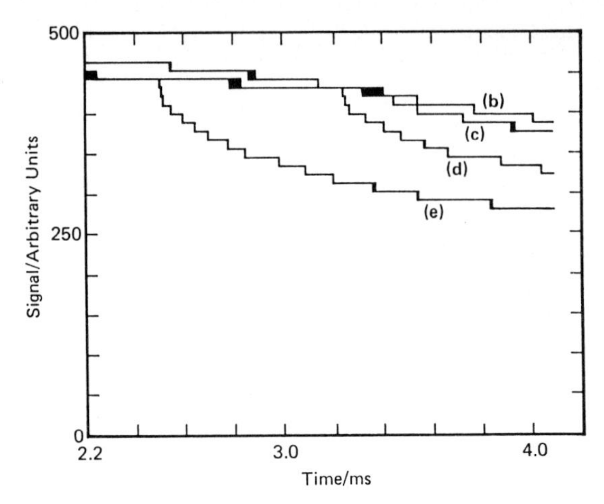


Fig. 4: Temperature during the transition from recrystallization to conduction in the solid state observed when annealing 30 nm thick Te-films with different laser fluences (b)-(e) as in Fig. 2.

however, not show any change in polarization. Repolarization of the depolarized thin surface layer upon cooling below the Curie temperature is conceivable as a consequence of the high electric fields generated by the hot, but still polarized bulk of the calorimeter.

## 3. Conclusion

In conclusion, the feasibility of calorimetric studies of thin films during laser annealing has been demonstrated. The data indicate the importance of the various relaxation processes for heating of the semiconductor film and different heat transport processes during the cooling phase. In addition boiling was identified as the prevalent mechanism for the loss of material in this experiment.

## 4. Acknowledgments

The authors would like to thank R. Grygier and L. Kelley for technical assistance. This work was supported in part by the Office of Naval Research.

## 5. References

[1] H. Coufal, *Appl. Phys. Lett.* **44**, 59 (1984).
[2] W. Lee and R. Geiss, *J. Appl. Phys.* **54**, 1351 (1983).

# Pulsed Laser Annealing of GaAs: A Comparison Between Calculation and Experiment

A. Rose
Division of Chemical Physics, Commonwealth Scientific and Industrial Research Organization, Lucas Heights Research Laboratories, PMB 7, Sutherland, NSW 2232, Australia

E.K. Rose
Applied Physics Division, Australian Atomic Energy Commission Research Establishment, Lucas Heights Research Laboratories, PMB, Sutherland, NSW 2232, Australia

Results from a thermal melting model for pulsed laser annealing of GaAs are presented and compared with laser dissociation measurements made as a function of absorbed laser energy.

Neutron activation is used to determine the number of As and Ga atoms lost from the surface by dissociation during the laser pulse. Surface temperatures are calculated on the basis of this measured loss. The model calculates temperatures significantly higher than previously reported, but in reasonable agreement with dissociation loss measurements.

## 1 Introduction

It is well known [1] that high power pulsed lasers can successfully anneal ion implantation damage in semiconductors. The main thrust of both experiment and calculation has centered on Si and the controversy [2-4a] on the physical mechanism of laser annealing seems to have been resolved in favour of thermal melting and recrystallization [4b].

More recently, interest in laser annealing of GaAs has grown and experiments by Aydinli [5] and Pospieszczyk [6] again cast doubt on the annealing mechanism. The former argue in favour of a non-thermal plasma heating model, while the latter are in favour of a thermal heating model. A number of dissociation loss measurements [6-8] have been reported and when these are considered we feel that the balance, as in the Si case, swings in favour of thermal melting. However, thermal melting model calculations of pulsed laser annealing of GaAs by Wood [9], Wang and Saris [10] and Boerma [8] predict surface temperatures which are too low if the experimentally determined As and Ga dissociation losses [6-8] are accepted. Using the experimental data on Ga loss [7] Pollock and Rose [11] argue that if vapour pressure data for Ga are taken into account the surface temperature of GaAs during laser annealing can exceed the boiling point of Ga.

Why then are the temperature predictions of the GaAs melting model calculations so low? A survey of previous models shows that they have relied on absorption coefficient values which are significantly smaller than that recently reported [5]. Using this recent data [5] we present a melting model calculation which predicts temperatures considerably higher than those of other models. We also report new measurements of Ga loss using the neutron activation technique of Rose [7] and compare temperatures predicted from vapour pressure considerations with our thermal model calculations.

## 2 Mathematical Model

For a pulsed laser beam incident normally along the z-axis of a target with the transverse (x,y) plane assumed infinite compared to the thickness, the problem of thermal diffusion may be treated by the one-dimensional equation

$$\frac{\partial T}{\partial t} = \frac{\partial}{\partial z}\left(\frac{K}{\rho c}\frac{\partial T}{\partial z}\right) + Q \tag{1}$$

where Q is the heat generation function due to the laser input energy and K, $\rho$, c are the thermal conductivity, mass density and heat capacity respectively of the target material. The solution of this equation can be found numerically by using the Crank-Nicholson finite-difference approximation

$$\frac{T_i^{n+1} - T_i^n}{\Delta t} = \frac{|\delta(\sigma\partial T)|_i^{n+1} + |\delta(\sigma\partial T)|_i^n}{2(\Delta z_i)^2} + Q_i^a \tag{2}$$

where the target is divided into M thin layers of thickness $\Delta z_i$ along the z-axis, with each layer assuming a definite temperature $T_i$ and thus a definite set of thermophysical properties $K_i$, $\rho_i$ and $c_i$ in each time interval $\Delta t$. $Q_i^a$ is the energy absorbed per unit area in the ith layer from the laser radiation and is defined as

$$Q_i^a = (I_i - I_{i+1})\frac{\Delta t}{\rho_i c_i \Delta z_i} \tag{3}$$

with $I_{i_o} = I_o(t)(1-R_i)$

$$I_{i+1} = I_i \exp(-\alpha_i \Delta z_i) \qquad i \geq i_o$$

and $I_o(t)$, the temporal intensity profile of the laser beam, is approximated by

$$I_o(t) = \begin{cases} \left(\frac{E_p}{t_p}\right)\left(\frac{t}{t_p}\right) & 0 \leq t \leq t_p \\ \left(\frac{E_p}{t_p}\right)\left(2 - \frac{t}{t_p}\right) & t_p < t \leq 2t_p \\ 0 & t > 2t_p \end{cases}$$

where $E_p$ is the incident laser energy per unit area, $t_p$ is the FWHM of the pulse, $R_i$ is the reflection coefficient of the material in the ith layer and $\alpha_i$ is the linear absorption coefficient for the laser radiation (both $R_i$ and $\alpha_i$ may take different values for the solid and molten states). Thus the equations to be solved at each time step are:

$$-\sigma^+ T_{i+1}^{n+1} + (1+\sigma^- + \sigma^+)T_i^{n+1} - \sigma^- T_{i-1}^{n+1} = Q_i^a + Q_i^d \tag{4}$$

where the right-hand side is a function of known quantities at time $t_n$ only. $Q_i^a$ is defined in (3) and $Q_i^d$ is the amount of heat received in the ith layer by thermal conduction from adjacent layers and given by

$$Q_i^d = \sigma^+ T_{i+1}^n - (\sigma^- + \sigma^+ - 1)T_i^n + \sigma^- T_{i-1}^n \tag{5}$$

with $\sigma^{\pm} = \frac{\Delta t}{2\rho_i c_i \Delta z_i}\left(\frac{K^{\pm}}{\Delta z^{\pm}}\right)$

$$K^{\pm} = \frac{K_i K_{i\pm1}(\Delta z_i + \Delta z_{i\pm1})}{K_i\, \Delta z_{i\pm1} + K_{i\pm1}\Delta z_i}$$

$$\Delta z^{\pm} = \frac{1}{2} (\Delta z_i + \Delta z_{i\pm 1})$$

To include the effects of material phase changes in the calculations which occur when

$$T_i^n \le T_i^m < T_i^{n+1} \qquad \text{(melting)}$$

$$T_i^{n+1} < T_i^m \le T_i^n \qquad \text{(solidification)}$$

and $$T_i^m < T_i^n < T_i^b < T_i^{n+1} \qquad \text{(vaporization)}$$

where $T_i^m$ , $T_i^b$ are the melting and boiling points of the material in the ith layer, the procedure of Jain et al. [12] was followed in order to incorporate the latent heats of fusion and vaporization respectively.

## 3 Computational Procedure

The finite-difference equation (4) may be rewritten as

$$-A_i T_{i+1} + B_i T_i - C_i T_{i-1} = D_i \tag{6}$$

where $A_i = \sigma^+$, $C_i = \sigma^-$ and $B_i = 1+A_i+C_i$, with the superscript n+1 deleted for simplicity, and $D_i = Q_i^a + Q_i^d$ at time $t_n$.

A very efficient and suitable method for automatic computation of any finite-difference approximation is the special adaptation of the Gauss elimination procedure reported by Richtmeyer and Morton [13] which seeks two sets of quantities $E_i$, $F_i$ such that

$$T_i = E_i T_{i+1} + F_i \tag{7}$$

with $$E_i = \frac{A_i}{B_i - C_i E_{i-1}}$$

$$F_i = \frac{D_i + C_i F_{i-1}}{B_i - C_i E_{i-1}} \qquad i \ge 1 \; .$$

By forward elimination of $E_i$ and $F_i$ with boundary conditions $E_0 = F_0 = 0$, the values of $T_i$ can be determined in order of decreasing i by backward substitution using the fact that $T_{M+1} = 293$ K (room temperature) for all timesteps. The efficiency of this method lies in the fact that it requires only three multiplications and two divisions per space point per time step, apart from computation of the coefficients.

## 4 Input Data

The thermal conductivity values K(T) for GaAs were obtained from Maycock [14] for $T \le 1000$ K, and assumed to follow the inverse law for $T > 1000$ K. Heat capacity c and mass density $\rho$ were held constant for all layers at 0.36 J $g^{-1}$ $K^{-1}$ and 5.32 g $cm^{-3}$ respectively. The melting point of GaAs was taken as 1511 K with the latent heat $L^m$ = 133 cal $g^{-1}$. As GaAs cannot be considered to have a boiling point, the boiling point of Ga was taken as 2510 K and used with latent heat $L^v$ = 533 cal $g^{-1}$. The reflection coefficients used were 0.33 and 0.67 for the solid and liquid phases respectively. The absorption coefficient has been measured [5] to rise to

$4 \times 10^5$ cm$^{-1}$ which is close to the expected value for a metallic liquid and much higher than for crystalline GaAs. Therefore, $5 \times 10^4$ cm$^{-1}$ was used below the melting point and $4 \times 10^5$ cm$^{-1}$ on melting. For these calculations a Gaussian shaped pulse with FWHM of 40 ns, which should approximate the ruby laser output used in the experiments, has been assumed. The thickness of the layer $\Delta z$ was held constant at 0.05 μm and the time interval $\Delta t$ was set at 0.1 ns.

## 5 Dissociation Experiments

The Q-switched homogenized ruby laser system and neutron activation technique used for these dissocation measurements has been described by Rose [7]. However, for the data reported here we measured absorbed energy by a calorimetric method in which each sample was an integral part of the calorimeter. The calorimeter was energy calibrated for each sample. As absorbed rather than incident energies were measured, we have used a reflectivity value of 0.33 to convert our measured absorbed energies to incident energies for comparison with other reported data.

Polished crystalline (100) GaAs samples were laser irradiated with a 40 ns pulse. Previous results [7] indicated that the lowest incident energy for Ga dissociation was 0.2 J cm$^{-2}$, hence a range of incident energies from 0.1 to 0.6 J cm$^{-2}$ were used. Dissociation measurements were also carried out on GaAs samples which had been implanted with Te. A summary of the measurements is given in Table 1.

Table 1 Experimental results

| Incident Energy J cm$^{-2}$ | Te Implant Dose cm$^{-2}$ | Ga Atoms cm$^{-2}$ |
|---|---|---|
| 0.44 | unimplanted | $1.49 \times 10^{13}$ |
| 0.51 | " | $1.52 \times 10^{13}$ |
| 0.58 | " | $9.70 \times 10^{14}$ |
| 0.50 | $5 \times 10^{15}$ | $5.30 \times 10^{15}$ |
| 0.51 | $1 \times 10^{15}$ | $2.28 \times 10^{15}$ |
| 0.61 | $8 \times 10^{14}$ | $4.79 \times 10^{15}$ |

## 6 Results and Discussion

From the model, calculated maximum temperatures as a function of laser energy are shown in Fig. 1. The maximum temperature increases steadily up to the melting point of GaAs at ∿0.4 J cm$^{-2}$. A plateau region exists from ∿0.4 to 0.5 J cm$^{-2}$ before a rapid climb to 0.76 J cm$^{-2}$ where vaporization takes place.

A similar pattern was reported by Pospieszczyk [6] in an elegant experiment using mass spectrometry to determine the temperature of Ga atoms evaporated during laser dissociation of GaAs. However, they [6] found the onset of Ga dissociation at 0.1 J cm$^{-2}$. In the present work Ga was detected at energies above 0.44 J cm$^{-2}$. From Table 1 the number of Ga atoms cm$^{-2}$ measured following laser irradiation of the unimplanted GaAs is constant for energies of 0.44 and 0.51 J cm$^{-2}$ then increases dramatically at 0.58 J cm$^{-2}$. This data also follows the trend shown in Fig. 1. Using the Ga dissociation

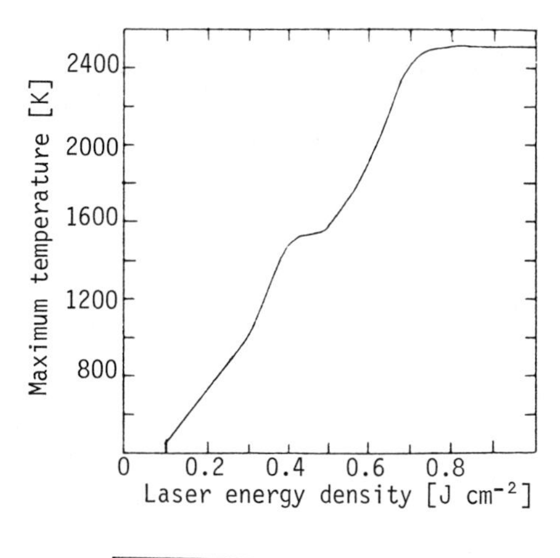


Fig. 1 Thermal model calculations of maximum surface temperatures reached as a function of incident laser energy

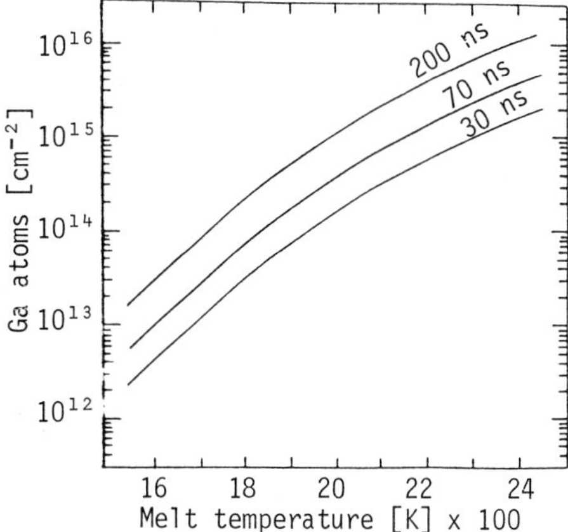


Fig. 2 Calculation of the number of Ga atoms $cm^{-2}$ vs melt temperatures

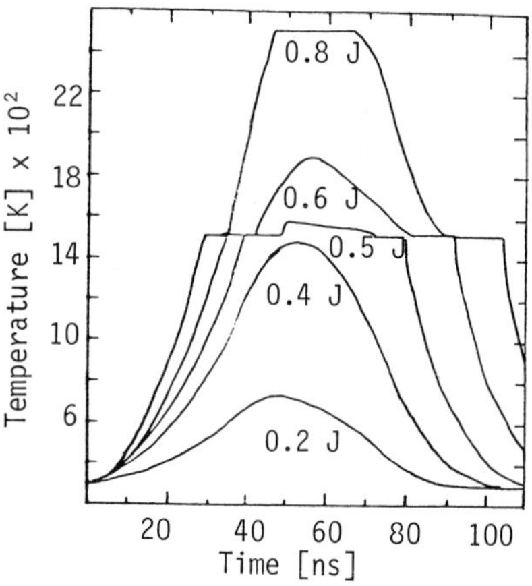

Fig. 3 Thermal model calculations of surface temperatures vs time

data in Table 1 and the calculated data in Figs. 2 and 3 estimates of the GaAs surface temperature can be made and compared with Fig. 1.

Figure 2, derived using Ga vapour pressure data [11,15], shows the number of Ga atoms $cm^{-2}$ as a function of melt temperature for different times after melting. The duration of the melting period for energies above 0.4 J $cm^{-2}$ is given in the computer model profiles of Fig. 3. It can be seen from Table 1 that laser energies of 0.44 and 0.51 J $cm^{-2}$ dissociate about $1.5 \times 10^{13}$ atoms $cm^{-2}$. If this value is used in Fig. 2 with a melt time of 40 ns from Fig. 3 a surface temperature of 1700 K is derived. Similarly, 0.58 J $cm^{-2}$ gives a melt temperature of 2200 K. From Fig. 1, the model predicts surface temperatures of 1580 and 1910 K, respectively.

These model-predicted temperatures are about 10-12% lower than those derived from the dissociation loss measurements, but give better agreement with the Ga dissociation data than do the predictions of earlier models [8,10].

The larger numbers of Ga atoms measured following annealing of Te implanted GaAs (Table 1) are interesting because it suggests an increase in absorption of laser energy with increasing implant dose. As the sample surface layer becomes more amorphous it is not expected [9] that absorption will increase. This is an area which merits further attention.

## 7 Conclusion

Using an absorption coefficient of $5 \times 10^4$ $cm^{-1}$ for crystalline GaAs and at the onset of melting increasing this to $4 \times 10^5$ $cm^{-1}$ has allowed a finite difference thermal melting model to predict surface temperatures of the order necessary to explain measured Ga dissociation losses.

## 8 Acknowledgement

Helpful discussions with J.T.A. Pollock are gratefully acknowledged.

## 9 References

1 J.F. Gibbons, L.D. Hess and T.W. Sigmon, eds., Proc. MRS Symp. on Laser and Electron-beam Solid Interactions and Material Processing (North-Holland, New York, 1981).
2 R.F. Wood and G.E. Giles, Phys. Rev. B 23 (1981).
3 R.F. Wood, J.R. Kirkpatrick and G.E. Giles, Phys. Rev. B23, 5555 (1981).
4a J.A. van Vechten, in Laser and Electron-beam Solid Interactions, edited by C.W. White and P.S. Peercy (Academic, New York, 1980), p. 53.
4b M.E.Thomson, G.I. Galvin, in Laser-Solid Interactions and Transient Thermal Processing of Materials, ed. by J. Narayan et al. (North Holland, New York 1983) Vol. 13, p.57.
5 A. Aydinli, A. Compaan, H.W. Lo and M.C. Lee, Phys. Lett. 86A (1981) p.199
6 A. Pospieszczyk and M. Abdel Harith, J. Appl. Phys. 54 (6) (1983).
7 A. Rose, J.T.A. Pollock, M.D. Scott, F.M. Adams, J.S. Williams and E.M. Lawson, in Ref.5, p. 633.
8 D.O. Boerma, H. Hasper and K.G. Prasard, Phys. Lett. 92A, 253 (1983).
9 R.F. Wood, D.H. Lowndes and W.H. Christie, (ref. 1), p. 231
10 Z.L. Wang and F.W. Saris, Phys. Lett. 83A, 367 (1981).
11 J.T.A. Pollock and A. Rose, "Laser and electron-beam processing", Boston MRS (1983). To be published.
12 A.K. Jain, V.N. Kulkarni and D.K. Sood, Appl. Phys. 25, 127 (1981).
13 R.D. Richtmeyer and K.W. Morton, Difference Methods for Initial Value Problems, 2nd Ed. (Interscience, New York, 1967).
14 P.D. Maycock, Solid State Electron, 10, 161 (1967).
15 "Selected Values of the Thermodynamic Properties of the Elements", American Society for Metals (1976).

# Melting Model for UV Lasers

S. Unamuno, M. Toulemonde[+], and P. Siffert

Centre de Recherches Nucleaires, Laboratoire Phase,
F-67037 Strasbourg-Cedex, France

The thermodynamic model we developed previously for ruby or YAG laser annealing of silicon has been applied to evaluate the melt depths in the same semiconductor under U.V. pulsed laser irradiation.

The optical parameters for this wavelength range and their temperature dependence, used in the calculations, have been estimated from available results in literature.

The calculated depths have been compared with some experimental results existing in the literature for XeCl laser annealing.

The rapid development of pulsed excimer lasers in recent years opens quite interesting capabilities in view of commercial applications of pulsed laser annealing. It is well known that ruby or YAG lasers have been successfully used to remove the lattice damage induced by ion implantation, but beam non-uniformity can give rise to some problems.

The excimer lasers present several advantages for commercial applications : they are able to show even a large rectangular annealing area within which the pulse energy is very uniform, in contrast with ruby lasers where the spatial beam distribution is, at best, Gaussian; furthermore the pulse repetition rate is greater for excimer lasers.

However, there is little experimental information on laser annealing of ion implanted silicon using pulsed ultraviolet wavelengths |1, 2, 3|. We think it is interesting to apply to the UV lasers the melting model |4, 5, 6, 7, 8|, widely and successfully used to describe experimental results for ruby lasers annealing, in order to determine the main characteristics of annealing procedure.

Following this model the photon energy is locally and instantaneously converted into heat : the heat flow in silicon can be represented by the one-dimensional diffusion equation.

$$C_s \rho \frac{\partial T(x,t)}{\partial t} = \frac{\partial}{\partial x}\left[ k \frac{\partial T(x,t)}{\partial x} \right] + S(x,t)$$

where $C_s$ is the specific heat, $\rho$ the density and k the conductivity of material. S (x, t) is the heat generation and T (x, t) the temperature : both S and T being functions of space x and time t :

$$S(x,t) = I(t)(1-R)\,\alpha\, e^{-\alpha x}$$

[+] Present address : CIRIL, BP 5133 - F-14040 CAEN CEDEX (France) where $\alpha$ is the absorption coefficient, R the reflectivity and I (t) the power density of laser.

The initial condition is : $T(x, 0) = T_0$

and the boundary conditions $|\partial T(x,t) / \partial x|_{x=0} = 0$

$T(L, t) = T_0$ (L being the sample thickness).

Due to the non-linearity of equation (1) we use the method of differences in order to solve it. Details of this method are given in (8 c).

## I Parameters used in the thermal model

In this work we apply the model to the annealing of silicon with a UV laser. The parameters that we used are as follows, for the various physical states of silicon during the heating :

### a) Crystalline silicon

Thermal parameters are the same as reported in (8 c) on annealing with a ruby laser : their values and temperature dependence are shown in Table 1.

Table 1: Calculation Parameters $\lambda$ = 308 nm

| PARAMETERS | | CRYSTALLINE SILICON | AMORPHOUS SILICON | LIQUID Si |
|---|---|---|---|---|
| Melting temperature (K) | | 1687 | 1420 | - |
| Latent heat of melting (cal/gr) | | 430 | 300 | - |
| Density ($gr/cm^3$) | | 2.32 | 2.32 | 2.52 |
| Thermal conductivity (cal/(s.cm.K)) | $T \leq 1200$ K<br>$T > 1200$ K | $364/T^{1.226}$<br>$2.15/T^{0.502}$ | 0.02 | 0.14 |
| Specific heat (cal/(gr.K)) | $T \lesssim 300$ K<br>$T > 300$ K | $0.044 \exp(4.5 \times 10^{-3} T)$<br>$0.166 \exp(2.375 \times 10^{-4} T)$ | 0.2 | 0.25 |
| Absorption coefficient ($cm^{-1}$) | $T \leq 1100$ K<br>$T > 1100$ K | $1.4 \times 10^6 \exp(\frac{T}{4545})$<br>$1.8 \times 10^6$ | $10^6$ | $1.46 \times 10^6$ |
| Reflectivity | | $0.59 + 4 \times 10^{-5}$ T | 0.60 | 0.69 |

Obviously, optical parameters depend on the light wavelength. Several measurements exist in the UV region |9-13| at various temperatures. For example, the measurements by JELLISON and MODINE |9| give the values of real ($\varepsilon_1$) and imaginary ($\varepsilon_2$) parts of dielectric constant of Si for photon energy ranging from 1.7 to 4.7 eV and for temperatures from 10 to 972 K.

We extrapolated their results up to the melting temperature of crystalline silicon by studying the evolution with T of peaks, slopes, knees, etc., in their curves $\varepsilon_1$, $\varepsilon_2$ versus $E_{photon}$. Therefore, we were able to "construct" the curves $\varepsilon_1$, $\varepsilon_2$ versus $E_{photon}$ for the silicon melting temperature.

From this, we can obtain, for a chosen $\lambda$, the variation of $\varepsilon_1$, $\varepsilon_2$, and therefore, of R and $\alpha$, with T varying from 10 K to melting temperature. The results are shown in Fig. 1 for a Xe Cl ($\lambda$ = 308 nm) laser, where the reflectivity and absorption coefficient are reported versus temperature. It appears that both parameters show little dependence on T.

b) Amorphous silicon

To our knowledge, there is no information in the literature on the reflectivity of amorphous silicon in this wavelength domain. However, as found elsewhere |8|, this value has negligible influence on model calculations because of the rapid melting of the surface, especially for E well over threshold.

In all calculations, we have considered : R = 0.6 .

For the absorption coefficient we used the curve from GATTUSO et al. |15|: they give the variation of $\alpha_a$ with the proton energy from 1 to 3.6 eV. There is a weak dependence on energy for $E \geq 3.2$ eV. We took $\alpha_a = 10^6 cm^{-1}$.

The amorphous Si parameters, for $\lambda$ = 308 nm are also reported in Table 1.

c) Liquid Silicon

The refractive index, and extinction coefficient were measured for $\lambda$ between 400 and 1000 nm by SVAREV et al. |14|.

The values for $\alpha$ and R from these measurements are shown in Fig. 1 (b) and can be parametrized as :

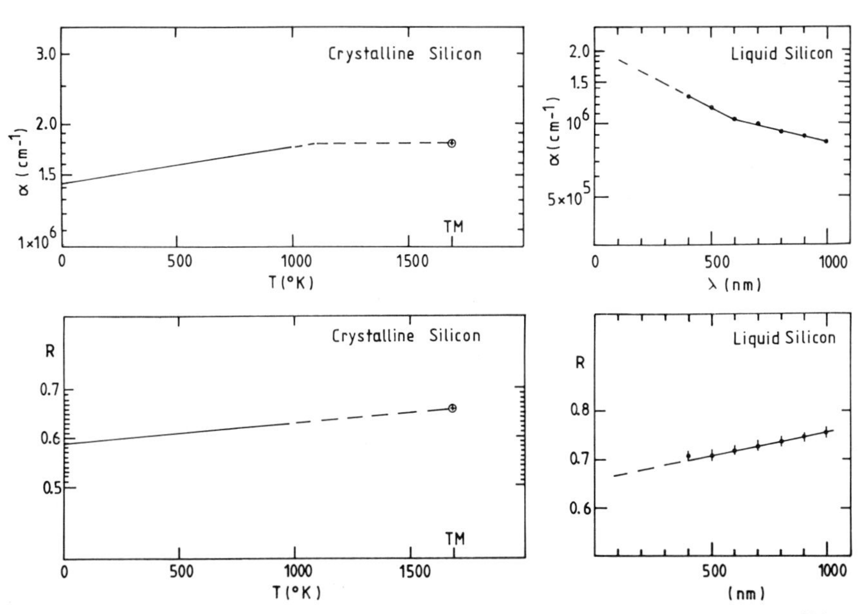


Fig. 1. a) Reflectivity and absorption coefficient of crystalline silicon for $\lambda$ = 308 nm versus temperature; b) Reflectivity and absorption coefficient for liquid silicon versus wavelength. Broken lines and ⊕ points are extrapolated values.

$$\alpha = 2.08 \times 10^6 \exp\left(-\frac{\lambda\ (\mathrm{nm})}{870}\right) \mathrm{cm}^{-1} \quad ; \quad (\lambda < 600\ \mathrm{nm})$$

$$R = 0.66 + 10^{-4}\ \lambda\ (\mathrm{nm}).$$

The parameters for liquid Si and $\lambda$ = 308 nm are shown in Table 1.

## II Results : Comparison with experimental values

Figure 2 shows the experimental results of WHITE |2| for melt depth versus laser energy, together with our calculations, for a Xe Cl ($\lambda$ = 308 nm) laser and pulses of 35 ns full width half maximum (FWHM) with a trapezoidal shape. We supposed in our calculations a rectangular shape and following observations can be made :

- a good agreement for amorphous silicon, if we take the conductivity of amorphous silicon $k_a$ = 0.02 cal/(s.cm.K) (which is much greater than the value we used (0.002) in another paper (8 c); if we take a Gaussian shape for the laser pulse the $k_a$ value giving the best agreement is $k_a$ = 0.009 cal/(s.cm.K);

- a reasonably (since only 2 experimental points are available) good agreement for crystalline silicon;

- the calculated values of threshold energy for melting are in good agreement with experimental values for both crystalline and amorphous silicon.

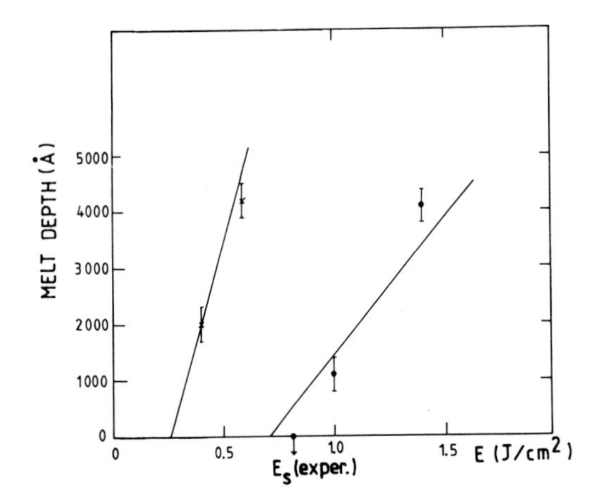


Fig. 2. Depth of melt versus laser irradiance: - White [2]; experimental points: x amorphous silicon; • crystalline silicon. Solid lines : model calculations

Figure 3 shows the experimental results of YOUNG et al. |3| for crystalline Si together with our calculations. As above our calculations have been performed with a rectangular shape of the laser pulse. It appears here that the experimental slope is smaller than calculated one. It should be noted that we have already found a similar discrepancy for the ruby laser annealing of As heavily doped crystalline silicon (8 c). No satisfactory explanation for this behaviour has yet been found.

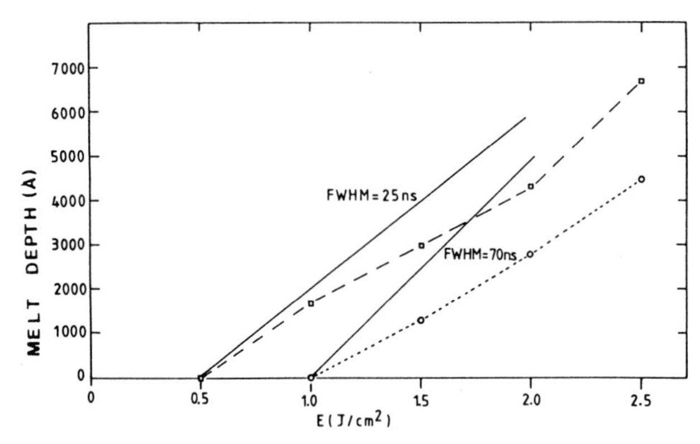


Fig. 3. Depth of melt versus laser irradiance. YOUNG [3] experimental points: FWHM = 25 ns; FWHM = 70 ns. Solid line : model calculations

## CONCLUSION

This investigation has shown that the thermal model is able to determine the effect of U.V. laser annealing of silicon. Reasonably good agreement has been found with the experimental data we have at our disposal. However, definitive conclusions may only be drawn when more experimental results become available.


1 D.H. Lowndes et al. Appl. Phys. Lett. 41, 938 (1982)

2 C.W. White. Journal de Physique C5-1983, page 145

3 R.T. Young et al. Sol. State Technology, 26, 183 (1983)

4 I.B. Khaibullin et al. Journ. Appl. Phys. 42, 5893 (1971)

5 P. Baeri et al. Journ. Appl. Phys. 50, 788 (1979)

6 A.E. Bell. RCA Review 40, 295 (1979)

7 R.F. Wood and G.E. Giles. Phys. Rev. B23, 2923 (1981)

8 a) M. Toulemonde, R. Heddache, S. Unamuno, P. Siffert, Strasbourg Rapport CRN-CPR 83-18
b) R.O. Bell, M. Toulemonde and P. Siffert, Appl. Phys. 19, 313 (1979)
c) M. Toulemonde, S. Unamuno, R. Heddache, M.O. Lambert, M. Hage-Ali and P. Siffert (to be published)

9 G.E. Jellison and F.A. Modine, Phys. Rev. B27, 7466 (1983)

10 A. Daunois and D.E. Aspnes, Phys. Rev. B18, 1824 (1978)

11 G.E. Jellison and F.A. Modine, J. Appl. Phys. 53, 3745 (1982)

12 H.R. Philipp and E.A. Taft, Phys. Rev. 120, 37 (1960)

13 H.R. Philipp and H. Ehrenreich, Phys. Rev. 129, 1550 (1963)

14 K.M. Shvarev et al. Sov. Phys. Solid State 16, 2111 (1975)

15 T. Gattuso et al. MIT-EL82-022 page 29

16 H.C. Weber et al. Appl. Phys. Lett. 43, 669 (1983)

17 E.P. Donoyan et al. Appl. Phys. Lett. 42, 698 (1983)

18 R.T. Young et al. IEEE, Electron Devices Letters, EDL-3, 280 (1982)

# Applications of Laser Annealing

J. Götzlich and H. Ryssel
Fraunhofer-Institut für Festkörpertechnologie, Paul-Gerhardt-Allee 42,
D-8000 München 60, Fed. Rep. of Germany

## 1. Introduction

Laser annealing has gained much interest in the last few years, and it was first widely thought that this new method would soon be a standard technique in semiconductor processing. This euphoric opinion, however, has to be scaled down to the real possibilities of this new and exciting technique.

In spite of the restrictions which have to be made in application, laser annealing offers new possibilities in comparison to furnace annealing. The heat treatment can be confined in both lateral ($\mu m^2$-$cm^2$) and vertical (0.1-some μm) dimensions and the time for which the temperature is applied can be varied from some psec to sec. The temperature range covers the region from approximately 600°-700°C (continuous lasers) to the melting point (pulsed lasers).

Laser annealing may fulfill essential demands of the VLSI technology such as shallower p-n junctions, higher dopant concentrations and lower defect densities. Due to the local confinement of the temperature treatment, negative feedback to those regions of the wafer in which other devices are already present can often be avoided.

This paper deals with the practical aspects of laser annealing in its stricter sense, that is the annealing of ion implantation damage and the activation of the implanted impurity atoms. First, the basic experimental concepts for laser irradiation of device structures will be described. Then, different problems influencing application are discussed. These problems are mainly the beam homogeneity and the different absorption caused by variation of dopant concentration and crystallinity. Another severe problem may arise by using structured dielectric layers or very high dopant concentrations in excess of the solid solubility limit. These dopant concentrations relax during subsequent thermal treatments and form clusters and precipitations. Finally, we will describe some devices which have been realized by laser annealing up to the present.

## 2. Basic Concepts

### a) Pulsed Laser Annealing

For the annealing of ion implanted layers by pulsed lasers, different Q-switched or mode-locked lasers with pulse lengths ranging between several psec to several 100 nsec are used. At first Nd:YAG and ruby lasers were mainly used but in the last years, very promising results were reported on annealing by excimer lasers (XeF, XeCl), which offer a very good beam homogeneity and a high pulse energy [1]. The wavelength region extends from 0.2 µm (Excimer) to 1.06 µm (Nd:YAG).

During the laser pulse, the surface is heated up to temperatures exceeding the melting point of the irradiated semiconductor. Thus, the annealing process involves the formation of a thin molten surface layer which recrystallizes starting from the substrate after the end of the pulse. The period of this high-temperature phase is in the order of 1 µsec. During this time, only little heat can diffuse from the surface to the substrate, so that the resulting temperature profile is very steep and shallow. Therefore, this mode of laser processing is often referred to as the adiabatic mode.

In Fig. 1, a typical arrangement for pulsed laser annealing is schematically shown. The samples are usually mounted on an x-y stage and annealed with overlapping pulses of various diameters, depending on the pulse energy. Depending on the absorption properties and pulselength, melt is initiated between 0.3 and several $J/cm^2$. Frequently, diameters between 40 µm and several mm, sometimes up to several cm, are used. For annealing implanted (and therefore often amorphous) layers, it is necessary to melt through to the undamaged substrate in order to facilitate a perfect epitaxial regrowth. Otherwise, only large polycrystals will form. Also, the overlap of different pulses has to be such as to avoid a polycrystalline zone between two annealed areas.

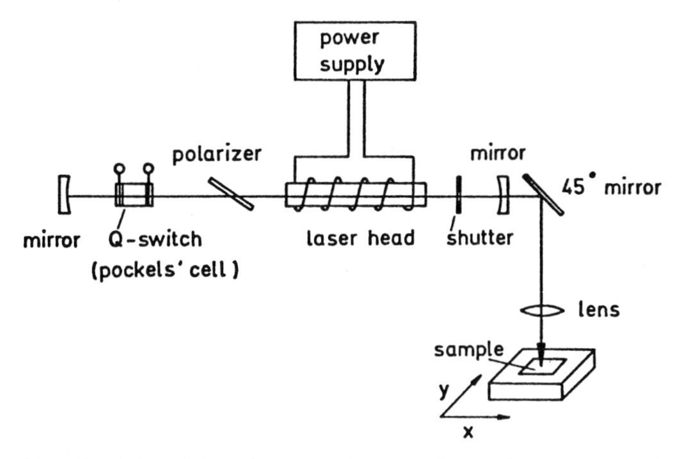


Fig. 1. Schematic diagram of experimental arrangement for pulsed laser annealing

b) CW Laser Annealing

In contrast to pulsed laser annealing, cw laser annealing is very similar to the well-known process of standard furnace annealing. The implanted layer is heated to such a temperature that a solid-phase epitaxial regrowth of the damaged layer takes place, starting from the undamaged substrate.

There are two different modes of CW laser annealing. The first is the thermal flux mode. In this case, a CW laser beam is focused and scanned over the surface of the wafer. The scanning is performed either by means of galvanometric mirrors or by moving the sample with a mechanical x-y stage (see Fig. 1). For annealing, beam powers between 2 and 20 W are used with argon lasers; Nd-glass lasers range up to 150 W; and $CO_2$ lasers up to 1 kW. Correspondingly, the dimensions of the beam vary from circular (with a diameter of 10 μm) to linear (2 cm x 1 mm). Usually, a heated stage with temperatures around 300 to 500°C is used to reduce the possibility of slip-line formation, which may occur with room-temperature anneals.

The dwell time is in the order of some msec, and is sufficiently long to allow the heat to flow completely through the whole thickness of the wafer. The temperature profile decreases monotonically with depth and can be calculated by solving the steady-state heat-flow equation [2]. The recrystallization process is temperature-dependent and can be described by the exponential law:

$$R(t) = R_o \exp(-E_a/kT) \tag{1}$$

found by Csepregi et al. [3]. ($R$ is the regrowth rate, $R_o = 3.22 \times 10^{-14}$ Å/s for undoped <100> silicon, and $E_a = 2.35$ eV). Equation (1) was first established for thermal recrystallization between 400 and 600°C. Growth rates obtained by laser annealing of implantation-amorphized silicon shown in Fig. 2 exhibit the behavior expected from Eq. (1), thus proving the solid-phase epitaxial nature of the recrystallization process [4]. In addition, Fig. 2 shows another interesting result of cw laser annealing. Due to the hemispherical nature of the heat flow, the surface temperature is a function of the power divided by the beam radius instead of the area.

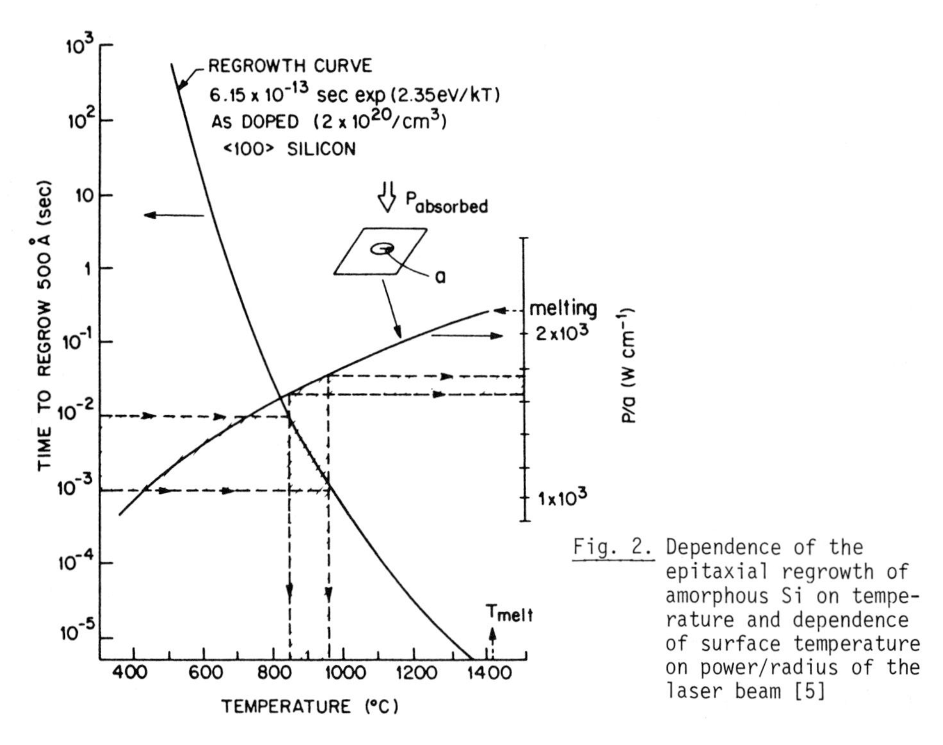


Fig. 2. Dependence of the epitaxial regrowth of amorphous Si on temperature and dependence of surface temperature on power/radius of the laser beam [5]

Since CW laser annealing does not result in melting and the heating periods are in the msec range, no diffusion of dopant atoms takes place. Therefore, the depth of the doping profile can be adjusted by the energy of the implanted ions. Moreover, a good dimensional control and a high reproducibility can be realized. Fig. 3 shows the carrier concentration profile after CW $CO_2$-laser annealing in comparison to the as-implanted LSS profile and the corresponding mobility profile.

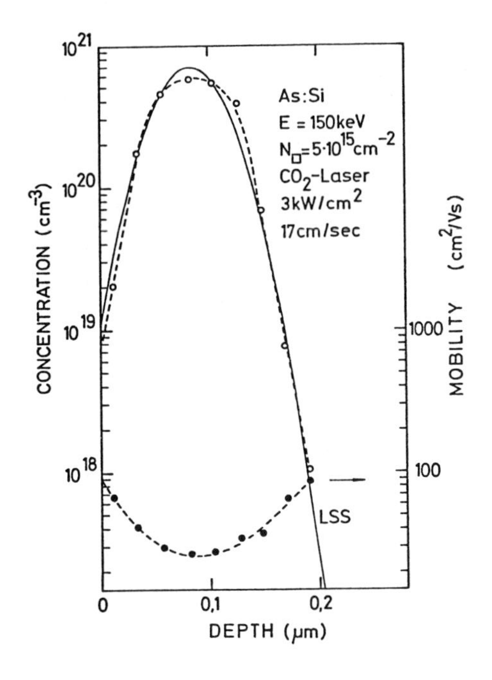


Fig. 3.
Carrier concentration and mobility profiles after As implantation and $CO_2$ laser annealing ($t_a \approx 5$ msec)

In the other CW annealing mode, the isothermal mode, the heating period is so long (1-20 sec) that the heat distribution is uniform throughout the whole sample thickness. This kind of annealing can mainly be performed by CW lasers with a high output power which allows to heat the sample homogeneously also laterally. For this purpose, $CO_2$ lasers can be applied very successfully. To minimize heat losses and temperature inhomogeneities the slice is often thermally isolated from the wafer holder.

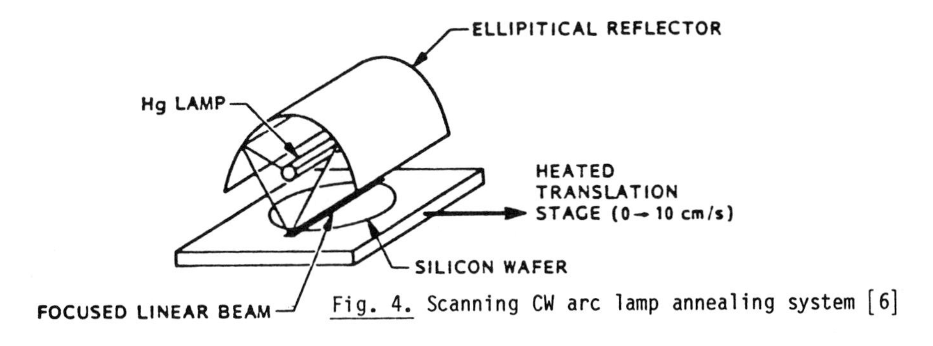


Fig. 4. Scanning CW arc lamp annealing system [6]

The isothermal laser annealing mode is very similar to another transient annealing technique which is performed by incoherent light sources. The main advantage of this last method lies in the low cost of the irradiation equipment. An example of a simple annealing system is given in Fig. 4 [6]. The light of a mercury arc lamp is focused by a long reflector into a narrow ribbon. The length of the ribbon can match the diameter of the wafer, so that the whole wafer can be annealed by one single scan with a scan rate of approximately 1 cm/sec. The results up to now, which are comparable to CW lasers, are very promising.

Another alternative to CW laser annealing is represented by fast thermal-annealing systems, consisting of a cavity which heats the whole wafer. In one system, the heating is performed by the absorption of the light of quartz halogen lamps which illuminate the wafer, as well as of the surrounding highly-reflecting cavity walls [7]. In another system, the walls of the cavity are heated to about 1200°C and act as a black-body radiator. In a production cassette-to-cassette automated system, a simple planar graphite heater is used to heat the wafers to 1200°C within several seconds. Experiments have shown that complete annealing of implantation damage can be achieved by this system [8]. This black-body irradiation and absorption mechanism is very similar to $CO_2$ CW laser annealing, since the energy absorption of the Si wafer mainly takes place through free carrier absorption.

## 2. Effects Influencing Application

### a) Beam Homogeneity and Reproducibility

In any application of laser annealing the electrical parameters of the annealed devices should fall within certain limits. Using pulsed lasers, the laser energy window which can be tolerated is only a few percent. The pulse-to-pulse energy reproducibility of a well-adjusted Q-switched laser is about 3-6%, but the spatial energy distribution of a Gaussian single-mode pulse can vary by about 30%, and that of a multimode pulse, which is often used, by even 60%. In addition, in solid state laser beams regions with high energy density (hot spots) occur, which cause a local overheating and evaporation of the semiconductor surface.

One method for the improvement of the beam homogeneity is the beam mixing technique. The initial laser beam is split spatially into many components and recombined at the surface to be processed. A system which was first applied by Cullis [9] consists of a curved and tapered quartz rod. At the matte input face, the beam is scattered into many angles and follows different paths through this optical guide to the polished output surface. This technique offers a very good rectangular shaped profile (homogeneity $\cong$ 5%) and a low energy loss ($\approx$40%).

Another method by which beam homogeneity problems may be overcome is the integration of multiple pulses by scanning and overlapping. Each pulse is displaced with respect to the previous pulse, thus producing a continuous line-shaped annealed region. If a laser wavelength is used at which amorphous (=not annealed) and single crystalline (=already annealed) material have comparable absorption coefficients, very flat surfaces without ripples can be obtained [10].

For CW laser annealing beam homogeneity is of minor importance because the lateral heat diffusion is nearly always faster than the movement of the beam spot on the wafer. Thus, possible spatial variations of the laser power can be equalized by thermal diffusion. Care must be taken, however, if x-y mirrors are used for laser beam scanning, because at larger scanning angles, a change of the beam spot area occurs and, therefore, the power/radius ratio is changed (see Fig. 2).

b) Differential Absorption

In annealing device structures often regions with different thermal and optical properties have to be irradiated by laser beams simultaneously. These properties may change due to different crystallinity and dopant concentration, or due to different reflection of the laser light in regions which are covered by dielectric layers.

Different crystallinity can be observed in regions where ions with different species or dose have been implanted. In addition, the crystallinity depends on the substrate temperature during implantation. In this case, a laser wavelength especially in the adiabatic processing mode by pulsed lasers, should be chosen which has a comparable absorption length in these different regions.

One special problem with laser annealing is the difference in the coupling of the laser light into the semiconductor due to oxide-passivation layers of different thickness, which can form an antireflective

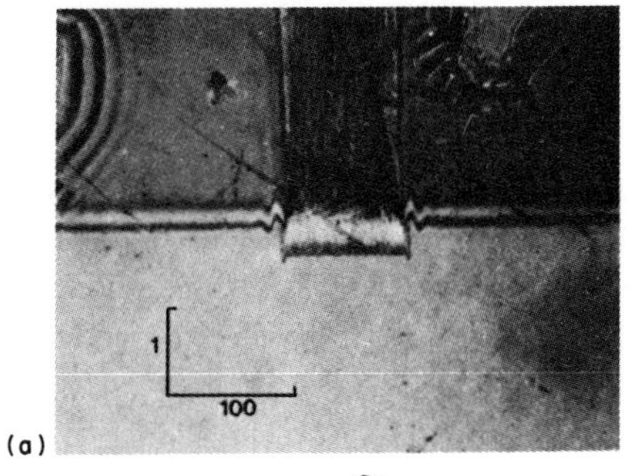


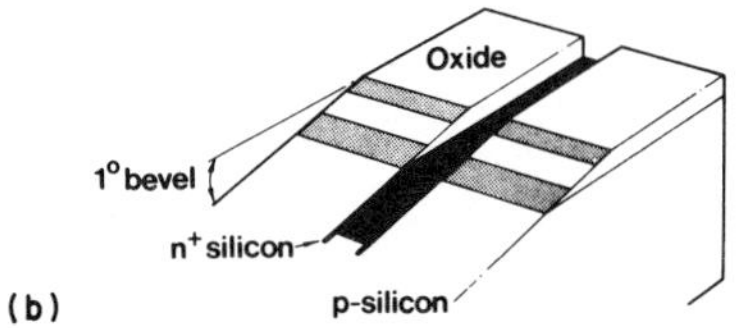


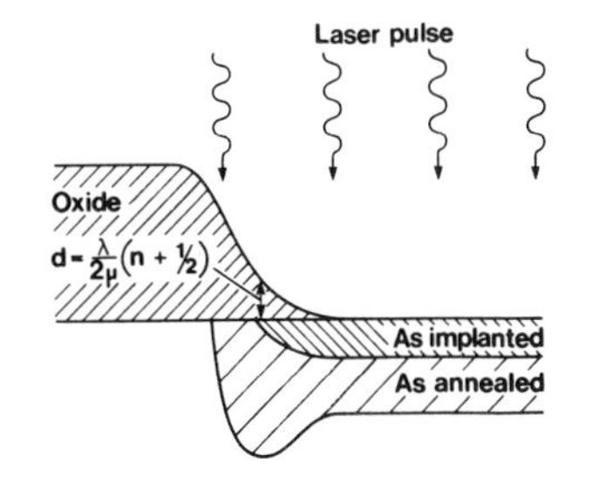


Fig. 5.
Effect of differential reflection at a $SiO_2$ window on Si [11]
a) stained bevel section
b) schematic view of the bevel section
c) schematic view of the window edge region

coating. This is especially important at the edges of windows cut into $SiO_2$ masks on silicon substrates. This inhomogeneous coupling is shown schematically in Fig. 5, and results in inhomogeneous junction depth. To circumvent this problem, a covering of the structured layer, e.g. with polysilicon, can be used to normalize the absorption.

c) Metastable dopant concentrations

If very heavily doped ion implanted layers are laser annealed, the solid solubility limit of these dopant atoms can be exceeded by orders of magnitude [12]. This procedure allows to form good ohmic contacts or regions with very low sheet resistivity in integrated circuits. Because of the metastable state of the excess dopant atoms, a relaxation of the carrier concentration to the thermal equilibrium value will take place during subsequent thermal processing [12-14]. Fig. 6 shows the carrier concentration profiles after phosphorus implantation and Nd:YAG laser annealing, as well as the corresponding profiles after a thermal post-anneal at temperatures between 600 and 900°C. This relaxation behavior can change the electrical characteristics of devices during subsequent technological steps such as LPCVD or evaporation processes.

## 3. Realized Devices

The problems described in the foregoing section indicate that the ideal structure for laser annealing would consist of a homogeneously doped flat surface with no lateral and only small vertical variation in the

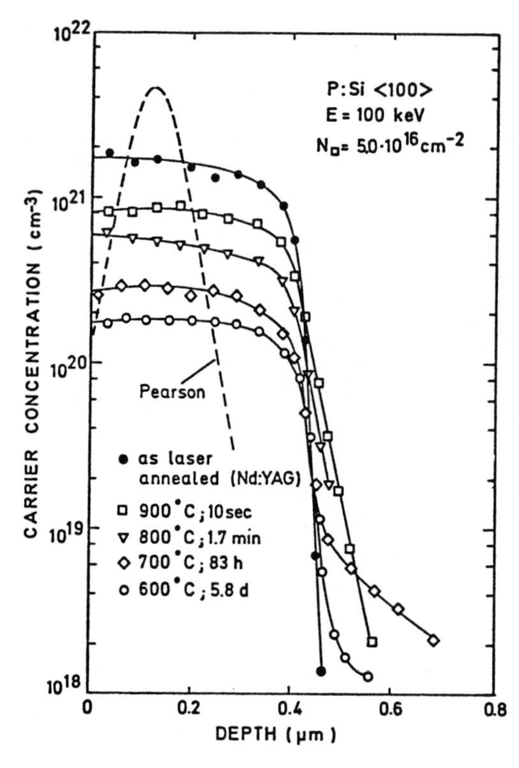


Fig. 6.
Carrier concentration profiles in Si after Nd:YAG laser annealing and subsequent thermal annealing at different temperatures

material properties. The simplest devices which fulfill these conditions are solar cells. Indeed, several authors [15-17] have shown that solar cells with improved efficiency up to 16 % can be obtained by pulsed laser annealing. In addition, it has been calculated that laser annealing may lower the total cost of solar cell fabrication [16].

Another relatively simple device successfully realized by laser annealing is double-drift impact diodes made by Hess et al. [18]. Hess reduced the interdiffusion of the doped layers and the contact resistance by laser annealing, thus improving the output power in CW diode operation by a factor of 10.

More complex devices such as oxide-passivated implanted diodes [19] and transistors [20] can also be satisfactorily laser annealed, but the laser induced degradation of the p-n junction at the $SiO_2$-Si interface requires a subsequent thermal annealing step of the devices at low temperatures (400-500°C) to remove the induced electronic levels.

Miyao et al. [21] fabricated short-channel MOSFETs by a self-aligned ion implantation and laser annealing technique. Fig. 7 shows the SEM micrograph of the cross section of the source-gate region. In contrast to the thermally annealed MOSFET (b), the laser annealed one (a) has a much smaller lateral (and vertical) diffusion of dopant atoms in the source region. Thus, a better control of the ratio of threshold voltage to gate length and a lower overlapping capacitance between gate and source (drain) were achieved. Making use of this reduced capacitance, Hess [22] improved the dynamic response of ring oscillators in CMOS-SOS structures. The delay time per oscillator stage thus could be reduced by 40% in comparison to devices which were annealed thermally.

## 4. Conclusions

Laser annealing offers many new possibilities for application in VLSI technology. Up to now, the main applications have been the production of very steep and shallow p-n junctions, the formation of good ohmic con-

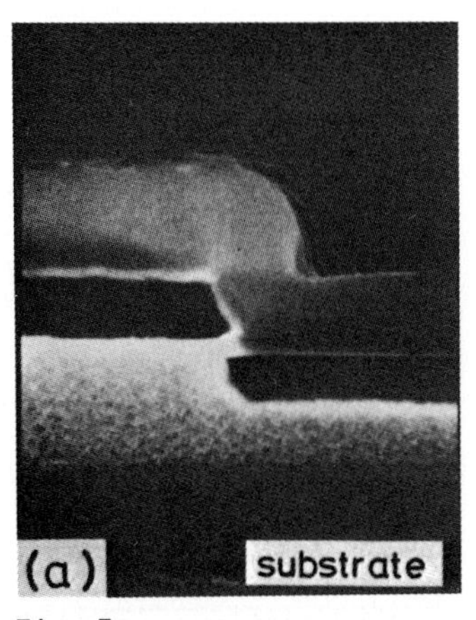


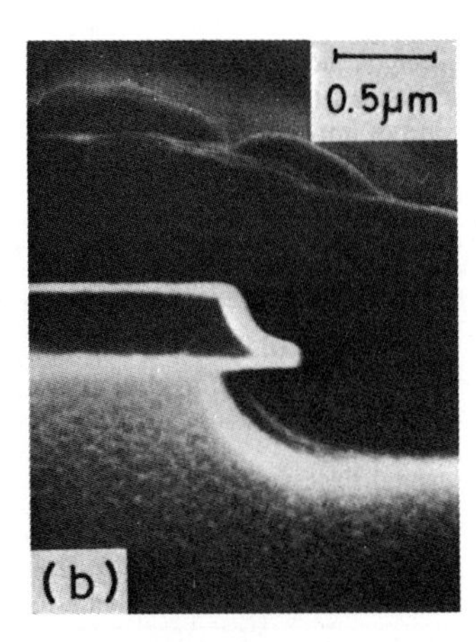


Fig. 7.
Cross section (SEM) of the source and gate region of MOS devices [21]:
a) after laser annealing (0,79 $J/cm^2$)
b) after thermal annealing (1000°C, 30 min)

tacts and the minimization of lateral diffusion, and thus the reduction of the parasitic capacitance in MOS structures.

In spite of these very promising results, some problems exist which have to be solved for each special application. The main factors influencing application are the laser beam homogeneity, the different absorption properties of the irradiated material and the thermal stability of the activated dopant atoms in excess of the solubility limit.

The first two of these problems can be overcome in part by the newly developed rapid optical and rapid thermal annealing methods. These new techniques could partly replace CW laser annealing, especially for full wafer applications, because of their lower cost and faster processing.

## References


[1] R.T. Young, J. Narayan, W.H. Christie, G.A. van der Leeden, J.I. Levatter, and L.J. Cheng, Solid State Technology, Nov. 1983, p. 183

[2] Y.J. Nissim, A. Lietoila, R.B. Gold, and J.F. Gibbons, J. Appl. Phys. 51, 1 (1980)

[3] L. Csepregi, J.W. Mayer, and T.W.Sigmon, Phys. Lett. 54A, 157 (1975)

[4] S.A. Kokorowski, G.L. Olson, and L.D. Hess, J. Appl. Phys. 53, 921 (1982)

[5] P. Baeri and S. Campisano in: Laser Annealing of Semiconductors (Eds. J.M. Poate and J.W. Mayer) p. 75, Acad. Press, New York (1982)

[6] J.F. Gibbons, in: Ion Implantation: Equipment and Techniques (Eds.: H. Ryssel and H. Glawischnig), Springer Series in Electrophysics, Vol. 11 (1983) p. 482

[7] R.A. Powell, T.O. Yep, and R.T. Fulks, Appl. Phys. Lett. 39, 150 (1981)

[8] D.F. Downey, C.J. Russo, and J.T. White, Solid State Technol. Sept. 1982, p. 87

[9] A.G. Cullis, H.C. Webber, and P. Bailey, J. Phys. E 12, 688 (1979)

[10] D.E. Aspnes, G.K. Celler, J.M. Poate, G.A. Rozgonyi, and T.T. Sheng in: Laser and Electron Beam Processing of Electronic Materials (Eds.: C.L. Anderson, G.K. Celler, and G.A. Rozgonyi), p. 414, Electrochem. Soc., Pennington, New Jersey

[11] C. Hill, in: Laser and Electron Beam Processing of Electronic Materials (see [10]) p. 26

[12] J. Götzlich, P.H. Tsien, and H. Ryssel, Proc. of the Mat. Res. Soc. Meeting, Boston 1983 (to be published)

[13] P.H. Tsien, J. Götzlich, H. Ryssel, and I. Ruge, J. Appl. Phys. 53, 663 (1982)

[14] J. Götzlich, P.H. Tsien, G. Henghuber, and H. Ryssel, in: Ion Implantion: Equipment and Techniques (see [6]) p.513

[15] R.T. Young, R.F. Wood, and W.H. Christie, J. Appl. Phys. 53, 1178 (1982)

[16] J.C. Muller and P. Siffert, Rad. Effects 63, 81 (1982)

[17] D.H. Lowndes, J.W. Cleland, W.H. Christie, R.W. Eby, G.E. Jellison jr., J. Narayan, R.D. Westbrook, R.F. Wood, J.A. Nilson, and S.C. Dass, in: Laser Solid Interactions and Transient Thermal Processing of Materials, (eds. J. Narayan, W.L.Brown, R.A. Lemons) p. 407, North-Holland, N.Y. (1983)

[18] L.D. Hess, G.L. Olson, C.R. Ito, and E.M. Nakaji, in: Laser and Electron Beam Processing of Materials (Eds. C.W. White and P.S. Peercy) p. 621, Acad. Press., N.Y. (1980)

[19] M. Lindner, Phys. Stat. Sol. A 57, 263 (1980)
[20] N. Natsuaki, T. Miyazaki, M. Ohkura, T. Nakamura, M Tamura, and T. Tokiyama in: Laser and Electron Beam Solid Interactions and Materials Processing (Eds. J.F. Gibbons, L.D. Hess, and T.W. Sigmon) p. 375, North-Holland, N.Y. (1981)
[21] M.Miyao, M. Koyanagi, H. Tamura, N. Hashimoto and T. Tokuyama, Jap. Journ. Appl. Phys. 19, Suppl. 19-1, 129 (1980)
[22] L.D. Hess, S.A. Kokorowski, G.L. Olson, Y.M. Chi, A. Gupta and J.B. Valdez, in: Laser and Electron Beam Interactions with Solids, (Eds. B.R. Appleton and G.K. Celler) p. 633, North-Holland, N.Y. (1982)

# Optical Regulation Using Crystalline Silicon

Ian W. Boyd, Thomas F. Boggess, Steven C. Moss, and Arthur L. Smirl

Center for Applied Quantum Electronics, Department of Physics,
North Texas State University, Denton, TX 76203, USA

The use of pulsed laser beams for transient thermal processing of various materials has increased dramatically over the past decade [1]. It is usually most desirable in such applications to control the processing parameters within specific limitations in order to achieve optimum reproducibility. In this respect, since the interaction of intense laser radiation with semiconductors and the subsequent energy redistribution mechanisms are usually highly nonlinear, it is important to minimize any shot-to-shot variations and to deliver essentially a constant beam fluence to the material [2]. In pulsed beam processing, unlike cw beam processing, the irradiation times are too short to allow any positive feedback techniques to operate in real-time. Therefore, a method for ensuring maximum reproducibility of the incident energy on the sample would be particularly desirable. In this paper we report a new picosecond nonlinear optical energy regulator for 1 micron radiation that effectively clamps the transmitted energy at a constant value for variations in incident energy of nearly two orders of magnitude. A potential application to short pulse laser beam processing is described.

The laser source for these studies was a mode-locked Nd:YAG laser that produced 48 ± 18 ps (FWHM) pulses at $\lambda = 1.06$ μm in a $TEM_{00}$ transverse mode. A single pulse was switched out from each mode-locked train and focused to a spot size of 150 μm (FWHM) on the surface of a 1 mm thick, high purity, single crystal silicon wafer. The sample was optically polished on both sides and antireflection coated on the back surface to minimize Fabry-Pérot effects. A portion of the beam was directed to calibrated pulsewidth and energy monitors so that the pulse duration and energy could be determined on a shot-to-shot basis. After passing through the sample the beam was collimated and directed onto a 2 mm diameter pinhole placed in front of a silicon PIN photodiode (see Fig.1). The transmission of the pinhole for low incident energies was 72%. A double stack of flashed opal glass placed directly in front of the detector provided a response that was insensitive to variations in spot size and position of the beam transmitted by the pinhole.

Figure 2 shows the total energy transmitted by the Si and pinhole in this geometry as a function of incident energy. Although not clearly resolved in this figure, the sharp low energy response is linear, corresponding to a transmission of 19% [3]. This is consistent with the previously determined pinhole transmission (72%) and a linear absorption coefficient of the Si of 10 $cm^{-1}$. However, for incident energies greater than 1 μJ, the transmission becomes nonlinear, and above 20 μJ the output energy is effectively clamped at 1.25 ± 0.25 μJ for a further increase in incident energy of nearly 2 orders of magnitude. Also shown in Fig.2 is the approximate fluence which imparted surface damage after 10 shots (A), which we define as the multishot damage threshold, and the single shot damage threshold (B) for these pulses [4]. Interestingly, for incident

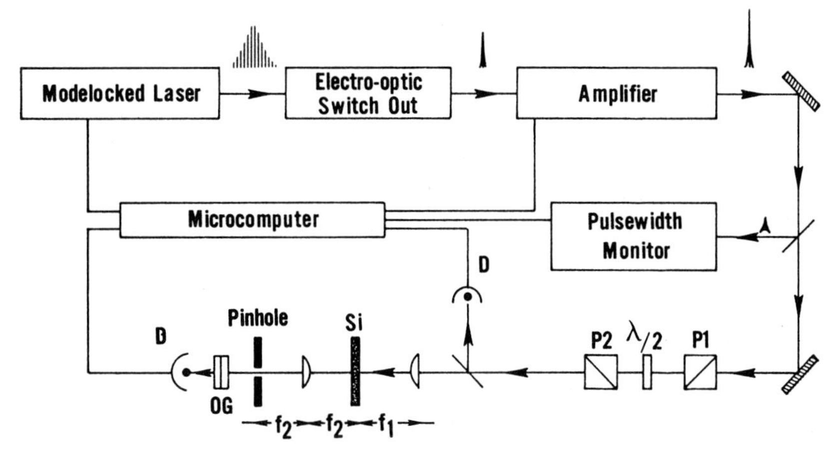


Fig.1 Schematic representation of the experimental set-up used to study energy regulation. P1, P2 = polarisers, λ/2 = half-waveplate, D = detector, OG = Opal Glass and $f_1$, $f_2$ = focal lengths of the lenses

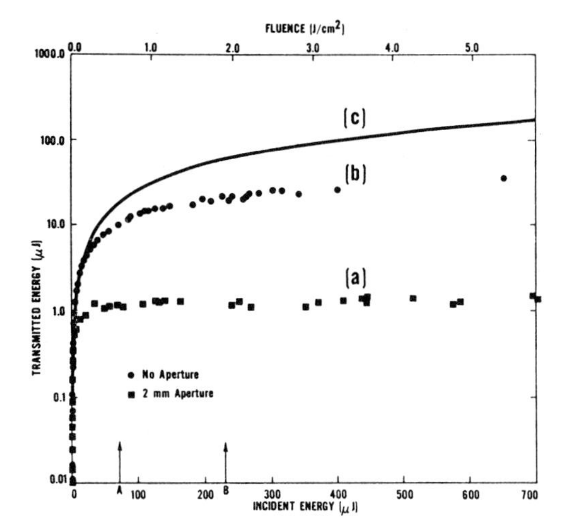


Fig.2 The energy transmitted by the geometrical configuration shown in Fig.1 (trace a) is compared to the energy transmitted by the Si alone without the limiting aperture (trace b), and with the expected energy transmitted for a constant linear absorption coefficient (trace c)

energies well above the single shot melting threshold the device continues to regulate the output. This is due to recrystallization of the melted layer which results in a near perfect reordering of the original phase. We have not yet quantified an upper limit to the number of shots the device can efficiently regulate at these high fluences. However, after only several shots at fluences far above (ten times) the single shot threshold, the low energy linear response is measurably degraded because of the gradual accumulation of surface damage.

The energy restricting nature of this device is due to changes in both the refractive index and absorption coefficient of the Si. The contribution of nonlinear absorption has been determined by removing the pinhole and, taking great care to collect all of the light, by measuring the energy transmitted through the Si (see Fig.2). We find at the highest input energies that nonlinear absorption reduces the transmitted energy by a factor of 5 over that expected by Beer's Law (also shown in Fig.2). The major contributions to the nonlinear absorption are free carrier absorption and temperature-dependent changes in the indirect absorption caused by lattice heating. The transmission of the pinhole is reduced by a factor of 40 as a result of self-lensing effects caused by nonlinear refraction that accompanies these absorption changes. For example, the photogeneration of free carriers leads to a reduction in the material index of refraction, and this induces gradual self-defocusing of the transmitted beam. This has indeed been confirmed for moderate fluences by monitoring the near field beam profiles immediately after the Si [3]. However, a positive change in refractive index with increasing lattice temperature, which would lead to self-focusing, will compete against this effect. To quantify the contribution of either is not a trivial matter. The interaction of intense picosecond pulses of 1.06 μm radiation with Si, unlike that of 0.53 μm radiation, is not well understood. An analysis of the energy deposition and redistribution mechanisms associated with 1.06 μm interaction with Si is under investigation.

There are potential applications of optical regulation devices as isolators in the area of device protection and as optical zener diodes. Devices similar to the one presently described have been demonstrated previously using thermal blooming in nitrobenzene [5], self-focusing in atomic sodium vapor [6], self-focusing and nonlinear absorption in $CS_2$ [7] and nonlinear absorption in various semiconductors [8]. However, unlike the majority of these devices, which are power regulators, our device exhibits energy clamping characteristics. We therefore propose a most appropriate application into the field of laser processing, where it is desirable to utilize a reproducibly constant energy (see Fig.3). In this case, unlike the applications mentioned above which operate in the linear regime and use the regulated characteristics only for protective means, the device will function in this "saturated" mode as a true regulator. In its present configuration, the device regulates at 1 μJ. However, the absorption of one micron radiation in c-Si is fluence dependent, and it is relatively straightforward to predetermine the clamping energy by changing the fluence incident on the silicon. Several approaches to this condition are currently being investigated. Since we use c-Si which is optically thin, the exact placement of the sample with respect to the focusing lens sensitively determines the precise device characteristics. For example, the transmission can be increased by placing the Si away from focus, by using a larger focused spot size on the sample, or by increasing the transmission of the aperture in front of the detector. A further consideration for designing the optimum configuration for obtaining usefully high clamped energy is the incident energy at which multishot or single shot damage

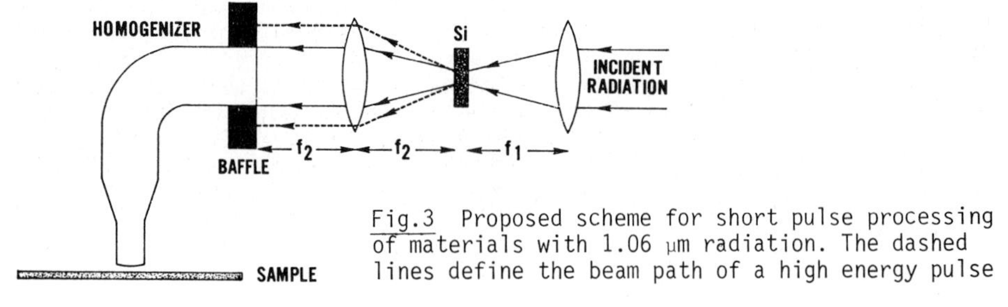


Fig.3 Proposed scheme for short pulse processing of materials with 1.06 μm radiation. The dashed lines define the beam path of a high energy pulse

occurs. Ideally, the device should exhibit optical limiting action well before the occurrence of any permanent surface degradation. Details of the device optimization are under study.

A possible drawback to the use of this regulating technique in laser processing is the distortion of the beam profile caused by the refractive self-action. This problem has previously been encountered for spatially nonuniform beams from ruby and $CO_2$ lasers. In these instances, beam homogenizers were used to average out the spatial (and temporal) variations in energy [9,10], although such uniformity was available only at ~1 mm from the exit face of the device. We propose the incorporation of such a homogenizer with the optical energy regulator to obtain reproducibly stable 1.06 μm picosecond pulses suitable for materials processing (Fig.3). The constant energy supplied by the regulator together with the spatial and temporal homogenizer would ensure a constant upper limit on the fluence incident on the sample for a wide range of incident energies. Since the absorption of 1.06 μm radiation in Si is fluence dependent [4], this technique can be used to regulate other, much longer pulsewidths in the same way. This limiting action has also been found for GaAs which is inherently much more transparent at 1.06 μm and hence gives a larger low energy transmission [11]. Additionally, with an appropriate choice of material, this technique can be extended for application towards regulation of other laser wavelengths.

In summary, we report an effective optical limiting device for picosecond 1.06 μm radiation that is suitable for application in materials processing. Advantages include extremely fast initiation times and completely passive operation. In the configuration reported here, energy transmitted by the device can be clamped at a predetermined value for a range of incident energies varying over nearly two orders of magnitude.

Acknowledgements

We are grateful to M. J. Soileau for many stimulating conversations. This work was supported by the Office of Naval Research, The Defense Advanced Research Projects Agency, The Robert A. Welch Foundation, and The North Texas State University Faculty Research Fund.

References

1. "Laser Annealing of Semiconductors," eds. J. M. Poate, James W. Mayer (Academic, New York, 1982) and references therein.
2. C. Hill, in ref. 1, p. 479.
3. T. F. Boggess, S. C. Moss, I. W. Boyd, A. L. Smirl, Opt. Lett., 9, 291 (1984).
4. I. W. Boyd, S. C. Moss, T. F. Boggess, A. L. Smirl, Appl. Phys. Lett., 45, 80 (1984).
5. R. C. C. Leite, S. P. S. Porto, T. C. Damen, Appl. Phys. Lett., 10, 100 (1967).
6. J. E. Bjorkholm, P. W. Smith, W. J. Tomlinson, A. E. Kaplan, Opt. Lett., 6, 345 (1981).
7. M. J. Soileau, W. E. Williams, E. W. Van Stryland, IEEE J. Quantum Electron., QE-19, 731 (1983).
8. J. M. Ralston, R. K. Chang, Appl. Phys. Lett., 15, 164 (1969).
9. A. G. Cullis, H. C. Webber, P. Bailey, J. Phys. E, 12, 688 (1979).
10. R. E. Grojean, D. Feldman, J. F. Roach, Rev. Sci. Instrum., 51, 375 (1980).
11. T. F. Boggess, A. L. Smirl, S. C. Moss, I. W. Boyd, E. W. Van Stryland, (unpublished).

# Optical and Electrical Properties of Laser Annealed Heavily Doped Silicon

A. Slaoui, E. Fogarassy, and P. Siffert

Centre de Recherches Nucleaires, Laboratoire Phase
F-67037 Strasbourg Cedex, France

## I INTRODUCTION

It's well established now that the laser annealing of high dose ion-implanted silicon allows one to obtain large concentrations of impurities well above the thermal solubility limit |1|, giving very low sheet resistivity, in the absence of microscopic defects. The fundamental properties of these extremely heavily doped layers have received considerable attention |2-5|. Much effort has been spent studying the effect of doping on the band structure of silicon using optical techniques such as optical absorption and ellipsometry measurements |2,3|. These effects can affect seriously the characteristics of devices.

In this paper, we report on some optical and electrical properties of ultraheavily doped silicon. The reflectivity in the UV and visible (2.5-5 eV) region gives information on the effect of doping on the band structure since the absorption coefficient in this region is very low compared to interband transitions. In the near infrared region, the effects of large concentrations are dominant. A change in the carrier effective mass follows. The electrical properties of these heavily doped layers have been focused essentially on the dark I-V characteristics trying to separate effects due to the high doping from those resulting from microscopic defects.

## II EXPERIMENTS

Several P-type silicon wafers, (100) orientation, having resistivities in the range 1-5 Ωcm, have been implanted with 80 KeV arsenic ions at doses ranging from $10^{15}$ to $10^{17}$ $cm^{-2}$. The activation of the dopants was done by laser annealing, using Q-switched Nd:YAG or Ruby lasers emitting pulses of 100 and 20 ns duration, respectively, at wavelengths of 0.530 and 0.69 nm, in an energy domain of 1.4 to 2.5 $J/cm^2$.

The experimental equipment we used has been described elsewhere |5,6|.

## III RESULTS AND DISCUSSION

### 1. Structural properties and electrical activity

We have previously shown |5,6| that the crystalline quality of the samples after laser annealing is perfect when observed by RBS, and the maximum dopant concentration is three orders of magnitude greater than the thermal solubility for an $5x10^{16}/cm^2$ implanted dose.

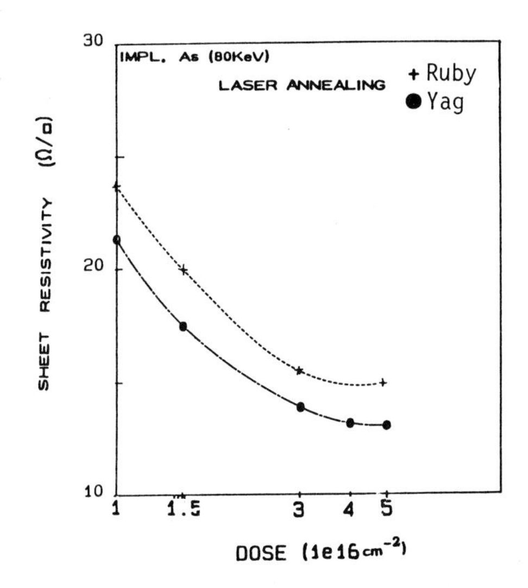


Fig. 1

Sheet resistivity vs. implanted dose determined by four-point probe technique. The values of $R_{\square}$ are very low, indicating a good electrical activity.

The electrical activity was determined by the four-point method. The sheet resistivity data $R_{\square}$ as function of dose are reported in Fig. 1 which shows a rapid decrease in $R_{\square}$ vs. dose with a saturation starting at about $3 \times 10^{16}$ $cm^2$.

There is a difference between Ruby and YAG because the melting depth is not the same for the two lasers.

## 2. Optical properties

As mentioned above, our optical measurements involve reflectivity spectra in the U.V.-visible as well as in the near IR region. The results are as follows :

### a) U.V.-visible reflectance

Accurate reflectivity spectra of substrate crystal and the doped silicon layer are shown on Fig. 2 in the range 2.5 to 6 eV. Two well known peaks at 3.4 and 4.5 eV are observed on the heavily doped crystal, denoted $E_1$ and $E_2$, respectively |2-6|. The reflectivity spectra of heavily doped Si are remarkably similar to those of undoped material except that the $E_1$ and $E_2$ structures are broadened and shifted to lower energies. In addition, the reflectivity coefficients are diminishing when the dopant dose is increased. The broadening is much larger for $E_1$ than for $E_2$. We have reported in Fig. 3 the threshold energy shift of the $E_2$ critical point with impurity concentration N, which indicates that $\Delta E_2$ varies as $N^{0.62}$. Previous data of Vina and Cardona |3| obtained from ellipsometric measurements are also reported on the same figure. They cannot conclude from their data whether an N or $N^{1/3}$ dependence law applies. Recently, several authors |2,7,8| have discussed which mechanisms induced by heavy doping can affect the threshold energies. The generally accepted view is that exchange and correlation effects produce an energy shift proportional to $N^{1/3}$, while screened electron-ion interactions provide a $N^{1/6}$ dependence |7|. Allen et al. |8|

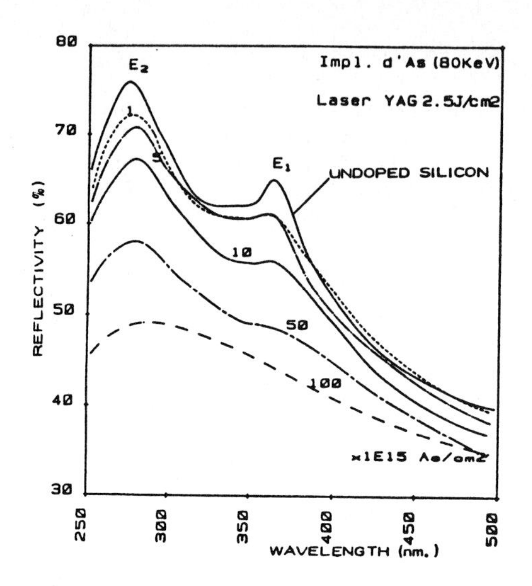


Fig. 2 UV-visible reflectivity spectra for undoped substrate (solid line) and heavy doped and laser annealed samples (dashed lines). The ion dose is the number multiplied by $10^{15}$ $cm^{-2}$.

predicted a linear dependence on N resulting from ensemble averages over form and structure factors for impurity atoms distributed at random sites over the lattice. Lately, Aspnes et al. |2| have shown, by determination of accurate dielectric constants, that threshold energies of the $E_1$ and $E_2$ critical points are linear with N, and attributed this behaviour to changes in the average or effective pseudopotentials of the Si-dopant lattice due to the presence of substitutional donors on the lattice sites. Our experimental data of $E_2$ are more consistent with a linear dependence with N, rather than a $N^{1/6}$ or $N^{1/3}$ law. This indicates that the dominant mechanism responsible for the shifts in our experiments is the effect of the random impurities on the crystal potential whose formalism has been given by Allen |8|.

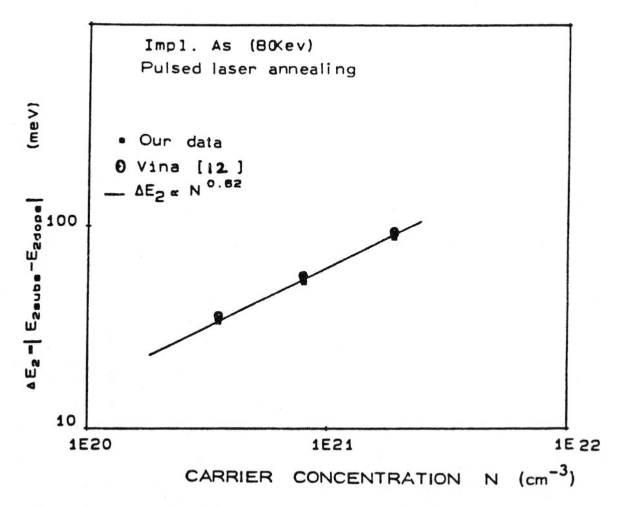


Fig. 3 Dependence on doping concentration of critical point energy for the $E_2$ singularity.

### b) Near IR reflectance - effective mass and relaxation time

Infrared techniques are commonly used in the semiconductor industry and in fundamental research laboratories because they allow determination of impurity level and provide information concerning the conduction band structure. In particular, transmittance and plasma reflectivity experiments have been used to determine the electron effective mass (m*) |4, 9, 10| of n-Si.

In the case of high-ion-implanted laser annealed silicon, the dopant distribution is strongly inhomogeneous. A theoretical model of the reflectance which accounts for this inhomogeneity is required. Here, we present two models |11|. The first is a single-layer model, i.e. the inhomogeneous layer is assumed to be a thin uniform film over a uniform substrate; the second model accounts for the asymetric and inhomogeneous depth distribution of carriers. We suppose

$$N(x) = N_o + N_{max} \quad \exp(-\alpha(x-d)^2) \quad \text{if } x > d,$$

and

$$N(x) = N_o + N_{max} \quad \exp(-\beta(x-d)^2) \quad \text{if } x < d$$

$N_o$ is the substrate doping, $N_{max}$ the maximum carrier concentration and d the depth at this maximum; $\alpha$ and $\beta$ are two adjustable parameters.

The determination of the reflectance coefficient using these models is founded upon the Drude model. We deduced the effective mass m* and the optical relaxation time from theoretical reflectivity spectra when they agreed with experimental reflectivity values.

The determined values of m* (Δ,□) and τ(⊕,o) as a function of carrier concentration N are shown in Fig. 4. In this figure, previously

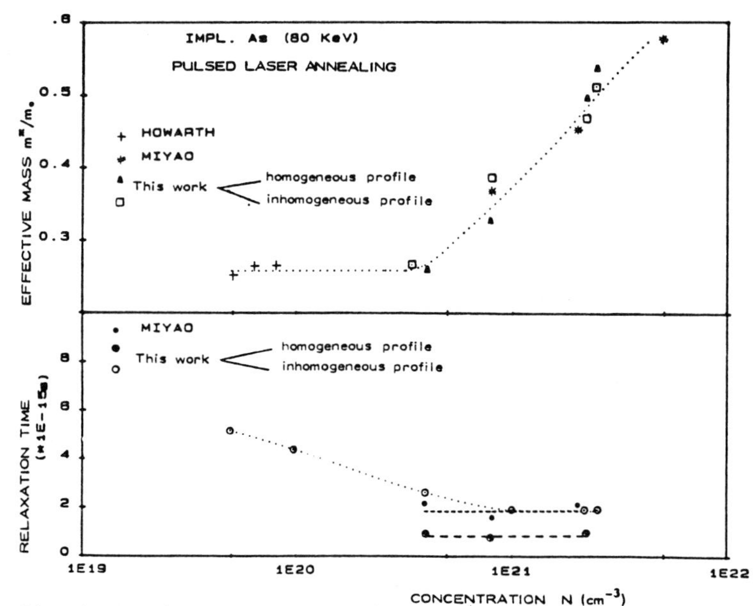


Fig. 4 Carrier concentration dependence of free electron effective mass (m*) and carrier relaxation time (τ)

reported results |4-10| for arsenic doped samples ($m^*$ (+,*) and $\tau$(•)). are also shown. The relaxation time is about constant at higher carrier concentrations, while the electron effective mass increases significantly from that in lightly doped Si |10|. Miyao et al. |4| have observed the same behaviour for $\tau$ and $m^*$. They explained the change in $m^*$ by the entrance into a new valley of electrons which have overflown the conventional valley on the Γ-X line. Indeed, the carrier concentration at which the Fermi level enters a new valley is $5 \times 10^{20}$ $cm^{-3}$, a value which is very close to the one at which we observed the increase in $m^*$.

## 3. Electrical properties

In Fig. 5, we report dark forward and reverse I-V characteristics of P-N junctions which have been ion implanted at different doses and laser annealed. Two slopes appear with a break at 0.35 V. We observed a degradation of the I-V characteristics (i.e. an augmentation of the current) when the dose was increased, particularly the leakage current which is the reverse current at - 1 volt. Three causes can be given to explain these facts :

a) the presence of recombination centres induced by the implantation tails in the depletion region;

b) the existence of recombination centres generated by laser treatment in the space charge region (SCR) and at the surface of the junction (surface states);

c) the high doping level due to the presence of large carrier concentrations.

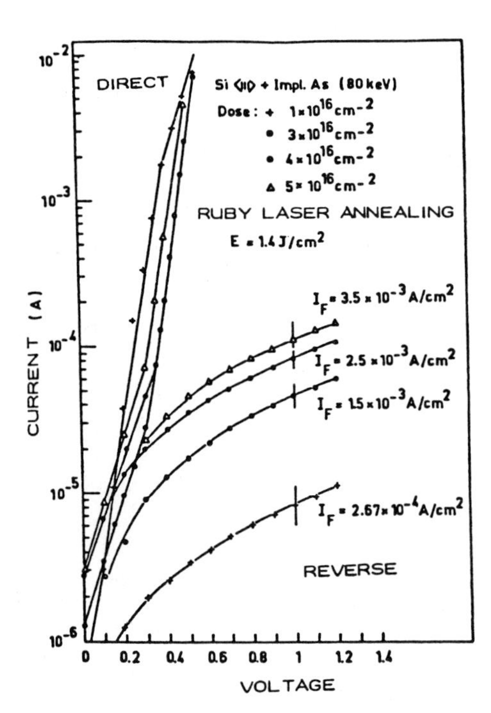


Fig. 5

Dark forward and reverse I-V characteristics after $As^+$ implantation at different doses and ruby laser annealing.

The first cause can be ruled out because when we performed a low temperature (600°C) thermal treatment on the junctions before laser annealing, to remove the residual defects due to the implantation tails in the depletion region |12|, we have observed similar behaviour of the currents with implanted doses |11|.

The presence of recombination centres created by the laser process has been demonstrated essentially by DLTS method |12|. Generally, quenching is employed to explain the observed defects. Kimerling et al. |13| have shown that the major observed defects act as electron traps which can play a compensating role in P-type materials.

It follows from the presence of these defects that the surface recombination velocity is increased and consequently higher dark currents than expected are observed.

The third cause involves many effects :

(1) the decrease of the carrier lifetime $\tau$ with emitter carrier concentration. In the frontal region, Auger recombination becomes dominant |14|. The current is then affected because $I_{OD}$ and $I_{OR}$ are inversely proportional to the square of $\tau'$ where $I_{OD}$ and $I_{OR}$ are the saturation currents.

(2) the energy-gap narrowing $\Delta E_g$, due to the presence of high carrier concentration, has been shown |7| to affect the performance of silicon bipolar devices.

Since the diffusion and recombination currents are proportional to the intrinsic carrier density $n_i$ squared and to $n_i$ respectively, a considerable increase of these currents follows from the change of $n_i$ by $n_{ie}$ because |15|

$$n_{ie}^2 = n_i^2 \exp\left(\frac{q \, \Delta \, E_g}{k \, T}\right) .$$

(3) the existence of a high gradient in the dopant distribution, as observed by RBS |5|, gives rise to electrostatic fields in the heavily doped region. Redfield |14| has shown that in this case there are no quasi-neutral regions and that minority carrier currents are controlled by electrical fields induced by the doping gradient rather than by a diffusion process. It follows that an increase in the saturation current of the diode would be observed.

## CONCLUSION

In this work, we have analyzed some optical and electrical properties of heavily doped Si prepared by implantation and laser annealing. We have shown that the major effects of heavy doping on UV-visible reflectance are a broadening of $E_1$ and $E_2$ peaks and a shift of the corresponding critical-points thresholds to lower energies due to the influence of the randomly substituted impurity potentials on the unperturbed lattice.

From near infrared reflectivity spectra, using two different models, we have deduced electron effective masses (m*) and relaxation times. The increase of m* with the number of free electrons has been attributed to the overflowing of the conventional valley by the majority electrons. The degradation of dark I-V characteristics has been explained by several mechanisms such as the presence of defects induced by implantation tails and/or laser treatment, and principally the effects of heavy doping which includes the preponderance of Auger recombination in the emitter region, the band-gap narrowing and the high doping gradient.

## REFERENCES


1 C.W. White, B.R. Appleton, S.R. Wilson : Laser annealing of semi-conductors, (Ed. by J.M. Poate and J.W. Mayer, Academic Press, p. 111, 1982)

2 D.E. Aspnes, A.A. Studna, E. Kinsbron : Phys. Rev. B, 29, 768 (1984)

3 L. Vina, M. Cardona : Physics, 117 et 118 B, 356 (1983)

4 M. Miyao, T. Motooka, N. Natsuaki, T. Tokuyama : Solid. Stat. Electron, 37, 605 (1981)

5 A. Slaoui, E. Fogarassy, P. Siffert, J.F. Morhange, M. Balkanski : Laser Solid Interaction and Laser Processing, Boston, U.S.A., Material Research Society Meeting (Nov. 1983)

6 A. Slaoui, E. Fogarassy, J.C. Muller, P. Siffert : Ref.12, p. 65

7 D.S. Lee, J.G. Fossum : IEEE Trans. Electron Devices, 30, 626 (1983)

8 P.B. Allen : Phys. Rev. B 18, 5217 (1978) and B. Chakraborty, P.B. allen : same reference, p. 5225

9 H. Engstrom : J. Appl. Phys. 51, 5245 (1980)

10 L.E. Howarth, J.F. Gilbert : J. Appl. Phys. 34, 236 (1963)

11 A. Slaoui : Thesis 3$^{th}$ Cycle, Université Louis Pasteur, Strasbourg (1984)

12 A. Mesli, J.C. Muller, P. Siffert : Laser-Solid Interactions and Transient Thermal Processing of Materials, J. de Physique, 44, C-5, p. 281 (1983), Strasbourg, Les Editions de Physique

13 L.C. Kimerling, J.L. Benton : MRS Symposium Processing of Laser and Electron Beam Processing of Materials (Ed. C.W. White and P.S. Peercy, p. 385, 1979)

14 D. Redfield : Solar Cells, 3, 63 (1980)

15 A.H. Marshak, M.A. Shibib, J.G. Fossum, F.A. Lindholm : IEEE Trans. Electron. Devives, 28, 293 (1981)

# CW-Laser Annealing of CdTe Epitaxial Layers

D.J. As, L. Palmetshofer, J. Schuller, and K. Lischka
Institut f. Experimentalphysik, Universität Linz
A-4040 Linz, Austria

## 1. Introduction

The potential of laser irradiation for the modification of semiconductor properties has been intensively explored and used in the last years. In silicon the basic mechanisms underlying the various applications from annealing of the lattice damage to crystal growth are now understood in principle [1,2]. In compound semiconductors, however, the understanding is meagre and the results are still somewhat contradictory. The laser treatment may change the surface composition because of the difference in vapour pressure of the components. This makes the results and their interpretation more complicated. On the other hand, laser annealing is an attractive alternative to overcome the problems inherent in conventional furnace processing of compound semiconductors like compound decomposition, compensation, limited solubility of dopants, etc.

In CdTe laser annealing has been used for the formation of p-n junctions [3] and ohmic contacts [4]. In these cases only electrical measurements have been performed. Other papers deal with defect reactions studied by luminescence [5] or with changes in the surface morphology [6] under the influence of laser irradiation without studying the electrical properties.

In this work we report on electrical measurements and photoluminescence studies of laser-annealed thin epitaxial layers of CdTe. The CdTe films, deposited on $BaF_2$ substrates by the hot-wall technique [7], are either nominally undoped (high resistivity) or doped with In. The laser treatment ('pulses' from a cw krypton-ion laser) is performed both on as-grown and ion-implanted films. The conductivity and the carrier concentration of CdTe:In increases by laser annealing, in contrast to thermal annealing. The increase in the carrier concentration is caused by an activation of the In donor as can be concluded from photoluminescence studies. The activation of the In masks doping effects in ion-implanted samples although the implantation damage is annealed out by the laser treatment.

## 2. Experiment

Epitaxial layers of CdTe were grown by the hot-wall technique on [111] surfaces of $BaF_2$ substrates [7]. The thickness of the films was (0.8 - 1.5) μm. The samples were either nominally undoped having a resistivity larger than $10^6$ Ωcm or doped with In. The In-doped samples were n-type with a resistivity of about 1 Ωcm, an electron concentration of $\approx 5\times10^{16}$ $cm^{-3}$ and a mobility of $\approx$ 100 $cm^2/Vs$ at room temperature. Details about the sample quality are given elsewhere [8].

In order to perform resistivity and Hall-effect measurements small Van der Pauw patterns [9] were etched by a common photolithographic technique.

Ohmic contacts were achieved by soldering with In. Resistivity and Hall-effect measurements were carried out in the dark.

Ion implantation was performed at room temperature with 300 keV ions of Ar, Ga (donor) and As (acceptor), respectively. The dose was varied between $10^{11}$ and $3x10^{15}$ $cm^{-2}$. The samples were aligned to the ion beam in a [111]-channel direction. This allows a deep penetration of the ions, comparable to the sample thickness ($\lesssim 1$ μm).

Laser annealing was carried out in ambient air with the radiation of a high-power cw krypton-ion laser operated in the $TEM_{00}$ mode at 647.1 nm. At this wave length the absorption coefficient of CdTe is about $6x10^4$ $cm^{-1}$, so that the laser light is well absorbed within the CdTe layer (≈1 μm thick); approximately 20% of the incident power is reflected [10]. The Gaussian shaped laser beam was focused onto the sample, the spot diameter (between $1/e^2$ points) was 1 mm. The samples were mounted on an X-Y stage and manually stepped with an increment of 0.1 mm providing a reasonable overlap of the individual spots. The irradiation time of each point was 2 s, the laser power was varied between 0.5 and 1.5 W. In order to prevent cracking of the $BaF_2$ substrates the samples were glued with thermal conductive paste onto a heat sink. For comparison some samples were conventionally annealed in a furnace. This thermal annealing was performed in vacuum at a temperature of 215°C.

Photoluminescence measurements were carried out at 4.2 K with the samples mounted in a helium flow cryostat. The luminescence radiation was excited by a $Kr^+$-laser ($\lambda$ = 647.1 nm), and the spectra were obtained with a grating spectrometer and a photon counting system in the energy range of 1.2 to 1.6 eV. The spectra shown in this paper were not corrected for the wave-length-dependent sensitivity of the S-1 (or GaAs) photocathode.

Several other techniques were used to observe the changes of the films caused by laser irradiation. The surface morphology was examined by optical and scanning electron microscopy and by a mechanical surface profilometer (Dektak). The composition was studied with an X-ray microprobe.

## 3. Results and Discussion

### 3.1 Surface Morphology

The surface morphology after laser irradiation was studied to find out the optimum anneal conditions. Up to a certain threshold value of the laser power the surface remains smooth without any change in composition. The threshold power is about 1.2 W, corresponding to a peak power density of 300 $W/cm^2$ (slightly dependent on the film thickness). At higher powers the surface deteriorates. At the center of the spot the film becomes thinner, while at the periphery it becomes slightly thicker. It appears that the film flows outward from the center of the laser spot. The composition of the film changes; at the center the Cd/Te ratio increases as compared to an unannealed film. Similar observations have been reported for CdSe [11].

For a laser power just below the threshold value the reflectivity of the CdTe changes slightly. The film appears darker after the laser irradiation. This region proved to be useful for laser annealing. The laser power is high enough to change the resistivity and to remove ion-implantation damage, but no deterioration of the film occurs. At still lower powers (<0.8 W) no changes in the physical properties of the films can be observed at all.

## 3.2 As-Grown Films

Laser annealing has a strong influence on the electrical properties of as-grown CdTe films doped with indium. In Fig. 1a the results are shown for a typical sample. The resistivity drops by an order of magnitude, both the carrier concentration and the mobility increase after a laser irradiation. Subsequent laser irradiation may continue this trend, but in general there is little influence on the electrical data. The most important result is the strong increase of the mobility. Mobilities around 300 $cm^2/Vs$ are the highest values obtained so far for epitaxial layers [8].

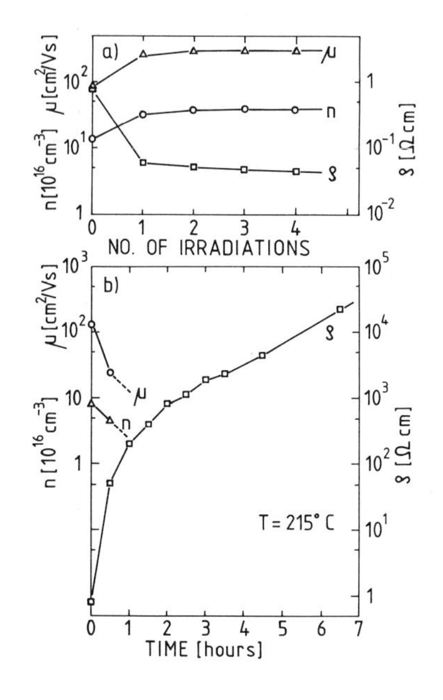


Fig.1: Carrier concentration n, mobility $\mu$ and resistivity $\rho$ of CdTe:In
a) after different numbers of laser irradiations,
b) after thermal annealing at T = 215°C as a function of the anneal time.

The temperature dependence (4 - 300 K) of both the carrier concentration and the mobility of laser-annealed films is similar to that of as-grown films. The carrier concentration is almost independent of the temperature (a slight increase at low temperatures is observed), the mobility decreases with decreasing temperature. This behaviour has been explained by a grain-boundary model [8,12], but might also be due to impurity-band conduction [13].

For comparison, some samples were thermally annealed. In order to obtain a reasonable temperature, a model calculation of the heating effect of the laser pulse was performed. Following the procedure given by LAX [14], a maximum temperature of 215°C was obtained for our parameters. The results for isothermal annealing at this temperature are shown in Fig. 1b. Contrary to laser annealing the resistivity increases strongly with the anneal time. Both the carrier concentration and the mobility decrease; because of the strongly increasing resistivity Hall-effect measurements could be performed only at the beginning. The contrasting results between laser and thermal annealing are not caused by the ambient air during laser annealing. Thermal annealing performed in vacuum and air, respectively, led to different results, but the general trend of increasing resistivity was the same.

Photoluminescence spectra of CdTe:In, recorded for the as-grown film and after laser and thermal annealing, respectively, are shown in Fig. 2. The spectra show only a single broad band peaking near 1.4 eV, which is typical for donor-doped CdTe. The luminescence is believed to result from transitions within complexes consisting of X-donor pairs, where X is an impurity atom (or $V_{Cd}$) and the donor is $In_{Cd}$ [5,15]. Compared to the spectrum of the as-grown film (full line), the luminescence intensity is strongly reduced after laser annealing (dotted line) and enhanced after thermal annealing (dashed line). This can be explained by the assumption that during laser annealing the complexes are dissolved and the In donors are activated. As a consequence, the free carrier concentration should increase and this is indeed observed (Fig. 1a). During thermal annealing, on the other hand, the reverse process takes place (among others).

Laser annealing of undoped CdTe produces almost no change in the resistivity of the films (about $10^6$ Ωcm). The effect on the photoluminescence spectra, which are dominated by exciton and edge emission, is discussed elsewhere [16].

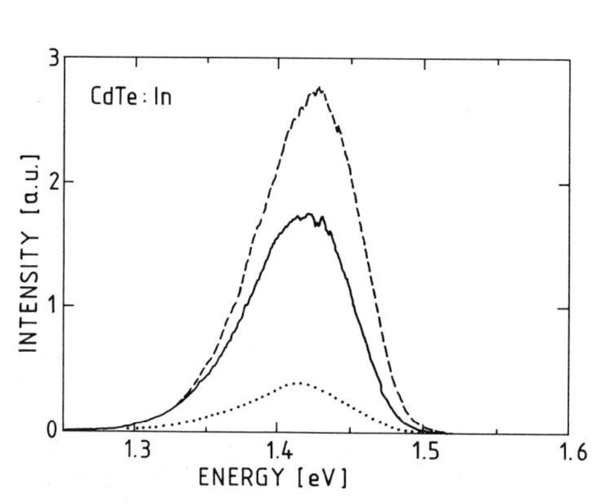


Fig.2: Photoluminescence spectra of an In-doped CdTe layer. The full, dashed and dotted lines correspond to as-grown, thermally annealed (T = 215°C, t = 30 min) and laser-annealed samples, respectively.

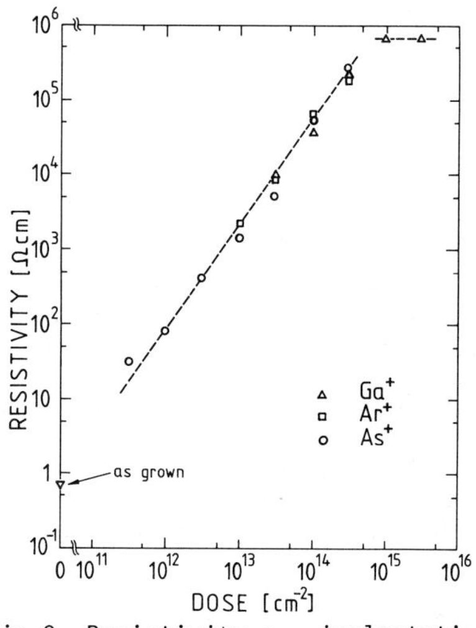


Fig.3: Resistivity *vs.* implantation dose for CdTe:In damaged with $Ar^+$, $Ga^+$ and $As^+$, respectively.

## 3.3 Ion-Implanted Films

The implantation damage enhances the resistivity of In-doped CdTe as shown in Fig. 3. The resistivity increases fairly linearly with the dose on a log-log scale (both the carrier concentration and the mobility are decreasing) until a saturation is observed at about $10^6$ Ωcm. The damage does not depend on the ion species; bombardment with donor ($Ga^+$), acceptor ($As^+$) and inert ions ($Ar^+$), respectively, results in about the same resistivity.

The photoluminescence is strongly quenched by the implantation damage as shown in Figs. 4 and 5. The full lines refer to as-grown samples, the dotted lines to damaged samples. In CdTe:In the luminescence spectrum is dominated by the band peaked near 1.4 eV (Fig. 4), in undoped CdTe the exciton peak at

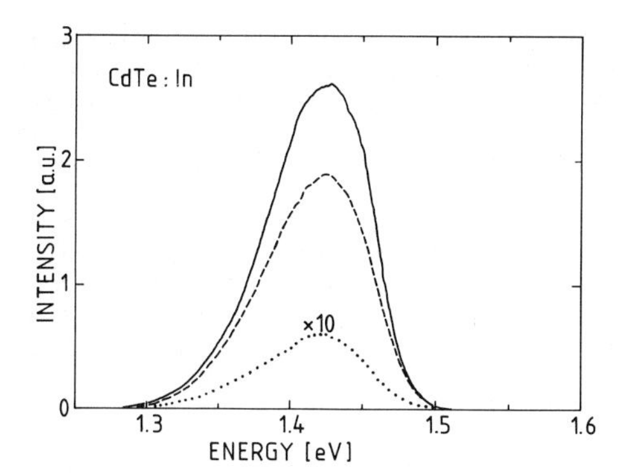


Fig.4: Photoluminescence spectra of an In-doped CdTe layer. Full line: spectrum obtained on the as-grown sample; dotted line: spectrum after implantation of $10^{14}$ $Ar^+$; dashed line: spectrum after laser annealing of the implantation damage.

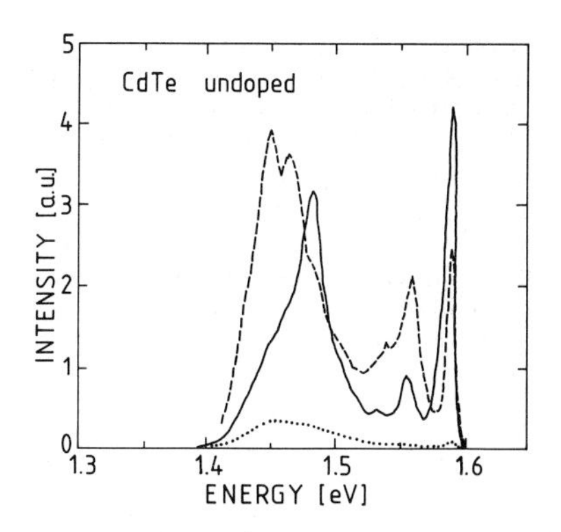


Fig.5: Photoluminescence spectra of an undoped CdTe film. Full line: spectrum obtained on the as-grown sample; dotted line: spectrum after implantation of $10^{13}$ $Ar^+$; dashed line: spectrum after laser annealing of the implantation damage.

1.59 eV and edge emission is typical (Fig. 5). (In Fig. 5 the emission below 1.4 eV is not shown because of the different sensitivity of the detector used).

Laser annealing recovers the luminescence spectra in both cases (dashed lines in Figs. 4 and 5). This is an indication that the implantation damage is removed. For CdTe:In the luminescence intensity after laser annealing is smaller than in the as-grown case. Further laser irradiation does not alter the intensity within experimental error.

The resistivity of ion-implanted CdTe:In also recovers during laser annealing giving additional evidence that the implantation damage is removed. This is shown in Fig. 6a for a $Ga^+$ implantation, but samples implanted with $As^+$ or $Ar^+$ behave in the same way. The resistivity after laser annealing is generally lower than in the as-grown case, further laser irradiations do not change the resistivity significantly. For comparison, in Fig. 6b the resistivity of a slightly damaged sample after thermal annealing at 215°C is shown. The resistivity does not decrease but increases similar to the unimplanted case (Fig. 1b). The similarity of the experimental results obtained on ion-

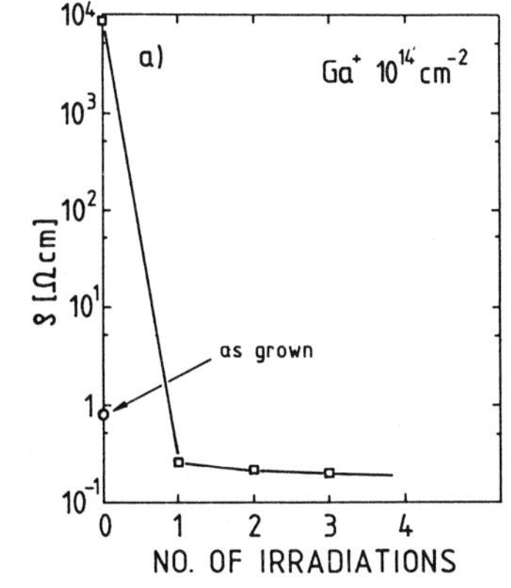


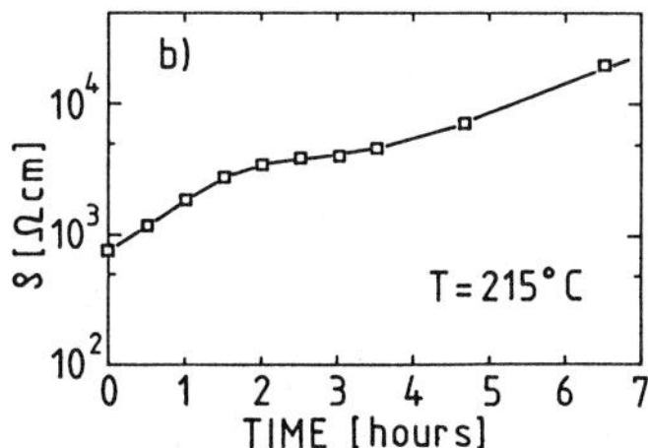


Fig.6: Resistivity of Ga-implanted CdTe:In a) after different numbers of laser irradiations, b) after thermal annealing in vacuum at T = 215°C as a function of the anneal time. The resistivity of the as-grown sample is shown for comparison.

implanted samples with those obtained on as-grown samples (Sect. 3.2) strongly indicates that any expected doping effect of the implanted impurities is outbalanced by the In-defect reaction and self-compensation mechanisms.

## 4. Conclusion

CdTe epitaxial layers grown by the hot-wall technique on $BaF_2$ substrates have been annealed by using a cw krypton-ion laser. In as-grown films doped with In the laser treatment led to an increase of both the carrier concentration and the mobility. The mobility values obtained are the highest reported so far for epitaxial layers. From photoluminescence measurements it has been concluded that the increase in the carrier concentration is caused by activation of the In donors. In ion-implanted films the damage has been removed by the laser annealing. Unfortunately, the In-defect reaction outbalances the doping effect of the implanted impurities in our samples. In order to obtain controllable electrical activation of the implanted impurities the implantation and anneal conditions have to be modified.

## References


1. M. Bertolotti, G. Vitali: "Laser Annealing of Semiconductors", in Current Topics in Materials Science, Vol. 8 (North Holland 1982), p 95
2. J. Götzlich, H. Ryssel: this volume
3. C.B. Norris, C.I. Westmark, G. Entine, S.A. Lis, H.B. Serreze: Radiat. Eff. Lett. 58, 115 (1981)
4. C. An, H. Tews, G. Cohen-Solal: J. Crystal Growth 59, 289 (1982)
5. C.B. Norris, P.S. Peercy: Radiat. Eff. 69, 267 (1983)
6. N.G. Blamires, D.H.J. Totterdell: J. Phys. D: Appl. Phys. 16, 2361 (1983)
7. A. Lopez-Otero: Thin Solid Films 49, 3 (1978)
8. W. Huber, A. Lopez-Otero: Thin Solid Films 58, 21 (1979)
9. L.J. Van der Pauw: Philips Res. Repts. 13, 1 (1958)
10. R.O. Bell, M. Toulemonde, P. Siffert: Appl. Phys. 19, 313 (1979)
11. R.M. Feenstra, R.R. Parsons, F.R. Shepherd, W.D. Westwood, S.J. Ingrey: J. Appl. Phys. 50, 5624 (1979)
12. W. Huber, A.L. Fahrenbruch, C. Fortmann, R.H. Bube: J. Appl. Phys. 54, 4038 (1983)
13. N.V. Agrinskaya, E.D. Krymova: Soviet Phys.-Semicond. 6, 1537 (1973)
14. M. Lax: J. Appl. Phys. 48, 3919 (1977), Appl. Phys. Lett. 33, 786 (1978)
15. C.B. Norris, K.R. Zanio: J. Appl. Phys. 53, 6347 (1982)
16. J. Schuller, D. As, W. Faschinger, K. Lischka, L. Palmetshofer, H. Sitter, W. Jantsch: Paper to be presented at the 13th Int. Conf. on Defects in Semiconductors, Coronado (1984)

# InSb Optical and Electrical Property Changes Induced by Multi-Pulsed TEA $CO_2$-Laser Irradiation

A.G. Vasiliev, V.I. Konov, A.B. Korshunov, A.A. Orlikovsky,
V.N. Tokarev, and N.I. Chapliev

Institute of General Physics, Moscow, USSR

The conductivity type conversion of InSb /1-3/ is among interesting effects induced on semiconductors by laser radiation. But it still remains practically obscure what processes are responsible for this effect.

The present paper gives some new experimental data on the subject. TEA $CO_2$ lasers are used as a light source. Optical properties (at $\lambda$ =10.6 μm), surface morphology, chemical composition and electrical properties of laser-irradiated initially p-InSb samples are investigated. Special attention is paid to the accumulation mechanisms (from pulse to pulse).

## 1. Experimental Set-up

The pulse shape was typical of TEA $CO_2$ lasers: leading spike and tail with total duration ≃1 μs. Linearly polarized or unpolarized radiation was focused in the air on the flat polished sample surface at the angle close to normal. The intensity distribution was near Gaussian and reproducible from shot to shot. The focal spot area is varied from 3 to 36 $mm^2$.

The samples with 0.5 mm thickness were made from p-InSb monocrystals with ⟨211⟩ and ⟨111⟩ orientation. Before and after laser irradiation the "cold" IR transmission spectrum and the surface morphology were examined by means of spectrometer and scanning electron microscope. In every shot by means of fast germanium photon-drag detectors the temporal behaviour of the mirror reflectivity R(t) and transmission coefficient T(t) were detected. The irradiated surface layer composition was analyzed by the Auger-spectrometer technique. According to /4/ the Hall effect measurements and conductivity type detection using thermoprobe were also performed.

## 2. Optical and Microscopic Investigations

Single-pulse irradiation. At $\lambda = 10.6\ \mu m$ the measured "cold" transmission coefficient $T=T_0$ was $\simeq 0.25$ (Fig.1, curve 1). This is in a good agreement with the literature data for InSb at low beam intensities when the sample heating is small and multiphoton absorption is negligible. But for laser experiments even at minimum energy density $E_s \simeq 0.5\ J/cm^2$ during pulse action T dropped to $T_{min} \simeq 0.04$. The $E_s$ growth till the surface plasma appeared ( $\simeq 8-9\ J/cm^2$) was accompanied by monotonous decrease of $T_{min}$ values. The obtained curves R(t) during laser pulse (in each shot a new sample area was irradiated) have shown the following: at $E_s \lesssim E_{th} \simeq 4\ J/cm^2$ R(t)=const and coincide with "cold" reflectivity $R_0 \simeq 0.3$. But if the threshold $E_{th}$ is passed R(t) functions show typical semiconductor behaviour /5/: at the beginning R(t) grows from $R_0$ level, reaches maximum, $R_{max}$, and then returns to the initial value. The dependence $R_{max}(E_s)$ is shown in Fig.2. One can see that for $E_s > E_{th}$ the reflectivity $R_{max}$ grows linearly with $E_s$. Note that for any fixed $E_s$ the temporal positions of $R_{max}$ and $T_{min}$ practically coincide.

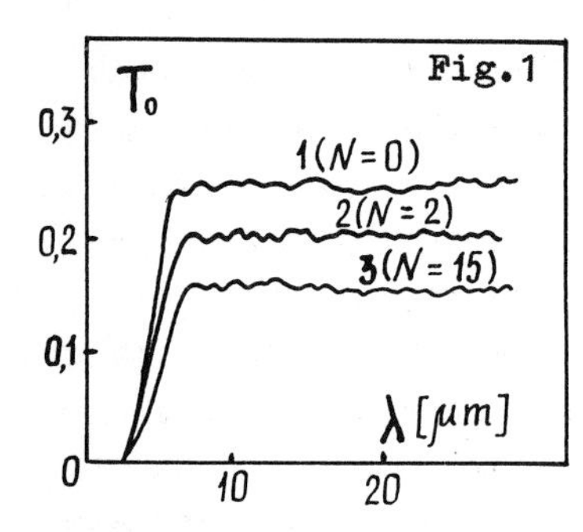


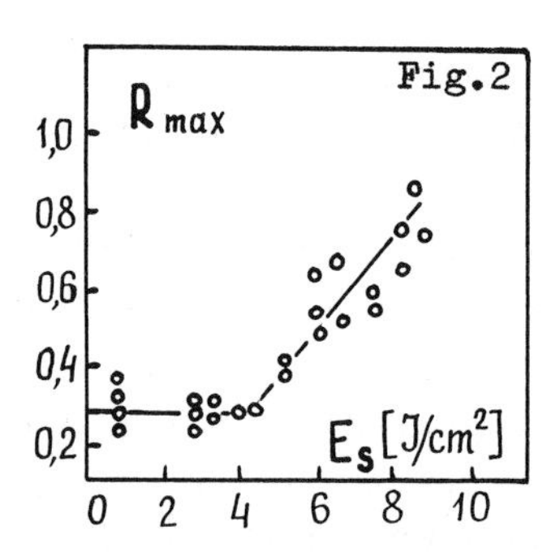


All these data can be explained on the basis of the well-known melting model (see, e.g./5/). Really, the higher $E_s$, the larger the surface area where melting point is reached and thus $R_{max}$ increases. This assumption is supported, first, by surface microscope analyses. In particular, for $E_s$ close to but larger than $E_{th}$ in the spot centre we observed disappearance of specially made grooves. Second, the possibility of InSb melting for $E_s > E_{th}$ follows from the calculations /6/.

Multi-pulse action. It was found that in case of single spot irradiation by a train of pulses (the repetition rate $f < 1$ Hz was small enough to let the sample completely cool between the pulses) $R_{max}$ values and R(t) dynamics depend on pulse number N. The effect had the threshold $E^{d}_{th}(N) \lesssim E_{th}$. The $E^{d}_{th}$ decreased with N and was $\simeq 3$ J/cm$^2$ for $N \lesssim 1000$. Typical curves $R_{max}(N)$ are given in Fig.3. In Fig.4 the laser pulse leading spike (curve 1) as well as R(t) functions for N = 2 (2), N = 29(3), N = 259(4) and $E_s = 4.5$ J/cm$^2$ are presented.

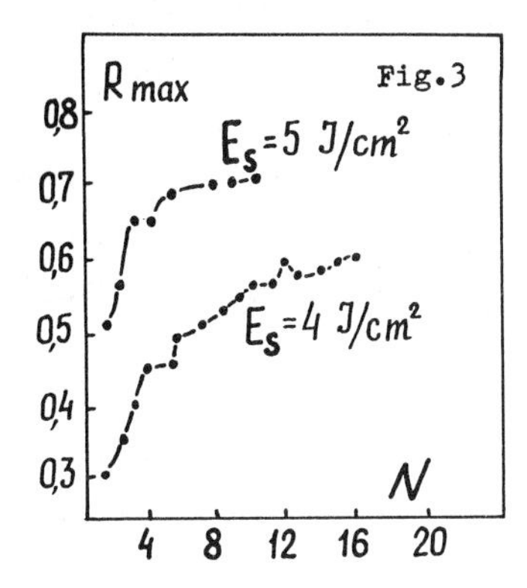


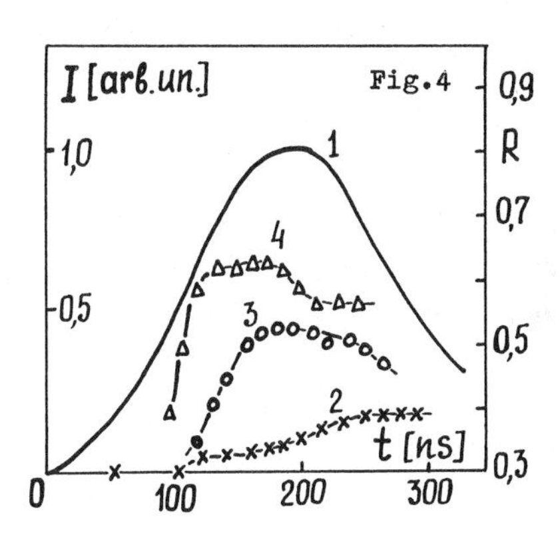


The surface morphology also depended on both $E_s$ and N. At low levels $E_s = 3$-$3.5$ J/cm$^2$ ($N \lesssim 100$) or for larger N and smaller $E_s$ no melting took place but surface cracking was observed. The increase of $E_s$ in linearly polarized beam was accompanied by appearance of surface ripples (see Fig.5). So, for $E_s \simeq 4 - 5$ J/cm$^2$ (Fig.5a) the well-known linear periodic structures (LPS) appeared. Such structures with a period of $\Lambda \sim \lambda$ are generated during the surface melting and can be frozen in the case of fast enough cooling. Moreover, the LPS amplitude increases in multi-pulse irradiation /7/. In their turn LPS may contain near spherical drops (Fig.5b). And, finally, at $E_s \simeq 8$-$9$ J/cm$^2$ two-dimensional PS could be formed (Fig.5c).

We would like to point out that the transition to unpolarized laser beams and longer pulses (both better) should block LPS development. At least in our experiments with unpolarized radiation at the same $E_s$ levels sufficient to cause R(t) changes we did not observe any surface degradation.

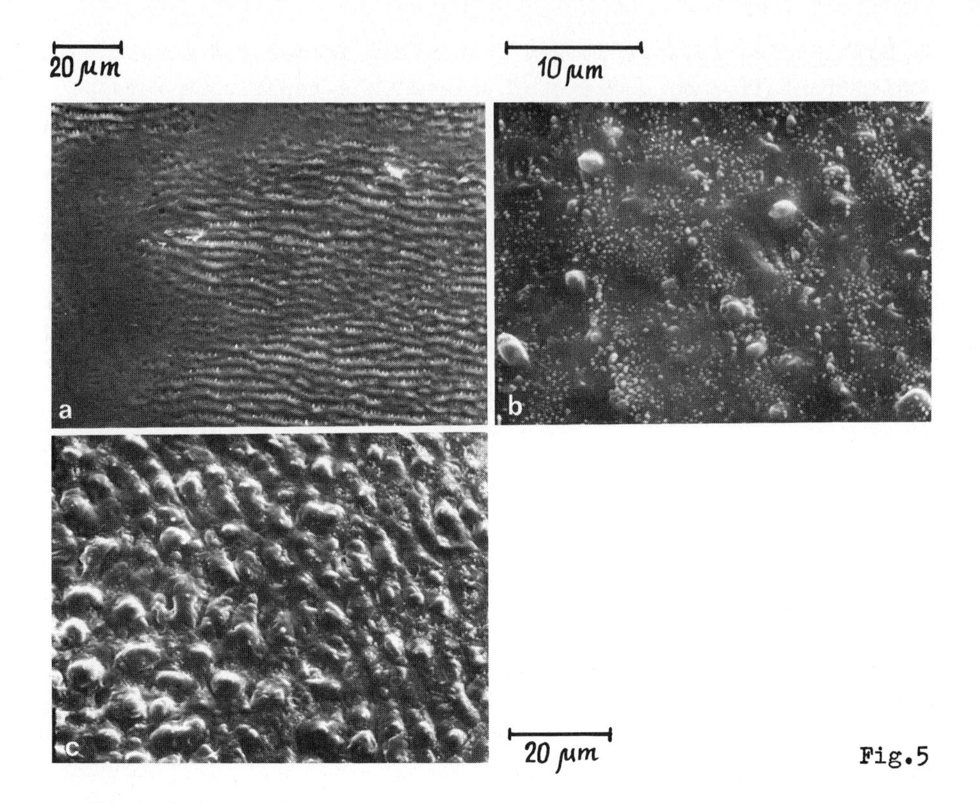

Fig.5

Now let us go back to the sample optical properties. From Fig.4 one can see that the heating speed increases for larger N. To explain this one must assume that every pulse at $E_s \gtrsim E_{th}^d$ causes irreversible increase of the surface layer absorption coefficient $\alpha$. To verify the proposed mechanism the control of experiment with unpolarized beam (to avoid surface degradation) was performed. The InSb plates were irradiated at $E_s > E_{th}$ and different N. After that $T_o$ was measured (Fig.1, curves 2,3). One can see that the N growth leads to a remarkable decrease of the plate transparency. To determine $\alpha$ through $T_o(N)$ detection we must know the exact thickness of the modified surface layer.

## 3. Irradiated p-InSb Electrical Properties

The measurements with unpolarized radiation have shown that for all N and $E_s > E_{th}$ the p - n conversion takes place. The electrical parameters - Hall coefficient $R_s$, layer conductivity $\sigma$, and efficient mobility $\mu = R_s \sigma$ - of the laser-produced n-layers are given in Fig.6. The correlation between $\sigma$ and carrier concentration $N_s = 1/eR_s$ (note that $R_s$ and $\sigma$ were obtained by independent measurements) is presented in Fig.7.

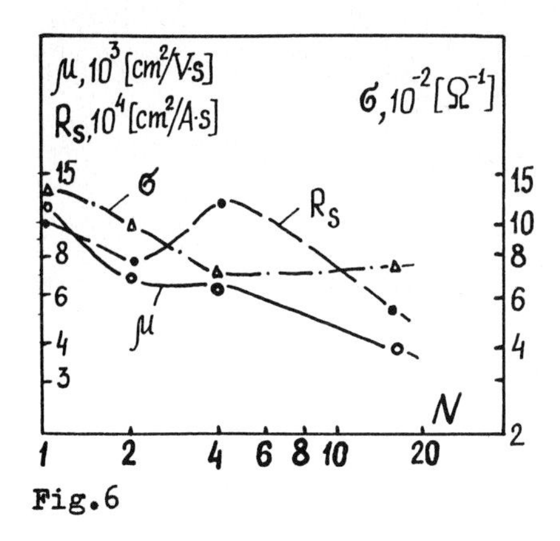


Fig.6

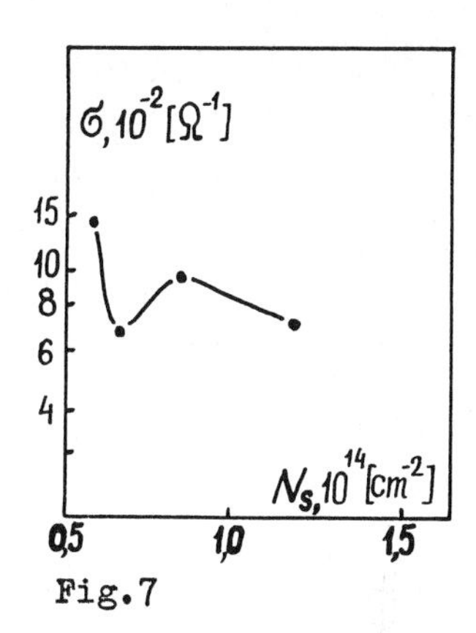


Fig.7

Two processes might be responsible for the observed irreversible change of InSb optical (by $\alpha$ ) and electrical properties: generation of new defects and surface chemical reactions (preliminary Auger analyses have shown that laser irradiation caused the increase of oxygen and decrease of antimony concentration and, evidently, indium oxide formation). Namely, oxidation could be responsible, in our mind, for p-n conversion. The joint action of the processes permits a qualitative explanation of the curves in Fig.6. Indeed, suppose that in spite of the rather small number of experimental points they truly reflect the real trends. Then for large $N \gtrsim 4$ the observed relation $\sigma =$ const can be explained if we consider that the laser-induced chemical action is saturated and the $\sigma$ behaviour is determined by the defect concentration $N_d$. Assuming $\mu \propto C_1/N_d$, $N_s \propto C_2 N_d$ ($C_1$, $C_2$ are constants) we obtain $\sigma = \mu N_s e = \text{Const.}$ For $N < 4$ the decrease of $\sigma$ (N) and monotonous $R_s$(N) behaviour might be the result of both processes appearing simultaneously. The final conclusions clearly need more detailed experimental data.

In conclusion note that the considered laser-induced effects on p-InSb can appear as well in the case of other conductors, namely, from $A^{III}B^{V}$ group.

References

1. V.A.Bogatyrev, G.A.Kachurin: Sov. Phys.-Semicond., 11, 56 (1977)
2. I.Fujiawa: Jap.J.Appl.Phys., 19, 2137 (1980)
3. L.N.Kurbatov, I.G.Stojanova, P.P.Trokhymchuk, A.S.Trokhin: Dokl. Acad. Nauk SSSR (in Russian), 268, 594 (1983)
4. A.B.Korshunov, G.M.Kuznetzov, A.G.Makarov, V.V.Olenin, I.V.Postnikov: Sov. Phys.-Semicond., 12, 554 (1978)
5. Current Topic in Material Science (ed. by E.Kaldis), 8 (North-Holland Publ. Comp., 1982)
6. J.R.Mayer, F.J.Bartoli, M.R.Kruer: Phys. Rev., B21, 1559 (1980)
7. V.I.Konov, A.M.Prokhorov, V.A.Sychugov, A.V.Tishenko, V.N.Tokarev: Zh. Techn. Fiz. (in Russian), 53, 2283 (1983)

# Laser Processing in Silicon on Insulator (SOI) Technologies

V.T. Nguyen and SOI Group

Centre National d'Etudes des Télécommunications, BP. 98,
Meylan Cédex, France

Silicon on insulator (SOI) technologies are an attractive alternative for VLSI circuit manufacturing, owing to such advantages as reduced parasitic capacitances, latch-up immunity and insensitivity to alpha particles. SOI technologies may be also viewed as a first but necessary step towards 3-D integration.

To produce SOI films, lasers among other energy beams have been used as heat sources to induce the recrystallization of silicon films deposited on insulating substrates. In this paper, we will describe briefly works on a special mode of laser recrystallization of amorphous Si thin films on glass substrates. These works have led to a comprehensive model of so-called "Explosive Recrystallization" (XCR), the results of which are now being considered for flat panel display applications. The recrystallized material obtained by XCR was still polycrystalline. Consequently, recent efforts were concentrated on the investigations of the laser-induced zone melting recrystallization (ZMR) of Si films for the fabrication of single-crystal silicon films on insulating substrates. Different techniques used in the laser-induced ZMR will be reviewed. Structural, electrical and device-application properties of crystallized films obtained by ZMR will be also discussed.

## Introduction

During the last several years, a great amount of interest has been generated in the growth of electronic quality silicon on insulators (SOI). The latter is very attractive for VLSI [1] integrated circuit and flat panel display applications.

For VLSI integrated circuit application, the speed of circuits built in SOI structures shown in Fig.1 is increased by elimination of interconnect-to-substrate capacitance and by the reduction of the junction capacitance. Dielectric isolation greatly reduces charges collection volumes, improving radiation hardness. Fewer masks are needed for CMOS on insulator because isolation diffusions are not required. Electrical latch-up of parasistic transistors, which imposes restrictions on the design of CMOS in bulk Si, is eliminated. Currently the silicon on sapphire (SOS) is being employed to provide dielectrically isolated silicon thin film for CMOS technologies but it is expensive and suffers from a high density of defects.

The second generic application of SOI is for flat panel displays. There, the requirement is for large area, transparent, inexpensive substrates with transistors on such substrates providing threshold switching for liquid crystal display elements and also decoding, multiplexing and line driver [2] circuitry. Fused silica and possibly glass plates are the most suitable insulating substrates (Fig.1a).

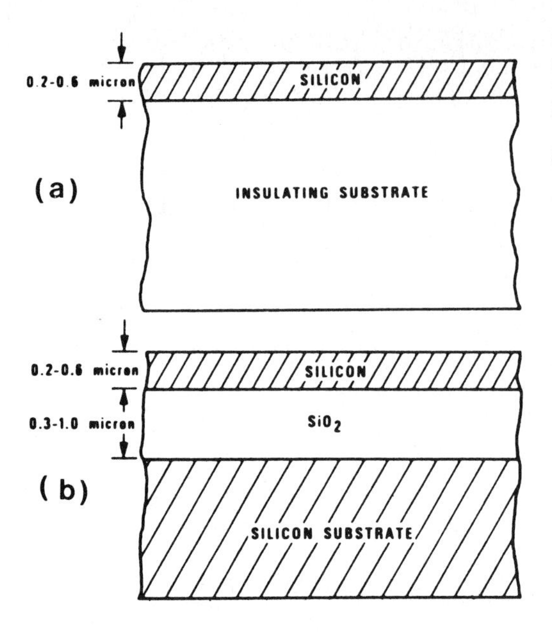


Fig.1 : Two basic silicon on insulator (SOI) structures
a) Insulator serves as entire substrate
b) Insulating film lies below a silicon substrate

Finally, it is clear that SOI technologies may be viewed as a first but necessary step towards three-dimensional integration [3] . Indeed, the possibility of depositing a layer of device-quality silicon on the top of an oxidized layer has provided the present stimulus for three-dimensional integrated circuit development.

Several recent approaches to obtain device worthy SOI structures have been demonstrated by using laser induced crystallization. Most of them rely on melting of amorphous or polycrystalline films and their controlled zone melting recrystallization (ZMR). Therefore, in this paper, we will first describe briefly a special mode of laser crystallization called "Explosive Recrystallization" (XCR) of amorphous Si on glass substrates. The rapidity of this process is attractive for some applications such as large flat panel displays. In the remainder of the paper, the emphasis will be on the CW laser induced ZMR of amorphous or polycrystalline Si films deposited on amorphous insulating substrates. Structural and electrical properties of crystallized films will be discussed and potential applications of crystallized films in microelectronics will be also reviewed.

## I. Laser induced explosive crystallization of silicon film

Rapid scanned laser crystallization has been first carried out by Fan et al. [4], for preparing Ge films on fused-silica substrates. Subsequently this technique has been intensively investigated by our SOI group in order to obtain low-cost large areas of crystallized Si films for fabricating transistor circuits for flat panel display devices. These works have led to a comprehensive study of a special mode of the laser crystallization process generally called "Explosive recrystallization" (hereafter XCR) of amorphous Si (a-Si) on insulators.

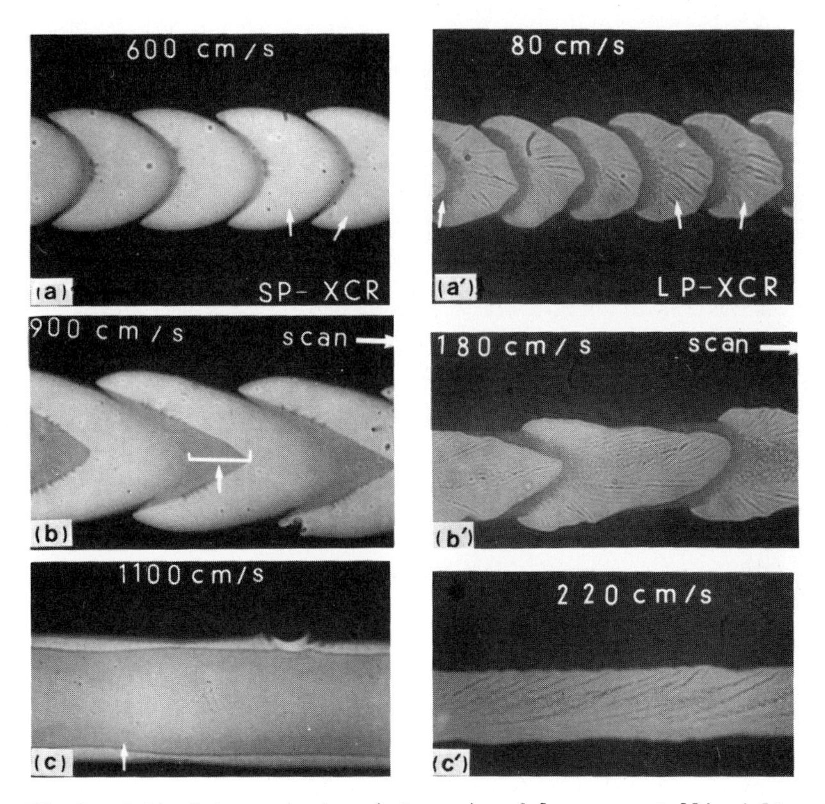


Fig.2 : Optical transmission photographs of laser crystallized lines at different laser scan speeds (a,b,c) in SP-XCR (a',b',c') in LP-XCR

XCR is a generic term which has been used to describe the rapid crystallization of amorphous materials due to free energy release during the amorphous to crystalline transition [5]. We have investigated this transition by studying the scanned laser crystallization of amorphous Si on glass substrates [6]. Amorphous silicon films of 500 nm thickness were prepared by CVD plasma deposition onto $Si_3N_4$ coated glass substrates. Our crystallization system utilized a CW argon laser with a computer controlled scanned beam having a typical diameter 2 W $\simeq$ 100 $\mu$m at the surface of the sample. With this system, it is possible, for a given scan speed, to determine precisely (within 2 %) the threshold power required to induce the surface optical damage indicative of melting [7]. Consequently, the laser scan speed is then the principal paramater that we have used to investigate all the phenomena of XCR [8,9] either in the so called solid phase (SP-XCR) or in liquid phase (LP-XCR). The most striking result of this study is that XCR in both phases occurs only for scan speeds above 30 cm/s [7] and exhibits periodic features whose spatial period increases with increasing laser scan speed (Fig.2 a,b,c. and Fig.2 a',b',c').

The difference between two SP-XCR and LP-XCR events in a-Si are more marked in their crystallographic behavior [10]. The LP-XCR crescent is composed by large grains ($\simeq 10\ \mu m \times 10\ \mu m$) and shows a surface roughness. In contrast with this, the SP-XCR crescent appears with a very smooth surface and is fine grained ($\simeq 0,5\ \mu m \times 1\ \mu m$). Changes in crystallinity between two phases of XCR are also correlated with the changes in electrical properties [10]. Thin film transistors (TFT) made in the different mode of crystallized silicon yield mobility values typically of 10 $cm^2/Vs$ for SP-XCR samples and of 70 $cm^2/Vs$ for LP-XCR films.

In conclusion, the high limit of scan speeds of 2 m/s and 10 m/s for obtaining continuous lines as shown in Fig.2c and Fig.2c' respectively is very attractive for producing large SOI area for flat panel display applications. However, cracks in LP-XCR samples and surface roughness in the LP-XCR regime present major problems which have to be solved.

## II. Zone melting crystallization of Si films on amorphous insulating substrates

### II.1. Crystallization of continuous unseeded Si films

Amorphous or polycrystalline Si films of typical SOI structures shown in Fig.1 (a) and (b) can be melted in their entire thickness with high power CW lasers. After removal of laser source, the liquid becomes cooled and starts solidifying. If the molten Si is in contact with an amorphous substrate, crystallites nucleate at the solid-liquid interface. To obtain single-crystal crystallized or large-grained Si films, lateral temperature gradients must be imposed to force the propagation of the crystallization front along the surface. Two principal methods of inducing lateral temperature gradients are the shaping of scanned laser beam and the selective annealing by patterning the film to obtain spatially varying optical properties.

#### II.1.a. Shaping of scanned laser beam

The temperature rise induced by a Gaussian CW laser beam is not uniform across the incident spot (it is hotter at the center of the spot than at its periphery). Therefore, after scanning a focused CW laser on the sample, a chevron-like crystallization pattern is observed (Fig.3a). The latter is caused by a convex liquid solid interface at the trailing edge of the molten zone. Crystallites grow along the thermal gradient (perpendicular to the trailing edge) from the borders of the scan line towards the center of the line. Grain boundaries arise between grains since crystallites grow from the existing randomly oriented polycrystalline Si located at the edge of the scan line.

On the other hand, concave trailing edges can be obtained by using modified beam shape such as the horseshoe-shaped spot [11] and the doughtnut-shaped beam [12] or by partly masking the incident beam [13,14]. In this last case, part of laser power is spoiled (Fig.3 b). When a concave trailing edge is produced, the temperature gradient shown in the Fig.3(a) is inverted, so that the growth proceeds from the center of the scan line outwards, as shown in Fig.3(b). Random nucleation arising from borders is thus ruled out, and long single crystals ($\simeq 20 \times 200\ \mu m$) can be grown.

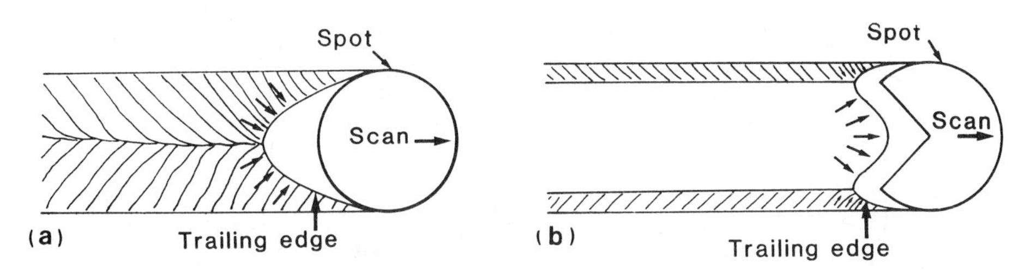


Fig.3 : Chevron-like and single-crystal grains grown using (a) a Gaussian or (b) a shaped beam. Arrows show the growth directions

II.1.b. Selective annealing

An alternative to beam shaping for tailoring the trailing edge is a modification of absorption or reflection of localized surface region. This technique has been demontrated for first time by Colinge et al. [15] by using an antireflecting material ($SiO_2$ or $Si_3N_4$) patterned atop of the silicon film which is to be crystallized. The resulting edge is shown in Fig.4. It is composed of a "row" of teeth. Except at the tips of the teeth, the trailing edge is always concave, provided that the spot size is large enough with respect to the antireflecting stripe periodicity (here the spot size is 120 $\mu$m and stripe periodicity is 20$\mu$m).

During the crystallization process, defects (mainly stacking faults) are swept towards the areas which are located beneath the antireflection stripes, i.e. those which are last to freeze. This is confirmed by an Electron Induced Current (EBIC) analysis [15] of crystallized Si film.

II.2. Crystallization of continuous seeded silicon films

It is worthwhile noting that, using the selective annealing technique for crystallizing continuous unseeded silicon films, grain boundaries form straight lines, and that they are located underneath the

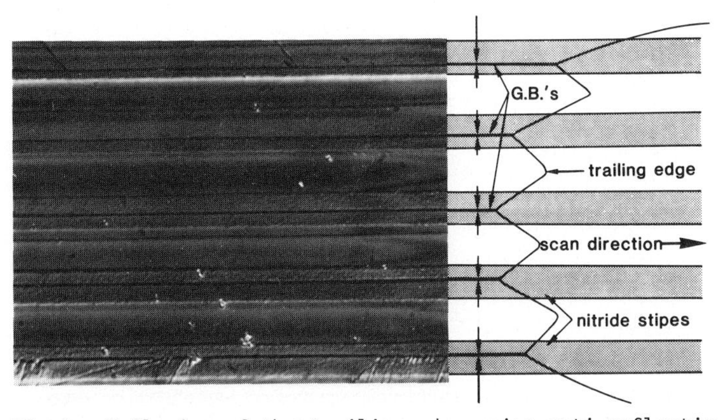


Fig.4 : Tailoring of the trailing edge using anti-reflection stripes and growth of large single crystals with control of grain boundary location

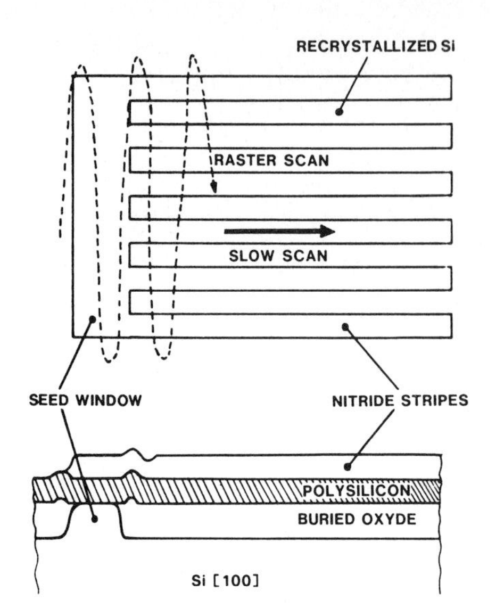


Fig.5 : Use of raster scan together with seeding and antireflectron stripes to grow large single crystals

anti-reflection stripes. Thus, location of grain boundaries can be determined by photolithography. Draw-back of this technique is that grain boundaries still appear between the nitride stripes in those regions of the silicon films where scanning lines are overlapped, due to the small and finite dimensions of the laser spot.

To eliminate the overlap problem, a new crystallization technique has been used [16,17]. This technique combines the selective annealing with the seeded oscillatory growth (Fig.5).

A circular or elliptical beam is scanned rapidly, perpendicularly to a regular array of AR nitride stripes, while advancing slowly along them. When the <100> aligned seeding windows are used, all crystallites grow with the same <100> orientation, and no grain nor subgrain boundaries appear between grains [16]. Single crystals as large as 3x0.5 $mm^2$ have been grown using this technique [16,17]. However some rotation of the crystal orientation is observed as the crystal propagates about 500 microns away from the seed.

II.3. Crystallization of patterned unseeded films

This technique is very important for obtaining single crystal silicon thin film on a non-silicon substrate such as fused quartz. In 1979 Gibbons et al.[18] have first demonstrated that small isolated islands of Si on $SiO_2$ can be melted in their entirety and crystallized into single crystal.

Subsequently, most of extensive works on crystallization of patterned unseeded films were carried out by Biegelsen et al.[19] by studying the role and utility of lateral heat flow in the growth of single-crystal silicon islands on amorphous substrates. They have demonstrated [19] that the thermal profile necessary for suppressing edge nucleation can be obtained by using a laser spot much wider and shorter than an island, and by controlling the optical absorption of laser radiations using various thin film structures (Fig. 6).

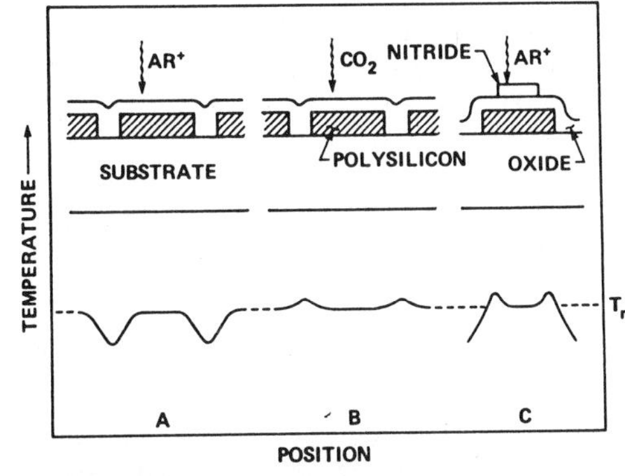


Fig.6 : Above : cross section of encapsulated silicon stripes on quartz substrates.
Below : corresponding temperature plats. (A) Argon laser radiation ; (B) $CO_2$ laser radiation ; (C) Silicon nitride dual dialectric control of visible absorption. $T_m$ is the melting temperature

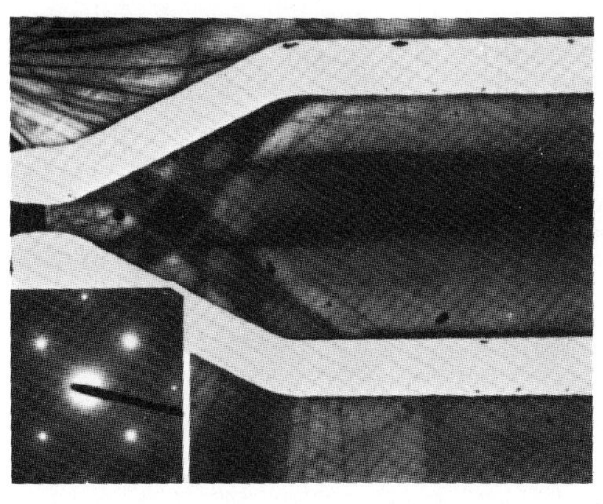

Fig.7 : Single-crystal "island" in patterned stripe ; insert shows diffraction diagram of the material

Utilizing the technique sketched in Fig.6(B), typical 20 $\mu$m-wide single crystalline island [19], as shown in Fig.7, has been obtained. The main defects are twinning and low angle grain boundaries. Otherwise, the material is surprisingly free of dislocations, stacking faults and precipitates. More recently, with a solidification front tilted relative to the direction of molten path, the defects shown in Fig.7 can be greatly reduced or even eliminated [20].

## III. SOI DEVICES

In 1979, the first MOS transistors were fabricated in laser crystallized silicon film on $SiO_2$ [21,22]. Since then, the literature pertaining to device characterisation of SOI films is rapidly expanding. Therefore, in this section, our emphasis is on the most recent and significant results of the study on the possibility of using laser crystallized silicon film in single-layer SOI devices and also in three dimensional (3D) structures.

### III.1. Single-layer SOI devices

In this class, devices are fabricated in a single layer of crystallized Si on an insulating substrate (Fig.1). Consequently, problems appearing in the fabrication of devices depend strongly on crystallization techniques.

III.1.a. Unseeded crystallization :

In this case, the crucial property that needs to be controlled is the interface charge at the bottom of the crystallized silicon. Unwanted fixed charge $Q_f$ at an $Si/SiO_2$ interface is specially serious when fabricating n-channel MOS transistor in crystallized silicon film since it can induce a parallel parasitic transistor at the bottom of the crystallized silicon film [23]. The presence of this parasitic transistor can influence the threshold voltage of the main transistor controlled primarily by the top gate electrode. With proper processing, values of $Q_f$ as low as $1x10^{11}$ $cm^{-2}$ appear to be reproducibly obtained [24].

The actual grain structure of crystallized silicon film has to be considered since grain boundaries, being the most electrically active among the defects, affect device performances. Grain boundaries occurring in heavily doped zones (source, drains) have no electrical activity and can therefore be neglected. In contrast to this, grain boundaries occurring in the channel of transistors have dramatic influence on device characteristics [25].

In the case where the grain boundary is parallel to current flow, grain boundaries act as paths of fast diffusion for source and drain doping impurities. Diffusion distances of 2 $\mu$m can be covered during source and drain dopant thermal activation. This causes exceedingly high leakage currents in devices having channel lengths of less than 4$\mu$m.

Figure 8 compares the output characteristics of two SOI transistors, one without any grain boundary, the other having a single grain boundary shorting source and drain through dopant diffusion.

If the grain boundaries are perpendicular to the current flow, carrier transport is impeded by potential barriers associated with the grain boundaries. Experimental measurements presented by Colinge et al. [26] show the influence of grain boundaries on the mobility which is typically half that of similarly doped single-crystal silicon. Therefore, the localisation of grain boundaries as described in section II-1 is necessary for aligning devices in those areas which are single-crystalline and defect-free [27]. N-channel enhancement and

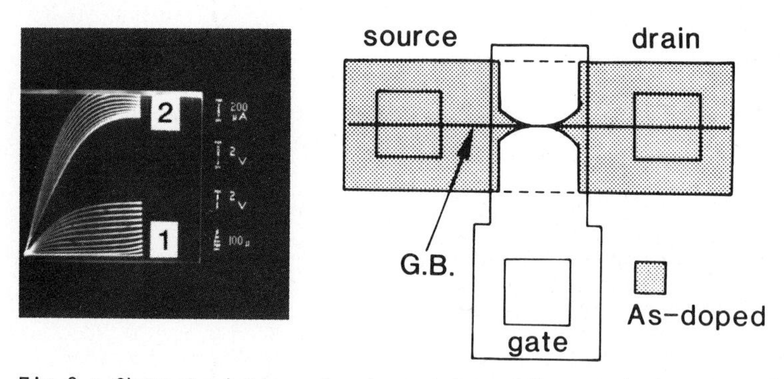


Fig.8 : Characteristics of a transistor with a grain boundary (GB) parallel to the current flow in the channel. (1) single crystal; (2) with a grain boundary

depletion transistors as well as ring oscillators have been fabricated in these areas. The transistors are self-aligned polysilicon gate devices, having a gate oxide of 60 nm. The source and drain are formed by arsenic implantation. Transistors with gate lengths ranging between 10 and 4 m have been realized. The inversion layer mobility is 650 $cm^2/Vs$, and the drain breakdown voltage is greater than 22 volts. The leakage current is in the 10 nA/$\mu$m range. However, by simply applying a negative bias of -5 volts to the substrate, which acts as a backside gate, this leakage current is reduced by a factor of 5000 (to a few pA/$\mu$m), suggesting that leakage is caused by a parasitic inversion layer due to $Si/SiO_2$ interface states [23] rather than by crystal defects within the junctions. More recently, short channel devices were fabricated in unseeded crystallized Si film, using thermal annealing for source and drain implant to avoid grain boundary diffusion [28]. For a 2$\mu$m design rule ring oscillator, a propagation delay per stage of 115 ps was obtained which is a factor 2 faster than the same circuit in bulk Si.

Patterned unseeded crystallization technique (section II-3) is also a powerful technique for producing single-crystalline and defect-free Si island on quartz substrate. Chiang et al. [20] have reported that MOS devices having channel mobilities of > 900 $cm^2/Vs$ and leakage currents 1 pA/$\mu$m have been fabricated in the single-crystal islands which were produced from patterned and encapsulated polysilicon films crystallized with a scanning $CO_2$ laser.

Finally, it is worthwhile noting that specific applications such as a new CMOS structure [29] and a dynamic RAM [30] have been also realized using unseeded crystallized Si film.

III.1.b. Seeded crystallization :

As it has been mentioned in section II-2, the seeded crystallization technique which combines the selective annealing with the seeded growth can produce a regular array of grain-boundary free single crystal silicon stripes of several hundred microns. MOS transistors formed in the single-crystal stripes have mobilities comparable to devices formed in bulk films [16,17]. Only drawback of the required size and spacing of these single-crystal stripes is that the wafer must be committed to a specific circuit (or at least a circuit of a certain chip size) before crystallization. Using the perimeter of the wafer for seeding avoids this disavantage. Unfortunately, defect-free single-crystal propagation in submicron films over the distances ranging from 1 to 10 cm has not yet been shown.

III.2. Three-dimensional (3-D) structures

Among new device designs emerging as a result of laser crystallization capabilities, the most exciting is the idea of fabrication 3-D integrated circuits. The concept of 3-D integration was first proposed from MIT in 1979 [31] and based on the realization that the present two-dimensional (2-D) integration will reach its limit of packing density in the near future. In fact, Gibbons and Lee [32] and subsequently Goeloe et al. [33] showed the feasability of a novel CMOS inverter with a single joint gate (JMOS) as shown in Fig.9a. The p-channel devices were fabricated in the bulk Si, followed by deposition and laser crystallization of an additional layer in which the whole complementary n-channel transistors were made. In that case, gate source and gate drain capacitances of the upper transistor show unacceptably

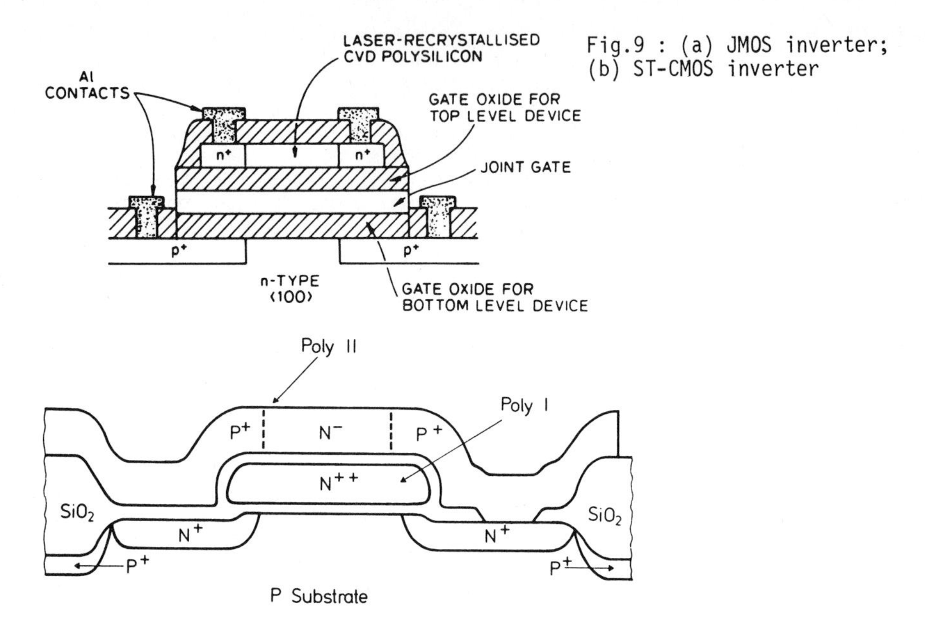


Fig.9 : (a) JMOS inverter;
(b) ST-CMOS inverter

large values due to the presence of the entire source and drain areas on the top of the gate. Therefore stacked transistor CMOS (ST-CMOS) have been made [34] in which advantage is taken of the fact that, in CMOS gates, the gate (and the drain for some configurations) is common to both p- and the n-channel transistor (Fig. 9b).

More recently, multilayer SOI structure, in which "SOI like" layers of devices are vertically stacked, the 0-th layer being the substrate, has been proposed [3]. However, up to now, only one layer has been stacked [35,36] on the top of the substrate (Fig.10 a and Fig.10 b).

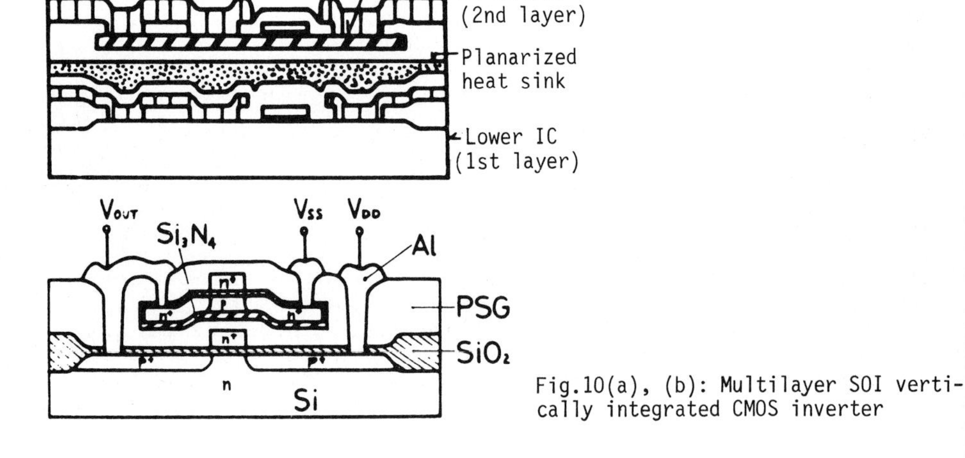


Fig.10(a), (b): Multilayer SOI vertically integrated CMOS inverter

CONCLUSIONS

Laser crystallization technique for producing SOI structures offers possibilities for new classes of devices, as well as improving more conventional circuitry. For large flat panel display applications, unseeded crystallized Si films should be satisfactory, but seeding will be required for high-performance, small geometry circuits. In addition to quality of the crystallized film (and also the substrate), the properties of the interfaces must be optimized.

Finally, in any 3-D structures, creating an upper active layer without damaging already fabricated underlying layers is unfortunately not the only key for 3-D integrated circuits. Other technological hot spots are : realization of interlevel connections, planarization, need for low temperature and shortime processes ....

REFERENCES


1 H.W. Lam, A.F. Tasch, JR., R.F. Pinnizzoto, in "VLSI Electronics : Microstructure Science", edited by N.G. EINSPRUCH (Academic Press, New York, 1982) vol. 4, pp. 1-54

2 D.J. Bartelink, in "Grain Boundaries in Semiconductors", edited by H.J. Leamy, G.E. Pike and C.H. Seager (North Holland, New York 1981) pp. 249-260

3 D.A. Antoniadis, in "Energy Beam-Solid Interactions and Transient Thermal Processing", edited by John C.C. Fan and N.M. Johson (North Holland, New York 1984)

4 J.C.C. Fan, H.J. Zeiger, R.P. Cale and R.L. Chapman, App. Phys. Lett. 36, 158 (1980)

5 G. Gore, Phil. Mag. 9, 73 (1855)

6 G. Auvert, D. Bensahel, A. Georges and V.T. Nguyen, App. Phys. Lett., 38, 613 (1981)

7 D. Bensahel, G. Auvert, V.T. Nguyen and G.A. Rozgonyi, in "Laser and Electron-Beam Interactions with Solids", edited by B.R. Appleton and G.K. Celler (North Holland, New York 1982), pp. 541-546

8 D. Bensahel and G. Auvert, in "Laser-Solid Interactions and Transient Thermal Processing of Materials", edited by J. Narayan, W.L. Brown and R.A. Lemons (North Holland, New York 1983), pp. 165-176

9 G. Auvert, D. Bensahel, A. Perio, V.T. Nguyen and G.A. Rozgonyi, App. Phys. Lett. 39, 724 (1981)

10 G. Auvert, D. Bensahel, A. Perio, F. Morin, G.A. Rozgonyi and V.T. Nguyen, in "Laser and Electron Beam Interactions with Solids", edited by B.R. Appleton and G.K. Celler (North Holland, New York 1982) pp. 535-540

11 D.K. Biegelsen, N.M. Johnson, D.J. Bartelink and M.D. Moyer, in "Laser and Electron Beam Solid Interactions and Laser Processing", edited by J.F. Gibbons, L.D. Hess and T.W. Sigmons (North Holland, New York 1981) pp. 487-494

12 J. Sakurai, M. Nakano and M. Tagaki, App. Phys. Lett. 40, 775 (1982)

13 T.J. Kamins, IEDM Tech. Digest, 1982, p. 420

14 T.J. Stultz and J.F. Gibbons, App. Phys. Lett. 39, 498 (1981)

15 J.P. Colinge, E. Demoulin, D. Bensahel and G. Auvert, Jap. J. of App. Phys. 22, Suppl. 22-1, 205 (1983) and also J.P. Colinge and E.D. Demoulin, in Proceeding of Sumer Course on "Thin Film Crystalline and Amorphous Silicon" edited by Ketholieke Universiteit Leuven, Belgium, 1984

16 J.P. Colinge, D. Bensahel, M. Alamome, M. Haond and J.C. Pfister, Electr. Lett., 23, 985 (1983)
17 C.I. Drowley, P. Zorabedian and T.I. Kamins, in ref. 3
18 J.F. Gibbons, K.F. Lee, T.J. Magee, J. Reng and R. Ormond, App. Phys. Lett. 34, 83 (1979)
19 D.K. Biegelsen, N.M. Johnson, W.G. Hawkins, L.E. Fennell and M.D. Mayer in ref. 8 , pp. 537-548
20 A. Chiang, M.H. Zarzyeki, W.P. Meuli and N.M. Johnson, in ref. 3

21 K.F. Lee, J.F. Gibbons, K.C. Sarawat and T.I. Kamins, App. Phys. Lett., 35, 173 (1979)
22 A.F. Tasch, Ir, T.C. Holloway, K.F. Lee and J.F. Gibbons, Electron. Lett., 15, 435 (1979)
23 T.I. Kamins, in "Proceeding of Material Research Society 1984 Spring Meeting", pp.
24 H.P. Le and H.W. Lam, IEEE Electron. Dev. Lett., 3, 161 (1982)
25 J.P. Colinge, Microelectron. J., 14, 58 (1983)
26 J.P. Colinge, H. Morel and J.P. Chante, IEEE Electron Dev., 30, 197 (1983)
27 J.P. Colinge, D. Bensahel, M. Alamome, M. Haond and C. Leguet, in ref. 3
28 K.K. Ng, G.W. Taylor, G.K. Celler, L.E. Trimble, R.J. Bayruns and E.I. Polilonis, in IEDM Technical Digest, 1983, pp. 356-359
29 T.I. Kamins, IEEE Electron Dev. Lett., 3, 341 (1982)
30 R.D. Jolly, T.I. Kamins and R.H. Mc Charles, IEEE Electron Dev. Lett., 4, 8 (1983)
31 M.W. Geis, D.C. Flanders, D.A. Antoniadis and H.I. Smith, in IEDM Tech. Dig., 9, 82 (1980)
32 J.F. Gibbons and K.F. Lee, IEEE Electron. Dev. Lett., 1, 117 (1980)
33 G.T. Goeloe, E.W. Maby, D.J. Silversmith, R.W. Mountain and D.A. Antoniadis, IEDM Tech. Dig, p. 554 (1981)
34 J.P. Colinge, E. Demoulin and M. Lobet, IEEE Electron. Dev., 29, 585 (1982)
35 S. Kawamura, N. Sasaki, T. Iwai, R. Markai, M. Nakano and M. Takgi, IEDM Techn. Dig. p. 364, (1983) and also in IEEE Electr. Dev. Lett., 4, 366 (1983)
36 S. Akiyama, S. Ogawa, M. Yoneda, N. Yoshii and Y. Terui, in ref. 32 p. 352

# Laser Recrystallisation of Silicon-on-Oxide

A.E. Adams and S.L. Morgan

GEC Research Laboratories, Hirst Research Centre,
Wembley, Middlesex, UK

The limitations of silicon-on-sapphire have led to considerable interest in alternative materials for silicon on insulator device technology. We have studied the use of a cw argon ion laser to recrystallise fine grain polysilicon deposited onto oxidised silicon wafers, utilising lateral seeding techniques to extend the area of recrystallised material. This paper describes in detail the results of this work. The design of a new line beam processor is also described.

## Introduction

A thin single crystal silicon layer grown on an insulating substrate is an ideal medium for MOS integrated circuit fabrication. The electric isolation between individual circuit elements offers the capability of increased packing densities and improved resistance to ionising radiation over bulk silicon structures, while deleterious effects such as parasitic capacitance and CMOS latch-up are eliminated. At present, the only silicon-on-insulator material available to the microelectronic industry is silicon-on-sapphire. However, this material is expensive, difficult to process, and the small mismatch between the $<1\bar{1}02>$ sapphire lattice parameter and the <100> epitaxial silicon parameter gives rise to a highly defective interface region. The reduction in crystal quality that occurs in the proximity of this region results in a concomitant decrease in effective carrier mobility which is likely to become more significant as thinner layers are required.

An alternative approach, which has been the subject of considerable interest over recent years, is to deposit a layer of fine grain polysilicon onto a standard silicon substrate which has previously been oxidised. A radiant heat source is then used to melt and recrystallise the polysilicon. Various schemes have been tried including lasers [1], graphite strip heaters [2], and electron beams [3]. However it has previously been shown [4] that unless some seeding or grain entrapment technique is also used all these recrystallisation techniques generally result in randomly orientated, large grain polysilicon layers, which are unsuitable for VLSI fabrication.

In this paper we examine the use of a well controlled, scanning spot cw laser processing facility and lateral seeding techniques which have previously been described elsewhere [5]. We also present results to indicate that this arrangement is non-ideal, and as an improved alternative the design of a line beam processor is discussed.

## Experimental

The experimental configuration used to process the polysilicon samples is shown in Fig 1 . The system consists of an 18 Watt argon ion laser

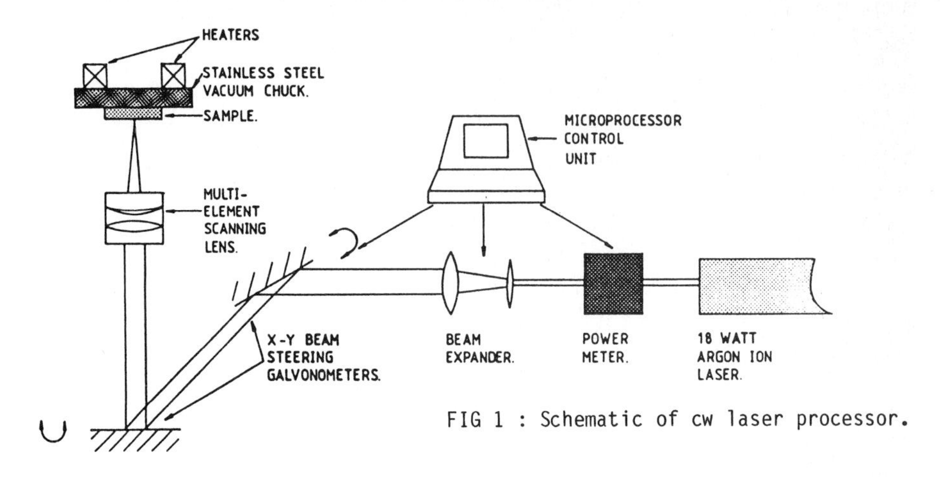


FIG 1 : Schematic of cw laser processor.

operating on all lines. After passing through an expanding telescope the beam is focused by a telecentric scanning lens which can scan a 10 cm field and is capable of producing a diffraction limited spot size of 20 μm; more typically a 35 μm spot is used. The beam is raster scanned across the sample surface with a velocity of 5 cm/s: after each successive scan the beam is stepped a distance of 9 μm. The polysilicon samples are mounted on a stainless steel vacuum chuck which can be heated to 650°C and the processing sequence is controlled by a desk top computer.

Various structures have been examined. The first consists of 0.5 μm and 1.0 μm of thermal oxide grown onto <100> silicon wafers. Seeding windows are then etched into the oxide using a mask set which has a variety of window sizes and spacings; a 1 μm layer of LPCVD polysilicon is then added. In other samples the oxide is recessed into the silicon substrate (LOCOS) so that the deposited silicon has a planar surface. The third type of structure examined has a regular area of seeding windows equally spaced 18 μm apart. To maintain the integrity of the polysilicon layer as it melts, all the structures are capped with 1 μm of $SiO_2$ followed by 500 Å of $Si_3N_4$.

The nature of the recrystallised layers has been investigated by anisotropic etching, SECCO etching and scanning electron microscopy.

## Results

All the various types of sample investigated show complete recrystallisation between windows spaced 20 μm or less apart, see for example Fig 2 . These areas extend for 600 μm along the length of the seeding windows in unrecessed oxide structures, but in the LOCOS samples lateral epitaxy has occurred along the entire length of the windows, that is 1.5 mm. It has been found that it is not necessary for the windows to be continuous. Single crystal material has been seen to seed from windows 300 μm x 50 μm linearly spaced by 20 μm, for as long as the structure is repeated. Anisotropic etching has been used to examine the maximum length which lateral epitaxy extends away from the seeding windows' edge,

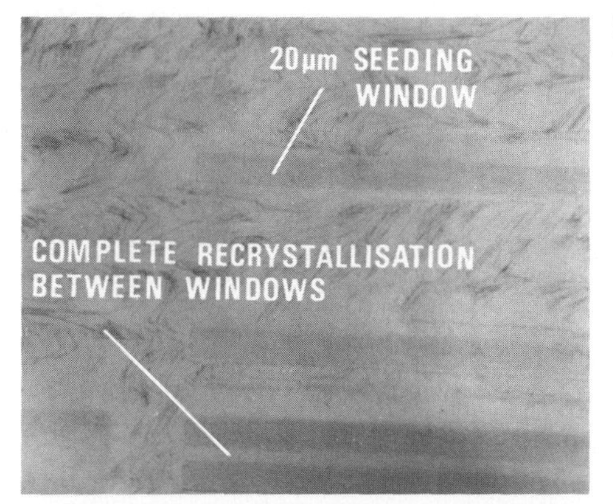


FIG 2 : Normaski micrograph of recrystallised polysilicon.

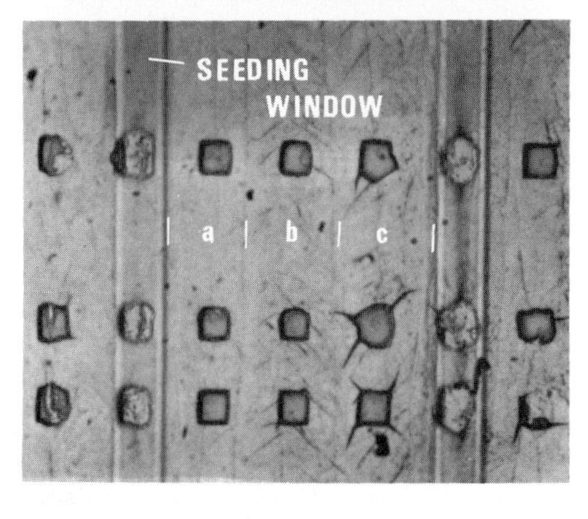


FIG 3 : Anistropically etched recrystallised layer, (a) laterally seeded region (b) low angle grain boundary area (c) randomly oriented polysilicon.

Fig 3 . The maximum range observed is about 50 µm; beyond this low angle grain boundaries are formed and the crystal growth direction begins to reorientate. After 100 µm the recrystallisation takes the form of randomly orientated large grain polysilicon with average grain sizes of 200 x 50 µm. Crystallites significantly larger than those usually present in regrown unseeded structures have been observed. Silicon grains as large as 25 µm x 2 mm have been regularly seen. The reason for such large growths has not yet been positively identified, but they are probably due to either the structure of these samples, or a greater degree of control available with this cw processor than others previously employed. Detailed examination has shown that recrystallisation of only the window edges is a necessary condition for lateral seeding to occur. No lower limit has been established for their dimension. However, the fact that they may be very narrow is important in applying this technique to practical device structures where seeding windows may need to be strategically placed between individual circuit elements.

Cross sectional scanning electron microscopy has been used to examine the interface region between the recrystallised layers and the original silicon substrate surface,see Fig 4 . No warping or cracking of the oxide layer has been observed. However, the original interface between the recrystallised polysilicon layer and the substrate is still visible. It is

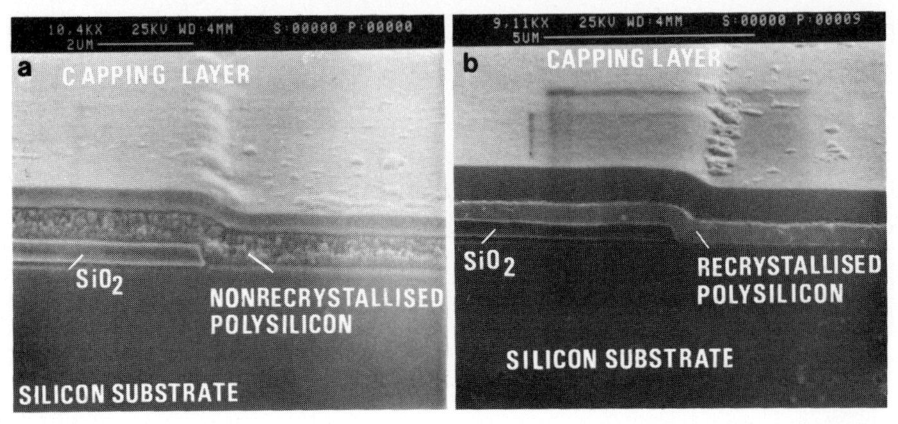


FIG 4a,b : Sample cross section after Secco etching showing: (a) Non-recrystallised silicon grains (b) Recrystallised layer and interface

clear that the pedestal temperature of 600°C was either insufficient or that the beam powers used were too low to allow the melt to penetrate into the silicon substrate which ultimately must limit the quality of the regrown material.

As well as limitations in the melt depths which are available with this type of processing arrangement, it is also believed that a scanning spot is a non-ideal geometry. As the focused spot is scanned across the sample surface, extreme temperature gradients are established which result in multi-directional resolidification and hence competitive nucleation fronts Fig 5a . To overcome these limitations, a new system has been designed and built to provide a line beam profile. This has the advantage of producing an undirectional resolidification front (Fig 5b) as in the case of the graphite strip heater. The system consists of a stainless steel cell with a quartz input window which houses a graphite substrate heater to raise the substrate to 1000°C,see Fig 6. The sample is placed in a quartz boat which is then mounted directly onto the heater. Oxygen-free nitrogen is flown through the cell to prevent the heater from burning up. Cylindrical optics are used to transform the laser beam into a line and focus it in one direction at the surface of the sample and the cell is mounted on an xy translation stage to enable the sample to be scanned under the beam. The system has only recently been commissioned and initial experiments have so far only produced results similar to those described above, but various aspect ratios of the beam dimensions and operating parameters are currently under investigation. However, recently published results have indicated [6] that there may be a fundamental limit to the distance away from seeding sites at which lateral epitaxy can occur due to oxygen incorporation from the $SiO_2$ layer. If this is so, modification of the temperature profiles would indeed have no effect on the regrowth range.

In conclusion, a cw argon laser processing facility has been used to examine lateral seeding phenomena in a variety of sample structures. For parallel windows spaced 20 μm or less apart, complete recrystallisation can be obtained. In order to investigate the effects of the laser beam profile on the quality of the regrown polysilicon layers a special beam processor has been designed and built.

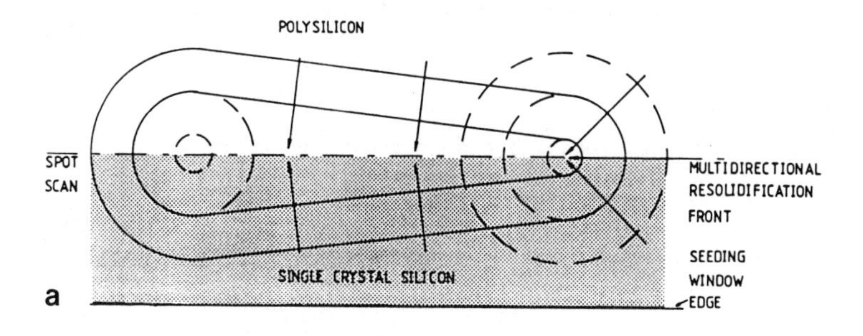


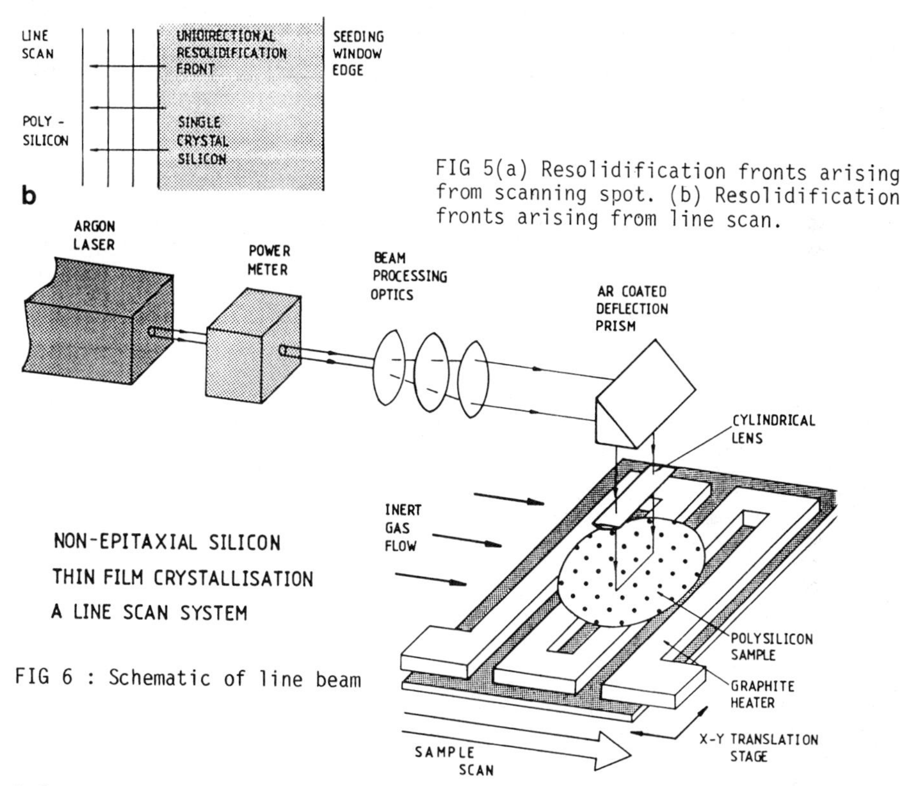


FIG 5(a) Resolidification fronts arising from scanning spot. (b) Resolidification fronts arising from line scan.

FIG 6 : Schematic of line beam

References

1 A. Gat, L. Gerzberg, J. Gibbons, et al: Appl. Phys. Lett., 33, 775 (1978)
2 J. Fan, M. Geis and B Tsaur: Appl. Phys. Lett., 38, 365 (1981)
3 J. Knapp and S. Picraux: MRS Proc., 'Laser-solid interactions and transient thermal processing of materials', Vol 13, Edit. J. Narayan W. Brown, R. Lemons, North-Holland 1983
4 M. Geis, et al: Ref.3, p.477
5 J. Davis, R. McMahon and H Ahmed: Ref.3, p.563
6 J. Fan, B. Tsaur, C. Chen, J. Dick and L Kaymerski: Appl. Phys. Lett., 44, 1086 (1984)

# Fundamentals of Laser Micromachining of Metals

G. Herziger and E.W. Kreutz

Institut für Angewandte Physik, Technische Hochschule Darmstadt,
Schloßgartenstr. 7, D-6100 Darmstadt, Fed. Rep. of Germany

Lasers as precise machining tools of high flexibility without wear out offer new possibilities for modification and processing of materials; there are already various applications such as drilling, cutting, welding, glazing, annealing and hardening. To understand and utilize laser microprocessing some of the physical processes involved are reported: intensity-dependent absorption, laser workpiece interaction by optical feedback, and plasma generation with all the drawbacks to different modes of operation. Investigations of the fundamentals of laser microprocessing are reported in order to achieve the processing results desired. It is necessary to match the laser parameters to the specific application so that the optimized processing parameters always create the same geometric and metallurgical properties of the processed materials.

## 1. Introduction

The unique temporal and spatial characteristics of directed energy sources such as lasers or electron beams with their high power allows the deposition of a great amount of heat into a selected region of a material. When the material is heated,making a transition of phase and structure, a beam-induced materials process is obtained. This may be hardening or annealing, melting and rapid solidification to form novel structures and alloys, or vaporization to remove material during abrasive machining such as cutting, drilling and shaping.

Lasers as precise machining tools of high flexibility without wear out have emerged in the last years for modification and processing of surface layers of metals, semiconductors and insulators /1-3/ for integrated circuit technology. Lasers have been used either for directed energy processing /2/ or for microprocessing machining /1,3/. In the former case lasers have become established as a useful method for annealing, alloying, solidification, and epitaxy of surfaces. In the latter case lasers have been employed for ablation and vaporization in fabricating circuit elements directly or for trimming components to desired tolerances by homogenization, maskless direct writing for personalization, drilling of deep holes for cooling, disconnection and via formation.

To utilize the advantages of laser microprocessing and for appropriate laser micromachining it is necessary to understand the underlying complex physical processes to a higher extent than for conventional machining. The present paper summarizes some investigations on the fundamentals of laser microprocessing in order to achieve the processing results desired.

## 2. Parameters of Laser Processing

A typical arrangement for laser materials processing /4/ is shown schematically in Fig.1. The laser radiation of power $P_L$ and divergence

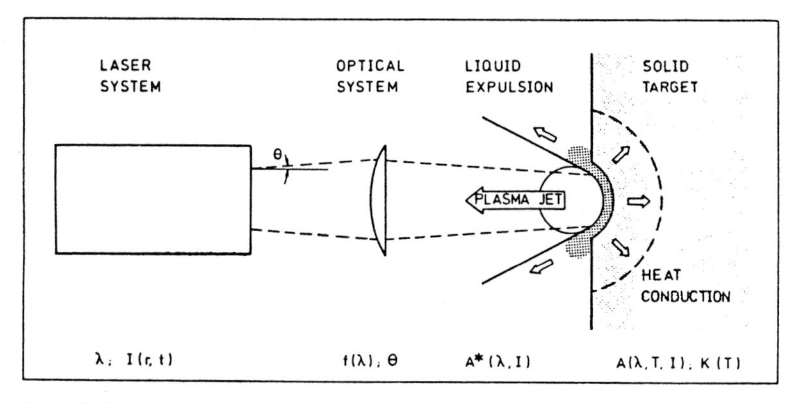


Fig. 1 Scheme of laser materials processing

angle $\Theta$ is focussed by an optical system of focal length f to yield the spatial and temporal intensity distribution I(r,t) at the surface of the workpiece, which is approximately determined by $P_L$ and the focal area. I(r,t) governs the energy density

$$\varepsilon = \frac{I(r,t)}{v} \quad , \tag{1}$$

which is necessary for a unique material processing at processing speed v. The focal area and also the intensity distribution as well depend on the mode configuration /5/, focussing optics and method of beam manipulation /6/ which are being used to produce suitable beam patterns at the workpiece surface.

Because of its symmetry it is frequently desirable to operate in the Gaussian $TEM_{oo}$ mode, where the intensity as a function of radius r from the center of the beam is given by

$$I(r) = I_o \exp(-2r^2/w_o^2) \quad , \tag{2}$$

where $I_o$ is the intensity of the beam at the center and $w_o$ is the beam waist, i.e. the radius at which the intensity is reduced from its central value by a factor of $e^2$. The maximum intensity

$$I_{max} = 2P_L/\pi r_F^2 \tag{3}$$

is governed by the focus radius

$$r_F = \frac{w_o f}{\sqrt{z_R^2 + (z-f)^2}} \quad , \tag{4}$$

where $z_R$ is the Rayleigh length and z is the distance from the beam waist showing a beam divergence angle smaller than for the higher-order transverse modes /5/. If not stated otherwise, the following considerations refer to Gaussian beams. A Gaussian intensity distribution might even be observed for multimode radiation, although there are strong fluctuations, which originate from the superposition of axial and transverse modes /7/, yielding a time-averaged Gaussian beam profile.

The laser parameters characterizing the processing properties are wavelength $\lambda$, polarization p, and intensity $I(r,t)$ at the surface of the workpiece. The spatial and temporal intensity distribution depends on the mode structure, and externally introduced modulation, or a combination of both. The intensity of the laser radiation in the area of interaction is the most relevant parameter governing working speed, efficiency, and quality of the processed materials.

The material properties which relate to laser processing are the absorptivity $A(\lambda,I,T)$, the thermal diffusivity $K(T)/\rho C$, and some threshold temperatures and the correlated transformation energies, which are typical for the individual treatment, such as the hardening temperature, melting temperature or boiling temperature. The absorptivity normally depends on wavelength, intensity and temperature of the material. Reflection of the incident radiation and heat flow in the material are the dominating loss mechanisms in materials processing, thus, the minimization of these losses is a main criterion for the determination of the appropriate intensity.

The laser energy absorbed in the material depends on the absorptivity, the intensity, and the available interaction time. The absorbed laser energy is converted to heat within the penetration depth of laser radiation with subsequent heat flow from the interaction volume into the material. A particular combination of intensity and interaction time defines a specific operational regime with the occurrence of a unique material processing effect. For a rough survey it is appropriate to distinguish between two intensity regimes, which are sharply determined by the threshold intensity of evaporation $I_v$.

At low intensities ($I<I_v$) lasers are employed for all kinds of heat treatment that do not alter the geometric shape of the workpiece, but rather improve or change the material properties at the surface of the workpiece. Common examples are transformation hardening, annealing, or alloying. The absorptivity A is independent of the incident intensity and the analytic treatment is based on the solution of the three-dimensional heat equation under conditions of temperature-dependent thermophysical properties.

High intensities ($I>I_v$) are the domain of abrasive processing, such as drilling and cutting as well as processes associated with material melting such as welding, glazing, and shock-hardening of surfaces. Characteristic phenomena of this intensity range are the appearance of a partially ionized plasma and an intensity-dependent absorption. The material is removed as liquid, vapour or plasma.

## 3. Special Features of Laser Processing

The tools of customary machines normally are not affected by materials processing, except for some more or less controllable wear out. Although laser machining shows no wear out, the system parameters of the laser tool are changed by optical feedback from the workpiece /8/. The laser and workpiece represent a system of coupled resonators with strong interactions between the dynamics of the laser and the workpiece. The workpiece controls the laser radiation depending on its reflectivity and location with respect to the focal plane. Tilting and moving of the workpiece, movements of the melt by capillary or acoustic waves, and changes of the absorptivity during processing can stimulate relaxation oscillations, mode instabilities or chaotic temporal behaviour which may result in stochastic fluctuations of the spatial and temporal intensity distribution. A controlled continuous operation may change into an uncontrolled pulse operation; this has been described in more detail elsewhere /7/. As further peculiarity the relevant material parameters change during material processing, due to temperature variation, to structure or phase changes, or to the generation of a laser-induced plasma in front of the workpiece. In addition, increases in peak intensities by superelevation relaxation oscillations, mode instabilities, and mode-locking phenomena due to the strong non-linearity of the laser-processing medium may generate a plasma in the surface region /9/, which affects the processing via shielding /10 to 11/, lensing, and recoil pressure /13/.

The main processes in laser material processing, which are summarized for microdrilling in Fig.2, are the losses due to reflection and heat conduction, the optical feedback, the material removal by vapour and melt expulsion as well as the influence of the laser-induced plasma. For microdrilling these processes must be adjusted with respect to given quality standards. Process adjustment /14/ by simple trial-and-error variation for parameter optimization must fail due to the gearing and mutual influence of the particular processes. Rather a physical description of the processing parameters is required including their mutual influences. Thus, the physical processes involved in laser materials processing necessarily have to be known in order to avoid uneconomic integration of lasers into production lines. In any case, laser beam diagnostics have to be performed in the arrangement for processing. The analysis of a free running laser beam is not sufficient for determining the spatial and temporal intensity distribution of a laser system for materials processing. Time and space resolution of the diagnostic system /7/ have to be adapted to the dynamical response of the materials processing effect.

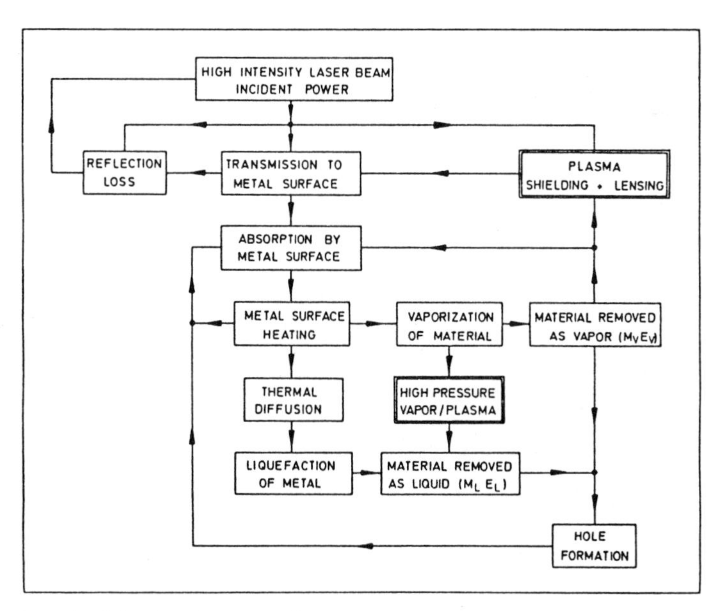


Fig.2 Block diagram for the main processes of material removal and their mutual influences

## 4. Absorption of Laser Radiation

In the low intensity range ($I<I_c$) the absorptivity A of a processing material for a given wavelength $\lambda$ is independent of intensity, but depends on variable surface conditions like surface finish and state of oxidation. The fraction of the laser power absorbed and the resulting machining efficiency are both proportional to A. Unfortunately, many of the materials which are interesting for laser machining are poor absorbers in the visible and infrared part of the electromagnetic spectrum. Thus, layers of high absorptivity frequently are deposited on the target surface /3/ in order to increase the absorbed laser power.

As the laser intensity at the surface of a workpiece approaches $I_c$, the absorption can instantaneously rise to nearly unity (anomalous absorption). The laser machining efficiency simultaneously increases markedly. The characteristic shape of A(I) has been verified for a large number of materials independent of the chosen wavelengths /15/. The threshold intensity $I_c$ of the anomalous absorption mainly depends on the interaction time $t_L$ (Fig.3). The onset of anomalous absorption ($I>I_c$) is accompanied by a laser-induced plasma generated in the surface region.

The plasma formation requires the vaporization of the material as a first step. Fig.3 shows a calculated plot of the threshold intensity $I_v$ versus $t_L$ on the assumption that a Gaussian beam is absorbed at an infinite plane surface. For short pulse durations there is no influence of transverse thermal conduction, and $I_v$ is independent of the focus radius. For longer pulse durations transverse thermal conduction becomes important. Thus, a beam with small $r_F$ requires higher intensities for vaporization. For comparison the threshold intensity of anomalous absorption /16/ measured with an Nd laser of $r_F$=40μm is given in Fig.3. As to be seen from Fig.3 the threshold values of vaporization and anomalous absorption are close together;
it also should be noted, that they are of the same order of magnitude as the threshold intensity $I_B$ for gas breakdown near a surface. Thus, for convenience $I_v$ is used as a common threshold intensity depending on the thermophysical properties of the material. Microprocessing normally has to be performed at a higher intensity level than macroprocessing.

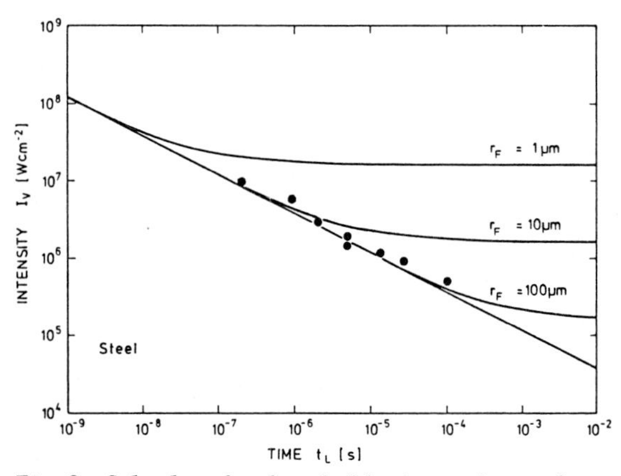


Fig.3 Calculated threshold intensity of vaporization versus interaction time. Measured values correspond to threshold intensity of anomalous absorption /15,16/

## 5. Plasma Formation and Materials Processing

Plasma formation originates from free electrons which exist at evaporation threshold in the surface of a processing material. Electrons inside the interaction volume are accelerated in the laser radiation field by inverse bremsstrahlung until their kinetic energy is high enough to ionize the ambient gas or the materials vapour; this increases the number of carriers by avalanche ionization. The classical model of plasma heating and generation by microwaves is applied approximately to energy transfer by inverse bremsstrahlung.

Using the rate equation for the electron density $n_e(t)$

$$\frac{dn_e}{dt} = R_i - R_{diff} - R_{rec} \tag{5}$$

$R_i$ ionization rate

$R_{diff}$ diffusion rate

$R_{rec}$ recombination rate

and the rate equation for the averaged electron energy $\bar{\varepsilon}$

$$n_e \frac{d\bar{\varepsilon}}{dt} = \alpha I - P_c - R_i(E_i + \bar{\varepsilon}) + R_{ee}(E_i - E_e + \bar{\varepsilon}) \tag{6}$$

$\alpha$ absorption coefficient

$P_c$ power losses by elastic collisions

$E_i$ ionization energy

$E_e$ excitation energy

$n_e$ and $\bar{\varepsilon}$ can be determined as a function of I /10/. The recombination rate

$$R_{rec} = R_{en} + R_{ee} \tag{7}$$

originates from three-body electron-ion recombination /17/. In this process, the excess internal energy of the recombination collision is removed by a neutral atom from the ambient or substrate ($R_{en}$) or by an electron ($R_{ee}$). The individual rates and constants are taken from the literature /18,19/. The substrate vapour density has been taken into account according to ref. /20/.

For $I > I_v$ the electron energy becomes higher within $t < 10^{-8}$s. If $\bar{\varepsilon} \geqq E_i$ the density of electrons increases exponentially by avalanche ionization /10/. $\bar{\varepsilon}$ remains constant /10/ similar to a phase transition of first order. The risetime and saturation density of a cw plasma depends on the intensity and the recombination rate /10,17/. The maximum electron density achievable can be deduced from the relationship,

$$\omega_L > \omega_p = (e^2 n_e / e_o m_e)^{1/2} \tag{8}$$

since for $\omega_L \leqq \omega_p$ the incident laser radiation is reflected by the plasma.

The vapour breakdown and the resulting plasma formation can be investigated by high-speed photography in the framing and streak mode of operation /10,11/. For low intensities an opaque plasma of nearly spherical symmetry is observed (Fig.4), which is confined to the surface region

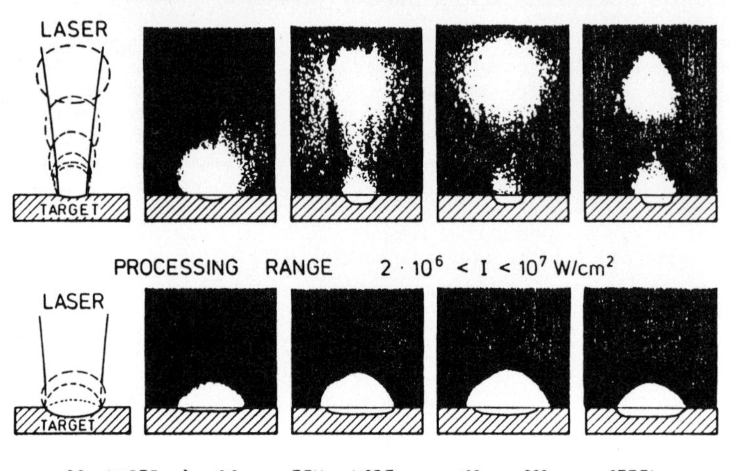


Fig.4 Plasma development shown by selected frames of high-speed photography

towards the laser. The plasma additionally determines the energy coupling into the workpiece. For high intensities (Fig.4) the plasma plume starts to decouple from the surface because of the attenuation of the incident radiation caused by the plasma absorption so that little laser energy was being delivered to the workpiece surface. The plasma plume leaves the surface and expands towards the laser with propagation speed $v_p \simeq 10^5$ cm/s. After complete decoupling, the optically dense plasma plume completely shields the workpiece surface, i.e. the vaporization and, consequently, the processing is interrupted (Fig.4). Since the substrate no longer supplies incandescent particles, and the plume begins to dissipate, yielding an optically thin plasma, its attenuation effect is diminished. In addition, the plume has propagated back towards the laser to a position where the intensity is lower. The transparency of the plasma plume becomes higher and plasma ignition starts again. The shielding of the substrate by a high-temperature plasma leads to the so-called laser-supported absorption (LSA) wave. The LSA wave is a plasma that is generated at the substrate surface and propagates back towards the laser, shielding effectively the substrate surface during its occurrence.

The observed interaction phenomena between laser radiation and plasma may be classified in three intensity regions /21/.

a) $I_v < I < I_B$

Vaporized material forms a plasma jet emerging towards the laser. The plasma is weakly ionized and almost transparent. Other than plasma lensing there is no considerable beam-plasma interaction.

b) $I_B < I < I_D$

The laser beam is partiallly absorbed by the material vapour, the surrounding atmosphere, or a mixture of vapour and atmosphere. The laserinduced plasma causes the formation of a laser supported combustion (LSC) wave.

c) $I > I_D$

The laser radiation is absorbed completely in a shock wave generated by the expanding plasma. This limiting case is characterized by the formation of a laser supported detonation (LSD) wave. The LSD wave moves towards the laser with supersonic velocity. A criterion for the onset of an LSD wave is

$$\alpha\lambda_c = 1, \qquad (9)$$

where $\lambda_c$ is the mean free path of the plasma ions. The material is shielded substantially by a thin strongly absorbing plasma layer. Material processing does not affect considerable material removal and is used only for special applications (shock hardening).

As a consequence of the sharp threshold for laser-induced gas breakdown material can be removed for $I<I_B$ without considerable absorption in the vapour. Exceeding the threshold intensity results in formation of an LSC wave (Fig.5). This can happen either in the surrounding atmosphere or in the plasma jet generated by the absorption of the laser radiation (Fig.4). The radiation is absorbed partly or completely, and the processing mode is not controlled entirely by the laser any more. At even higher intensity $I>I_D$ (threshold intensity of detonation) and with a smaller absorption length the limiting case of an LSD wave will occur. Instantaneously with the onset of the anomalous absorption a plasma of high luminosity develops from the surface. With increasing laser intensity the laser radiation is absorbed substantially in a thin plasma sheath travelling with supersonic speed towards the incident laser beam (Fig.5). The high degree of ionization of the detonation wave front yields an increased shielding of the substrate from the incident laser light.
In the limit of a fully developed LSD wave the plasma sheath approaches the velocity /22/

$$v_D = \{ 2(\gamma^2 - 1)/\rho\}^{1/3}(\beta\delta I)^{1/3}, \qquad (10)$$

where $\gamma$ is the adiabatic coefficient, $\beta$ corrects for the emission and transparency of the plasma and $\delta$ takes into account the radial expansion of the LSD wave. Because of the strong plasma absorption the target is

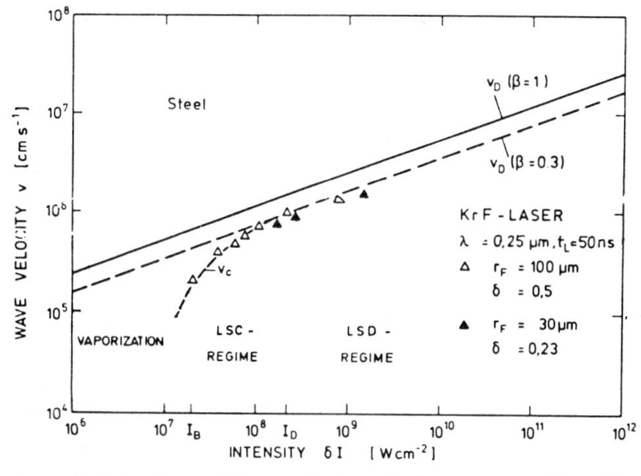


Fig. 5 Velocity of laser-induced plasma expanding from the substrate

completely shielded and the machining is interrupted. Optical feedback from the target also is modulated by the lensing and absorption features of the laser-induced plasma. As a consequence, diagnostics of the laser beam must be performed on line during processing, otherwise there is no correlation between the properties of the laser beam and the processing results. The pressure at the surface is strongly enhanced due to the recoil of the expanding plasma sheet. In the limit of detonation the pressure can reach the value behind a detonation wave /22/

$$p \leq p_D = \left( 4\rho(\gamma-1)^2/(\gamma+1) \right)^{1/3} (\beta\delta I)^{2/3} \tag{11}$$

which is for $I \simeq 10^8 W/cm^2$ and $\lambda = 10.6\ \mu m$ in the range $10^2 < p|bar| < 10^3$ and can be increased to values $p \simeq 10^6$ bar by increasing the laser intensity resulting in any case in a rigorously uncontrolled expulsion of molten material. At a corresponding intensity the pressure load for a short wavelength laser is considerably below these values due to the wavelength dependence of laser plasma interactions. The expelled liquid is splattered around the crater edges of the processed area. By proper shaping of melt depth, intensity and pressure these unwanted effects can be largely suppressed. Multimode operation exhibits an irregular pressure distribution, fluctuating in time, which often results in chaotic splattering at the edges of the processing area.

The laser-induced plasma changes dramatically the processing conditions. In the limit of weak absorption the plasma plume lenses the original beam geometry. In the limit of strong absorption the plasma completely absorbs the incoming radiation. In either case, the processing is no longer controlled by the laser parameters, but rather by the generated plasma plume influencing the processing results and - by optical feedback - intensity and mode structure of the laser itself. The working process may become totally irregular. For controlled and reproducible machining the laser parameters have to be matched to the properties of the induced plasma /10/.

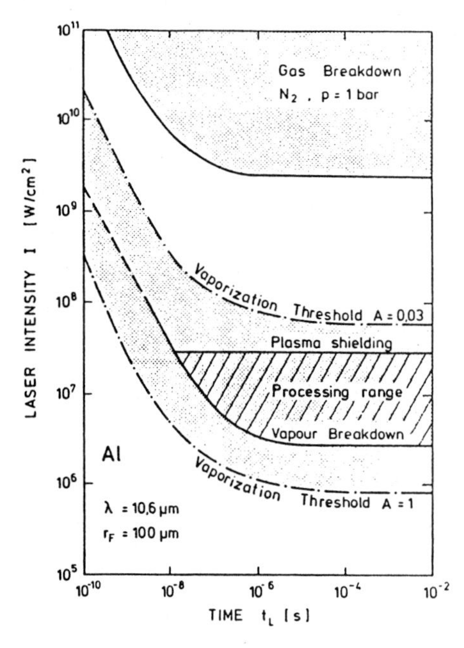


Fig. 6 Processing diagram showing calculated threshold intensities for vaporization, critical intensity for laser-induced plasma in metal vapor, plasma shielding and range of free gas breakdown

Figure 6 shows a processing diagram for laser welding /10/. Dashed-dotted lines are threshold intensities for surface vaporization at various absorptivities. The screened part of the graph indicates threshold intensities of surfaces in manufacturing environments. The dotted line, which is in agreement with experimental observations (Fig.4), is the calculated critical intensity for generation of a laser-induced plasma near the processing surface following the formalism above. The straight line for plasma shielding has been taken from the investigations by high-speed photography. The optimum laser parameters for high efficiency machining are within the shaded region (processing range). At intensity levels exceeding $2\times10^7 W/cm^2$ continuous machining is periodically interrupted due to plasma shielding, yielding quasi pulsed processing at time scales that are governed by the time constants of the plasma. Average processing intensities of cw-$CO_2$ lasers, for example, normally do not exceed $1\times10^7 W/cm^2$. But, because of feedback effects and mode instabilities local or temporal intensity peaks may occur that exceed these levels considerably /7,9/. The pulse separation has to be chosen for pulsed laser machining in a way that the plasma absorption has diminished between two successive pulses, and the pulse halfwidth has to be adjusted so that there is not complete absorption during the interaction time.

## 6.1 Surface Heat Treatment

Lasers inherently offer highly localized, high heating and cooling rates for a chemically clean and high-intensity heat treatment process with easy handling in an atmosphere of desired composition that produces a localized heat-treated zone of arbitrary geometry in complex workpieces. Distortions are low due to self-quenching by heat conduction into the surrounding material and improved hardness, wear, and fatigue properties for many materials are achieved. Conventional heat treatment data generally are not applicable to laser processing without modification. An illustrative example which represents various types of heat treatment is laser transformation hardening: the hardening temperature is well above that of induction hardening resulting in a characteristic difference in the dependence of carbon content of the material on temperature. The probability of nucleation and the velocity of diffusion of the carbon atoms differs from conventional data.

Since laser heat treatment is performed below the threshold of anomalous absorption effects, coatings are often applied /3/ to the surface to increase the absorbed power for transformation hardening. Usually, these coatings have a rather poor electrical and thermal capacity, however. Consequently, the laser energy absorbed in the layer is transferred to the target with poor efficiency.

The independent process parameters /3,23/ which affect the laser heat treatment are incident laser power, incident beam diameter, beam energy distribution at the workpiece, surface absorptivity of the material, processing speed across the surface, and thermophysical and metallurgical properties of the material. The dependent process parameters /3,23/ are the depth of hardness, the microstructure and the geometry of the heat-affected zone (HAZ), and the metallurgical properties of the heat-treated, and possibly transformed material. The absorptivity and the thickness of the coating additionally have to be taken into accouunt for materials covered by a coating. If the coating is too thick, excessive power is required to burn through the coating, and the resulting plasma plume will absorb too much power (Section 5). Among others paints are often used as coatings because of their ease of application /3/. Paints which have a high content of pigment and fillers and a low content of organics are superior /24/. The organics will only burn away, thus creating a plasma which must be controlled and removed (Section 5).

Analytical models of heat treatment are based on the solution /24,25/ of the heat conduction equation /26/ in the approximation of three-dimensional temperature distribution as a function of time for a flat semi-infinite and finite body under conditions of temperature-independent thermo-physical properties and different beam profiles. The analytic heat treatment model /24,25/ allows calculation of the isotherms in the workpiece (Fig.7) in combination with the TTT diagram by gauging with metallurgical and geometric investigations of the HAZ. Heat transfer into the substrate also is quantitatively described /23/ as a function of thermophysical properties of coating and substrate as well as laser processing parameters. As seen from Fig.7 the calculations represent the geometry of the HAZ with reasonable agreement for a semi-infinite body (hardened depth<<thickness of the workpiece) and for a finite body (hardened depth $\simeq$ slab thickness).

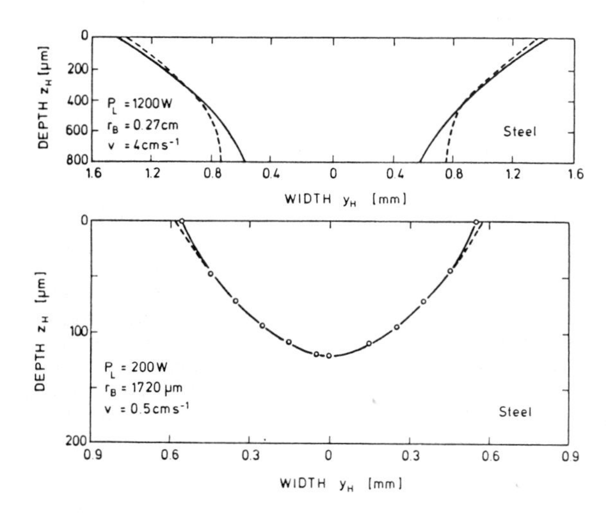


Fig. 7 Experimental (-o-) and calculated (---) hardening geometry for finite and semi-infinite body ($r_B$ beam radius)

The absorptivity, thermal stability, and the thermal conductivity of surface coatings have to be matched to the metallurgy of the substrate for an optimization of laser heat treatment as a function of the processing parameters in combination with coating handling and economics of pre or post heat treatment procedures. Molybdenum disulfide exhibits a high absorptivity /24/ but a low heat transfer into the substrate /23/. For paints with high absorptivity /25/ but low boiling temperature the energy coupled in has a tendency to decrease with increasing laser power (Fig.8) because of substantial destruction of the coating due to evaporation.

## 6.2 Abrasive Machining

The removal of material during cutting and hole drilling involves melting and vaporization. Before boiling the surface must first start to melt. Because of the fast temporal development of boiling ignition, there is not

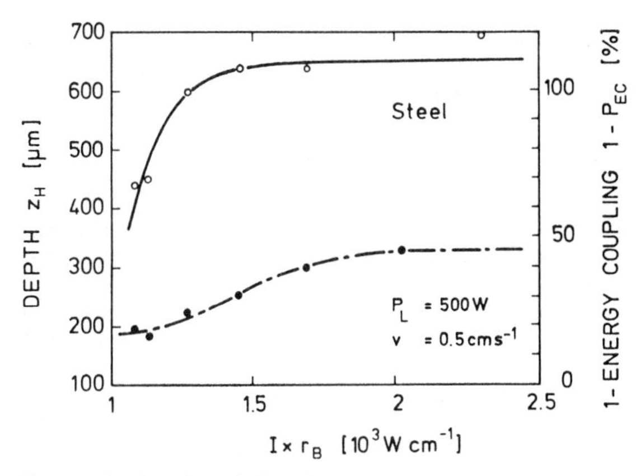


Fig. 8 Hardened depth $z_H$ and energy coupling $P_{EC}$ versus scaling parameter $I \times r_B$. $P_{EC}$ is determined by gauging of calculated temperature distributions with metallurgical investigations

time for much material to melt. Thus, at high intensities $I>10^6 W/cm^2$, the dominant process is vaporization, and the role of melting tends to be less significant. For $I<I_c$ the vaporized material flows away from the area of interaction without further interaction with the laser beam. For $I>I_c$ the vaporization material becomes partially ionized by the laser radiation resulting in the formation of a laser-induced plasma (Section 5). In both cases the laser continues to deliver more energy to the surface at vaporization temperature, which is supplied as latent heat of vaporization carrying material away from the workpiece as vapour and plasma, respectively. The vaporization occurs at a continually retreating surface. Following this consideration the thickness of the molten layer decreases with the laser intensity. According to the magnitude of the vaporized volume a melt front moves into the material at a velocity v, which depends on the intensity of the incident radiation. The practical meaning of v is that of a drilling or cutting speed.

The dependence of the drilling velocity on laser intensity, as it is observed for various materials, typically shows a characteristic increase of the working speed at a certain intensity level. It is appropriate to distinguish four intensity regimes /4/:

a) Threshold regime: material processing starts at the threshold distinguished by evaporation from the surface. The processing velocity v increases with intensity ($v \sim I$) where the slope is dominated by the thermophysical properties of the processing material.

b) Liquid expulsion regime: due to hole formation the vapour builds up a pressure that causes an additional flow of molten material along the face of the crater, removing some of the mass as unvaporized droplets. Since the mass removal is larger, then if only vaporization occurs, the processing speed is further increased.

c) Regime of anomalous absorption: the absorption increases by plasma formation and changes of surface topography (cratering, multi-reflection). Accordingly, the evaporation rate increases with increasing power and the thickness of the melt decreases. Without melt expulsion the processing velocity approaches the upper theoretical limit as given by equation (1).

d) Shielding regime: the plasma absorption dominates with increasing intensity (Section 5). The material is heated indirectly by radiation and heat transfer from the plasma. The plasma controls the efficiency of the material being removed and the quality of processing (Fig.9 and 10).

The material removal starts by vaporization after a material-dependent heating time. An abrupt increase of absorptance simultaneously is observed by on-line measurements of reflectance /16/ due to plasma formation and changes of surface geometry. The laser power is coupled almost totally into the material. The processing velocity increases steeply /27/ to a material dependent value (Fig.9). The plasma absorption at first lowers v, but a slight enhancement is observed by the plasma-assisted drilling and the increased transparency for high intensities. A detailed description has to consider the particular processes involved (Fig.2).

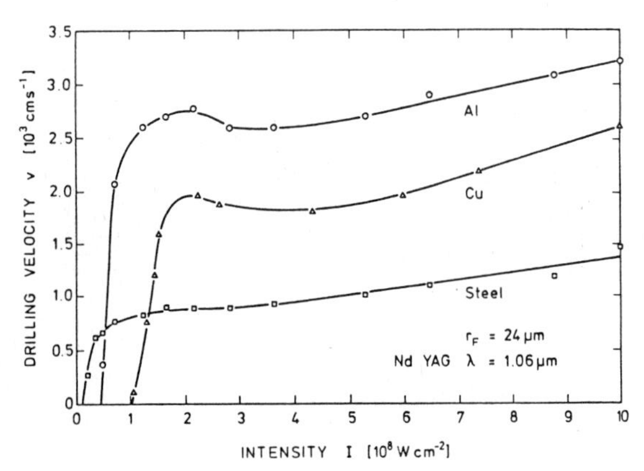


Fig. 9 Processing velocity as a function of intensity

The difference between laser- and plasma-controlled material removal is demonstrated by the correlation of processing workpiece and laser parameters /10/.

The drilling efficiency, defined as

$$\eta = \frac{V\varepsilon_V}{It_L \pi r_F^2} , \qquad (12)$$

where V is the volume of removed material and $\varepsilon_V$ is the vaporization energy density, is plotted in Fig.10 versus intensity; micrographs of the surface are also shown. Processing with intensities $I_M<I<I_V$, where $I_M$ is the threshold intensity of melting, just melts the material without vaporization. The area of interaction is smaller than expected from the beam geometry (micrograph 1 Fig.10). For $I_V<I<I_B$ the generated plasma

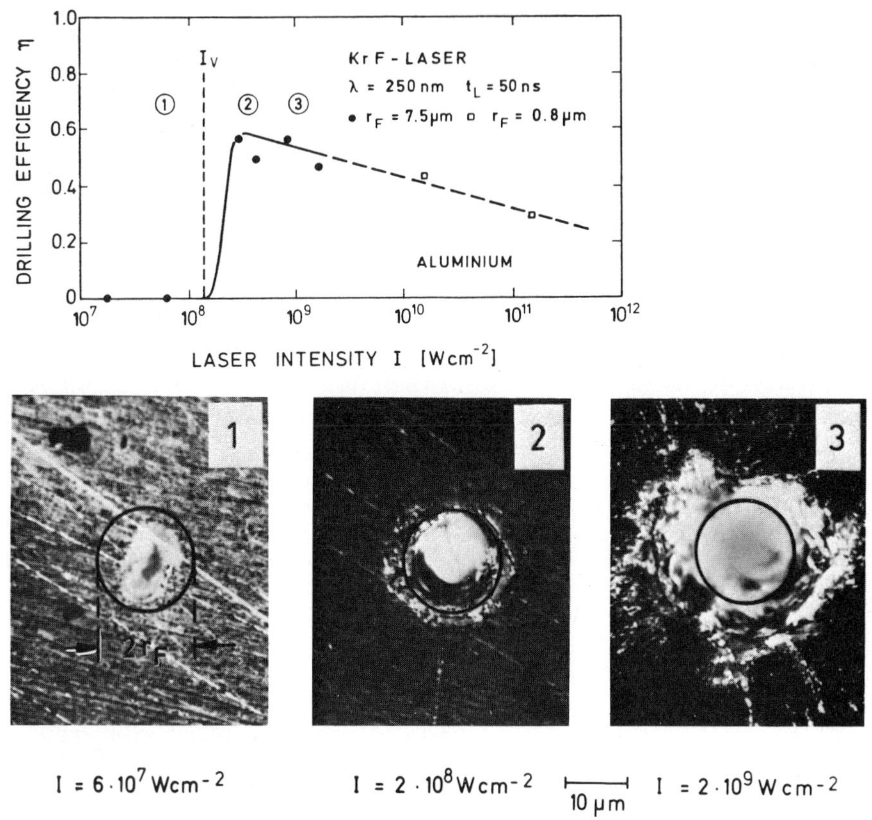


Fig. 10 Efficiency of material removal versus intensity

(Section 5) causes in deflection of the beam by lensing and even in absorption of the beam under certain conditions. For $I > I_B$ the plasma heating and further absorption increases the absorption of radiation. The efficiency increases steeply with a maximum value corresponding to the matching of the processed area and the beam geometry. The diameter of the hole and the beam diameter coincide (micrograph 2 Fig.10). If the intensity is further increased, $\eta$ decreases due to the plasma shielding. The processing geometry is governed by the feedback of the plasma expansion (Fig.5) to the molten pool. The hole diameters are about an order of magnitude larger than the beam diameter (micrograph 3 Fig.10).

Working efficiencies scaling from 0.1 to unity are obtained during laser processing even for those materials which do not seem appropriate for easy laser machining because of their extremely high thermal conductivity and high reflection or transmission, for instance, $CO_2$-laser processing of copper, or Nd-laser machining of diamond or sapphire. In any case, the laser parameters have to be adjusted in order to achieve proper quality of laser processing. During abrasive machining a tailored pulse program assures that neither melt nor vapour expulsion from the processing area optically influence the incident radiation. Furthermore, the exact tuning of the absorbed radiation to losses by heat flow balances the movement of the interface of the liquid-solid phase transition.

## 6.3 Surface Modelling

In both the limits of low ($I<I_V$) and high ($I>I_V$) intensities with intensity-independent and intensity-dependent absorption, respectively, laser processing typically impresses spatially periodic microscopic surface structures on a wide variety of opaque and transparent materials /28 to 30/.

For intensities $I_M<I<I_V$ above the intensity of melting $I_M$ surface transformations are produced by pulsed illumination showing a complex dependence on polarization and angle of incidence of the laser radiation (Fig.11). The properties of the spontaneous periodic surface structures are discussed on the basis of interference effects /31,32/ with respect to the dependence on angle of incidence, wavelength of laser, dispersion relation with polarization of light, and multiple subthreshold illumination /33/.

For intensities $I>I_V$ surface irregularities are generated during pulsed laser irradiation in the area of interaction (Fig.12). The concentric surface structures, which are strongly dependent on the fluence and the pressure of the ambient, originate from capillary waves on the laser molten material /33/, the structure of which is conserved by fast cooling.

## Conclusion

The independent parameters which affect laser microprocessing are incident laser power, beam diameter, beam energy distribution at the workpiece,

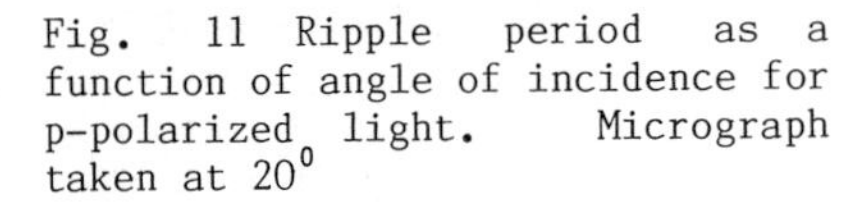

Fig. 11 Ripple period as a function of angle of incidence for p-polarized light. Micrograph taken at $20^0$

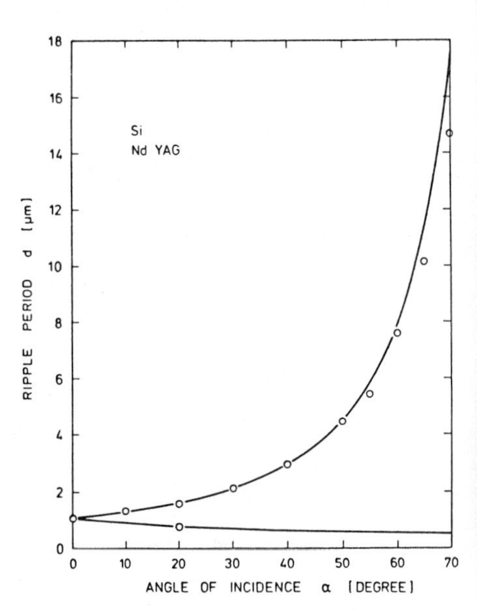


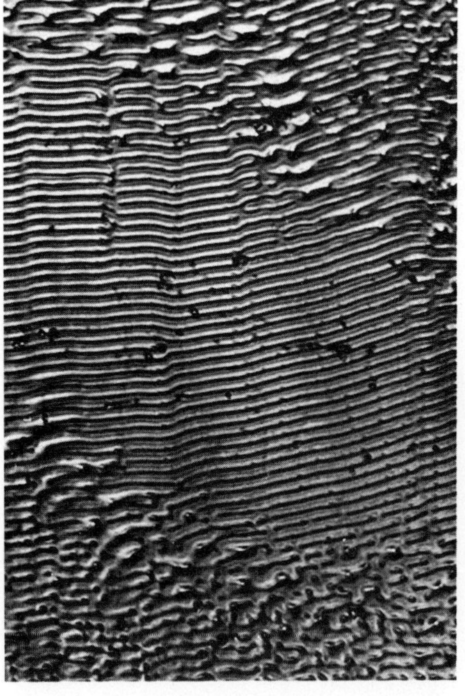

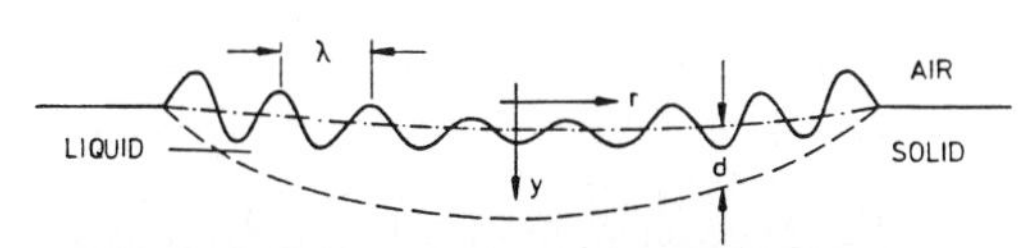


Fig. 12 Schematic representation and micrograph of capillary waves

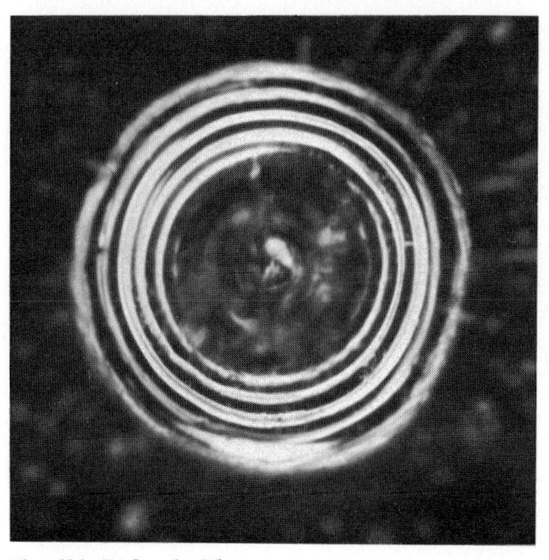

Al, Nd:YAG, 1.06 μm ├──────────┤ 100 μm

processing time, absorptivity, thermophysical and metallurgical properties of the material. Poor optical absorptivity of most materials is of minor importance because the absorption can be increased by application of either absorptive coatings or appropriate choice of the laser parameters. The losses by heat flow, reflection or transmission also can be minimized so that a particular combination of intensity and interaction time defines a specific operational regime with the occurrence of a unique material processing effect.

The efficiency of material removal and the quality of processing necessarily require the matching of intensity-dependent absorption, optical feedback, and plasma dynamics. The adjustment of the intensity for the plasma-induced state of high absorption, the control of the optical feedback in the laser workpiece interaction by on-line diagnostics and the plasma assisted transport of processing material as vapour or melt have to be optimized with respect to characteristic time constants of the physical processes involved following the outline of the paper presented.

## References


1 J.F. Ready: Industrial Applications of Lasers (Academic Press, New York, San Francisco, London, 1973)
2 J.M. Poate and J.W. Mayer, Eds.: Laser Annealing of Semiconductors (Academic Press, New York, San Francisco, London, 1982)
3 M. Bass, Ed.: Laser Materials Processing (North Holland, Amsterdam, New York, Oxford, 1983)
4 G. Herziger: Feinwerktechnik + Meßtechnik 91, 4 (1983)
5 G. Ripper and G. Herziger: Feinwerktechnik + Meßtechnik in press

6 D.N.H. Trafford, T.Bell, J.H.P.C. Megaw, and A.S. Brandsen: "Heat Treatment Using a High-Power Laser", in Heat Treatment 1979, The Metal Society, London, pp.32-38

7 P. Loosen, L. Bakowsky, G. Herziger, and F. Rühl: "Diagnostic of High Power $CO_2$-Lasers", in Optoelectronics in Engineering 1984, Springer-Verlag, Berlin, Heidelberg, New York, Tokyo, pp.247-253

8 H. Eichler and G. Herziger: Zeitschrift Angew. Phys. 23, 297 (1967)

9 E. Beyer, A. Donges, P. Loosen, and G. Herziger: "Optical Feedback during Laser Materials Processing" in Optoelectronics in Engineering 1984, Springer-Verlag, Berlin, Heidelberg, New York, Tokyo, pp.259-263

10 E. Beyer, L. Bakowsky, R. Poprawe, and G. Herziger: "Formation and Influence of Laser Induced Plasma during $CO_2$-Laser Welding" in Optoelectronics in Engineering 1984, Springer-Verlag Berlin, Heidelberg, New York, Tokyo, pp.367-372

11 R.L. Stegmann, J.T. Schriempf, and L.R. Hettche: J.Appl.Phys. 44, 3675 (1973)

12 E. Beyer, K. Wissenbach, and G. Herziger: Feinwerktechnik + Meßtechnik 92, 3 (1984)

13 D.W. Gregg and S.J. Thomas: J.Appl.Phys. 37, 2787 (1966)

14 M.K. Chun and K. Rose: J.Appl.Phys. 41, 614 (1970)

15 E. Kocher, T. Tschudi, J. Steffen, and G. Herziger: IEEE J. Quantum Electr. QE-8, 120 (1972)

16 H.G. Treusch and K. Wissenbach: Verh. DPG 3, 372 (1983)

17 E. Beyer: to be published

18 W.A. Fabrikant: J.Exp.Theor.Phys. 8, 35 (1938)

19 G. Weyl, A. Pirri, and R. Root, Am.Inst.Aeronautics and Astronautics J. 19, 461 (1981)

20 O.N. Krokhin: Laser Handbook, Vol.2 (North Holland, Amsterdam, New York, Oxford, 1972)

21 R. Poprawe, E. Beyer, L. Bakowsky, G. Brumme, and G. Herziger: "Limitation of Laser Processing Intensity by Laser Induced Gas Breakdown", in Optoelectronics in Engineering 1984, Springer-Verlag, Berlin, Heidelberg, New York, Tokyo, pp.361-366

22 Yu.P. Raizer: J.Exp.Theor.Phys. 21, 1009 (1965)

23 K. Behler, A. Gillner, G. Herziger, E.W. Kreutz, and K. Wissenbach: "Optical Properties of Surface Coatings for Laser Heat Treatment", in Proc. Materials Research Society 1984, Strasbourg

24 K. Wissenbach, L. Bakowsky, and G. Herziger: Feinwerktechnik + Meßtechnik 91, 7 (1983)

25 K. Wissenbach, L. Bakowsky, H.G. Treusch, and G. Herziger: "Laser Hardening Process Parameters", in Optoelectronics in Engineering 1984, Springer Verlag, Berlin, Heidelberg, New York, Tokyo, pp.312-316

26 N.N. Rykalin: Berechnung der Wärmeleitung beim Schweißen (Technik, Berlin, 1957)

27 H.G. Treusch, L. Bakowsky, K. Wissenbach, and G. Herziger: "Metal Drilling with Lasers" in Optoelectronics in Engineering 1984 Springer Verlag, Berlin, Heidelberg, New York, Tokyo, pp.383-388

28 M. Birnbaum: J.Appl.Phys. 36, 3688 (1965)

29 F. Keilmann and Y.H. Bai: Appl.Phys. A29, 9 (1982)

30 J.F. Young, J.S. Preston, H.M. van Driel, and J.E. Sipe: Phys.Rev. B27, 1155 (1983)

31 J.E. Sipe, J.F. Young, J.S. Preston, and H.M. van Driel: Phys.Rev. B27, 1141 (1983)

32 P.M. Fauchet and A.E. Siegman: Appl.Phys. A32, 135 (1983)

33 E.W. Kreutz, M. Krösche, H.G. Treusch, and G. Herziger: these proceeedings

# Surface Modelling During Laser Microprocessing

E.W. Kreutz, M. Krösche, H.G. Treusch, and G. Herziger

Institut für Angewandte Physik, Technische Hochschule Darmstadt,
Schloßgartenstr. 7, D-6100 Darmstadt, Fed. Rep. of Germany

The spatially periodic surface structures impressed during laser material processing on metals and semiconductors are investigated as a function of intensity, pulse duration, polarization, and angle of incidence. The threshold intensity for the formation of the surface damage pattern is determined with respect to illumination conditions and material parameters. The initial and the laser-induced microroughness of the surface influence the evolution of the damage.

## 1. Introduction

In some laser materials processing applications heat treatment is required and takes advantage of the high power and good focusability of laser beams to deposit heat into a selected region of a target. A particular combination of power density and interaction time defines a specific operational regime within the various interaction processes between a laser beam and a target surface resulting in the occurrence of a unique materials-processing effect. There are two intensity regimes ruled by the threshold intensity of evaporation $I_V$/1/. In the limit of low intensities ($I<I_V$) with intensity-independent absorbance the material properties within the surface region are improved or changed by the processing heat. In the limit of high intensities ($I>I_V$) with intensity-dependent absorbance, the material is removed during abrasive processing as liquid, vapour, or plasma. In both intensity regimes laser processing typically impresses spatially periodic microscopic structures on the surface of many materials /2,3/.

Laser-induced damage of solids is of high importance in the interaction of high-intensity optical radiation with matter, and of prime interest for the fabrication of components with optimum optical properties for the handling of high-intensity laser beams. In addition, lasers have been used either for directed energy processing /4/ or for microprocessing machining /5/. In the former case lasers have been established as a driving force for the motion of a crystallizing interface for the processing and modification of surface layers of semiconductors during annealing and device fabrication. In the latter case lasers are accomplished for hardening, melting and rapid solidification to form quite novel structures and alloys, or vaporization to remove material during abrasive machining as cutting, drilling, and shaping. The study of laser-induced damage as a function of material properties as well as laser parameters allows a complete characterization of the damage process in terms of intrinsic or extrinsic material properties.

For intensities $I_M<I<I_V$ above the intensity of melting $I_M$ we report on spontaneous periodic surface structures in semiconductors (InSb,Si) and metals (Al,Pb,steel) produced by pulsed laser radiation.

For intensities $I > I_V$ we present concentric surface structures in metals (Al,steel,brass) obtained during pulsed laser irradiation. The results are discussed in view of the laser-induced damage process and of the optimum surface finish achievable by laser microprocessing /6/.

## 2. Experimental

We used InSb (110), Si (111) and Si (100) single crystalline wafers grown by different pulling techniques. The other samples are prepared from Al, Pb, brass, and steel as provided from the stock. Standard procedures have been used for preparation of surfaces with different finish such as polishing, sandblasting, and machining.

Irradiation was provided by an Nd:YAG laser, which produces a 1.06 µm fundamental beam. Square pulses are formed with a Pockels cell outside the resonator giving with the pulse duration $(25 < t_L |\mu s| < 400)$, the focus radius $(10 < r_F |\mu m| < 300)$, and the laser power $(240 < P |W| < 300)$ a laser radiation intensity $I < 10^7 W/cm^2$. Fluence levels were measured using Si photodiodes. Beam diagnostics were performed by scanning with a wedge /7/ in combination with a Si photodiode. The focused low order mode $TEM_{oo}$ of Gaussian distribution was fitted to the beam radius using the $1/e^2$ point of the beam pattern. An optical microscope with a maximum magnification of 1100 X allows the surface topography to be viewed.

## 3. Experimental Results

For $I_M < I < I_V$ Fig.1 shows a plot of the single-pulse threshold intensity as a function of pulse duration for the generation of spatially periodic surface structures on Si(111) surfaces of different preparation (Section 2). The polished surfaces of mirror-like finish exhibit a higher threshold intensity $I_T$ than the sandblasted surfaces of averaged roughness of 4 µm (Fig.1). The threshold intensity is lower for Si (100) surfaces of the

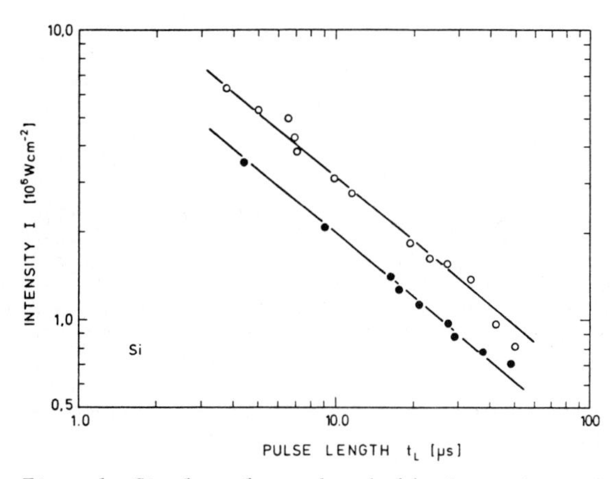


Fig. 1 Single-pulse threshold intensity versus pulse length for the generation of periodic surface structures on Si(111) surfaces of different finish (o polished, • sandblasted)

corresponding surface treatment. Multiple-pulse illumination with pulse energy below this threshold also produces these periodic surface structures /3,8/. Qualitatively similar results are obtained for InSb, Al, Pb, and steel surfaces with the threshold depending on the thermophysical and metallurgical properties of the material.

Fig.2 shows a comparison between the experimental (Fig.1) and calculated threshold intensities. The calculations as a function of pulse duration and focus radius are based on the assumption that a Gaussian beam is absorbed at an infinite plane surface and the absorbed laser power density required for surface melting to begin. The calculations have been done with constant temperature-independent optical and thermophysical properties neglecting any carrier diffusion. Experimental and calculated threshold curves show reasonable agreement (Fig.2).

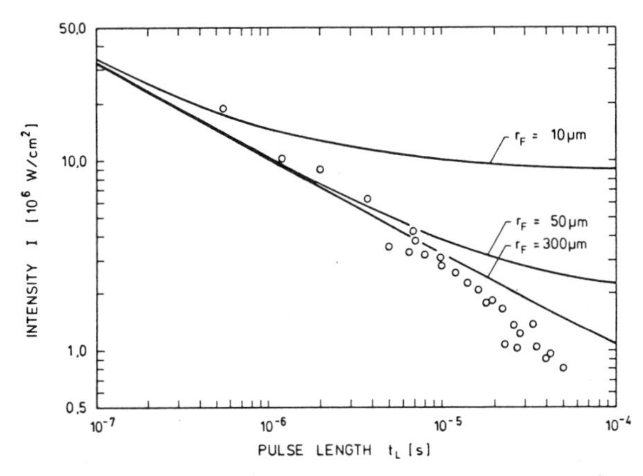


Fig. 2 Experimental (o) and calculated (——) single-pulse threshold intensities versus pulse length for the generation of periodic surface structures on polished Si(111) surface

For p-polarized light the laser-induced surface damage consists of two superimposed sets of periodic structures with the spacings $1.06/(1\pm\sin\alpha)$ µm (Fig.3) in agreement with the observations of other authors /9/. For s-polarized light the laser-induced surface damage consists of a single set of periodic structures /9/ with a spacing $1.06/\cos\alpha$ µm (Fig.3). The periodic structures are perpendicular to the polarization. The threshold intensity is higher for s polarization /9,10/. There is only a narrow range of intensities for the generation of periodic surface structures. Namely, for $I \simeq I_V$ the surface anneals to a very smooth finish in the central region with periodic structures generated in a narrow band around the perimeter, or the microprocessing of the surface starts by vaporization and ablation /6/.

For $I > I_V$ Fig.4 shows concentric surface structures after single-pulse laser illumination as a function of pressure ($10^{-1} < p|Pa| < 5\times10^4$) and fluence ($10 < E|mJ| < 10^3$). At low pressures the spacing becomes higher with increasing fluence for steel and Al (Fig.4). At very high fluence levels the structures are destroyed with the onset of laser-induced materials processing. The concentric surface structures also are obliterated with

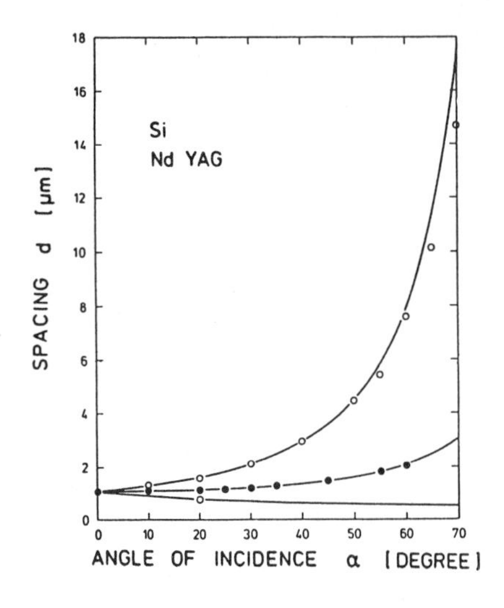


Fig. 3 Spacings of the periodic surface structures on Si(111) surfaces with p(o)- and s(•)- polarized light as function of the angle of incidence. The curves are plots of the functions given in Section 3

Fig. 4 Micrographs of concentric surface structures on metals at normal incidence as a function of fluence and ambient pressure

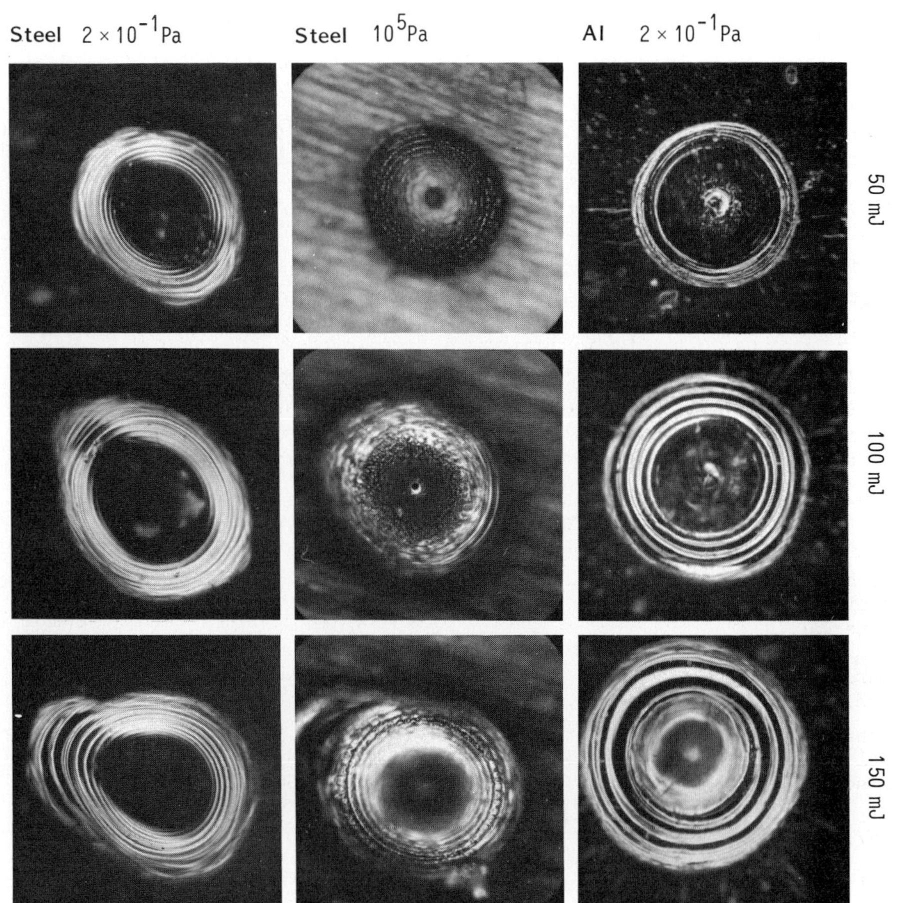

increasing pressure (Fig.4) with a material-dependent speed of reaction. The obliteration is stronger for Al. For brass no concentric surface structures are observed in the range of investigation. In any case laser-induced materials processing is observed via hole formation and more or less splattering around the crater edges of the molten material flow within the crater.

## 4. Discussion

The periodic structures (Fig.3) result from an interference /11,12/ between the incident laser beam and a surface scattered wave /11/ which originates from scattering of the incident polarized coherent radiation at the microroughness of the surface /2/. A universal theory /11/ has been developed by van Driel et al., which considers a non-radiative surface field, so-called radiation remnants, accounting for all the ripple spacings, orientations, material and polarization dependences, that have been observed for a variety of materials. In addition, various excitation mechanisms like transverse electromagnetic waves, surface plasmon polaritons, or surface phonon polaritons have been suggested, which may contribute to the development of the periodic structures.

For an isotropic surface the incident beam assumingly should scatter in all directions across the surface. The geometric location of the periodic structures (Section 3) dominating for p-polarization at small angles of incidence (Fig.3) indicates that the incident beam preferentially scatters in the forward and backward directions from the randomly rough surface. The appearance of the structures running parallel to the plane of incidence for the case of p-polarized light also at large angles of incidence indicates that the beam preferentially scatters along the surface along the plane of incidence. In general, the interference between the incident wave and the surface-scattered wave would be characterized by grating vectors $\vec{k}=\pm(\vec{k}_i-\vec{k}_s)$, where $\vec{k}_i$ is the component in the surface plane of the wave vector of the incident beam and $\vec{k}_s$ is the wave vector of the surface scattered waves.

When the pulsed laser beam (Fig.1) interacts with the surface, material removal involves conventional melting and vaporization /1,6/. Under typical conditions , the melting temperature is reached in very short times for $I_M<I<I_V$. The threshold intensity decreases with $t_L$, as to be seen from Fig.1. The important parameter is the energy density in the surface region, in the range of investigation (Fig.1) a steep increase at small pulse durations is followed by a slow increase at large $t_L$. If the energy density is high enough that the peak intensities in the interference pattern of the incident and the scattered waves exceed the damage threshold of the material, the periodic surface corrugations are generated. The dependence of threshold intensity on the microroughness and material properties is partially explained by the reflectivity. Metals exhibit a larger specular reflectivity so that $I_T$ necessarily is higher. The rough surface shows an enhanced diffuse reflectivity. Multiple reflection within the surface selvedge becomes more probable, when the laser radiation is more strongly absorbed resulting in a lowering of $I_T$ (Fig.1). The threshold intensities for gas breakdown near a surface qualitatively also show this behaviour /8/. Another important factor is the latent heat of melting. $I_T$ is lower for materials with a lower latent heat of melting. The appearance of the

surface corrugations also occurs at lower threshold intensities, if the atomic positions of surface atoms allow an easier propagation of the scattered waves in order to generate the surface corrugation, i.e. $I_T$ is lower (≃30%) for the Si (100) surface (unit mesh: square) than for the Si (111) surface (unit mesh: rhombus). In any case, the actual damage patterns produced for a given wavelength, polarization, angle of incidence, and surface conditions then provide a mapping of the relative strength with which the incident beam scatters in any given direction across the surface.

Figure 2 shows a calculated plot of $I_M$ versus $t_L$. For short pulse durations, there is no time for transverse thermal conduction, and $I_M$ is independent of the focus radius. For longer pulse durations transverse thermal conduction becomes important, and heat is conducted out of the focal area more rapidly because of the higher thermal gradients. Thus, a small $r_F$ requires higher intensities for melting. The intensity-dependent absorption and the assumed absorption within the surface plane may account for the deviations in experimental and calculated threshold intensities. Nevertheless, there is some open discussion on the homogeneous /2/ and inhomogeneous /13,14/ melting of the surface, respectively, prior to the formation of the periodic surface structure. After two consecutive laser pulses the area on the surface covered by corrugations is larger and the corrugations themselves are more pronounced compared to a single-pulse. This result is difficult to understand under the assumption of a uniform molten surface layer.

The modulation of the incident power depends on the exact nature of the scattering center in the surface selvedge. Feedback may amplify the modulation enhancing simultaneously the growth of the surface corrugation. Significant feedback is possible only during the interaction time. These considerations favour an inhomogeneous intensity distribution which probably originates in non-uniformly molten layer responsible for the stimulated surface scattering. The corrugations assumingly have no influence on laser macroprocessing. The dynamics of the melt during welding, for example, changes the phase of the scattered beams continuously preventing any formation of surface damage patterns. However, the corrugations may influence laser microprocessing. Since the thermal losses increase with decreasing $r_F$ (Fig.2), laser microprocessing has to be done at higher intensities than laser macroprocessing. The electron concentration near the surface is enhanced by field emission at the laser-induced corrugations. Both the effects increase the probability for the ignition of a laser-induced plasma /6/ with all its drawbacks on the laser materials processing to different modes of operation.

Material removal by pulsed laser beam is done mainly by vaporization for $I > I_V$ /1,6/. Losses by heat flow are in equilibrium with the laser power absorbed and vapour pressure approximately equals the surface pressure of the boiling melt. The removing vapour and plasma govern by recoil the processing geometry /15/. Above a critical thickness of the melt concentric surface structures are observed (Fig.4), which might be due to gravity or capillary waves. The experimentally observed wavelengths ($1 < \lambda|\mu m| < 15$) claim for capillary waves in agreement with a theory /8/ developed for the coupling of the laser power into the melt at the surface. The wave structure is frozen in, if the time for solidification after switching off the laser radiation is far below the duration of the wave period. For fluences such that the metal surfaces melt very quickly to a significant depth, the incident laser beam can scatter from initial surface roughness on the melt and produce capillary waves, i.e. the mechanism of excitation is the same as for the development of the periodic surface corrugations. For materials like brass with the high partial vapour pressure of Zn the evolution of the capillary waves is prevented and true processing starts by ablation and vaporization. On the other hand, the surface tension, the ambient pressure, chemical reactions, and the dynamics of the laser-solid interaction altogether determine the complex development of the concentric surface corrugations, which will be described elsewhere /8/.

In order to obtain optimum surface finish during microprocessing or annealing the laser-induced development of any surface structure must be prevented /8/. During abrasive machining the laser delivers energy, which is supplied as latent heat for the removal of the material involving melting and vaporization. The thickness of the molten layer decreases with I. Following these considerations high surface quality might be achieved either by intensities $I \gg I_V$ with very short $t_L$ or by intensities $I > I_M$ with prolonged $t_L$ depending on the operative materials-processing effect. In the former case the melting depth is well below the structural spacing, in the latter case the duration of the structural transformations is well below the time constant of freezing. Hence, after switching off the laser irradiation attenuation of surface structures will occur.

## 4. Summary

The spatially periodic structures produced by pulsed laser irradiation on metal and semiconductor surfaces arise from the interference of the incident laser light and induced waves scattered spontaneously along the surface. The concentric structures produced by pulsed laser irradiation on metal surfaces originate from capillary waves. For optimum and reproducible surface finish during laser materials processing the laser intensity, the interaction time, and the material properties have to be optimized preventing the evolution of the surface damage.

## References

1 G. Herziger: Feinwerktechnik + Meßtechnik 91, 4(1983)
2 H.M. van Driel, J.Y. Young, and J.E. Sipe: Mat.Res.Soc.Symp. Proc.13,197 (1983) and references therein
3 P.M. Fauchet, Z. Guosheng, and A.E. Siegman: Mat.Res.Soc.Symp. Proc.13,205 (1983) and references therein
4 J.M. Poate and J.W. Mayer, Eds.: Laser Annealing of Semiconductors (Academic Press, New York, San Francisco, London 1982)
5 M. Basse, Ed.: Laser Materials Processing (North Holland, Amsterdam, New York, Oxford, 1983)
6 G. Herziger and E.W. Kreutz: these proceedings
7 P. Loosen, L. Bakowsky, and G. Herziger: Feinwerktechnik + Meßtechnik 92,11 (1984)
8 E.W. Kreutz: to be published
9 J.F. Young, J.S. Preston, H.M. van Driel, and J.E. Sipe: Phys.Rev.B27,1155 (1983)
10 M. Krösche, diploma work, 1984, Technische Hochschule Darmstadt
11 J.E. Sipe, J.F. Young, J.S. Preston, and H.M. van Driel: Phys.Rev.B27,1141 (1983)
12 P.M. Fauchet and A.E. Siegman: Appl.Phys.A32,135 (1983)
13 S.R.J. Brueck and D.J. Ehrlich: Phys.Rev.Lett.48,1678 (1982)
14 S.R.J. Brueck and D.J. Ehrlich: Appl.Phys.Lett.41,630 (1982)
15 R. Poprawe, E. Beyer, L. Bakowsky, G. Brumme, and G. Herziger: "Limitation of Laser Processing Intensity by Laser Induced Gas Breakdown", in Optoelectronics in Engineering 1984, Springer-Verlag, Berlin, Heidelberg, New York, Tokyo, pp.361-366

# Part 2

# Photophysics and Chemistry of Molecule - Surface Interactions

# Electronic Structure of Adsorbed Layers

A.M. Bradshaw

Fritz-Haber-Institut der Max-Planck-Gesellschaft, Faradayweg 4-6,
D-1000 Berlin 33, Fed. Rep. of Germany

## 1. Introduction

Surface processes such as photodesorption, electron-stimulated desorption, photoluminescence, photocatalysis and photolytic decomposition rely on the population of excited electronic states in the adsorbate layer. A satisfactory description of both the excited and the ground state electronic structure of the adsorbate-substrate system is thus a necessary prerequisite for understanding these phenomena. This article attempts to explain simply some of the more important aspects of the adsorbate-substrate interaction and to describe how surface electronic structure can be probed spectroscopically.

The interaction of an atom or a molecule with a clean metal surface leads to a perturbation of the electronic structure in the surface region. If the atom or molecule is inert only physisorption will occur: the attractive interaction is of the van der Waals type (so-called dispersion forces) and very weak, giving rise to an adsorption energy of less that 30 $kJmol^{-1}$ (0.3 eV/particle). Although the wavefunctions of the adsorbate are barely modified, a change in the electrostatic potential at the surface occurs which in turn influences substrate electronic properties such as the work function and the surface states. A reactive atom or molecule will form a chemical bond to the metal surface,i.e. a sharing of electrons results. We then speak of chemisorption. Chemisorption energies range typically from 30 to 200 $kJmol^{-1}$ (0.3 - 2.0 eV/particle). Here of course a change in surface electrostatic potential also occurs, but additionally a strong perturbation of the valence levels on both substrate and adsorbate takes place. The hitherto discrete atomic or molecular orbitals of the adsorbate give rise to a new set of electronic energy levels which are broadened and shifted relative to those of the free atom or molecule. Degeneracies may also be lifted due to the lower symmetry of the surface complex. This new set of adsorbate-derived energy levels contains considerable substrate character. They are usually referred to as adsorbate-induced surface states, or, if they couple to Bloch states of the bulk crystal as adsorbate-induced surface resonances. At finite coverages of the adsorbate atom or molecule lateral interactions will also play an important role. In the case of an ordered overlayer the adsorbate-induced levels will form two-dimensional Bloch states. In the next section the chemisorption case will be examined in more detail. In particular, we will examine whether it is possible to account not only qualitatively but also quantitatively for the position and width of adsorbate-induced levels. The role played by lateral interactions will also be briefly considered. More detailed accounts are to be found in the appropriate books and review articles [1-4].

## 2. The Surface Chemical Bond

To begin this discussion we take the example of atomic adsorption of oxygen in a threefold symmetric site on a single crystal metal surface (e.g.

O/Al(111)). The point group of this system is $C_{3v}$ [5]. The three 2p orbitals of the oxygen will give rise to adsorbate-induced states belonging to the $A_1$ and E irreducible representations. If we take the z axis to be in the surface normal, the $p_z$-derived state belongs to $A_1$; the $p_x$, $p_y$-derived states distributed in the plane of the surface remain degenerate and belong to E. The lower symmetry of the surface thus only partially lifts the degeneracy of the oxygen 2p orbitals. Treating the semi-infinite substrate as a giant molecule, symmetry considerations tell us that only those substrate levels of $A_1$ and E symmetry can interact with the adsorbate levels and form the chemisorption bond. If we assume, however, that only one substrate level of each representation participates in the bond, four molecular orbitals would be formed - two bonding and two anti-bonding. Such molecular orbital energy diagrams are used in discussing chemical bond formation in molecules. However, unlike a molecule, the substrate has a near-infinite number of electrons. The oxygen 2p orbitals thus interact with a semi-infinite continuum of levels and the simple picture of a discrete molecular orbital scheme has to be extended. (We will, however, return to this picture later when we discuss cluster models). The former discrete levels of the adsorbate will shift towards lower energy due to the attractive potential of the metal but, at the same time, are substantially broadened (Fig. 1a). This interaction involves hopping of electrons between substrate and adsorbate orbital; the width of the level is now inversely proportional to the dwell time of the electrons on the adsorbate. In an equivalent description these broad levels are referred to as adsorbate-induced resonances: electrons incident from the bulk are scattered at the adsorbate. Without the adsorbate the standing wave resulting from the incident wave and the wave reflected at the potential barrier has a node at the surface. An adsorbed particle modifies the reflection properties by shifting the phase of the reflected wave. On the low energy side of the resonance the phase shift is such that charge is accumulated along the axis between adparticle and substrate, indicating that these states are bonding in character. On the high energy side of the resonance the states are cor-

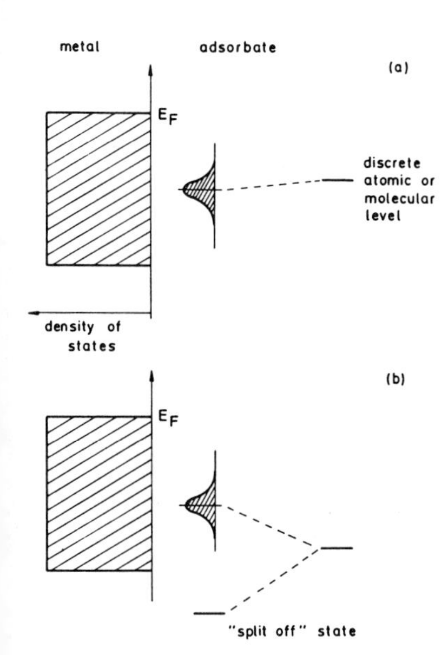


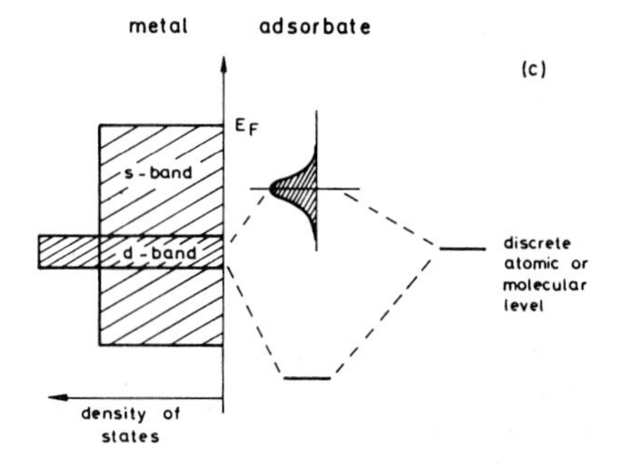


Fig. 1 a) Schematic representation of a discrete level interacting with the surface of a nearly free electron metal. b) Stronger interaction resulting in a "split-off" bonding level below the metal valence band. c) Split-off states formed by strong directional bonding as on a transition metal surface.

respondingly anti-bonding in character. If the interaction with the substrate is very strong, however, the adsorbate-induced resonance will be pulled down below the valence band, becoming again discrete in nature (the "split off" state). A corresponding broad, anti-bonding resonance will appear in the valence band (Fig. 1b). A similar bonding-anti-bonding splitting is obtained when strong directional bonding occurs such as might be the case on a transition metal surface with a narrow d-band. This situation is illustrated schematically in Fig. 1c.

The above considerations on the interaction of atoms and molecules with nearly free-electron-like substrates derive from the work of LANG and others [3,6,7] using the "jellium" model. In this picture the lattice of ion cores is replaced by a semi-infinite constant background of positive charge. A treatment of the interacting electron gas using the density functional formalism in the local density approximation enables not only the total energy of the system but also the electronic charge density and effective potential, $V_{eff}(\rho)$, at the surface to be calculated. The only parameter characterising the jellium substrate is the positive charge density. The semi-infinite jellium model is the simplest approximation to a metal surface. It is, however, a reasonable approximation for nearly free-electron-like metals, such as magnesium and aluminium, and has been extended to include the lattice of discrete ion cores and even, more recently, to transition metals. For semi-conductors and insulators the jellium model is not applicable.

Figures 2-4 present some results from jellium calculations for substrate charge densities corresponding to aluminium. Figure 2 shows how the electron density decays exponentially outside the metal surface giving a "spill-out" of electrons into the vacuum and the formation of a surface dipole layer [8]. Inside, the electron density approaches the constant bulk value in an oscillatory way. These Friedel oscillations are more strongly pronounced in a less dense electron gas (dashed curve). The change in electron density induced by a homogeneous adsorbate layer at high and low coverage is depicted in Fig. 3. A positively charged slab (simulating the adlayer ion cores and corresponding to Cs) has been placed on the semi-infinite positive background [9]. The adsorbate-induced electronic charge is peaked at the interface, indicating that electron density is transferred in some degree to the substrate. An alkali metal layer thus gives an additional (adsorbate-induced) dipole with the positive end pointing away from the surface. Compared to the clean metal a reduction in total dipole moment, and

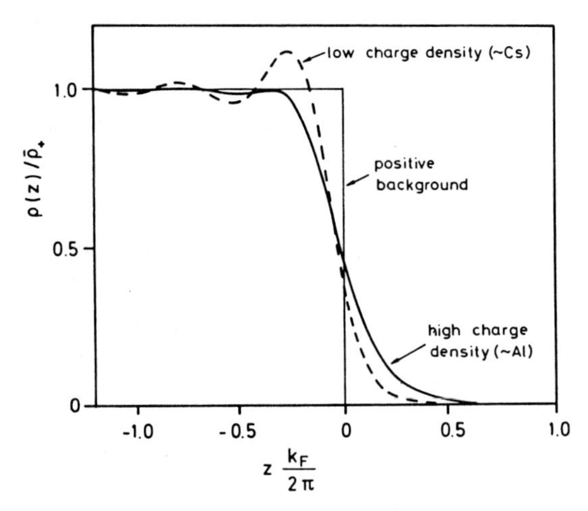


Fig. 2 The electron density at a metal surface calculated in the jellium approximation for two substrate charge densities. After LANG [8].

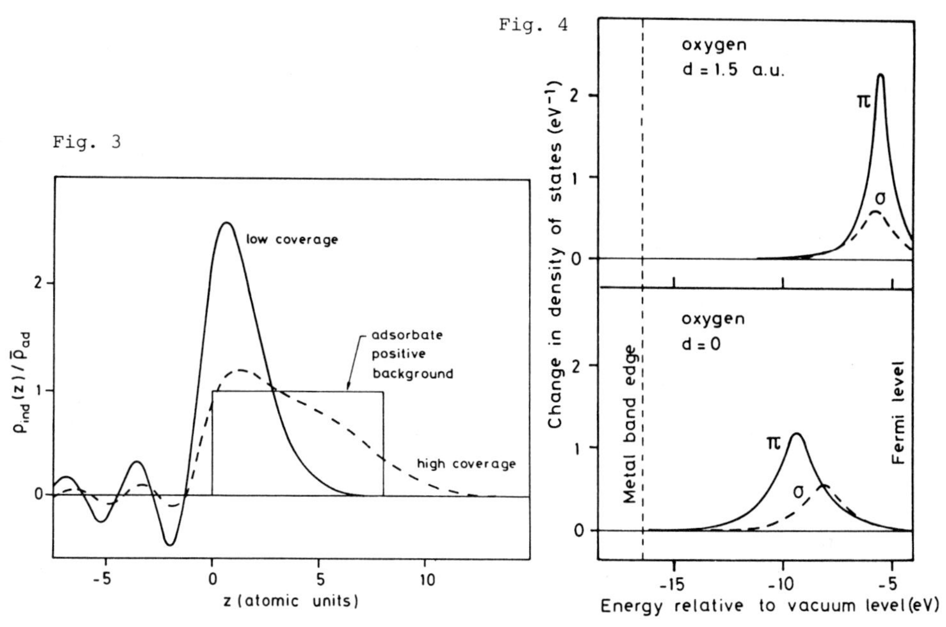


Fig. 3 Change in electronic charge density induced by an adsorbed ionic layer (corresponding to Cs) adsorbed on a jellium substrate (corresponding to aluminium). Both adsorbate and substrate are treated in the uniform background model. After LANG [9].
Fig. 4 The $\sigma$ (O $2p_z$) and $\pi$ (O $2p_{x,y}$) components of the density of states due to chemisorption of a single oxygen atom on a jellium surface corresponding to aluminium. After LANG and WILLIAMS [10].

thus a reduction in work function, occurs. The reverse situation occurs when a net electronic charge transfer towards the adsorbate takes place as in the case of an oxygen adlayer. LANG and WILLIAMS [10] have calculated the effect of a single oxygen atom on a jellium surface. In order to link up with the simple molecular orbital picture discussed above, it is convenient here to look at the adsorbate-induced changes in the density of states. Figure 4 shows the energy spectrum of the oxygen-induced levels at two metal-adatom distances. The calculated equilibrium distance for the jellium substrate lies between these two cases at d = 0.58 Å (1.1 a.u.). We notice that the two peaks corresponding to the two different representations are split only very little at d = 1.5 a.u. (0.79 Å). The peak labelled $\sigma$ is due to the O $2p_z$ interaction with the substrate and the $\pi$-peak to the O $2p_x$, $p_y$ interaction. As explained above the low energy tail of each peak is due to bonding states and the high energy tail to antibonding states. We see that charge transfer has taken place towards the oxygen atom so that the anti-bonding levels of the O $2p_z$ as well as of the O $2p_x$, $p_y$ induced resonance are largely filled. If the adatom comes even closer to the surface, the width of both peaks increases and the splitting is enhanced; they shift to lower energy and further antibonding states become filled.

At sufficiently high coverages adparticles can become sufficiently near such that covalent interactions between orbitals on neighbouring species occur. When the overlayer is ordered the system forms two-dimensional Bloch states defined by their reduced $\vec{k}_{\parallel}$ vector (in the surface Brillouin zone) as well as by their energy. This problem can be treated illustratively in

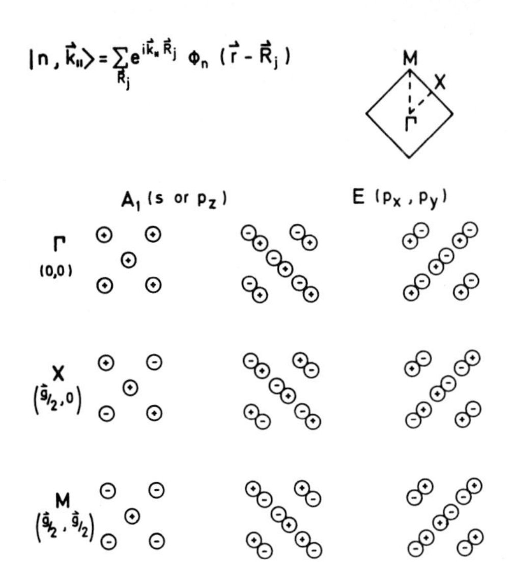


Fig. 5 Schematic representations of the two-dimensional Bloch states formed from atomic or molecular wave functions belonging to $A_1$ ($p_z$) and E ($p_x$, $p_y$) at the three high symmetry points of the surface Brillouin zone from a square array of adparticles. After SCHEFFLER [11].

a simple tight binding picture [11,4]. We consider $p_x$-, $p_y$- and $p_z$-type atomic (or molecular) wave functions, $\phi_n$, in a square array on a metal surface, but do not allow them initially to interact with the substrate. Figure 5 is a schematic representation of the Bloch states at $\bar{\Gamma}$, $\bar{X}$ and $\bar{M}$ in the corresponding surface Brillouin zone (also depicted above). The $R_j$ are the two-dimensional lattice vectors in real space and g is the adlayer reciprocal lattice vector. The figure has been constructed by putting orbitals of the appropriate symmetry at the nearest neighbour sites around one adparticle with the phase factors $e^{ik_\parallel R_j}$ corresponding to the appropriate point in the surface Brillouin zone. An analysis of this diagram already gives the qualitative band structure which is depicted in Fig. 6a. At $\bar{\Gamma}$ ($\vec{k}_\parallel$=o) the $p_z$-derived 2D Bloch state is completely bonding, at $\bar{M}$ it is completely anti-bonding and at $\bar{X}$ somewhere between. The energy of the $p_z$-derived band will thus be lowest at $\bar{\Gamma}$ and highest at $\bar{M}$. Similar conside-

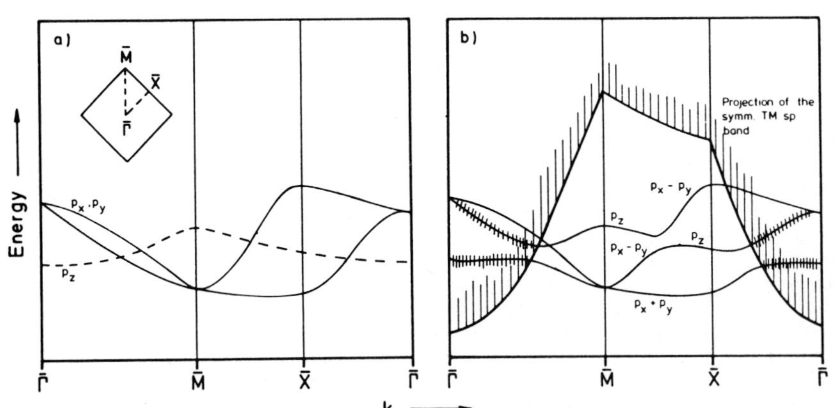


Fig. 6 a) Schematic representation of the surface band structure deriving from a (hypothetical) isolated square array of adparticles with an np valence shell. b) As in (a), but here the interaction with the substrate has been turned on.

rations apply to the $p_x$-, $p_y$-derived bands. Note the lifting of the degeneracy of this band at points other than $\bar{\Gamma}$ and $\bar{M}$. $C_{4v}$ symmetry pertains at the latter, $C_{2v}$ at $\bar{X}$ and $C_s$ along $\bar{\Gamma}\bar{M}$ and $\bar{\Gamma}\bar{X}$ and $\bar{M}\bar{X}$ . When the interaction with the substrate is switched on, two things happen. Bands along the main symmetry direction belonging to the same representation can no longer cross, giving rise to so-called hybridisation gaps. Secondly, adsorbate bands can interact (bond, or hybridise) with substrate states of the same energy and $\vec{k}_{\parallel}$. This is shown schematically in Figure 6b. The importance of these "surface band structures" for experimentalists should not be underestimated: as will be mentioned again below, photoemission may be used here as a direct probe.

The examples shown in this section have so far been primarily of illustrative character and have served to demonstrate some of the simple concepts germane to this article. However, sophisticated self-consistent calculations of chemisorption systems are possible and generally fall into two classes. Slab calculations have recently produced very promising results for ordered adsorbate overlayers. They all use the density functional formalism in the local density approximation. It is becoming possible not only to calculate total energy, work function and the $\vec{k}_{\parallel}$-resolved density of states but also to find the adsorption site by minimising the total energy. Examples of various approaches are to be found in the literature: APW [12], LCAO [13] and pseudopotentials [14]. An alternative approach - the extended layer KKR [15] - is not self-consistent but does allow the direct calculation of the photoemission spectrum. The comparison of slab calculations with photoemission data (see section 3 below) is difficult because the matrix elements are not known; nor are relaxation effects at present accounted for. The same is of course true of cluster calculations. The cluster is a small metal particle with bulk interatomic spacings to which the adatom or admolecule is bonded at an appropriate site. The whole is treated as a molecule and calculated with self-consistent quantum chemical methods (e.g. SCF-CI [16] or GVB [17]) to obtain the total energy and the eigenvalues. The latter, even those with mainly substrate character, are of course discrete. The method has, however, been quite successful in describing the relative positions of adsorbate-induced levels. The size of the cluster is normally determined by the amount of computational time required for the calculation. Relaxation effects in photoemission have to be accounted for in some kind of ΔSCF approach and this has already been done for one or two cases [18]. In the following, an example of each sort of calculation will be discussed.

KLEINMAN and co-workers [19] have recently calculated the electronic structure of the (1x1) oxygen monolayer on an Al(111) surface. They have made a self-consistent linear combination of Gaussian orbitals (SCLCGO) energy band and binding energy calculation for oxygen overlayers at various z values on a six-layer Al(111) slab. The oxygen atom is placed over the three-fold site. A minimum in the total energy was obtained for z = 0.60 ($\pm$ 0.10) Å in agreement with EXAFS data [20]. For this separation another calculation with an 18 layer aluminium slab was performed in order to study more accurately the surface state bands. The results are shown in Fig. 7. The filled area represents the Al sp bands projected onto the surface Brillouin zone; because of the finite slab thickness this area is not a continuum as would be obtained by projecting the three-dimensional band structure. The strong O 2p-derived surface state bands and surface resonances are highlighted. The degeneracy of the O $2p_x$, $p_y$-derived state at $\bar{\Gamma}$ is lifted along $\bar{\Gamma}\bar{M}$; the symmetrical component hybridises with the substrate bands emerging again as a split-off band towards the $\bar{M}$ point. The $p_z$-derived band hybridises very strongly with the substrate and is only

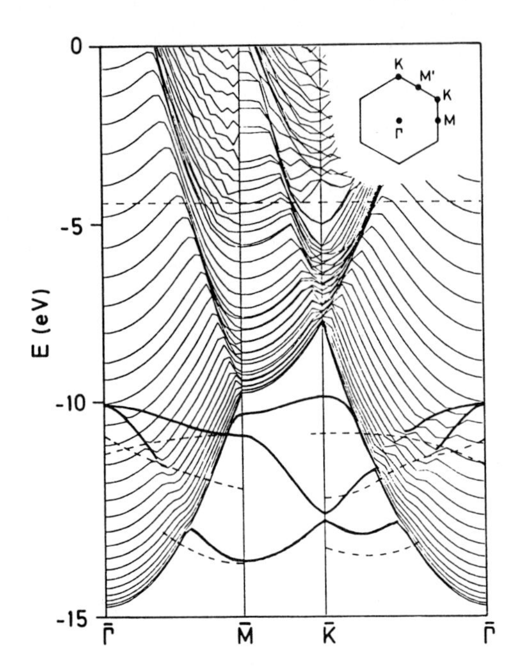


Fig. 7 The energy bands of an 18 layer Al(111) film terminated on each face by (1x1) oxygen overlayers. The dashed curves represent experimental data obtained by angle-resolved photoemission. After KLEINMAN et al. [19] and HOFMANN et al. [21].

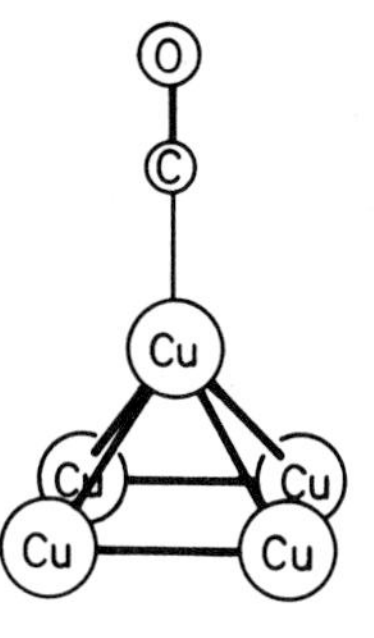


Fig.8 The $Cu_5CO$ cluster used to model the bonding of CO to a Cu(100) surface by BAGUS et al. [22].

visible near the zone edge along $\overline{MK}$. The dashed lines result from angle-resolved photoemission experiments [21]. The agreement is relatively good; the $p_z$-derived surface resonance is, however, clearly visible in the spectra along both $\overline{\Gamma M}$ and $\overline{\Gamma K}$.

BAGUS and co-workers have recently treated a $Cu_5CO$ cluster using the Hartree-Fock self-consistent field (SCF) method [22]. The arrangement of copper atoms (Fig. 8) is intended to model a Cu(100) surface. In particular, a special procedure (termed the constrained space orbital variation method) was adopted in order to analyse the various contributions to the interaction energy, $E_{int}$. The latter is defined as the difference in the energy of the cluster with CO and the sum of the energy of the separated units; it thus corresponds to the adsorption energy. The SCF equilibrium bond distances were found to be r(Cu-C) = 2.07 Å and r(C-O) = 1.13 Å; $E_{int}$ = 0.48 eV and the C-O stretch frequency was 2143 $cm^{-1}$ (lowered by 127 $cm^{-1}$ compared to the SCF free molecule value). The major contribution to $E_{int}$ is dπ-pπ back-bonding where charge is transferred into the CO 2π* antibonding orbital. Also important are the contributions provided by charge polarisation on the metal moiety and the CO ligand. Charge donation from CO 5σ to the metal is not very significant, contributing a factor of three less to the interaction energy than the dπ-pπ bonding. A multiconfiguration SCF calculation on the same cluster which included correlation in the π space gave r(Cu-C) = 1.96 Å, r(C-O) = 1.13 Å and $E_{int}$ = 0.67 eV.

## 3. Probing Surface Electronic Structure

The most successful technique for probing the electronic states of an adsorbate-covered surface has been photoemission, or photoelectron spectroscopy [4,23]. A photon is absorbed by the N particle system and the energy of the photoemitted electron, $E_{kin}$, is measured at a detector far away from the surface. The electron binding energy (also referred to as the ionisation energy or ionisation potential) is given by

$$E_B = \hbar\omega - E_{kin} = E^{N-1} - E^N$$

and, for a given $E_{kin}$, corresponds to an N-1 particle state of the system. In the one-electron picture (Fig. 9) the binding energies can be identified with the single particle energies of the ground state. Each electronic energy level of the system then gives rise to one feature in the photoelectron spectrum, I(E), its energy being given by the energy balance. In practice, photoemission is more complicated: the removal of an electron from the system changes the effective potential. The other electrons can thus rearrange in response to the creation of the hole, thereby lowering the energy of the N-1 system. The energy difference, termed the relaxation energy, is passed onto the photoelectron which is measured at a higher $E_{kin}$. Furthermore, due to the dynamics of the change in potential the photoionisation can be accompanied by the excitation of phonons, molecular vibrations, surface plasmons and bound-to-bound electronic transitions. The photoelectron can thus be emitted from an excited state of the N-1 system and will be found at a different $E_{kin}$ in the spectrum as a satellite. On a surface there are additional possibilites for promoting relaxation, or for "screening", compared to the free molecule. Since relaxation effects, in a first approximation, will be similar for all adsorbate-induced states or bands, the relative position of levels can still be compared with ground state calculations or, if appropriate, with the corresponding photoelectron spectrum of the gas phase species. These problems will be illustrated by the system CO/Cu discussed below.

We noted above how high coverage ordered overlayers of adsorbate give rise to the formation of two-dimensional Bloch states. In photoelectron emission it is generally assumed that the parallel component of electron momentum is conserved in the emission process. Since $\vec{k}_\parallel$ can be determined experimentally from

$$k_\parallel = (2mE_{kin})^{1/2}\sin\Theta/\hbar,$$

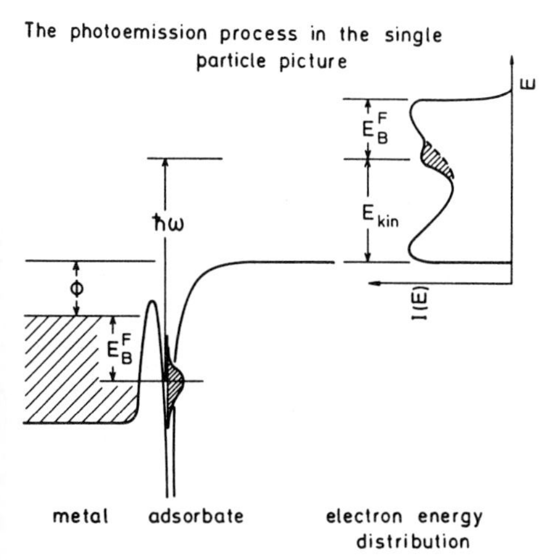


Fig. 9 The photoemission experiment applied to an adsorbate-covered surface.

where $\Theta$ is the polar emission angle, it is clear that the dispersion relationship $E_B^F(\vec{k}_{\parallel})$ for different directions in the surface Brillouin zone can be determined directly with angle-resolved photoemission. Results obtained for the (1x1) ordered overlayer formed by atomic oxygen on Al(111) have already been shown in Fig. 7.

The unoccupied states of the adsorbate-substrate system (or, more accurately, the affinity levels) can be probed with the technique of Bremsstrahlung isochromat spectroscopy (BIS), or inverse photoemission [24]. In this method a radiative transition occurs in which an electron is incident on a metal surface and decelerated, occupying transiently an empty level above the Fermi energy. The Bremsstrahlung radiation is then collected energy selectively at a suitable detector. In practice the spectrum is obtained by varying the electron energy, $E_{el}$, at a fixed photon detection energy, $\hbar\omega$. Figure 10 shows this schematically: at the threshold at $E_F$ the electron energy $E_{el}$ is equal to $\hbar\omega$. $E_{el}$ is then increased but only photons with energy $\hbar\omega$ are detected, thus probing the states above $E_F$. This method has only just begun to be applied to adsorbate systems. The discussion above concerning relaxation in photoemission applies equally well to inverse photoemission. The final state in the BIS experiment is an N+1 particle system. The energy of an unoccupied level or band deriving from a ground state calculation will not in general correspond to the difference in energies of the N and N+1 systems.

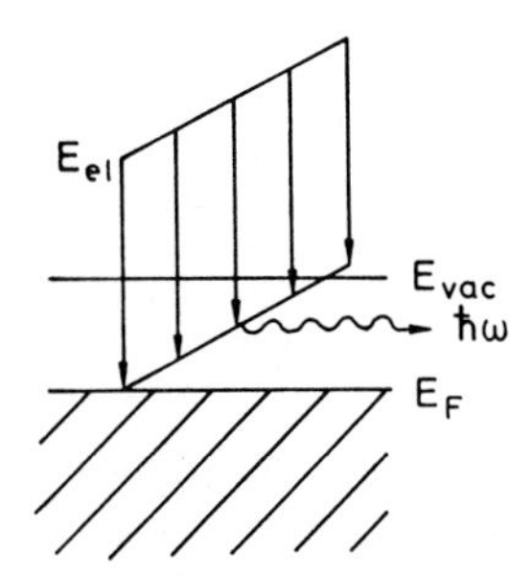


Fig. 10 Schematic representation of Bremsstrahlung isochromat spectroscopy (or inverse photoemission).

A third technique for studying surface electronic structure is optical spectroscopy. So far this appears only to have been used once in the VUV region necessary for adsorbates such as CO [25]. More studies have been performed, however, with electron loss spectroscopy (ELS) where essentially similar results should be obtained in the limit of zero momentum transfer [26]. One important difference is that under appropriate conditions symmetry and spin-forbidden transitions can be observed in electron loss. Whereas energy loss studies of metals give excitation energies for critical points in the Brillouin zone that agree reasonably well ($\sim$1 eV) with the corresponding energy separations in a band structure calculation, we should not necessarily expect this to be the case for an adsorbate system. The excitation energy in a free molecule can be many eV lower than the corresponding difference in the Hartree-Fock orbital energies (or indeed than the sum of the ionisation potential and the affinity energy). The reason lies in the importance of the "self-Coulomb interaction" between excited electron and hole in the molecular system.

In the following we look at an adsorption system - CO/copper - in somewhat more detail and discuss the information that can be obtained from these spectroscopies.

## 4. An Example: The Adsorption System CO/Copper

Numerous investigations of this adsorption system have been performed with a variety of techniques. Some of the results are summarised in the following. The initial adsorption energy for CO on the three simplest faces - (111), (100) and (110) - has a value of ∿0.7 eV. It will be remembered that the MSCF calculation of BAGUS gave 0.67 eV for the interaction energy. Low energy electron diffraction (LEED) investigations have shown that ordered overlayer structures are formed with unit meshes that are simply related to the unit meshes of the copper surfaces. The first ordered structure to appear on Cu(100) is c(2x2), on Cu(111) it is $(\sqrt{3}x\sqrt{3})R30^{o}$ and on Cu(110) it is p(2x1). (For a description of the nomenclature, see for example [27].) Further adsorption to saturation coverage gives diffraction patterns that are most readily interpreted in terms of "compression structures", or incommensurate overlayers; there is, however, some controversy about the correct interpretation [28,29]. The compression structures are accompanied by drastic decreases in the adsorption energy. A LEED structure analysis of the c(2x2) overlayer on Cu(100) by ANDERSSON and PENDRY [30] has indicated that the CO molecules are bonded through the C atom in a vertical geometry directly over the Cu atoms (the "on-top" site). The Cu-C and C-O distances were found to be 1.90 and 1.15 Å, respectively. Reflection IR measurements by PRITCHARD and co-workers on the three simplest faces gave C-O stretching frequencies between 2079 and 2104 $cm^{-1}$ at low coverages [31], also indicative of the occupation of "on-top" sites.

Many photoemission studies of CO chemisorbed on transition metals have appeared in the literature. In general, two peaks are observed in the photoelectron spectrum, at 7-8 eV and at 11-12 eV below $E_F$. The first one is assigned to emission from the $\tilde{5\sigma}$ and $\tilde{1\pi}$ orbitals and the second to emission from the $\tilde{4\sigma}$ orbital. The tilda indicates that there are adsorbate-derived (in this case "split-off") states modified by the interaction with the metal surface. The corresponding spectrum for CO on copper is more complicated, exhibiting more than two features,e.g. [32]. HORN and co-workers have recently re-investigated this system [33] and discussed the origin of the additional features. Figure 11 shows their data at a photon energy of 32 eV. The peaks $P_1$ and $P_2$ appear at a similar energy to those on other metal surfaces and are attributed to the "well screened" (see be-

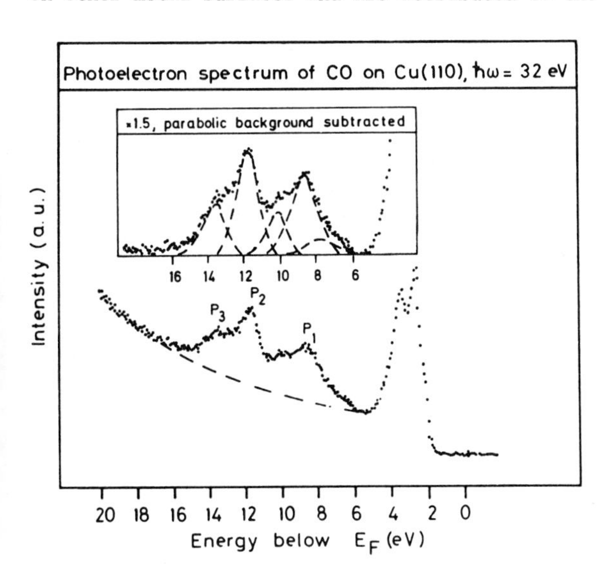


Fig. 11 The photoelectron spectrum of CO adsorbed on a Cu(110) surface at 80 K and saturation coverage. Photon energy, ħω = 32 eV. Curve resolving reveals the presence of two satellites, one on each of the main features $P_1$ and $P_2$. $P_1$ is also seen to be composed of two features, probably corresponding to the slightly different ionisation energies of $\tilde{5\sigma}$ and $\tilde{1\pi}$. After HORN et al. [33].

low) $\tilde{5\sigma}/\tilde{1\pi}$ and $\tilde{4\sigma}$ hole states, respectively. It is interesting to consider the position of these features relative to the corresponding ionisation energies in the free CO molecule. The latter have values, relative to the Fermi level of the clean Cu surface, of 9.5 eV ($5\sigma$), 12.5 eV ($1\pi$) and 15.2 eV ($4\sigma$). Clearly a stabilisation of the $5\sigma$ orbital relative to the $1\pi$ orbital takes place, whereas the $1\pi$-$4\sigma$ separation remains approximately the same. This reflects a strong interaction between $5\sigma$ and the substrate although, as we learnt above, the $d\pi$-$p\pi$ bonding interaction is probably more important. The expected changes in the Cu d band corresponding to this interaction with the $2\pi^*$ orbital have not yet been observed. In addition, an overall upward shift of ~3 eV has occurred due to additional relaxation processes. Since we know that all the orbitals will also be pulled down due to the attractive potential of the substrate, it is clear that this relaxation shift is actually larger than is at first obvious. Two additional relaxation mechanisms are available on the surface: image charge screening, whereby the energy of the hole state is lowered by the dielectric response of the metal conduction electrons, and charge transfer screening, whereby an unoccupied adsorbate orbital is pulled down below $E_F$ and charge flows into it from the metal. The peaks $P_1$ and $P_2$ in Fig. 11 correspond to the well-screened situation where metal electrons have been transferred into the $\tilde{2\pi}^*$ orbital, thus screening the positive hole. The higher binding energy satellites (that on $P_2$ ($\tilde{4\sigma}$) is designated $P_3$ in this picture) are the corresponding unscreened features. "Unscreened" here refers only to charge transfer screening; image charge screening is still operative. On a metal such as nickel, where the CO chemisorption bond is stronger, the overlap with the $2\pi^*$ state is greater, the charge transfer screening mechanism is more effective and nearly all the intensity is found in the well-screened peak. Figure 11 illustrates one of the problems of interpreting photoemission data: whereas relative shifts of adsorbate-derived features are easy to explain qualitatively, it is difficult, if not impossible, because of relaxation effects to compare the data with absolute values from calculated ground state energy level schemes.

The BIS technique has recently been applied to the chemisorption system CO/Cu (110) by ROGOZIK et al. [34]. Here one is particularly interested in probing the energy and width of the $\tilde{2\pi}^*$ level. A recent photoemission experiment had indicated that in the c(2x2) CO layer on Cu(100) the $2\pi^*$-derived band disperses downward and drops below $E_F$ away from the centre of the surface Brillouin zone [35]. Inverse photoemission spectra for CO/Cu (110) are shown in Fig. 12. The $2\pi^*$-derived feature is found 3.4 eV above $E_F$ and its halfwidth varies from 1.9 eV at low coverage to 2.6 eV at high coverage. To what extent does the position of this feature give the energy of the $2\pi^*$-derived level(s) in the ground state? (We are also entitled to ask whether the energy of an unoccupied state actually has any physical signifance at all!) In the case of a molecule the situation is quite clear: relaxation will ensure that the measured affinity level will be lower in energy than the corresponding Hartree-Fock orbital energy. In CO, for example, the calculated $2\pi^*$ level lies 3.15 eV above $E_{vac}$ and the electron affinity is 1.5 eV relative to $E_{vac}$. On a surface an additional relaxation channel, namely, image charge screening, is available. This appears, however, only to be a few tenths of an eV for an adsorbed $CO^-$ transient, as electron scattering experiments have shown [36]. It would appear from the width of the feature in the present data that a very strong interaction with the substrate occurs and, at high coverages, lateral interactions in the adlayer also take place. Under such conditions the radiatively captured electron will find itself in a metallic-like band and be rapidly delocalised. Image charge screening will be of even less importance in this situation. We might thus expect the BIS experiment to probe essentially the energy of the $2\pi^*$-derived band just as in the application of the technique to

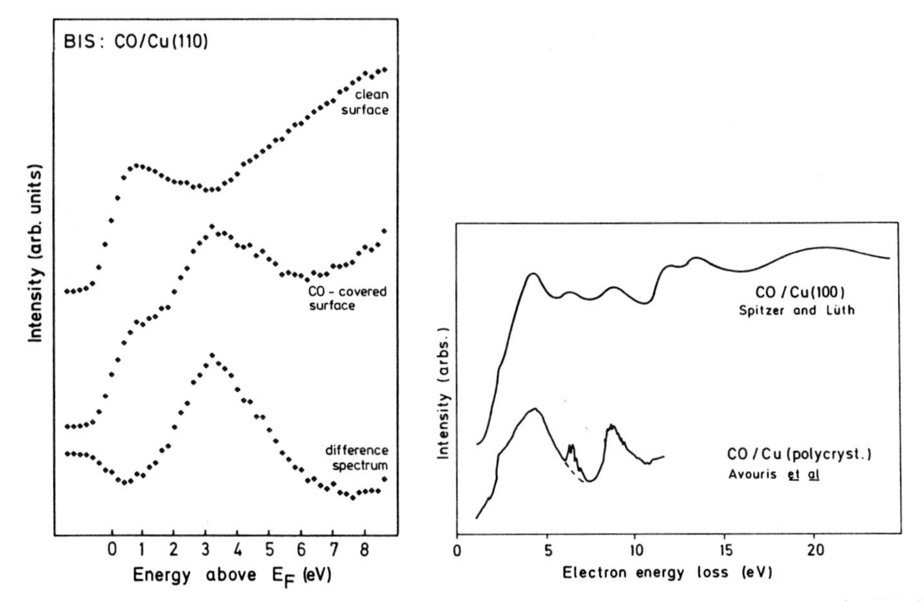


Fig. 12 Bremsstrahlung isochromat spectra of the adsorption system CO/Cu(110). The spectrum of the CO-covered surface corresponds to saturation coverage at the substrate temperature of 170 K. After ROGOZIK et al. [34].

Fig. 13 Valence region electron energy loss spectra from CO/copper. After [26] and [38].

structure studies of metals. In the corresponding photoemission experiment it is not possible to neglect relaxation, but here the charge to be screened is more localised and an additional mechanism, namely, charge transfer screening, is available. The strong lateral interactions affecting the $2\pi^*$ level have been indicated by the observation of dispersion in the c(2x2) CO layer on Cu(100) [37].

It remains for us to discuss the optical excitation spectra of this system. Figure 13 shows two sets of electron loss data from SPITZER and LÜTH [38] for CO/Cu(100) at a primary energy of 40 eV and from AVOURIS et al. [26] for CO on polycrystalline copper at a primary energy of 14 eV. The latter spectrum corresponds to approximately two monolayers, i.e. there is an additional physisorbed layer on top of the chemisorbed layer. The features at ~2 eV and ~4 eV derive from the substrate. A chemisorbed layer gives rise to additional features at ~6 eV and ~8.5 eV, roughly corresponding to the peaks in the upper spectrum. For coverages higher than one monolayer (as shown) these two features are more prominent and that at ~6 eV develops vibrational fine structure. For the chemisorbed layer investigated at 40 eV primary energy (upper spectrum) further adsorbate-induced features are observed at 11.9 eV and 13.5 eV. Surprisingly enough, there is considerable disagreement as to the interpretation of these spectra. AVOURIS et al. claim that the features at ~6 eV and ~8.5 eV are due to the $5\sigma \rightarrow 2\pi^*$ transition which can result in either a triplet or a singlet final state. If this interpretation were correct (and the careful observation of the transition to multilayer formation support this) then these transitions occur at almost exactly the same energy as in the free CO molecule. SPITZER and LÜTH claim that the 6 eV feature is substrate-derived and that the 8.5 eV feature is due to a d(Cu) $\rightarrow$ $2\pi^*$ charge transfer transition; they ascribe the higher energy losses to $5\sigma \rightarrow 2\pi^*$ and other intramolecular transitions in CO. Other authors have come up with alternative assignments for the similar spectra obtained for CO adsorbed on other metal surfaces. It is indeed extraordinary that the features in these spectra have not yet been conclusively assigned. Nor does it presage well for our understanding of photoinduced processes on surfaces for which these excitations constitute the primary processes.

## 5. Some Concluding Remarks

In this article I have tried to give a brief overview of the qualitative features of the adsorbate-substrate interaction and of the spectroscopic methods that can be applied to help elucidate surface electronic structure. Before concluding it is appropriate in the context of these Proceedings to examine briefly the ramifications for photoeffects in adsorbed layers. This is best done by taking the case of photodesorption which has attracted considerable attention in recent years [39]. Photodesorption in the VUV is believed to occur via a valence excitation to a repulsive neutral or ionic state, $M+A \rightarrow (M+A)^*$ [40]. In the case of desorption of neutrals the excitation energy is transformed into nuclear kinetic energy via transfer onto the non-repulsive potential energy surface of another excited state $M^*+A$. If "recapture" (or de-excitation) does not occur, despite the availability of metal conduction electrons, desorption will result. In the case of ionic desorption, excitation to the repulsive part of an ionic curve, $M^-+A^+$ occurs. If A is a molecule, photofragmentation via similar mechanisms can also occur. More recently the occurrence of so-called multi-electron excitation (similar to the shake-up satellites observed in photoemission spectra) has been identified as an additional mechanism in the VUV. Electronically promoted desorption of CO on metal surfaces gives rise to $CO^+$, $O^+$ and neutral CO. A recent study of CO on ruthenium [41] shows thresholds at 3-6 eV and 14 eV thought to be due to a $d\pi \rightarrow 2\pi^*$ excitation and a multielectron excitation characterised by the final state $5\sigma^{-1}$ $d\pi^{-1}$ $2\pi^*$, respectively. The corresponding $CO^+$ thresholds at 14 eV and 22-27 eV are similarly attributed to multielectronic excitations. It is thus clear that an understanding of surface electronic structure is a necessary condition for explaining such phenomena: threshold energies, recapture rates and indeed the complete dynamics of the desorption process are dependent on the energy level scheme. It should not go unsaid that the same will be true for laser-induced photolytic decomposition at metal surfaces.

## Acknowledgements

I thank M. SCHEFFLER and M. SUNJIC for useful discussions and K. HORN for a critical reading of the manuscript.

## References

1. The Nature of the Surface Chemical Bond, T.N. Rhodin and G. Ertl eds. (North Holland, Amsterdam, 1979).
2. Theory of Chemisorption, J.R. Smith ed. (Springer-Verlag, Berlin, 1980).
3. N.D. Lang in Theory of the Inhomogeneous Electron Gas, D. Lundqvist and N.H. March eds. (Plenum Press, New York, 1983) p. 304.
4. M. Scheffler and A.M. Bradshaw in Chemical Physics of Solid Surfaces and Heterogeneous Catalysis, D.A. King and D.P. Woodruff eds. (Elsevier, Amsterdam, 1983) Vol. II p. 165.

5. See for example, A.M. Bradshaw, Z. Phys. Chemie NF 112 33 (1978).
6. N.D. Lang in Solid State Physics, H. Ehrenreich, F. Seitz and D. Turnball eds. (Academic Press, New York, 1973) Vol. 28 p. 225.
7. E.g. O. Gunnarsson, H. Hjelmberg and B.I. Lundqvist, Physica Scripta 11 97 (1975); Phys. Rev. Letters 37 292 (1976); Surface Sci. 63 348 (1977) and 68 (1977).
8. N.D. Lang, Solid State Commun. 7 1047 (1969).
9. N.D. Lang, Phys. Rev. B 4 4234 (1971).
10. N.D. Lang and A.R. Williams, Phys. Rev. B 18 616 (1978).
11. M. Scheffler, Dissertation, TU Berlin (1978); A.M. Bradshaw and M. Scheffler, J. Vac. Sci. Technol. 16 447 (1979).
12. P.J. Feibelman, D.R. Hamann and F.J. Himpsel, Phys. Rev. B 22 1734 (1980).
13. F.J. Arlinghaus, J.G. Gay and J.R. Smith, Phys. Rev. B 21 2055 (1980).
14. S.G. Louie, K.M. Ho and M.L. Cohen, Phys. Rev. B 19 1774 (1979).
15. A. Liebsch, Phys. Rev. B 17 1653 (1978); R. Hora and M. Scheffler, Phys. Rev. B, in press.
16. P.S. Bagus, K. Hermann and M. Seel, J. Vaci. Sci. Technol. 18 435 (1981).
17. T. Upton and W. Goddard III, CRC Critical Reviews in Solid State and Mathematical Science 10 261 (1981).
18. K. Hermann and P.S. Bagus, Phys. Rev. B 16 4195 (1977).
19. L. Kleinman and K. Mednick, Phys. Rev. B 23 4960 (1981); D.M. Bylander, L. Kleinman and K. Mednick, Phys. Rev. Letters 48 1544 (1982).
20. D. Norman, S. Brennan, R. Jaeger and J. Stöhr, Surf. Sci. 105 L 297 (1981).
21. P. Hofmann, C. von Muschwitz, K. Horn, K. Jacobi, A.M. Bradshaw, K. Kambe and M. Scheffler, Surf. Sci. 89 327 (1979)
22. P.S. Bagus, C.J. Nelin and C.W. Bauchschlicher, Jr., J. Vac. Sci. Technol. A 2 905 (1984).
23. W. Eberhardt and E.W. Plummer, Adv. Chem. Phys. 49 533 (1982).
24. V. Dose, Progr. Surf. Sci. 13 225 (1983).
25. G.W. Rubloff and J.L. Freeouf, Phys. Rev. B 17 4680 (1978).
26. Ph. Avouris, N.J. DiNardo and J.E. Demuth, J. Chem. Phys. 70 491 (1984).
27. G. Ertl and J. Küppers, Low Energy Electrons and Surface Chemistry (Verlag Chemie, Weinheim, 1974).
28. J. Pritchard, Surf. Sci. 79 231 (1979)
29. J.P. Biberian and M. Van Hove, Surf. Sci. 118 443 (1982).
30. S. Andersson and J.B. Pendry, Phys. Rev. Letters 43 363 (1979).
31. K. Horn and J. Pritchard, Surf. Sci. 55 701 (1976); P. Hollins and J. Pritchard, Chem. Phys. Letters 75 378 (1980) and Surf. Sci. 134 91 (1983).
32. C.L. Allyn, T. Gustafsson and E.W. Plummer, Solid State Commun. 23 (1977) 531.
33. C. Mariani, H.-U. Middelmann, M. Iwan and K. Horn, Chem. Phys. Letters 93 308 (1982).
34. J. Rogozik, H. Scheidt, V. Dose, K.C. Prince and A.M. Bradshaw Surf. Sci., in press.
35. C.F. McConville, C. Somerton and D.P. Woodruff, Surf. Sci. 139 75 (1984).
36. J.E. Demuth, D. Schmeisser and Ph. Avouris, Phys. Rev. Letters 47 1166 (1981).
37. J. Rogozik, V. Dose, K.C. Prince and A.M. Bradshaw, to be published.
38. A. Spitzer and H. Lüth, Surf. Sci. 102 29 (1981).
39. Desorption Induced by Electronic Transitions, N.H. Tolk, M.M. Traum, J.C. Tully and T.E. Madey, eds., (Springer-Verlag, Berlin, 1983)
40. E.g. R. Gomer, in [39], p. 40.
41. D.E. Ramaker, in [39], p. 70.

# Laser Photochemistry of Molecular Systems Involving Gas-Surface Interactions

K.L. Kompa

Max-Planck-Institut für Quantenoptik,
D-8046 Garching, Fed. Rep. of Germany

## Introduction

The scope of this report may be described by the concept of examining ideas and methods which proved to be applicable to gas phase laser photochemistry and extending them to surface photochemistry. Although this field is still largely unexplored many new and unexpected observations have already been made. It has also become apparent that more than in other types of laser chemistry technical applications of the observed effects are conceivable.

In which way does a laser chemist look at surface processes? Obviously the questions he likes to ask have to do with the dynamics and the selectivity in thermal versus laser induced surface phenomena. In general terms this means to look for chances to enhance reaction rates and alter reaction routes. This approach is based then on the success and popularity of ideas in general laser chemistry like the following:

1) The selective activation and probing of molecules by lasers has yielded very detailed insight into gas phase reaction mechanisms.
2) High laser radiation powers have given access to multiphoton excitation of molecules on a practical scale.
3) The high directionality of laser radiation has made it possible to spatially confine reaction initiation and to accomplish non-perturbative measurements of gas transport and concentration over considerable distances.
4) Short laser pulses have dramatically extended the timescale of dynamic and spectroscopic studies.

All four of these features also appear to be of interest for surface studies. In the following some discussion will be devoted to points 1) and 2) with some consideration of 3). Results concerning point 4), however, are left out since this is a very large and complex research area which cannot be adequately treated here.

## Phenomenological description of laser-influenced surface interactions

To illustrate some molecule-surface interactions Fig. 1 may be used as a guideline. It is appropriate to distinguish in this context between laser photophysics and photochemistry but it is also necessary to point out the links between the two related areas.

It should be clear that the selection of examples is not systematic here and does not include all possible cases of interaction. It rather reflects the current interest in the literature.

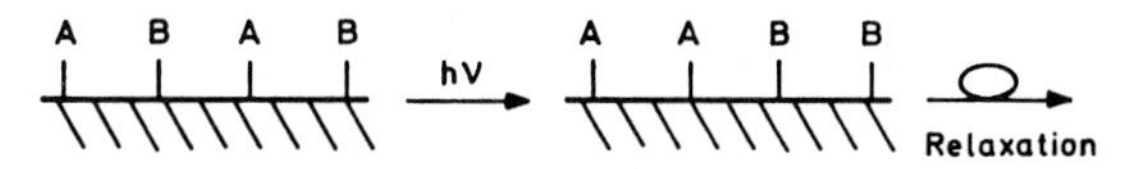


(I) Adsorbate mobility and lateral diffusion

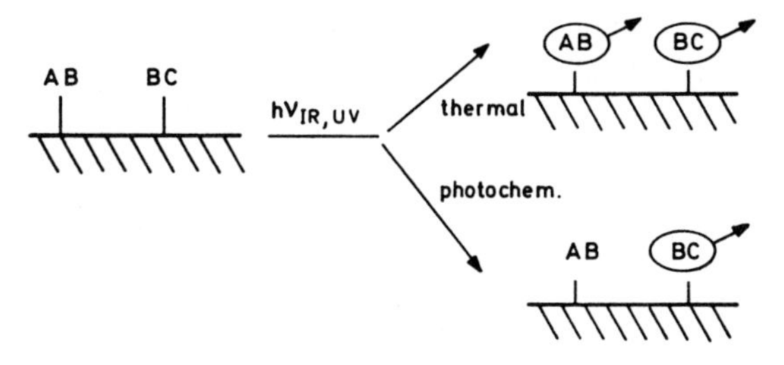


(II) Laser thermal and photochemical desorption

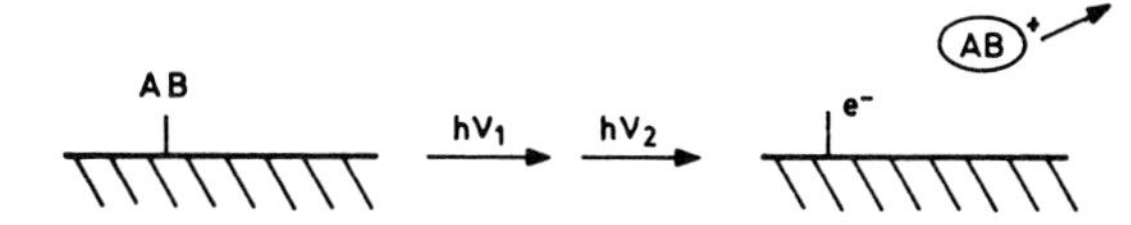


(III) Laser photoionization and subsequent desorption

Fig. 1a: Some types of laser-induced surface physical processes (for explanations see text)

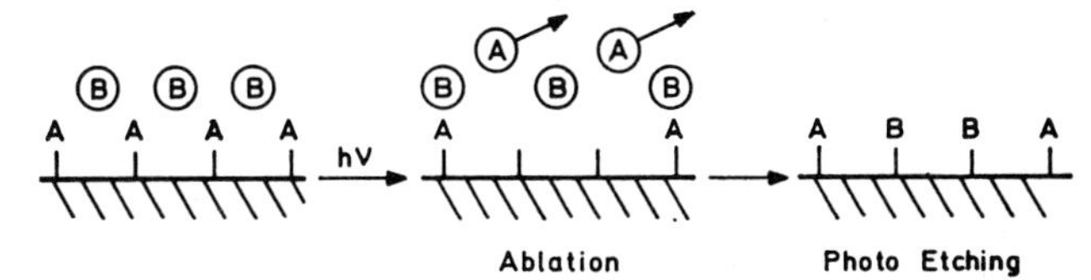


(1) Removal of surface material: Etching, polymer degradation. For example:

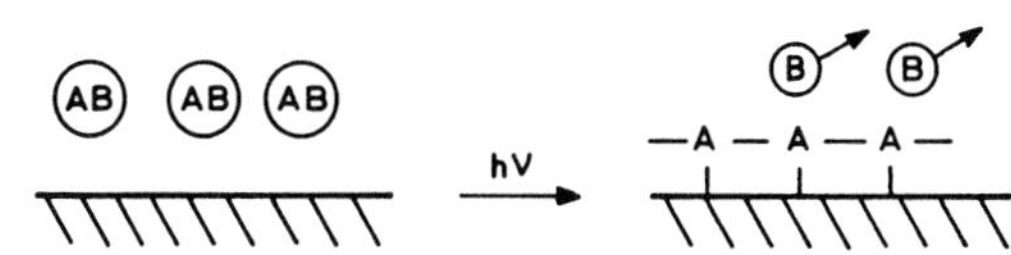


(II) Modification of surface structure/properties by chemical conversion of surface species. For example:

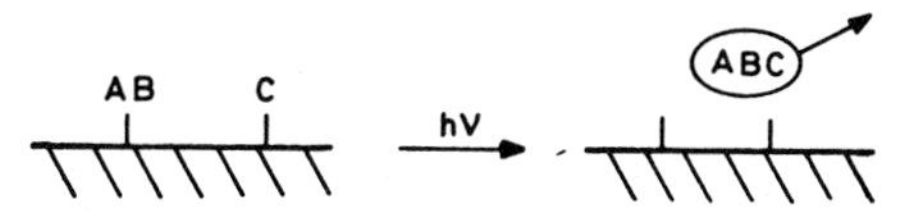


(III) Catalysis. For example:

Fig. 1b: Some types of laser surface photochemical processes (for details see text)

In laser thermal desorption substrate phonons are excited by pulsed laser interaction and as a result the surface temperature is raised with heating rates in the range of $10^8$-$10^{11}$ $Ks^{-1}$. Desorption occurs molecularly via energy transfer into the adsorbate-surface bond, with a characteristic translational temperature of the desorbed species. Since the pioneering study by Ertl and Neumann [1] on the adsorption systems $H_2$/Ni(100) and CO/Pd(111) in 1972 this method has been advanced considerably and among other applications can be used to detect transients from surface reactions. Very detailed insight into surface-molecule energy transfer can also be obtained by molecular beam scattering experiments where the (generally short) residence time of the molecules on the surface can be varied [2]. In contrast photochemical desorption by infrared lasers is accomplished by coupling laser energy resonantly into internal vibrations of adsorbates and condensates. Experiments were performed using the $CO_2$ laser frequency range which imposes some limitations on the choice of adsorption systems. First desorption of $SF_6$ by vibrationally exciting the $\upsilon_3$ mode - a process well known from the multitude of IR-multiphoton excitation studies on this molecule in the gas phase [3] - was carried out by Heidberg et al. [4]. Resonance and intensity dependence as well as the quantum yield of laser-induced desorption of $CH_3F$ from NaCl by multiphoton $CO_2$ laser excitation was determined by the same group [5]. A third system which was studied by Chuang et al.[6] concerns the desorption of $NH_3$ from Cu(100) by $CO_2$ laser excitation.

UV laser-induced desorption is initiated by nuclear displacement due to electronic excitation of the adsorbate-substrate complex into some higher state potential. Although this has been studied for a long time the general conclusion seems to be that the excitation rarely can remain localized in the excited complex and that desorption effects are mainly thermal in nature [7,8]. A new look at this subject may be taken again because of the variety of laser emission lines available now in the UV spectral range.

Related to this concept is the desorption of photo-ions reported for the first time by Letokhov et al. [9,10]. Here molecular ions are displaced from molecular crystals upon pulsed UV laser irradiation at $\lambda$ = 249, 308 and 337 nm while still retaining their chemical identity (see Fig. 1a (III)). The experiment was performed in a time of flight mass spectrometer and showed initial velocities of the desorbing ions up to 1 eV. Not only were molecular crystals employed but biomolecules deposited on metallic substrates were also studied. Among these molecules were five nucleic bases. Almost no fragmentation took place, a result very different from similar experiments in the gas phase. This phenomenon has strong interest as a potential method for the determination of molecular structures of macromolecules. A laser ion projection scheme was proposed. For a more detailed discussion of the results the reader is referred to [10].

In addition it should be noted that pulsed infrared lasers can also yield ions under certain conditions. Hess et al. [12] found laser induced isotopically selective ionization of methanol from thick layers of co-condensed isotopic mixtures.

This brief overview shows that indeed laser studies have just scratched the surface of desorption phenomena and more work can be expected in the near future. This situation also prevails for surface processes involving chemical changes of adsorbates to be discussed with regard to Fig. 1b.

Laser photo-deposition of reactive species has been used to chemically etch patterns on GaAs and InP [13] and Si and Ge [14]. Halogenated silicon surfaces by a variety of halogen donors ($XeF_2$, $Br_2$, $CH_3Cl$, $Cl_2$, $SF_6$) have been effectively etched. This work has recently been reviewed [15].

In this context surface activation and bond breaking in organic polymer films deserves mentioning. In such materials UV radiation is effectively absorbed in layers of less than 3000 Å. At low light intensity (i.e. with steady mercury lamps) the material is significantly removed only in the presence of oxygen (etching). At high light intensities, as from a UV excimer laser, ablative photodecomposition takes place and leads to spontaneous removal (opposite to oxidative etching) of material from the surface by a non-linear non-thermal process [16]. This may be looked upon as a photolithographic process without the need for development.

The light source of most interest here is the ArF excimer laser at 193 nm. Since the radiative lifetimes of polymer species are on the order of 0.1 ns bond breaking must occur on a timescale shorter than this if the process is considered to be photochemical rather than thermal. This is indeed the conclusion reached by the author [16] who reports on quantum yields of $\phi = 0.1 - 1.0$, again a surprising result. While no melting is observed at this wavelength some combination of photochemical and thermal ablation seems to exist at $\lambda = 248$ and 308 nm. Fig. 2 reproduces typical results.

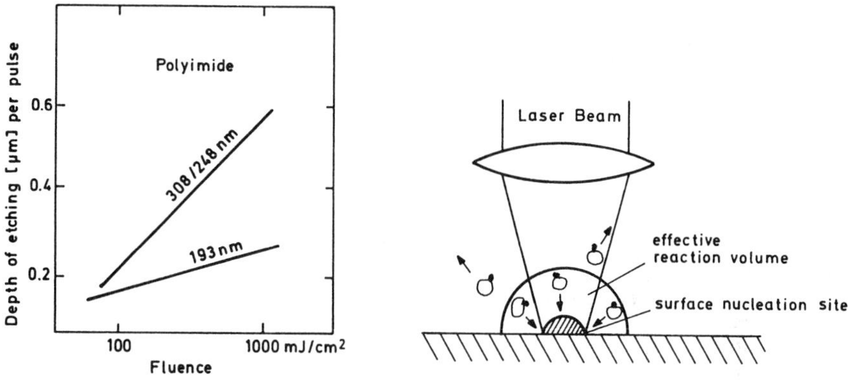


Fig. 2: Polymer ablation and dry etching due to UV laser radiation [16]

Fig. 3: Geometry of laser induced surface microreaction [18]

As to the second topic of Fig. 1b,we may look at three distinct subject areas namely metal deposition, surface oxidation and polymer coatings. UV-laser photodecomposition for metal deposition has been pioneered by Ehrlich, Osgood and Deutsch [17]. It has been shown that by the use of tightly focussed UV laser beams it is possible to excite highly localized microchemical reactions on surfaces. Both vapor/solid and liquid/solid interfaces may be considered for treatment. Direct writing in connection with semiconductors and insulators has been demonstrated with sub-μm spatial resolution. The spot size or line width may be controlled by the laser or the reaction characteristics (e.g. diffusion). The case of most interest here is the deposition starting with a volatile organometallic compound in contact with the surface according to the geometry shown in Fig. 3.

A two-step mechanism is often applicable to describe this process. The first step then is the decomposition of adsorbed organometallic molecules to form critical nuclei followed by gas phase partial fragmentation and completion of the fragmentation on these active surface sites. This is discussed for instance by Schröder et al. [19] in another paper at this conference for the case of platinum deposition. There is obviously a catalytic enhancement of the reaction rate on the small metal features initially formed. Other authors have also reported that both shiny metallic films as well as black particulate films were obtained depending on the deposition geometry [20]. Many different materials with good physical properties have been laser-deposited in this way with a look at applications in semiconductor processing [21]. Related to this concept is the work on laser pyrolysis at short wavelength to grow metal and insulator structures on various substrates. This was pioneered by Bäuerle et al. and is discussed in another chapter of this volume [22]. The formation of oxide films on surfaces can be accomplished by deposition of oxides in a way related to the metal deposition mentioned above [17,20] or by inducing an oxidation reaction in the first surface layer. Various laser types have been employed here as for instance a $CO_2$ laser for niobium oxidation [23], a Nd-glass laser for chromium oxide formation [24] or rare gas ion lasers for copper and cadmium oxide [25], to mention just a few examples.

The last example out of this group of laser applications aiming at a modification of surface properties has to do with polymer coatings and the initiation of polymerization by lasers. This is a research subject which may open very far reaching technical and scientific applications. It can, however, be discussed only very briefly here. While conventionally such polymerizations need a chemical initiator to start, lasers may open the possibility to avoid this admixture and activate the process by direct absorption in the monomer [26]. Not much work has been published in connection with surface coatings but the principle has been demonstrated [27].

A very important type of adsorbate photochemistry is connected to the concept of heterogeneous catalysis of chemical reactions. Lasers can aid here in particular in an improved mechanistic understanding by identifying and analysing intermediates and products. An illustrating example is provided by the work of Lin [28] on hydrogen/hydrocarbon oxidation on platinum looking at the product hydroxyl radical. However, lasers may also be used here as a synthetic tool to prepare reagents and increase reaction rates. Khmelev et al. [29] observed IR photon induced $NH_3$ decomposition on Pt and Umstead and Lin [30] observed on the same metal a sensitivity of catalytic conversion rates of formic acid HCOOH to $CH_2$ + $H_2$ and CO + $H_2O$ to the influence of $CO_2$ laser wavelengths. A strong effect was found on the resulting $[CO_2]/[CO]$ ratio. The mechanism remains uncertain, awaiting further experimental study. C.T. Lin et al. [31] studied the bimolecular reaction of $BCl_3$ with $H_2$ catalysed by titanium and initiated by a $CO_2$ laser. Isotopic selectivity was reported as function of the initiating laser line which could be used to enrich $^{11}BCl_3$ in the remaining unreacted gas. Also new compounds were produced. For a detailed discussion of the rather complex situation arising in such isotope separation experiments reference is made to [4]. Bass et al. [32] conclude that vibrationally excited $N_2O$ (001) exhibits a 5000 fold increase in reaction probability over $N_2O$ (000) when colliding with a copper surface at 363 K in the reaction $N_2O + Cu \rightarrow N_2 + CuO$. Again a detailed discussion of all the possible energy transfer and partitioning phenomena conceivable in the adsorbate-surface complex is not possible here. The authors point out that the vibrational mode excited (the $\upsilon_3$ mode) is indeed the one involved in breaking the N-O bond.

## Conclusion

What are the answers to the questions posed initially concerning the extension of laser chemistry to surface reactions? A general evaluation of molecule-surface interactions involving electronically excited states appears not to be possible at this point. As to other degrees of freedom vibrational non-equilibrium effects are seen in many systems. This points to chances for reaction kinetics with no complete equilibration between various adsorbates and between adsorbates and surface layers. Surely lasers can play an important role here. In addition the products of laser-driven surface interactions, e.g. laser CVD, appear to be of considerable interest for their material properties. A systematic perspective of this field, however, has not been reached yet.

## References


1 G. Ertl, M. Neumann: Z. Naturforschg. 27a, 1607 (1972)
2 W. Krieger, H. Walther in "Laser Applns. in Chem.", Eds.: K.L. Kompa, J. Wanner: Plenum Press, New York, London 1984 p. 215 and literature quoted therein
3 W. Fuß, K.L. Kompa: Progr. Quant. Electr. 7, 117 (1981)
4 J. Heidberg, H. Stein, A. Nestmann, E. Hoefs, I. Hussla in "Laser Solid Interactions and Laser Processing". AIP Conf. Proc. 50, Eds.: S.D. Faris, H.J. Leamy, J.M. Poate. For further discussion see also J. Heidberg et al. in "Surface Studies with Lasers", Eds.: F.R. Aussenegg, A. Leitner, M.E. Lippitsch: Springer Verlag, Berlin 1983, p. 226
5 J. Heidberg, H. Stein, E. Riehl: Phys. Rev. Lett. 49, 666 (1982)
6 I. Hussla, T.J. Chuang: to be published
7 R.S. Lichtman, D. Shapira: CRC Critical Rev. Solid State Mat. Sci. 8, 93 (1978)
8 P. Kronauer, D. Menzel in "Adsorption-Desorption Phenomena", Ed.: F. Ricca: Academic Press, New York 1972, p. 313
9 V.S. Antonov, V.S. Letokhov, A.N. Shibanov: Appl. Phys. 25, 71 (1971)
10 V.S. Antonov, V.S. Letokhov, A.N. Shibanov: Pisma Zh. Exp. Teor. Fiz. 31, 471 (1980)
11 V.S. Letokhov: this Volume
12 P. Hess in "Laser Applns. in Chem.", Eds.: K.L. Kompa, J. Wanner: Plenum Press, New York and London 1984, p. 207
13 D.J. Ehrlich, R.M. Osgood, T.F. Deutsch: Appl. Phys. Lett. 26, 916 (1980)
14 I.M. Beterov et al.: Sov. J. Quant. Electr. 8, 1310 (1978) L.L. Sveshnikova et al.: Sov. Phys. Techn. Phys. Lett. 3, 223 (1977)
15 T.J. Chuang: J. Vac. Sci. Technology 21, 798 (1982)
16 R. Srinivasan: J. Rad. Curing, October 1983, p. 12 see also R. Srinivasan, this volume
17 D.J. Ehrlich, R.M. Osgood, T.F. Deutsch: IEEE J. Quant. Electr. QE-16, 1233 (1980)
18 D.J. Ehrlich, J.Y. Tsao in "Laser Diagnostics and Photochem. Processing for Semicond. Devices", Eds.: R.M. Osgood, S.R.J. Brueck, H.R. Schlossberg: North Holland, New York 1983, p. 3
19 H. Schröder, I. Gianinoni, D. Masci, K.L. Kompa: this volume
20 P.K. Boyer et al.: Ref. 18, p. 119
21 I.W. Boyd: this volume T. Tokujama, S. Kimura, T. Warabisako, E. Murakami, K. Miyake: this volume
22 D. Bäuerle: Ref. 18, p. 19

23 R.F. Marks: J. Chem. Phys. 78, 4270 (1983)
24 S. Metev et al.: J. Phys. D 13, L 75 (1980)
25 R. Andrew et al.: Ref. 18, p. 283
26 I.N. Kalvina et al.: Sov. J. Quant. Electr. 4, 1285 (1975); A.P. Aleksandrov et al.: Sov. J. Quant. Electr. 7, 547 (1977)
27 R. Bussas, K.L. Kompa: to be published
28 L.D. Talley, W.A. Sanders, D.J. Bogan, M.C. Lin: J. Chem. Phys. 75, 3107 (1981)
29 Khmelev et al.: Sov. J. Quant. Electr. 7, 1302 (1977)
30 M.E. Umstead, M.C. Lin: J. Phys. Chem. 82, 2047 (1978)
31 C.T. Lin et al.: J. Appl. Phys. 48, 1720 (1977)
32 H.E. Bass, J. R. Fanchi: J. Chem. Phys. 64, 4417 (1976)

# Selective Laser-Induced Heterogeneous Chemistry on Surfaces

C.T. Lin

Instituto de Química, Universidade Estadual de Campinas
13100, Campinas, SP, Brazil

## 1. Introduction

The effects of laser radiation on the heterogeneous catalytic processes depend upon the nature of the surfaces, the electronic and vibrational structures of the adspecies/surface system, and the characteristics of the laser beam. Depending upon the chemical and physical states of the excited species, there are several ways in which laser radiation can influence the heterogeneous processes. In the past few years, at least three types of laser-stimulated surface processes have been reported: 1) laser excitation of reactants in the gas phase located in the volume above the surface. The laser radiation was used to overcome or compensate the reaction barrier, thus the rate of laser-catalyst chemistry was enhanced [1-3]; 2) Laser excitation of reactants adsorbed on a solid surface. Djidjoev et al.[4] showed that the actions of laser radiation on the adsorbed molecules, such as hydroxyl groups and amino groups $NH_2$ and NH on silica surfaces, are quite different from oven heating. The mechanisms of activation of heterogeneous reactions by laser radiation have been shown [5,6] theoretically to result from the stimulation of simultaneous electron-vibrational transitions in neighboring adsorbed groups, due for example, to electron transfer; and 3) Laser heating of substrate, i.e., a combination reaction of the pyrolytic (substrate heating) and photolytic (dissociation or excitation of the reactants) processes has been studied in laser-induced chemical vapor deposition [7], laser annealing [8], laser photochemical doping [9], laser-activated photooxidation [10] and laser-induced etching [11] with applications to microelectronics. The advantages of laser-activated processes over the conventional methods in the area of device fabrication for microelectronics and integrated optics are: i) the laser technique is a highly selective [12], dry and single step direct writing process; ii) the surface rate processes have been observed [13] to increase as much as $\geq 10^4$ times; and iii) the spatial resolution of the microscopic pattern achieved [13] was as small as $\simeq 1$ µm.

In this communication, we will describe two types of laser-induced heterogeneous chemistry on surfaces. First, surfaces act as a catalyst where the selective laser photochemistry is enhanced but the surfaces do not participate in the heterogeneous reactions as a reagent. Emphasis will be given to the effects of laser power density on the reaction pathway and dynamics. Second, surfaces are actually involved in the laser-induced heterogeneous reactions as reagents. In this case, the reaction intermediates and mechanisms on the surfaces will be detected and discussed.

## 2. Results and Discussions

### 2.1. Surfaces Act as a Catalyst

We studied the $CO_2$ laser-induced heterogeneous photochemistry of $BCl_3$ (20 torr) and $H_2$ (40 torr) on surfaces of Ti and Pb as catalysts. The experimental set-up is similar to that reported earlier [1]. A pulsed $CO_2$ laser ($\lambda = 10.55$ μm) beam is focussed into the reaction systems in a parallel fashion adjusted ~1 mm above the catalyst surfaces. Since the adsorption of $H_2$ on the Ti surface is a chemisorption process whereas that on the Pb surface is a physical adsorption, thus the effects of laser radiation on the adsorption strength of hydrogen on metals can be expressed as

$$H_2 + 2Pb \rightarrow H_2 \cdots\cdots 2Pb \xrightarrow{nh\nu} H_2^{**} + 2Pb \tag{1}$$

and

$$H_2 + 2Ti \rightarrow 2\,(H\text{-}Ti) \xrightarrow{nh\nu} H_2^{*} + 2Ti\,. \tag{2}$$

It was shown [6] that the selective laser-assisted bond breaking in a heterogeneous system is due to the surface-enhanced local field acting on the adspecies. The desorption rate, $P_D$, of the adspecies may be enhanced by laser-stimulated surface process as shown in the last step of equations (1) and (2). Since $P_D$ and local electric field ($E_{loc}$) are governed by $P_D \propto (E_{loc})^2$, then the desorption probability could be enhanced by a significant factor when $E_{loc}$ is increased due to the laser-initiated surface effects.

$CO_2$ laser multiphoton excitations and dissociations of $BCl_3$ have been studied by various researchers [14-16]. The effects of laser radiation on the $BCl_3$ molecules in the gaseous phase located in the volume above the surfaces give principally the excited $BCl_3$ or $BCl_2\cdot$ under our experimental conditions. Following the molecular transport equation, the laser excited species, $BCl_3^*$, can diffuse to the metal surface with a flux, $J_{iz}$, in moles cm$^{-2}$ sec$^{-1}$. It was demonstrated [17] that the specified molecules absorbing laser photons have a faster diffusive movement than those in the ground state.

Since the dependence on laser power density of $P_D$ ($H_2$) is quadratic whereas that of $J_{iz}$ ($BCl_3$) is linear, thus we will expect to have $J_{iz}$ ($BCl_3$) >> $P_D$ ($H_2$) for the low laser power density of $< 3 \times 10^6$ w/cm$^2$, likewise $P_D$ ($H_2$) >> $J_{iz}$ ($BCl_3$) for some high level of laser power ($> 1 \times 10^9$ w/cm$^2$). Figure 1 shows the experimental results for both power levels. The left-hand figure shows the observed (top) and computed (bottom) mass spectra of the $CO_2$ laser photochemistry of $BCl_3$ and $H_2$ using Ti and Pb as catalysts. The principle reaction products were identified [1] as $B_2H_2Cl_4$ and $B_2Cl_4$ for the systems of $BCl_3/H_2/Ti$ and $BCl_3/H_2/Pb$, respectively, i.e., the heterogeneous reaction occurred predominately at the metal surfaces. The right-hand diagram of Fig. 1 gives the IR spectra of the reaction products that resulted from the $CO_2$ laser photochemistry of both $BCl_3/H_2/Ti$ and $BCl_3/H_2/Pb$ under the laser power density of > 1 GW/cm$^2$. The new bands appeared at 880-920 cm$^{-1}$ ($\nu_5$, HBCl in-plane deformation), 1080-1110 cm$^{-1}$ ($\nu_4$, B-Cl asymmetric stretching) and 2617 cm$^{-1}$ ($\nu_2$, B-H stretching) are clearly identified to originate from $BHCl_2$ [18] which is similar to that observed in the surface free reaction of Rockwood and Hudson [19]. Moreover, the reaction yields ($\Phi$) of $BHCl_2$ at ~1 GW/cm$^2$ were found to have: i) $\Phi(BCl_3/H_2/Pb) \cong 1.5\,\Phi(BCl_3/H_2/Ti)$ and ii) $\Phi(BCl_3/H_2/Ti) \cong 2\Phi(BCl_3/H_2)$. The observation (i) is expected because the heat of

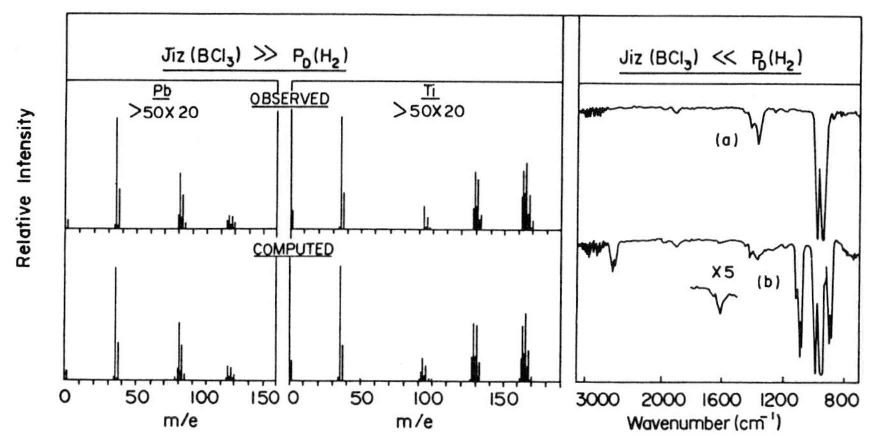


Fig. 1. Left: The observed (top) and simulated (bottom) mass spectra for the catalytic $CO_2$ laser photochemistry of $BCl_3$ (20 torr) and $H_2$ (40 torr) using Ti and Pb as catalysts with power density < 3 x $10^6$ w/cm$^2$. Right: IR spectra for the same laser catalytic reactions but with power density > 1 x $10^9$ w/cm$^2$.

adsorption for $H_2$ on Pb is smaller than that for $H_2$ on Ti, i.e., $P_D$ ($H_2$/Pb) > $P_D$ ($H_2$/Ti). The observation (ii) might be explained by the fact that $BCl_3^* + H_2^* \rightarrow BHCl_2 + HCl$ is energetically more favorable than that of $BCl_3^* + H_2 \rightarrow BHCl_2 + HCl$. This result provides direct evidence of the effects of a catalyst on the speed of laser photochemistry.

## 2.2. Surfaces Involved as Reagents

We studied the laser-induced photooxidation of niobium surfaces. The detailed experimental arrangements have been reported elsewhere [10]. We observed two distinct laser wavelength dependent mechanisms which give the $Nb_xO_y$ layers of different stoichiometry, thickness and film quality. Figure 2 shows the ESCA and electron microprobe spectra of the $Nb_xO_y$ distributions and the $Nb_2O_5$ thickness with respect to the number of laser pulses, $\lambda = 193$ nm (left) and $\lambda = 10.6$ µm (right). Since UV radiation (e.g., ArF laser: $\lambda = 193$ nm, KrF laser: $\lambda = 248$ nm and XeCl laser: $\lambda = 308$ nm) is highly absorbed [20] by Nb metal (absorptivity is ~60% at $\lambda = 308$ nm) and reflected by niobium oxide, the laser energy heats and melts the niobium surfaces, and oxygen diffuses into and reacts with the molten Nb metal. The resultant heating of the metal/oxide interface causes significant interdiffusion and formation of suboxide at the metal oxide interface (see the inserted XPS spectra in the left-hand diagram of Fig. 2). Moreover, the $Nb_2O_5$ thickness increases with respect to the number of laser pulses and a thickness of ≈1100 Å was obtained after 500 laser shots.

In contrast, IR radiation ($\lambda = 10.6$ µm) is highly reflected [20] by the niobium metal . The $CO_2$ laser pulse focussed upon the metal surface is absorbed by the oxide and initiates a plasma in the oxygen ambient which then further absorbs the IR laser pulses as the plasma intensifies. Reactive species in the plasma diffuse through the oxide layer, react with the niobium metal and produce a sharp metal/oxide interface with very low valence defect ($\delta$) of $Nb_2O_{5-\delta}$ [10] (see the inserted XPS spectra of the

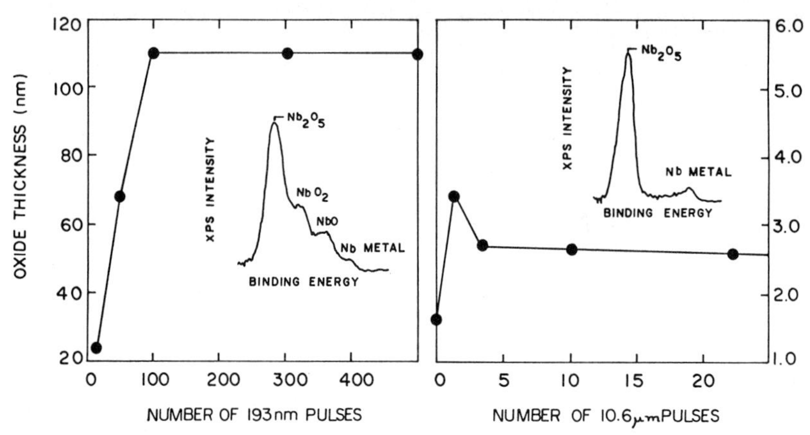


Fig. 2. Plots of the number of laser pulses and $Nb_2O_5$ thickness. Inserted diagrams: XPS spectra of the $Nb_xO_y$ distributions at two excitation wavelengths.

right-hand diagram of Fig. 2). One notes that the niobium metal in one atmosphere oxygen demonstrates a single-pulse, self-limiting oxide growth induced by the pulsed $CO_2$ laser.

In order to understand the reaction mechanisms of the laser-induced photooxidation of Nb surfaces, we recorded the yellow emissions that originated from the metal surfaces during the laser-activated oxidation of niobium foil. Figure 3 shows the observed emission spectra using $\lambda = 193$ nm excitation (top) and $\lambda = 10.6$ μm excitation (bottom). The top spectrum seems quite complicated at a first look, however, all observed spectral peaks can be assigned easily as NbO* emission by using the known literature data [21-22]. The spectral ranges of 420-520 nm are the vibronic transitions of $G(^4\Sigma^-) \rightarrow X(^4\Sigma^-)$ and F → X systems with origins at G(0,0) = 465 nm and F(0,0) = 484 nm. The spectral peaks, between 560 nm and 670 nm in Fig. 3, are the vibronic bands of B → X, C → X, D → X and E → X systems with origins at B(0,0) = 653 nm, C(0,0) = 641 nm, D(0,0) = 606 nm and E(0,0) = 658 nm, respectively. The vibronic bands that appear between 520 nm and 560 nm probably belong to the second blue system of NbO* with an origin at 547 nm. For 10.6 μm laser irradiation , the emission spectrum consists of some resolvable vibronic peaks ranged only from 420 nm to 520 nm. The frequency assignments show that the bottom spectrum of Fig. 3 corresponds well with the G → X and F → X systems of the top spectrum. However, it is found that the $G(^4\Sigma^-) \rightarrow X(^4\Sigma^-)$ emission system resulting from the $\lambda = 10.6$ μm irradiation has a Franck-Condon maximum built on the G(1,0) and G(0,1) but not on G(0,0), which is different from the ArF laser excitation in our experiment and also from the earlier literature reported [21-22].

The observed NbO* but not $NbO_2$* emission might suggest that it is the atomic oxygen and not the molecular oxygen that is active in the laser-induced photooxidation of niobium surfaces. To verify the above findings, we studied the effects of laser wavelengths and reagents on the film quality produced. $Nb_2O_5$ of 1100 Å thickness were obtained by the reaction of $O_2$ and Nb after 500 laser shots of ArF laser (~25 MW/cm$^2$). The individual oxide grain size decreased with increasing thickness. It remained, however, larger than 10 μm even for the thickest films of ~1500 Å. Better film quality (grain size and smoothness) was obtained by $\lambda = 193$ nm rather

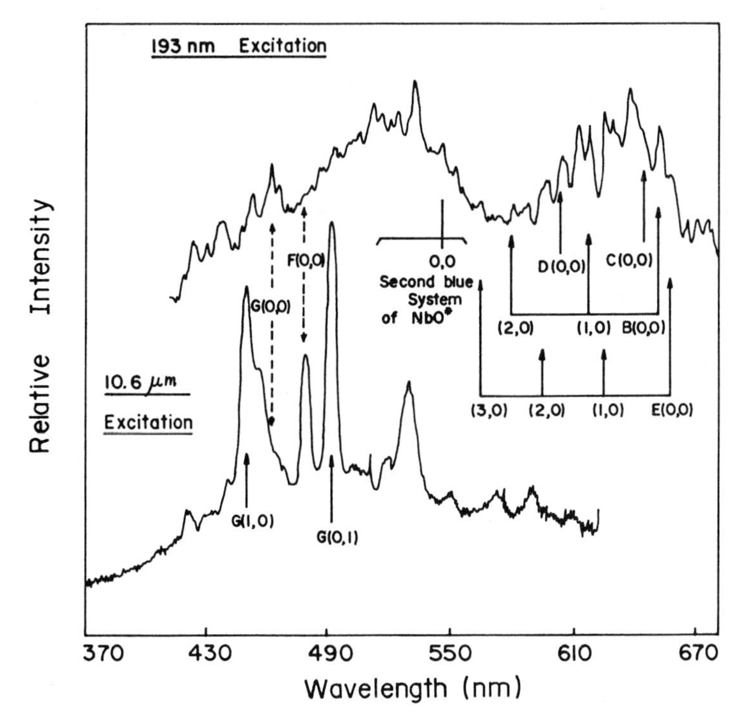


Fig. 3. Emission spectra of laser-initiated photooxidation of niobium surfaces. Top: UV excitation. Bottom: IR excitation.

than by $\lambda = 248$ nm irradiation. Better quality films at 248 nm were obtained by using $O_3$ (which absorbs the 248 nm light) instead of $O_2$ (which only absorbs the 193 nm light). These observations suggest that a photochemical component, perhaps the atomic oxygen in $^1D$ state, is the primary thermal chemistry.

## 3. Remarks

We have illustrated two types of selective laser-induced heterogeneous chemistry on surfaces. It is found that laser power density can be used to control the dynamics of the heterogeneous catalytic processes and alter their reaction paths. For laser-induced photooxidation of niobium, we showed that IR irradiation gives a thin (~50 Å), sharp interface oxide film which is essential for the preparation of $Nb/Nb_2O_5/Nb$ Josephson junctions. Emission and film quality studies suggest that the atomic oxygen but not molecular oxygen is predominately responsible for the laser-initiated photooxidation of niobium surfaces.

## Acknowledgments

The author thanks IBM Brasil and FAPESP for the financial support. The second part of this work was carried out in the IBM T.J. Watson Research Center.

References


1. C.T. Lin and T.D.Z. Atvars, J. Chem. Phys., 68, 4233 (1978).
2. M.E. Umstead and M.C. Lin, J. Phys. Chem., 82, 2047 (1978).
3. T.J. Chuang, J. Chem. Phys., 74, 1453 (1980).
4. M.S. Djidjoev et al.: in Tunable Lasers and Applications, Proceedings of the Loen Conference, Norway, 1976, edited by A. Mooradian, T. Taeger and P. Stokseth, Springer Series in Optical Sciences, Vol. 3, P. 100.
5. M.S. Slutsky and T.F. George, J. Chem. Phys., 70, 1231 (1979).
6. M.S. Dzhidzhoev, A.I. Osipov, V.Ya. Panchenko, V.T. Platonenko, R.V. Khokhlov and K.V. Shaitan, Sov. Phys. JETP, 47, 684 (1978).
7. T.F. Deutsch, D.J. Ehrlich and R.M. Osgood, Jr., Appl. Phys. Letters, 35, 175 (1979).
8. A. Gat, L. Gerzberg, T.F. Gibbons, T.J. Magee, J. Peng and J.D. Hong, Appl. Phys. Letters, 33, 775 (1978).
9. T.F. Deutsch, D.J. Ehrlich, R.M. Osgood, Jr. and Z.L. Lian, Appl. Phys. Lett., 36, 847 (1980).
10. R.F. Marks, R.A. Pollak, Ph. Avouris, C.T. Lin and Y.L. Thefaine, J. Chem. Phys., 78, part II, 4270 (1983).
11. D.J. Ehrlich, R.M. Osgood, Jr. and T.F. Deutsch, Appl. Phys. Lett., 38, 1081 (1981).
12. G.L. Loper, "UV Laser-induced radical-etching for microelectronic processing", SPIE meeting, Los Angeles, 1984.
13. D.J. Ehrlich, R.M. Osgood, Jr. and T.F. Deutsch, Appl. Phys. Lett., 36, 698 (1980).
14. N.V. Karlov, Appl. Opt., 13, 301 (1974).
15. R.V. Ambartzumian, N.V. Chekalin, V.S. Doljikov, V.S. Letokhov and E.A. Ryabov, Chem. Phys. Lett., 25, 515 (1974).
16. P.L. Houston, A.V. Nowak and J.I. Steinfeld, J. Chem. Phys., 58, 3373 (1973).
17. T. Arisawa, M. Kato and Y. Nasuse, Chem. Phys. Lett., 86, 91 (1982).
18. C.D. Bass, L. Lynds, T. Wolfram and R.E. DeWames, J. Chem. Phys., 40, 3611 (1964).
19. S.D. Rockwood and J.W. Hudson, Chem. Phys. Lett., 34, 542 (1975).
20. G.J. Sayag and A. Sepher, Thin Solid Films, 55, 191 (1978).
21. K.P. Huber and G. Herzberg, "Molecular Spectra and Molecular Structure, IV. Constants of Diatomic Molecules", Van Nostrand Reinhold Company, 1979, P. 446.
22. R.W.B. Pearse and A.G. Gaydon, "The Identification of Molecular Spectra", John Wiley & Sons, Inc., New York, 1976, Fourth Edition, P. 251.

# Spectroscopy of Adsorbates by Transient Laser Calorimetry

H. Coufal, T. J. Chuang, and F. Träger*

IBM Research Laboratory 5600 Cottle Road, K34/281
San Jose, California 95193 U.S.A.

The status of photothermal surface spectroscopy is reviewed. The importance of real time compensation techniques is underlined. Most recent results demonstrating sensitivities of hundredths of a monolayer of adsorbate are reported.

## 1. Introduction

In photothermal spectroscopy, the sample under investigation is excited with a modulated or pulsed light source [1-3]. Via radiationless decay part of the absorbed light is released in the sample as heat. With the incident energy being either modulated or pulsed the heat generation will also show a corresponding time dependence. Thermal waves are therefore generated and due to thermal expansion acoustic waves are induced. These waves can be detected with suitable transducers, such as pyro- or piezoelectric transducers. Only the *absorbed*, and *via* radiationless decay into heat converted fraction of the incident light energy contributes towards the photothermal signal. The fact that the absorbed energy is determined directly and not as the difference of incident and reflected or transmitted light energy makes photothermal techniques particularly suitable for weakly absorbing samples, such as adsorbates. Combined with laser excitation this detection method therefore offers a unique combination of advantages such as high sensitivity, high spectral resolution, high time resolution and instrumental simplicity.

For adsorbates on an ideal, not light absorbing substrate, be it a perfect mirror or a completely transparent substrate, the amount of adsorbate that is detectable is in principle limited only by the available light intensity: the incident light intensity has to be made large enough to generate a detectable increase in temperature in the sample. Nonlinear optical processes and even more so non-ideal substrates, reduce, however, the sensitivities obtainable in a typical experiment. The signal from a non-ideal substrate can be greatly suppressed by real time compensation techniques, making this technique applicable to many combinations of adsorbates and substrates in various environments. This detection method permits recording of vibrational or electronic spectra at coverages of a fraction of a monolayer under well-controlled UHV conditions, *in situ* in an electrolyte, at atmospheric conditions or under high pressure. Despite the complicated signal generation process involving optical and thermal, and in the case of acoustic detection even acoustic properties of the sample, these techniques offer many advantages over conventional surface analytical methods because of their sensitivity and simplicity and their time- and spectral resolution.

*Permanent address: Physikalisches Institut der Universität Heidelberg, Philosophenweg 12, D-6900 Heidelberg, Federal Republic of Germany.

## 2. Experiments and Results

### 2.1 Detector

In this report the experimental considerations to obtain high surface sensitivity and some recent results are presented. Ferroelectric ceramic or polymeric materials were used as transducer materials. Discs made from PZT 5A® or SONOX P51® ceramics with a diameter of 10 mm and a thickness of 1 mm, metallized on both sides and sealed around the perimeter with a glass film to prevent outgassing served as detectors in UHV experiments requiring high temperatures during bakeout or annealing. $PVF_2$ films (Pennwalt KYNAR®) with a thickness of 9 $\mu$m were employed in the most recent experiments [4,5]. These films were coated with an adhesion layer of Al and on top of that an Ag thin film electrode. Due to its organic nature this material can sustain only temperatures up to 100°C and is therefore only of limited use in UHV experiments. The excellent time resolution of the organic thin film detector - tens of nanoseconds have been achieved [4], as compared to typically microseconds for ceramic materials [2] - makes this material, however, a prime candidate for pulsed excitation or time resolved experiments.

Both types of materials can be used in a pyroelectric mode, detecting only the thermal wave, or in the piezoelectric mode, detecting sound waves. Thermal waves are critically damped diffusive waves, *i.e.*, within one wavelength the amplitude is attenuated by $e^{-2\pi}$. A typical value for the wavelength of a thermal wave with a frequency of 1 MHz is 1 $\mu$m [2]. A thermal wave detector has, therefore, to be in direct contact with the sample; a delay line will delay and at the same time also attenuate the signal appreciably. Sound waves of the same frequency have wavelengths in the order of mm and are basically unattenuated. Taking the acoustic impedance of various materials into account transmission lines can, therefore, be utilized to couple the sound wave from the sample, where it is generated, over a long distance to a detector. Sample and detector can be separated in this detection mode and can be at different temperatures, pressures, *etc.* Furthermore the transmission line introduces a time delay between excitation and detection, allowing to distinguish between electromagnetic interference during the excitation, which propagates with the velocity of light, and the acoustic signal. A purely thermal detector is insensitive to acoustic noise and vibrations. No mechanical resonances occur and therefore a ringing free signal is observed. In addition a thermal detector can easily be calibrated in absolute units using conventional calorimetry. These virtues of the pyroelectric detector [4] make it an interesting alternative to piezoelectric detection. In both detection modes the sample under study is a thin film deposited on a substrate. In the pyroelectric mode the detector itself serves as substrate, whereas in the piezoelectric mode the substrate is for example a sapphire rod used as a transmission line to the detector.

The sample under study was mounted in an UHV system ($1 \times 10^{-10}$ Torr) equipped with an ESCA-Auger spectrometer or a quartz microbalance to determine the amount of surface coverage. Simultaneous photoacoustic and X-ray photoemission or microbalance measurements allow after a suitable calibration to evaluate the photoacoustic signal as a function of surface coverage.

### 2.2 CW Excitation

CW $CO_2$-lasers line-tunable in the infrared spectral region between 9 and 11 $\mu$m with an output power in the order of 1 W were used to excite vibrational transitions of adsorbed molecules. The unfocused beam was incident at 80° from the surface normal and covered the entire sample area about 7 mm in diameter. The light beam was intensity modulated at frequencies of typically 10 Hz. The signal was detected by two-phase lock-in analyzers (EG&G 5206). Without employing signal averaging techniques a sensitivity corresponding to a surface coverage of 0.002 of a monolayer of $SF_6$ on silver was achieved. That high a sensitivity can be readily obtained for nonabsorbing, highly reflecting or transparent substrates using a *stabilized laser* of sufficient output power. Time-dependent phenomena like the adsorption/desorption cycle of $SF_6$ on silver [6] or the adsorption of $NH_3$ [7] were readily observed. In addition, vibrational spectra from submonolayer to multilayer coverages have been obtained; they indicate distinctive adsorbate-substrate interactions and a nonlinear relation between PA signal and coverage.

### 2.3 Pulsed Excitation

For pulsed excitation and highly time resolved studies an Excimer laser pumped dye laser system (Lambdaphysik EMG 201, FL 2002) and suitable transient digitizers (Dataprecision D6000, Tektronix 7912) were employed. The laser system provided pulses with up to 60 mJ pulse energy at 12 ns half width, tunable over the wave length range 575 nm - 605 nm. A Raman cell is being prepared to shift this output into the IR. For the time being only electronic spectra of $Nd_2O_3$ in the wavelength domain covered by the existing system can be reported [4]. As shown in Fig. 1 for a sample containing $0.8\times10^{15}$ $Nd_2O_3$ molecules isolated in a 10-$\mu$m-thick poly(methyl methacrylate) matrix, corresponding approximately to a one monolayer coverage of $Nd^{3+}$-ions, a spectrum can be obtained at a sensitivity of hundredths of a monolayer with the existing system.

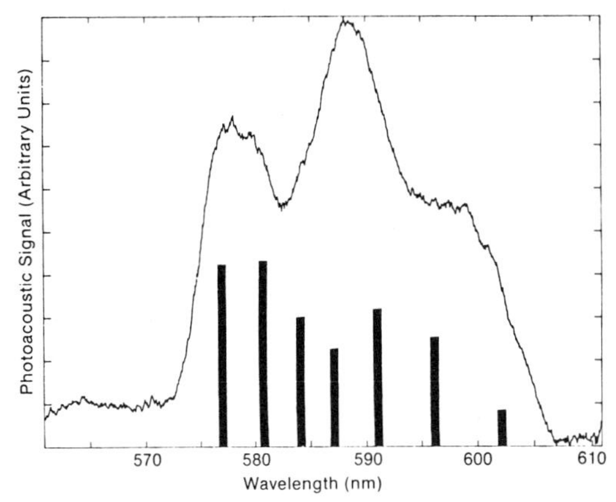


Fig. 1: Photothermal absorption spectrum of $0.8\times10^{15}$ $Nd_2O_3$ molecules isolated in a 10 $\mu$m thick PMMA matrix.

### 2.4 Compensation Techniques

With absorbing substrates, and at a high enough sensitivity every substrate starts to absorb an appreciable fraction of the incident light intensity, a background signal due to the substrate is superimposed on the signal originating from the material on the surface. Fluctuations of the incident light intensity translates then directly into fluctuations of the background signal,*i.e.*, noise. This effect limits the detection of adsorbed species on the surface of a light absorbing substrate. This background problem cannot be overcome by electronic techniques like zero suppression. If one, however, could suppress this background signal the detection sensitivity could be largely enhanced or an unstabilized light source could be used.

We have, therefore, explored a new scheme of general applicability which permits almost complete background suppression for a large variety of experimental purposes [8]. It has been shown [9] to permit ultrahigh sensitive photoacoustic probing (0.002 of a monolayer) of adsorbate materials on light absorbing substrates. Substrate and adsorbate are excited by a suitable modulated light source thus generating a thermal wave; a second source with an appropriate amplitude and phase is used to generate a thermal wave with an amplitude identical to that one due to the substrate but with a 180° phase shift. This second thermal wave adds to the first thermal wave. Contributions due to the substrate therefore result in a DC heating of the sample and cannot contribute to the AC signal detected by a lock-in amplifier. The thermal wave due to the adsorbate, however, still causes an AC signal which is no longer buried by the background originated from the substrate. Amplitude and phase adjustment of the compensation source is achieved by zeroing the signal of the uncovered substrate.

In the pulsed mode another approach proved successful. It is not possible to generate heat pulses with different polarities. It is, however, no problem to generate two identical heat pulses in two identical samples and detect them with two pyroelectric detectors with opposing polarizations, but otherwise identical properties. The electric signals from both detectors have identical amplitude and pulse shape, but different polarities. Both signals cancel and the difference signal is zero. If this symmetry is disturbed, for example, by a thin film on one of the substrates, a net signal is observed.

Several versions of this compensation scheme have been tested successfully illustrating that the scheme can be realized in many different ways to achieve the same goal, *e.g.*, by applying a single light beam or in a two-beam arrangement. In addition, different physical principles can be used to generate a second heat source.

In the first one an adsorbate on a metallic substrate was studied. A particular surface property was used here: the difference in absorption between s- and p-polarized light is different for the substrate and the adsorbate. Therefore, by illuminating the substrate with alternating polarizations (*i.e.*, s- and p-polarized light waves phase shifted by 180°) the relative amplitude of the electric field vector for the two polarizations was adjusted in such a way as to obtain a zero substrate signal. With the intensities for s- and p-polarization being different, this results in an overall intensity modulation which causes a photoacoustic signal originating only from the adsorbate layer. Figure 2 shows the

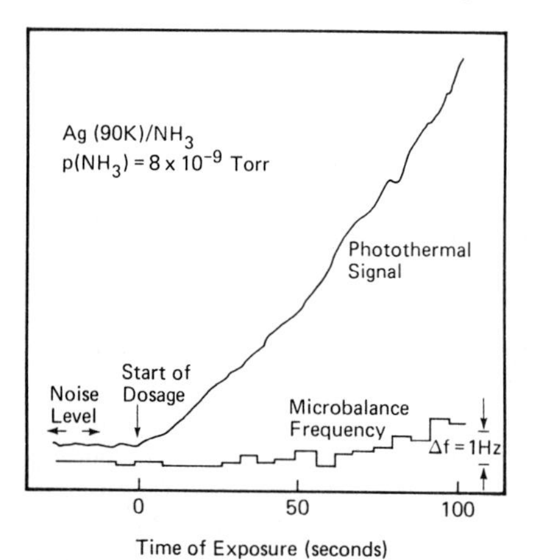


Fig. 2: Photothermal signal and microbalance read out as a function of time as ammonia molecules are slowly adsorbed on the cold silver substrate. A 1 Hz change in the microbalance reading corresponds to a coverage of 0.7 monolayers.

photothermal signal as a function of time as ammonia molecules are slowly adsorbed on a silver substrate at 90 K. The *unstabilized* CW $CO_2$ laser is tuned to a wavelength of 9.30 $\mu$m, corresponding to the $\nu_2$ mode of $NH_3$. The laser power at the sample is approximately 1 W. Simultaneously the microbalance reading is recorded. The ammonia partial pressure in the system is $8 \times 10^{-9}$ Torr during the dosage. The maximum coverage as determined from the change in the frequency of the microbalance and independently from partial pressure and sticking probability is 0.8 of a monolayer. From the signal to noise ratio a sensitivity of a few thousandths of one monolayer is estimated.

In another experiment the thermal wave due to the substrate was cancelled by a second thermal wave generated at the backside of the sample with a suitable amplitude and phase shift to achieve zero substrate signal. The thermal wave from the adsorbate on the front side, however, is not cancelled and causes a photoacoustic signal. Using the same laser to excite both thermal waves eliminates long term drifts efficiently and therefore lowers the requirements for laser stabilization. Using two lightsources with different wavelengths [10] does not have this advantage but instead allows to take advantage of differences in the absorption of substrate and adsorbate and to measure deposition rates differentially. Preliminary experiments on conducting substrates showed that instead of undergoing the formidable task of stabilizing a laser, essentially the same sensitivity can be achieved by resistance heating of the substrate. The phase of the current and the gain of the feed back loop is adjusted prior to the adsorption; during the exposure the fluctuations of the laser are compensated efficiently by the feed back loop.

## 3. Conclusion

In conclusion, the feasibility of photothermal spectroscopy at submonolayer coverages and under ultrahigh vacuum conditions has been demonstrated. It has been shown that these sensitivities can be obtained with CW or pulsed excitation. This new surface analytical technique, alone or in combination with the compensation schemes that are under further development, is not only able to provide important information at high sensitivity and spectral resolution but should also have a high potential for applications to chemical systems in various environments, whether in vacuum or not.

## 4. Acknowledgments

The authors would like to thank J. Goita, R. Grygier, L. Kelley and L. W. Welsh, Jr. for technical assistance. This work was supported in part by the Office of Naval Research.

## 5. References

[1] Y.-H. Pao, *Optoacoustic Spectroscopy and Detection* (Academic Press, New York, 1977).
[2] A. Rosencwaig, *Photoacoustics and Photoacoustic Spectroscopy*, (Wiley, New York, 1980).
[3] A. C. Tam, in *Ultrasensitive Spectroscopic Techniques*, edited by D. Kliger (Academic Press, New York, 1983).
[4] H. Coufal, *Appl. Phys. Lett.* **44**, 59 (1984).
[5] H. Coufal, *Appl. Phys. Lett.*, to be published.
[6] F. Träger, H. Coufal, and T. J. Chuang, *Phys. Rev. Lett.* **49**, 1720 (1982).
[7] T. J. Chuang, H. Coufal, and F. Träger, *J. Vac. Sci. Technol.* **A1**, 1236 (1983).
[8] H. Coufal, T. J. Tuang, and F. Träger, *J. Physique Colloque* **C6** 297 (1983).
[9] H. Coufal, T. J. Chuang, and F. Träger, *Surf. Sci.*, to be published.
[10] H. Coufal and J. Pacansky, *IBM Tech. Disclosure Bull.* **22**, 4681 (1980).

# Laser Vaporization of Clean and CO-Covered Polycrystalline Copper Surfaces

R. Viswanathan* and Ingo Hussla**

Department of Chemistry, Northwestern University,
Evanston, Illinois 60201, U.S.A.

Data and results of experiments on the ablation of clean and CO-covered polycrystalline copper surfaces by 248 nm KrF excimer laser pulses of moderate peak power densities (300 MW/cm$^2$ – 1 GW/cm$^2$) are presented. Temperatures of the vaporized copper species were determined from velocity distributions obtained by real time resolved quadrupole mass spectrometry. It was found that the temperatures of neutral copper species (22000 K – 27000 K) in the vapor were significantly higher than the boiling point of copper (2855 K), even near the vaporization threshold for clean polycrystalline copper (300 MW/cm$^2$). Submonolayer coverages of CO on the copper surfaces caused a significant increase in the vaporization threshold absorbed laser power density (> 400 MW/cm$^2$).

## 1. Introduction

Surface ablation effects are of interest in the context of processes occurring in Laser-Induced Thermal Desorption (LITD) [1-4], which has emerged as a new tool in the study of desorption dynamics and chemical reactions at surfaces. Etching of semiconductor, ceramic and metal surfaces by pulsed laser beams has been shown to have potential applications in the preparation of electronic circuitry in integrated circuits [5]. This paper describes an extension of the time-resolved quadrupole mass spectrometric technique used in LITD to a study of laser-induced vaporization processes. Specifically, results of experiments involving pulsed UV laser vaporization of clean and CO-covered polycrystalline copper under controlled conditions in ultra high vacuum are presented and discussed in the context of models developed for the description of laser vaporization phenomena [4,6-8].

## 2. Experimental

Figure 1 is a schematic diagram of the apparatus [9] used in our experiments. A focussed pulsed KrF excimer laser beam (15 ns FWHM, 248 nm maximum single pulse energy=250 mJ, Lambda Physics EMG 101) was utilized to vaporize the copper surface. The intensity profile of the laser beam was mapped using a photodiode array and was found to be uniform within 5% over the entire cross-sectional area [9]. A laser-in arrangement was utilized to avoid spurious effects due to light scattering within the chamber. The experiments were carried out with the copper sample cooled to 90 K. Copper species, formed in the vapor phase by surface ablation, were detected in real time by a UTI-100C quadrupole mass spectrometer equipped with a custom-designed fast electrometer amplifier (rise time=3 $\mu$s). The amplified signal was digitized and stored by a high speed (100 MHz) digitizer (Biomation 8100) interfaced to a signal averager

*Present address: Department of Chemistry, Beloit College, Beloit, Wisconsin 53511, U.S.A.

**Present address: IBM Research Laboratory San Jose, California 95193 U.S.A.

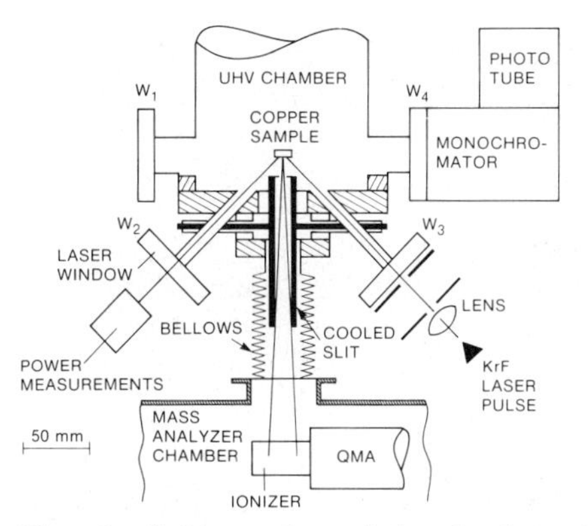


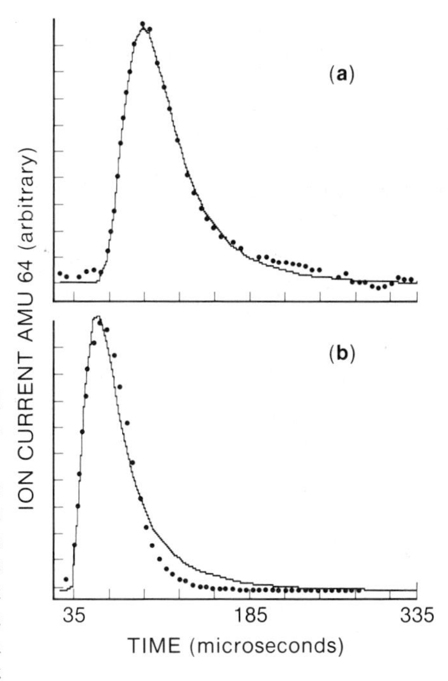


**Fig. 1 (left).** Laser-induced thermal desorption apparatus with fluorescence detection. Further details see [9].

**Fig. 2 (right).** Time-resolved mass spectrometric signal of copper species (amu 64) ablated from a polycrystal Cu surface by the KrF laser pulse. Points are the actual data, while the solid line is the least squares fit signal shape obtained from a fit of the data to a Maxwell-Boltzmann distribution. (a) Neutral copper emission at 300 MW/cm$^2$ absorbed laser power; (b) Cu(+1) ions, detected at 550 MW/cm$^2$ absorbed laser power with the electron impact ionizer switched off.

(Nicolet 1170). The time-of-flight (TOF) distance from the surface to the mass spectrometer was 218 mm, the detection angle being coincident with the surface normal. Copper species ablated from the surface were also detected by monitoring the characteristic fluorescence from excited electronic states (centered in the green region of the visible spectrum) using a photomultiplier (RCA 1P28) and grating monochromator (Jobin Yvon) arrangement placed next to the window W4 (Fig. 1). A detailed description of the apparatus and technique will be presented in a forthcoming paper [9].

## 3. Results

Surface ablation of clean polycrystalline copper surfaces occurs at absorbed laser power densities greater than 300 MW/cm$^2$, as indicated by the detection of neutral copper species (amu 64) by the mass spectrometer. A typical time-resolved signal is shown in Fig. 2a. Scanning Electron Microscope pictures of the copper surfaces before and after exposure to excimer laser pulses are reproduced in Figs. 3a and 3b. At higher laser power densities (550 MW/cm$^2$) two distinct peaks appear in the TOF spectrum. The two peaks are assigned to copper (+1) and copper neutral species respectively. In order to confirm this assignment, the TOF peak times were compared with the single peak TOF time for copper (+1) ions obtained after switching the electron impact ionizer of the mass spectrometer off, with the absorbed laser power density remaining unchanged (Fig. 2b). The temporal intensity distributions for the various copper species obtained from the TOF spectra were fitted to a Maxwell-Boltzmann distribution [9,10]. The translational

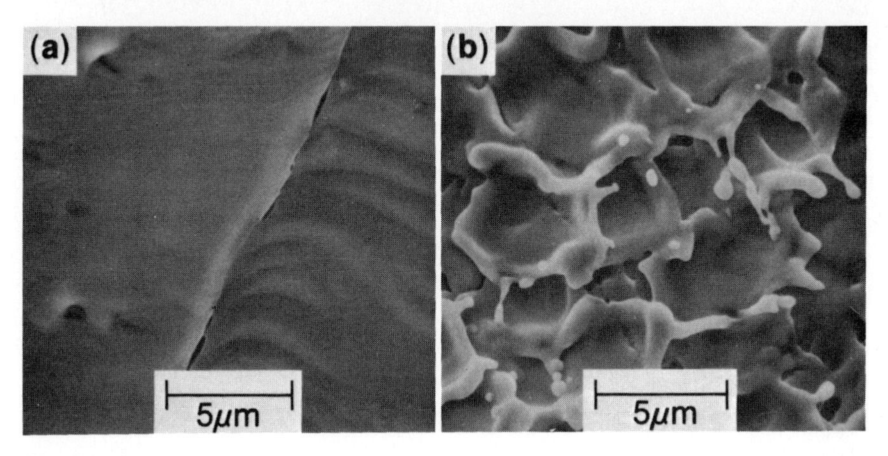


**Fig. 3** . Scanning electron micrographs of a polycrystalline copper surface. (a) Before exposure to KrF excimer laser pulse; (b) after exposure to a single laser pulse with peak absorbed power density ≈300 MW/cm$^2$ [17].

temperatures obtained from the fit of data at different absorbed laser power densities range from 22000 (1000) K at 300 MW/cm$^2$ to 27000 (1500) K at 550 MW/cm$^2$ for neutral copper species. The ionized copper (+1) species at 550 MW/cm$^2$ has a much higher temperature of approximately 81000 (4000) K, or about 7 eV. Copper dimer and trimer species were also detected at the appropriate mass peaks. The threshold for dimer formation was approximately 360 MW/cm$^2$. The ratio Cu:$Cu_2$:$Cu_3$ changes from 100:12:1 at 500 MW/cm$^2$ to 100:3:0 at 1 GW/cm$^2$. No ionized dimer and trimer and no multiply ionized copper monomer species were detected over the absorbed laser power density range (300 MW/cm$^2$ – 1 GW/cm$^2$) at which the experiments were carried out.

The vaporization of copper surfaces with a saturation coverage of CO at 90 K was also studied as a function of the absorbed laser power density. Figure 4a shows the LITD time-resolved signal of CO from Cu(100) at a low laser power density of 44 MW/cm$^2$. At low laser power densities (10–50 MW/cm$^2$), both single crystal and polycrystalline copper surfaces show no evidence of surface damage or reconstruction and only the normal LITD signal of desorbed CO (with translational temperatures in the region of 300 K) is obtained [1]. However, in the present work, performed at power densities greater than 300 MW/cm$^2$, a second very energetic CO species (Peak I, Fig. 4b) was also detected, in addition to the normal CO desorption (peak II, Fig. 4b). A similar effect has been observed in the case of CO desorbed from tungsten using a Q-switched pulsed ruby laser [11]. The characteristic neutral copper TOF spectrum (detected at amu 64) appeared only at absorbed laser power densities greater than 400 MW/cm$^2$, indicating that this was the vaporization threshold for CO-covered polycrystalline copper surfaces. Interestingly, the normal CO desorption peak disappeared at laser power densities greater than 400 MW/cm$^2$ (Fig. 4c), with only a peak corresponding to the very fast CO desorption being observed. Thus, it appears that even sub-monolayer coverages of CO molecules on the copper surface cause a significant change in the ablation properties of the surface, the specific effect in this case being to raise the absorbed laser power density threshold for vaporization.

Figure 5 shows a typical low resolution optical emission spectrum of copper species in the vapor phase obtained at very high absorbed laser power densities (>600 MW/cm$^2$). The spectrum is complex and consists of a number of discrete lines, with a cluster centered

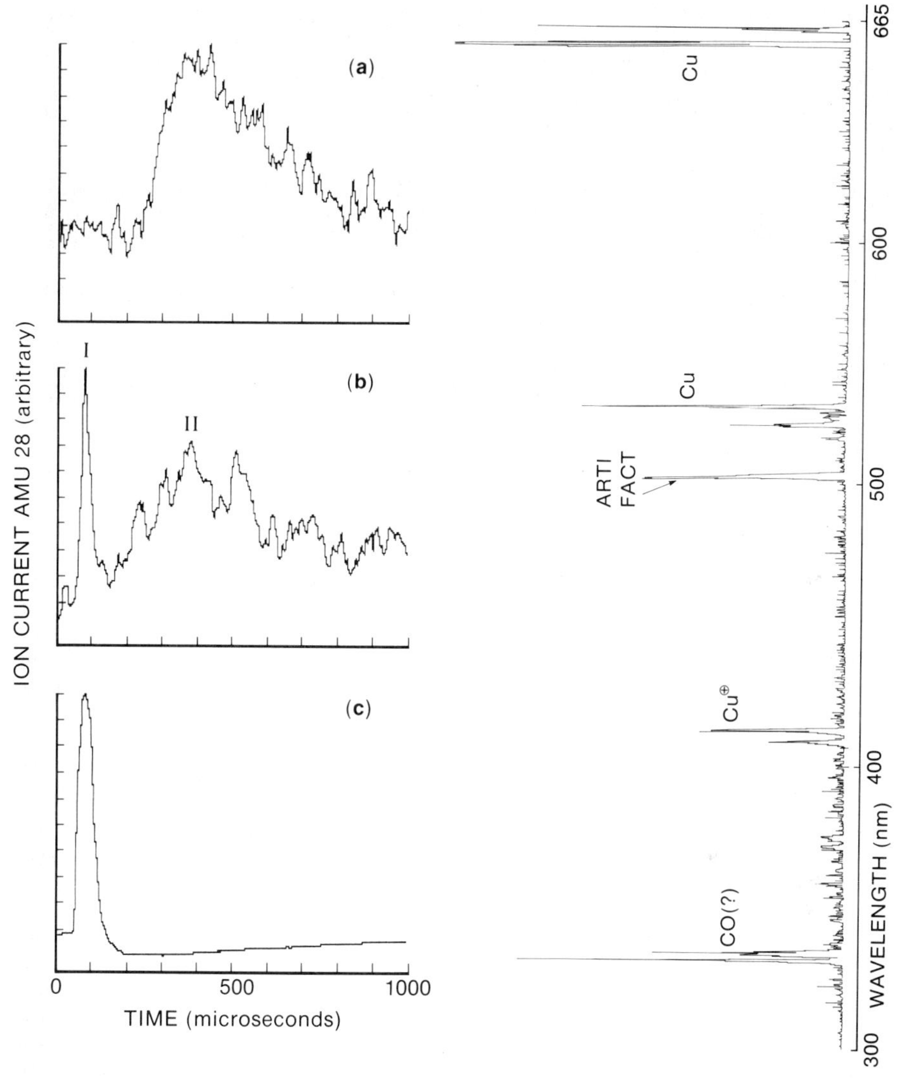


**Fig. 4 (left).** Time-resolved mass spectrometric signal of CO species removed from CO-covered copper surfaces by KrF excimer laser pulses as a function of absorbed laser power density. (a) LITD desorption signal obtained at 44 MW/cm$^2$; (b) Desorption signal obtained at 350 MW/cm$^2$; (c) Desorption signal obtained at 550 MW/cm$^2$.

**Fig. 5 (right).** Low resolution optical emission spectrum of copper species in the vapor phase after laser-induced ablation from a polycrystalline copper surface cover with CO at an absorbed laser power density of 600 MW/cm$^2$. Band assignment after [18]; transition at 504 nm is an artifact caused by the monochromator. Abscissa expanded from 600 to 665 nm.

in the green region of the visible spectrum. A preliminary analysis of the spectrum indicates that the lines may mainly arise from Cu neutral and Cu(+1) states of the copper species [18] and that transitions from the higher ionization states are not present in accordance with the mass spectroscopic findings reported here.

## 4. Discussion

The quadrupole mass spectrometer utilized in our experiments is a true mass filter and detects species of one particular charge-to-mass ratio, regardless of their momenta. The temporal distribution of the species detected by the spectrometer represents the true velocity distribution and enables accurate calculation of translational temperatures of the vaporized species. We believe that the excellent fits (see Fig. 2a) of the time-resolved signals to a Maxwell-Boltzmann distribution, especially in the absorbed laser power density range in the vicinity of the threshold for vaporization (300 $MW/cm^2$ – 400 $MW/cm^2$) yield correct values for the translational temperature of the neutral copper species in the vapor. It is interesting to note that these temperatures (22000 K – 27000 K) are much higher than the normal boiling point of copper (2855 K). This is in qualitative agreement with models [7,8,12] for laser vaporization which use a temperature at the moving boundary between the vapor and solid interface that is higher than the ordinary vaporization temperature. Such models predict temperatures substantially larger than the boiling point for the vaporized species, especially at laser flux densities such as those employed in the present work. The least squares fit for Cu(+1) ions (see Fig. 2b) is not very good, the normalized width [1] being 1.11 as opposed to 1.0 for a Maxwell-Boltzmann distribution. However, it must be noted that the fit is better than in the case of velocity distributions of ions obtained by conventional TOF mass spectrometric techniques [13]. Since the present experiments were performed in a uhv chamber [9] specifically designed to eliminate spurious wall desorption effects due to laser light scattering and the possibility of plasma-induced desorption [14] in the mass spectrometer housing, we believe that temperatures for copper species obtained from our data are good estimates of the true thermal energies.

The SEM photograph of the copper surface after vaporization has occurred (Fig. 3b) shows that the surface is roughened in a uniform fashion after exposure to the excimer laser pulses. This effect may be of some importance in surface enhanced Raman spectroscopic studies [15] carried out in ultra high vacuum, since it provides an in situ method of roughening a specific small position of the surface by exposing it to a laser pulse. It is also interesting to note that there is no evidence of surface annealing after vaporization, presumably because of the ultra-fast cooling, which is estimated to be of the same order of magnitude as the heating rate of approximately $10^{10}$ K/s.

Excimer laser-induced ablation of metal surfaces is a much more efficient process than ablation of metal surfaces using infrared lasers, *e.g.*, $CO_2$ lasers. This is primarily because of the enhanced light absorptivity of metals in the ultra-violet, as opposed to their high reflectivities in the infrared [6,16]. In addition, the comparatively short pulse width (15 ns FWHM) of the excimer laser ensures that any ablation effects are constrained to regions in the vicinity of the surface [4]. We have demonstrated that excimer laser-induced ablation of a copper surface can be carried out at moderate peak absorbed laser power densities, easily obtainable with an excimer laser that typically has a single pulse energy of 250 mJ.

Finally, we would like to point out that the significant change in threshold for vaporization from 300 $MW/cm^2$ to 400 $MW/cm^2$ which results when the clean copper surface is covered with a saturation (submonolayer) coverage of CO indicates that surface cleanliness may be an important factor in laser surface processing techniques such as those that are being presently developed in the semiconductor industry [5,19].

Acknowledgments

We would like to thank the Office of Naval Research for support of this work under ONR contract No. N00014-79-C-0794. One of us (I.H.) would like to thank the Deutsche Forschungsgemeinschaft for granting fellowship Hu 339/1-1. We are thankful to Professor Eric Weitz and Professor Peter Stair for providing laser and ultra high vacuum facilities. Thanks to D. R. Burgess, Jr. for friendly help.

References

1. D. R. Burgess, Jr., R. Viswanathan, I. Hussla, P. C. Stair, and E. Weitz, *J. Chem. Phys.* **79**, 5200 (1983).
2. G. Wedler and H. Ruhmann, *Surf. Sci.* **121**, 464 (1982).
3. G. Ertl and M. Neumann, *Z. Naturforsch.* **279**, 1607 (1972).
4. J. F. Ready, *Effects of High Power Laser Radiation*, Academic Press, New York (1971).
5. T. J. Chuang, *Surf. Sci. Reports* **3**, 1 (1983); T. J. Chuang, *J. Vac. Sci. Technol.* **21**, 798 (1982).
6. N. Bloembergen in "Symposium Laser-Solid Interaction and Laser Processing - 1978," p. 1, S. D. Ferris, H. J. Leamy, and J. M. Poate, eds., *American Institute of Physics Conference Proceedings No. 50*, New York (1979).
7. A. K. Jain, V. N. Kulkarni, and D. K. Sood, *Appl. Phys.* **25**, 127 (1981).
8. S. I. Anisimov, *Zh. Tekh. Fiz.* **36**, 1273 (1966); English Transl.: *Sov. Phys.-Tech. Phys.* **11**, 965 (1967).
9. I. Hussla, R. Viswanathan, D. R. Burgess, Jr., P. C. Stair, and E. Weitz, *Rev. Sci. Instrum.*, submitted for publication (April 1984).
10. D. R. Burgess, Jr., unpublished work.
11. L. P. Levine, J. F. Ready, and E. Bernal, *IEEE J. Quantum Electron.* **QE-4**, 18 (1968).
12. See Ref. 4., Chapter 3.
13. E. Bernal, J. F. Ready, and L. P. Levine, *IEEE J. Quantum Electron.* **QE-2**, 480 (1966).
14. S. E. Egorov, V. S. Letokhov, and A. N. Shibanov, in "Surface Studies with Lasers," *Springer Series in Chemical Physics* **33**, F. R. Aussenegg, A. Leitner, and M. E. Lippitsch, eds., Springer-Verlag, New York (1983), p. 156.
15. See, *e.g.*, H. Seki, *J. Chem. Phys.* **76**, 4412 (1982). J. F. Evans, M. Grant, A. Albrecht, D. M. Ullevic, and R. M. Hexter, *J. Electroanal. Chem.* **106**, 209 (1980). P. F. Liao, J. G. Bergmann, D. S. Chemla, A. Wokaun, J. Melngailis, A. M. Hawryluk, and N. P. Economou, *Chem. Phys. Rev.* **82**, 355 (1981).
16. H. Ehrenreich and H. R. Philipp, *Phys. Rev.* **128**, 1622 (1962).
17. I. Hussla and R. Viswanathan, *Surf. Sci.*, **144**(1984), in press.
18. National Bureau of Standards, Spectral Tables in *Monograph* **53**, 1963.
19. T. J. Chuang, I. Hussla, and W. Sesselmann, these proceedings.

# Laser Investigation of the Dynamics of Molecule-Surface Interactions

J. Häger[1], Y.R. Shen[1*], and H. Walther[1,2]

[1]Max-Planck-Institut für Quantenoptik, D-8046 Garching, Fed. Rep. of Germany

[2]Sektion Physik der Universität München
D-8046 Garching, Fed. Rep. of Germany

## 1. Introduction

In the past decade the interest in the dynamics of the interaction between molecules and clean and well-characterized solid-state surfaces has steadily increased [1]. Most information has been obtained from angular and velocity distribution measurements in surface scattering experiments, giving a complete insight into the dynamics only where atoms are involved. For molecules, however, it is necessary to have additional information on the internal state distribution. It was recently demonstrated that the population distribution of the rotational and/or vibrational states of the scattered molecules can be investigated by laser-induced fluorescence and laser-induced resonance ionization [2-12]. Furthermore, resonance ionization in connection with time-of-flight measurements gives information on the velocity distributions of the scattered particles [13]. As these measurements are angle and state-selective, they yield a full description of the average energy and momentum exchange between the molecules and the surface. Such investigations were performed in our laboratory for the NO/Pt system as well as for the weak inelastic NO/graphite system and are discussed in the following.

## 2. Experimental

An ultrahigh vacuum (UHV) chamber with a pulsed molecular beam was developed for measuring the angular, rotational and velocity distributions of surface-scattered NO molecules. Figure 1 shows the experimental arrangement equipped for the measurement of velocity distributions. Apart from a modification of the detection scheme, it is quite similar to the setup which was used for the angular and rotational distribution measurements [2]. The UHV chamber was kept at a pressure of $2 \times 10^{-10}$ mbar. The supersonic NO beam was produced by a 200 µm pulsed nozzle with a back pressure of 1 bar. This led to a mean velocity of 750 m/s, a rotational temperature of about 35 K, and a beam spread of 2 mrad. The beam was directed onto a clean Pt(111) or smooth graphite sample mounted on the rotatable axis of a manipulator. The angular distribution of the molecules scattered from the surface could be measured by a rotatable mass spectrometer with an angular resolution of 5°. On the other hand, the velocity of the scattered molecules could also be analyzed by the resonant two-photon ionization scheme in the following way. A cylindrical cage 17 mm in diameter and 6 mm in height made of metal wire mesh at ground potential was set in front of the sample. An excimer-laser-pumped dye laser beam was frequency-doubled and propagated along the cage axis in synchronization with the molecular beam.

---

* permanent adress: Physics Department, University of California, Berkeley, California

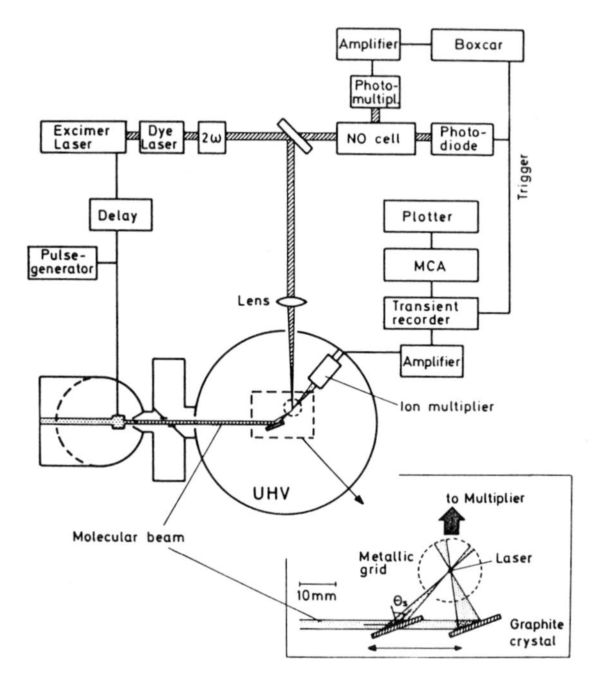


Fig. 1: Experimental setup for the measurement of state-selective velocity and angular distributions.

The molecules in a particular energy state were selectively ionized by a two-photon transition via the intermediate $X(^2\Pi) \rightarrow A(^2\Sigma)$ resonant excitation. The ions produced should move in the cage with the velocity of the parent molecules. As soon as they emerged from the cage, they experienced a strong electrostatic field generated by the negative plate of the ion multiplier biased at 2.9 kV at a distance of 5 cm from the cage. They were then pulled towards the multiplier and properly detected. The time-of-flight spectrum of the ions could be recorded with a multichannel analyzer. It was found that both the time of flight of ions outside the cage and the fringe field effects inside the cage are of no significant influence. Consequently, the observed spectrum was also the time-of-flight spectrum of the state-selected scattered molecules, from which the velocity distribution of such molecules could be deduced. Scanning the laser excitation also allowed us to measure the internal energy distribution of these molecules (calibrated against the laser-induced fluorescence spectrum from a NO cell at room temperature). The scattering angle in this case was determined by the relative position of the cage with respect to the sample. The angular distribution of the state-selected scattered molecules could thus also be measured by displacing the sample along the molecular beam direction.

## Results

The adiabatic expansion of the NO molecular beam in the nozzle causes an increase of the average velocity in the beam direction and, simultaneously, a strong reduction of the rotational temperature and the velocity spread. The molecules in our supersonic beam had an average velocity of ~750 m/s, a velocity spread (FWHM) of ~ 140 m/s and a rotational population distribution corresponding to about 35 K [2]. The beam hit the surface at a selectable incidence angle of between 30° and 70°. An important parameter in the scattering experiments is the molecule-surface potential. Therefore, our investigations concentrated on two systems, the NO/Pt and the NO/graphite system, having an interaction potential depth of 1.4 and 0.1 eV, respectively.

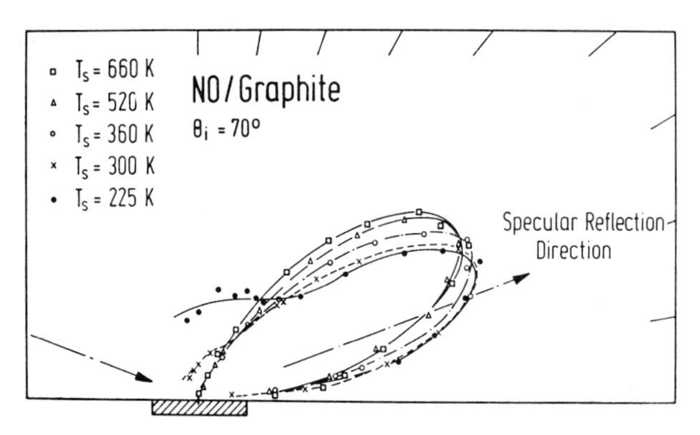


Fig. 2: Angular distributions (normalized mass spectrometer signals) of NO molecules scattered from a graphite surface at different temperatures $T_s$.

Figure 2 shows the angular distributions of NO molecules scattered from the graphite surface at an incidence angle of 70° for different surface temperatures $T_s$. The data were derived directly from the rotatable mass spectrometer signals corresponding to the density of the particles. To obtain the molecular flux, the data have to be corrected for the particle velocities at different scattering angles. It is obvious that the distributions are generally composed of a quasi-specular scattering or lobular part peaked at a scattering angle $\theta_s$ significantly less than the specular reflection angle and a diffusive scattering or cosine distribution part at low $T_s$. With increasing surface temperature the diffusive part decreases relative to the specular part together with a shift of the specular lobe to lower scattering angles. This can be interpreted as a weakly inelastic scattering process with an increasing trapping/desorption contribution for decreasing temperature. This behaviour is well correlated with the behaviour of the velocity distributions of the scattered NO molecules, as will be discussed later.

The angular distributions of NO scattered from a Pt(111) surface yielded (for all surface temperatures) cosine distributions slightly distorted in the direction of specular reflection [2,14]. These results suggest that most of the particles scattered from the surface had their mean translational energy accommodated to the surface temperature. This was supported by the direct determination of velocity distributions of the scattered NO molecules by time-of-flight measurements [14]. The NO/Pt interaction is clearly dominated by trapping/desorption processes.

Tuning the laser wavelength leads to fluorescence or ionization spectra of the scattered molecules with signal heights correlated to the population of the corresponding ground-state rotational levels. In both

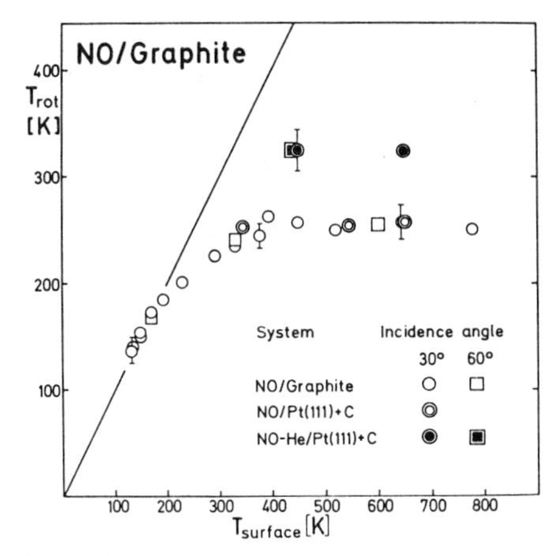


Fig. 3: Scattering of NO molecules from a pyrographite crystal and a carbon-covered Pt(111) surface. The rotational temperature of the scattered molecules is plotted versus the surface temperature for two different incidence angles and translational energies of the incoming particles.

cases, for the NO/Pt as well as for the NO/graphite system, the rotational-state populations could be fitted approximately to Boltzmann distributions with a characteristic rotational temperature $T_{rot}$ [2]. In addition, it was found that the population distribution in the electronic states $^2\Pi_{1/2}$ and $^2\Pi_{3/2}$ could be described by the same $T_{rot}$. Even the overall population ratio $N(^2\Pi_{1/2}) : N(^2\Pi_{3/2})$ is given roughly by $\exp(-\Delta E/kT_{rot})$, where $\Delta E$ is the fine-structure splitting.

The dependence of $T_{rot}$ on the surface temperature for the NO/graphite system is shown in Fig. 3. The solid line corresponds to complete accommodation of the rotational degree of freedom to the surface temperature. While the experimental points follow this line closely up to a surface temperature of about 170 K, they deviate at higher temperatures. At $T_s$ higher than 350 K, $T_{rot}$ approaches a constant value of about 250 K. The results characterized by open symbols were obtained at an incoming energy of about 80 meV; increasing the average kinetic energy of the incoming NO molecules to about 200 meV (NO seeded in He) led to a somewhat higher rotational temperature (solid points).

The corresponding measurements for the NO/Pt(111) system gave qualitatively the same results: rotational accommodation to the surface temperature at $T_s < 350$ K and a $T_{rot} < T_s$ for higher surface temperatures [2]. For example, a $T_s$ of 800 K leads to a rotational temperature of ~ 450 K. Contrary to the NO/graphite system, a larger kinetic energy of the incoming beam did not cause an increase in $T_{rot}$. Instead, the rotational energy of the scattered molecules was clearly independent of the incoming translational energy (between 80 and 200 meV). The molecules lost their translational energy to the surface during their very long residence time, which could be measured to be ~ 3s at $T_s$ = 400 K and ~ 5 x $10^{-7}$ s at $T_s$ = 800 K [2].

The velocity distribution of both the scattered and the incoming particles could be investigated by ionizing the NO molecules, starting

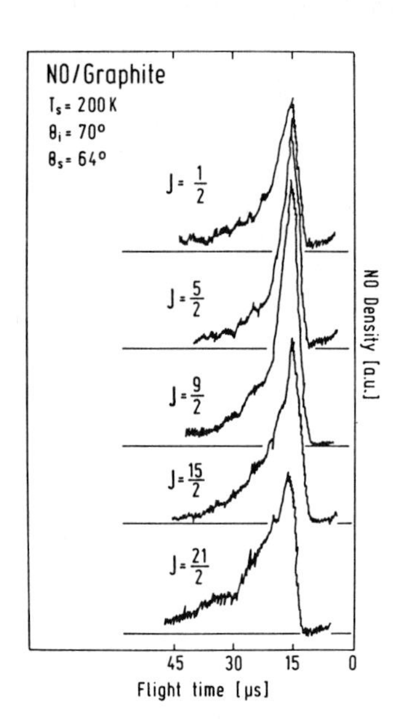


Fig. 4: Time-of-flight spectra of NO molecules in different rotational states, scattered from a 200 K graphite surface with a scattering angle of 64° (incidence angle 70°).

from specific rotational states and measuring the time-of-flight of the ions [13]. Since the translational energy is conserved during photoionization, the time-of-flight spectra can easily be transferred into velocity distributions of the scattered neutral particles. Changing the position of the surface in the direction of the incoming molecular beam allows molecules scattered at the different angle to be ionized. In our experiment the incidence angle of the particles was fixed at 70°; the scattering angle was varied between 2° and 64°, i.e. between the nearly normal direction and nearly specular reflection direction.

Figure 4 shows time-of-flight spectra of NO molecules scattered from a 200 K graphite surface at an angle of 64°, i.e. into the nearly specular reflection direction. The spectra reflect the velocity of the scattered molecules in different rotational states, from J = 1/2 to J = 21/2 with a rotational energy of about 1 $cm^{-1}$ and 200 $cm^{-1}$, respectively. The time-of-flight spectra of the scattered molecules in various J states are quite similar and are composed of a very high quasi-specular peak and a longer tail resulting from the diffusively scattered particles. The two contributions can be more clearly observed if the scattering angle is changed (see Fig. 5). From the spectra in Fig. 4 it is obvious that the high J states have a stronger diffusive part than the low J states. Increasing the surface temperature reduces the tail of slow molecules more and more corresponding to the decreasing diffusive part of the angular distributions.

Time-of-flight spectra of NO molecules scattered at various angles (from $\theta_s$ = 2° to $\theta_s$ = 64°) are presented in Fig. 5. In this case the scattered molecules are in the J = 9/2 rotational state and are scattered from the 200 K graphite surface with an incidence angle of 70°. The quasi-specularly scattered part decreases with decreasing scattering angle and, instead, the diffusive tail increases. It is obvious that the flight time in the normal direction is much longer than in the specular direction, and that the width of the distribution is narrower than the

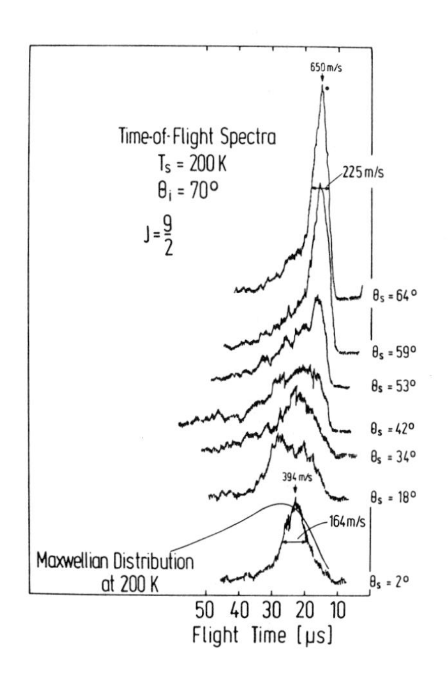


Fig. 5: Time of flight spectra of NO molecules in the J = 9/2 rotational state scattered at different angles from a 200 K graphite surface. The spectrum of the molecules in the normal ($\theta_o$ = 2°) direction is compared with the flight time expected from a 200 K Maxwellian distribution.

specular width and is nearly identical to the width of the incoming velocity distribution (the relative velocity spread, however, increases from 20 % to 40 %). Comparing the time-of-flight spectra of molecules in different rotational states yields the same dependence on the scattering angle, but, as was shown in Fig. 4, the diffusive part for the higher rotational states is stronger than that of the specular part. This means that the diffusively scattered molecules gain more rotational energy during the scattering process. The diffusive and specular parts of the scattered molecules can be characterized by two different rotational temperatures. For $T_s$ = 200 K, the quasi-specularly reflected part (evaluated at $\theta_s$ = 64°) has a rotational temperature $T^{qs}_{rot}$ = 180 ± 20 K, and the diffusive scattering part (evaluated at $\theta_s$ = 2°) has a $T^{d}_{rot}$ = 230 ± 30 K. The latter appears to be larger than $T_s$, but this could be the result of experimental inaccuracy. In any case, it is clear that $T^{d}_{rot} > T^{qs}_{rot}$. Similar measurements at $T_s$ = 250 K and $T_s$ = 300 K yielded $T^{qs}_{rot}$ = 190 K, $T^{d}_{rot}$ = 250 K and $T^{qs}_{rot}$ = 200 K, $T^{d}_{rot}$ = 250 K, respectively.

From the time-of-flight spectra of Fig. 4 and Fig. 5 it is possible to calculate (with the known dimensions of the cage) the velocity distributions of the scattered molecules and to compare them with the incoming velocity distribution. Such distributions are shown in Fig. 6 for NO molecules in the J = 9/2 rotational state. The peak velocity of the incoming particles (solid points) is 750 m/s with a velocity spread of 145 m/s. After scattering from a 550 K graphite surface into the specular direction ($\theta_s$ = 64°) the molecules exhibit a peak velocity slightly less than and a spread nearly double (open points) as that of the incoming beam. The form of the distribution is nearly symmetric around the peak velocity, since at this high surface temperature there is only a minor contribution of diffusive scattering. The velocity distribution of the molecules scattered from the 200 K surface (crosses) shows a much slower peak velocity than that of the incoming beam. This distribution is cal-

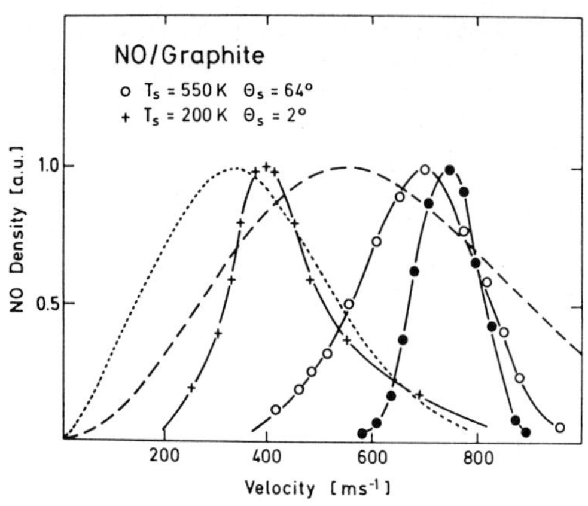


Fig. 6: Velocity distributions of incoming NO molecules (solid points) of specularly scattered molecules ($\theta_s$ = 64°, $T_s$ = 500 K, J = 9/2) and of diffusively scattered molecules ($\theta_s \leq$ 2°, $T_s$ = 200 K, J = 9/2). Maxwellian distributions of 550 K (---) and 200 K (····) show that there is no accommodation of the molecular velocity distributions to the surface temperature.

culated from the $\theta_s$ = 2° time-of-flight spectrum shown in Fig. 5. As mentioned above, the spread (FWHM) is nearly identical to that of the incoming beam despite its large translational energy loss to the surface. The distributions in Fig. 6 are normalized to the same height; the real intensity ratio, however, is about 1:3, corresponding to the data of Fig. 2 and Fig. 5. With increasing $T_s$, the peak intensity associated with diffusive scattering diminishes; in addition, the scattering angle of the lobular maximum decreases, so that the maximum in the time-of-flight spectrum appears at decreasing $\theta_s$. We found, interestingly enough, that the peak velocity of the quasi-specular peak, measured in the direction of the lobular maximum, increases with increasing $T_s$ (650 m/s at $T_s$ = 200 K, 685 m/s at $T_s$ = 300 K, 710 m/s at $T_s$ = 470 K, and 750 m/s at $T_s$ = 660 K, as compared with 750 m/s for the peak incoming velocity). In addition, we found, more pronounced at higher $T_s$, an increasing particle velocity with decreasing $\theta_s$ (710 m/s at $\theta_s$ = 64°, 770 m/s at $\theta_s$ = 59°, 820 m/s at $\theta_s$ = 53°, and 850 m/s at $\theta_s$ = 48° at a surface temperature $T_s$ = 470 K and the peak incoming velocity at 750 m/s).

## 3. Discussion

With our experimental setup it was possible to measure the angular and rotational distributions as well as the state and angle-selective velocity distributions of NO molecules scattered from a graphite surface. In addition, the rotational and angular distributions of the NO/Pt(111) scattering system were investigated. The interaction of NO with the Pt surface is a typical trapping/desorption process with a cosine angular distribution and accommodation of the velocity to the surface temperature. A surprising result was the lack of accommodation of the internal degrees of freedom, which, however, has also been found for other trapping/desorbing systems and can be explained by the model of a desorbing hindered rotor [15,16]. The weak inelastic scattering of NO molecules from the graphite surface seems to be more complicated. Here the interaction with phonons in the normal and tangential directions during the very short interaction time appears to influence the angular, rotational and velocity distributions, as well as the coupling of the translational and rotational motions of the scattering molecules. The results of the investigation of the NO/graphite system can be summarized as follows:

- The angular distributions show broad lobes of specular reflection and a small diffusive part. With decreasing temperature the diffusive part increases while the specular part decreases: at low surface temperatures the molecules undergo partly trapping/desorption and partly quasi-elastic scattering, whereas quasi-elastic scattering is predominant at high $T_s$.

- The rotational distributions show Boltzmann-like behaviour and can be characterized by a rotational temperature $T_{rot}$. This $T_{rot}$ is nearly equal to $T_s$ for low $T_s$; at higher surface temperatures, however, $T_{rot}$ is lower than $T_s$. The rotational temperature reaches a limiting value which depends on the translational energy of the incoming particles [2]. Diffusively scattered molecules exhibit a slightly higher $T_{rot}$ than the specularly scattered particles [13].

- The velocity distributions of scattered NO molecules in different rotational states are nearly identical, also for varying $\theta_s$. At low surface temperatures there are two scattering channels: one corresponds to quasi-specularly reflected molecules with a velocity slightly lower than the incoming velocity, the other corresponds to diffusively scattered particles with a much lower velocity. The peak velocity of the quasi-specularly scattered molecules increases with increasing $T_s$ and with decreasing $\theta_s$ [13].

The above results provide useful information about the molecular energy and momentum exchange with the graphite surface. For low surface temperatures the rotational energy gained by the quasi-specularly scattered molecules is actually comparable to their translational energy loss. At $T_s$ = 200 K, the average rotational energy gain per scattered molecule is ~100 $cm^{-1}$, while the translational energy loss is 170 $cm^{-1}$. (The average internal energy gain per scattered molecule is 130 $cm^{-1}$, considering excitation of the $^2\Pi_{3/2}$ state of NO). For the diffusively scattered molecules, the translational energy loss per molecule is 500 $cm^{-1}$ at $T_s$ = 200 K, which is much larger than the internal energy gain per molecule in the scattering process. The larger amount of energy deposition by the diffusively scattered molecules in the solid (~ 380 $cm^{-1}$ per molecule) is a manifestation of the trapping/desorption process.

The mean velocity of the diffusively scattered molecules is not as low as that expected for molecules desorbed from a surface at $T_s$ = 200 K, and the velocity distribution ($\theta_s$ = 2° in Fig. 3) is not broader than that of the incoming beam and is much narrower than the Maxwellian distribution at 200 K. Thus, the diffusive scattering part cannot arise from an equilibrium trapping/desorption process, but is more likely the result of a transitional trapping/desorption process, in which the molecules bounce around on the surface in the trapping well before desorption. The residence time is short compared to the time required for complete thermal equilibrium between the molecules and the surface. This is analogous to the case of gas-phase molecular collisions through a transitional bound-state. The residence time at this low surface temperature is long enough for complete accommodation of the internal degrees of freedom, but apparently not long enough for translational accommodation of the diffusively scattered particles.

The quasi-specular scattering, especially at higher surface temperature, is believed to be a single-collision process. Here, the molecule-surface interaction time is so short that accommodation of the velocity distribution to the surface temperature seems impossible. The energy transfer to the molecular rotational degree of freedom, however, is still quite efficient.

At low $T_s$ (< 300 K), the quasi-specular part has a significantly smaller mean velocity than the incoming beam, corresponding to a net momentum loss along the surface. This momentum loss corresponds roughly to the increase of the rotational energy of the molecules, as discussed above. Another interpretation would be a molecule-surface interaction which allows the molecules to impart to the solid a net average momentum along the surface. This, however, would be contrary to the assumptions of the hard cube model [17]. Nevertheless, the translational energy exchange in normal direction between the molecules and the surface should be more or less determined by this hard cube model. There is a net momentum transfer to the molecules scattered in the normal direction; however, only at a sufficiently high surface temperature, can the molecules gain a net translational energy from the surface in the quasi-specular direction. For example, the fact that the peak velocity of the scattered molecule increases with decreasing $\theta_s$ at high $T_s$ is a clear indication of momentum and energy transfer from the surface to the molecules in the surface-normal direction.

Summarizing the results on the overall energy balance for the NO/graphite system, we find that the diffusively scattered NO molecules gain some rotational energy, but transfer much more translational energy to the surface, so that the energy balance is considerably negative. For the specularly scattered molecules, energy loss and gain are nearly balanced at low surface temperatures, but with increasing $T_s$, the translational energy of the scattered molecules increases while the rotational energy stays constant, resulting in a substantial energy transfer from the surface to the scattered NO molecules.

Acknowledgement

One of the authors (Y.R.S.) sincerely thanks the Alexander von Humboldt Foundation for a senior Humboldt award.

REFERENCES

1. See for example F.O. Goodman and H.Y. Wachman, "Dynamics of Gas Surface Scattering", (Academic Press, N.Y., 1976).
2. a) F. Frenkel, J. Häger, W. Krieger, H. Walther, C.T. Campbell, G. Ertl, H. Kuipers, and J. Segner, Phys. Rev. Lett. 46, 152 (1981);
b) F. Frenkel, J. Häger, W. Krieger, H. Walther, G. Ertl, J. Segner, and W. Vielhaber, Chem. Phys. Lett. 90, 225 (1982):
c) G. Ertl, H. Robota, J. Segner, W. Vielhaber, F. Frenkel, J. Häger, W. Krieger, and H. Walther, Surf. Sci. 131, 273 (1983).
3. a) G.M. McClelland, G.D. Kubiak, H.G. Rennagel, and R.N. Zare, Phys. Rev. Lett. 46, 831 (1981);
b) G.D. Kubiak, J.E. Hurst, Jr., H.G. Rennagel, G.M. McClelland, and R.N. Zare, J. Chem. Phys. 79, 5163 (1983).
4. a) A.W. Kleyn, A.C. Luntz, and D.J. Auerbach, Phys. Rev. Lett. 47, 1169 (1981);

b) A.C. Luntz, A.W. Kleyn, and D.J. Auerbach, J. Chem. Phys. 76, 737 (1982);
c) A.C. Luntz, A.W. Kleyn, and D.J. Auerbach, Phys. Rev. B 25, 4273 (1982);
d) A.W. Kleyn, A.C. Luntz, and D.J. Auerbach, Surf. Sci. 117, 33 (1982).

5. a) M. Asscher, W.L. Guthrie, T.H. Lin, and G.A. Somorjai, Phys. Rev. Lett. 49, 76 (1982);
b) H. Asscher, W.L. Guthrie, T.H. Lin, and G.A. Somorjai, J. Chem. Phys. 78, 6992 (1983).
6. H. Zacharias, M.M.T. Loy, and P.A. Roland, Phys. Rev. Lett. 49, 1790 (1982).
6. J.S. Hayden and G.J. Diebold, J. Chem. Phys. 77, 4767 (1982).
8. a) J.W. Hepburn, F.J. Northrup. G.L. Ogram, J.C. Polanyi, and J.H. Williamson, Chem. Phys. Lett. 85, 127 (1982);
b) D. Ettinger, K. Honma, M. Keil, and J.C. Polanyi, Chem. Phys. Lett. 87, 413 (1981).
9. R.R. Cavanagh and D.S. King, Phys. Rev. Lett. 47, 1829 (1981).
10. J. Misewich, C.N. Plum, G. Blyholder, P.L. Houston, and R.P. Merrill, J. Chem. Phys. 78, 4245 (1983).
11. a) D.E. Tevault, L.D. Talley, and M.C. Lin, J. Chem. Phys. 72, 3314 (1980);
b) L.D. Talley, W.A. Sanders, D.J. Bogan, and M.C. Lin, Chem. Phys. Lett. 78, 500 (1981).
12. J.B. Cross, and J.B. Lurie, Chem. Phys. Lett. 100, 174 (1983).
13. J. Häger, Y.R. Shen, and H. Walther, submitted for publication in Phys. Rev. Lett.
14. W.L. Guthrie, T.H. Lin, S.T. Ceyer, and G.A. Somorjai, J. Chem Phys. 76, 6398 (1982).
15. J.W. Gadzuk, U. Landman, E.J. Kuster, C.L. Cleveland, and R.N. Barnett, Phys. Rev. Lett. 49, 426 (1982).
16. S.E. Bialkowski, J. Chem. Phys. 78, 600 (1983).
17. a) R.N. Logan, and R.E. Stickney, J. Chem. Phys. 44, 195 (1966).
b) W.L. Nichols, and J.H. Weare, J. Chem. Phys. 63, 379 (1975).

# Part 3

# Photoassisted Chemical Processing

# 3.1 Deposition

## Laser-Induced Chemical Vapor Deposition

**Dieter Bäuerle**

Angewandte Physik, Johannes Kepler Universität
A-4040 Linz, Austria

### 1. Introduction

Laser-induced chemical vapor deposition (LCVD) is a new technique for single-step local deposition or direct writing of thin films of metals, semiconductors or insulators [1,2]. The lateral dimensions of these films can at present be varied from about 0.5 µm up to several centimeters. Holographic methods may permit single-step deposition of complete patterns. In pyrolytic LCVD, the deposition rates are so high that three-dimensional structures can be produced.

Flat structures with widths down to micron size are needed in many areas of technology, such as microelectronics or integrated optics. Such structures are now produced by standard chemical vapor deposition (CVD) [3] together with sequential application of mechanical masking or lithographic methods. These standard techniques, which require several production steps, are well established for large area planar substrates. On the other hand, these techniques are not very suitable for deposition of structures on nonplanar substrates. Furthermore, the increasing complexity and miniaturization of systems require controlled area coating techniques which avoid thermal or chemical cycling of entire partially fabricated devices. In such cases, LCVD is an extremely promising technique.

Applications of complex three-dimensional structures produced by pyrolytic LCVD can only be speculated on. In this new and fascinating field only the first steps have been taken: recently, rods of single crystalline Si have been grown within the beam of a laser - without any crucible and in an otherwise cold atmosphere [4]. The possibility of producing non-equilibrium materials or materials which form only under extreme conditions, e.g. at high temperatures together with high pressures, or high electric or magnetic fields, is obvious.

LCVD can be based on reactions which are initiated mainly pyrolytically or mainly photolytically or a combination of both. Pyrolytic LCVD is based on local substrate heating by laser light which is not absorbed by the gaseous molecular species. Apart from the initial phase of nucleation, the microscopic mechanism for decomposition is the same as in conventional CVD, namely thermal activation of the chemical reaction. Therefore, the wide variety of deposition reactions used in conventional CVD can be applied to LCVD. The situation is quite different for photolytic LCVD. In this case the laser radiation breaks chemical bonds directly, i.e. nonthermally.

Another mechanism would be to transfer the bond breaking energy via an intermediate species as, e.g., in photosensitization. Since most molecular bond energies are several eV, ultraviolet (UV) laser light is generally required. Besides dissociative electronic excitation, dissociation of molecular species can also be achieved by selective multiphoton vibrational excitation with infrared (IR) laser light of suitable frequency.

In this review we concentrate on pyrolytic LCVD by means of visible, mainly cw $Ar^+$ and $Kr^+$ laser light. Deposition by means of infrared laser light and laser photochemical deposition with frequency doubled cw $Ar^+$ or frequency multipled pulsed Nd:YAG lasers and with excimer lasers is described in the following contributions in this chapter.

## 2. General Remarks and Survey

The analysis of the microscopic mechanisms in the initial phase of growth is very complicated. In the phase of nucleation, we have to consider two cases: first, the case of strongly absorbing substrates, and second, the case of transparent substrates which do not or only very slightly absorb the laser light. In the first case the molecules are thermally dissociated near the hot spot which is produced on the substrate by the absorbed laser light. The free atoms form clusters which provide nucleation centers for further film growth. The time for nucleation, $t_n$, is very small compared to laser beam illumination times, $t_i$, henceforth considered. The main differences from nucleation in large area thin film growth techniques, e.g. standard CVD [5], arise from the confinement of the temperature distribution and the related strong temperature gradients which are produced on the substrate surface. A further difference from CVD is based on the rapid change in the local laser-induced temperature distribution due to changes in reflectivity and thermal conductivity provided by the nuclei. For transparent substrates, the situation is even more complex. Here, nucleation may be initiated by atoms which result from non-thermal (single- or multiphoton) dissociation of adsorbed molecules [1,6,7]. It is clear that in such cases changes in the electronic properties of molecules due to adsorption, especially a shift and a broadening of the dissociative continuum, are of fundamental importance [8,9,10]. Because of the high density of adsorbed molecules, the free atoms may form clusters which, even when of subcritical size, may strongly absorb the laser radiation. Such hot clusters will then provide nucleation sites and film growth will proceed mainly thermally. In this case $t_n$ depends strongly on the laser wavelength and may last several seconds or even minutes. The first evidence for such processes has been obtained in the deposition of Cd, Al and Ni from the alkyls and carbonyls, respectively [6,7,11]. At present, however, we are a long way from an understanding of these initial dissociation and nucleation processes in LCVD.

As in standard CVD, deposition in pyrolytic LCVD is characterized by two temperature regimes: the kinetically controlled regime, in which the deposition rate strongly increases with temperature, and at higher temperatures, the transport limited regime, where the rate is nearly independent of temperature but is affected by the geometry of the reactor, the flow rate, etc. In the kinetically controlled regime, the thickness and width of the deposit is given by

$$h(r,t_i) = A \int_{t_n}^{t_i} dt\, k_0\left(T(r,t),\, p_i\right) \exp\left\{ -\Delta E_j / RT(r,t) \right\} \tag{1}$$

where the temperature distribution $T(r,t)$ is an implicit function of the geometry of the deposit $h(r)$, which itself influences the heat transport through the substrate material (see Sect. 3). $\Delta E_j$ is the apparent chemical activation energy which characterizes the slowest step in the chemical kinetics involved in the deposition process. The preexponential factor $k_0$ also depends on temperature and on the partial pressures of reactants and reaction products. A is a constant. In direct writing of microstructures, the local temperature rise also depends, in principle, on the scanning velocity of the laser beam and therefore the integral must be extended from $-\infty$ to $+\infty$.

The confinement of the chemical reaction in LCVD, compared to standard CVD $(T \neq f(r,t))$, has some further consequences. For example, controlled deposition can be performed at much higher partial pressures of reactants, resulting in deposition rates which are orders of magnitutes higher. Furthermore, three-dimensional diffusion of molecules to and from the reaction zone is possible. Therefore, transport limitation becomes effective only at much higher temperatures, i.e. (1) will be valid over a wider temperature range. It is clear that these consequences are more significant as the temperature distribution becomes more localized. As well as investigating the temperature dependence of the deposition rate, some evidence of the dominant decomposition mechanism in LCVD can in some cases be more easily obtained from the influence of the laser wavelength. For strongly absorbing materials, e.g. metals with constant absorbance in the visible spectral region, the total absorbed laser power and therefore the temperature distribution is independent of the laser wavelength. In this case thermally activated deposition should remain unchanged.

A quantitative analysis of the deposition process requires detailed knowledge of the laser-induced temperature distributions. During deposition of thin films, direct temperature measurements have not yet been performed with reliable accuracy. However, as we have shown previously [12,13], many features in pyrolytic LCVD of flat structures can be qualitatively - and in some cases even quantitatively - explained from calculated temperature distributions. The essential features of the model calculations are presented in the following section. Then, after a short description of a typical experimental setup (Sect. 4), we analyze and discuss the experimental results for the deposition of flat structures in the form of spots (Sect. 5.1) and for steady growth of stripes (Sect. 5.2) on the basis of calculated temperature profiles. Under special conditions, namely during steady growth of rods, the temperature distribution can be held constant with respect to time and the relevant temperature can be directly measured during the deposition process. The results are summarized in Sect. 6. In Sect. 7, finally, we will comment on the morphology and on the physical properties of the deposited material.

## 3. Temperature Distributions

In the calculations presented in this section we do not consider the problems in the phase of nucleation, as discussed in Sect. 2, but assume that after a time $t_m$ the semi-infinite plane substrate is already covered with a thin film of the deposited material within the area exposed to the focussed laser beam. As we have shown in related papers [12,13], the temperature distribution induced by the cw laser radiation absorbed on the surface of such a combined structure is strongly affected by the heat transport through the deposited material itself. This is especially true in cases where the thermal conductivity of the deposited material, $k_D$, is higher than that of the substrate, $k_S$. Fig. 1 shows model structures for the deposition of circular spots. The deposit (diameter d, height h) repre-

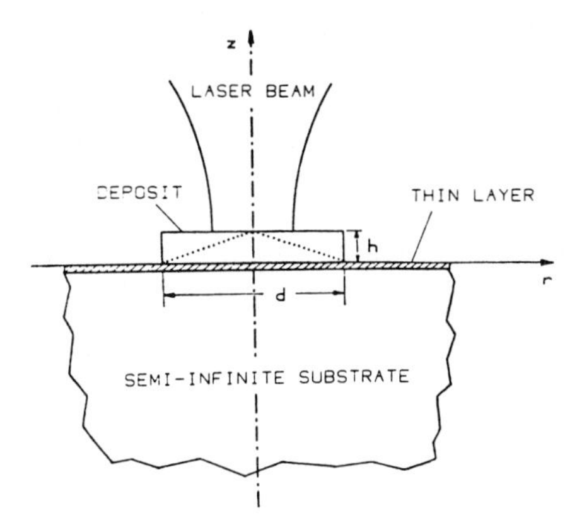


Fig. 1. Model structures for which temperature distributions have been calculated. The dash-dotted line is an axis of symmetry. The deposit is represented by a circular cylinder (full) or a circular cone (dotted)

sented by a circular cylinder (full lines) or by a circular cone (dotted), is placed on an extended plane substrate ($k_S$) covered with a thin layer ($h_L$, $k_L$). The laser beam is assumed to be Gaussian and at normal incidence to the center of the deposit (see Sect. 4). In the calculations we do not include the temperature dependence of the thermal conductivities, k, and of the surface reflectivity of the deposit $R_D$. Heat losses to the gas phase and latent heat effects (heat of formation) which occur in real LCVD are also neglected. The stationary heat equation which describes the spatial dependence of the temperature T can be written as

$$- \vec{\nabla}^2 T = \frac{Q}{k} \tag{2}$$

where k is the thermal conductivity of the deposit, the thin layer, or the bulk substrate, as appropriate. Q is the source term arising from the absorption of the incident laser light. Assuming no light penetration into the deposited material - which is valid for metallic structures in the visible spectral region - Q can be written for the cylindrical deposit in the form

$$Q = 2P(1-R_D)/\pi w_0{}^2 \cdot \exp\left\{-2r^2/w_0{}^2\right\} \cdot \delta\,(z-h) \tag{3}$$

and correspondingly for the circular cone. P is the total effective laser power and $2w_0$ the diameter of the laser focus (see Sect. 4). To solve (2), in cylindrical coordinates, we have employed a numerical finite element procedure [14]; the elements were triangles in the rz plane. The boundary conditions were:

1) vanishing temperature gradient normal to the gas-solid interface, and
2) zero temperature rise $\Delta T \equiv T-T_\infty$ at infinity.

The approximation was made that at sufficient distance from the irradiated surface, the temperature rise ΔT is determined by radial heat conduction (spherical symmetry) only.

Fig. 2 shows temperature profiles calculated for three different ratios of thermal conductivities $k_D$, $k_L$, $k_S$. The parameters used correspond to Ni spots on glass covered with 4000 Å a-Si (Fig. 2a), to Ni on Si covered with 4000 Å $SiO_2$ (Fig. 2b) and to Ni on Si (Fig. 2c). All curves except the dense dotted one (Fig. 2a) refer to the model of the circular cylinder. The full curves were calculated for equal center temperature, $T_C$ = 530K, which of course requires different absorbed laser powers, namely 10 mW, 56 mW and 120 mW in cases a), b) and c), respectively.

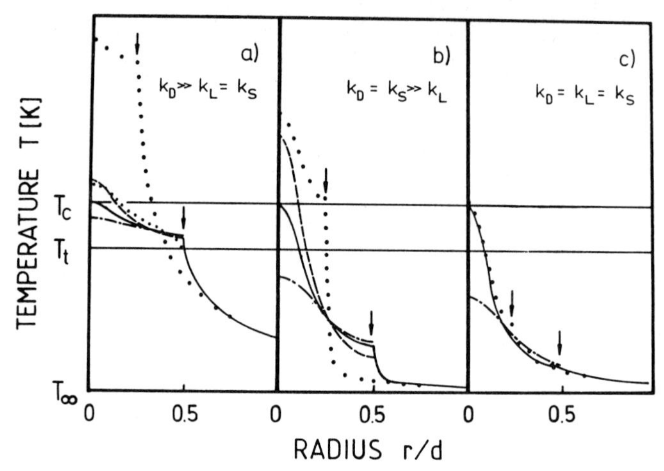


Fig. 2. Temperature distributions calculated for the model structures shown in Figure 1. The edges of deposits with different diameters are marked by arrows. Circular cylinder: —— $h = d/20$, $2w_0 = d/3$; --- $h = d/40$, $2w_0 = d/3$; -·- $h = d/20$, $2w_0 = 2d/3$; · · $h = d'/20$, $2w_0 = d'/3$, $d'=d/2$. Circular cone: ···· $h = d/20$, $2w_0 = d/3$; a) $k_D$ (Ni) = 70 W/Km, $k_L$ (a-Si) ⌊16⌋ ≈ $k_S$ (glass) = 1.3 W/Km, b) $k_D$ (Ni) ≈ $k_S$ (Si) = 70 W/Km, $k_L$ = 1.3 W/Km, c) $k_D = k_L = k_S$ = 70 W/Km. $T_\infty$ = 300K, $T_c$ = 530K

For the case of Fig. 2a and constant spot diameter, d, the temperature at the edge of the deposit, T(d/2), depends only very slightly on the geometry of the deposit (compare full, broken and dense dotted curves). Actually, in this case, the temperature rise $\Delta T$ (d/2) scales approximately inversely with d and can be described to a good approximation by the simple equation $\Delta T\ (d/2) = P\ (1-R_D)\ /\ (2\ d\ k_S)$ ⌊17⌋ (compare full and sparse dotted curves). It is therefore not surprising that $\Delta T$ (d/2) is not very sensitive to changes in $k_D$ as long as $k_D \gg k_S$; e.g., using instead 70 W/Km $k_D$ = 30 W/Km, $\Delta T$ (d/2) decreases only by about 5%. A further point is that $\Delta T$ (d/2) is independent of the laser focus diameter, as long as $d \gg 2w_0$ (see full and chain-dotted curves). In Fig. 2c the temperature distribution is nearly independent of the diameter of the deposit and is very similar to that for a plane substrate; significant differences occur only near the edge of the deposit. Note the strong influence of a change in laser focus diameter. Fig. 2b represents the intermediate case.

Temperature profiles for stripes were calculated in ⌊12⌋ for $k_D = 30\ k_S$ and $k_D = k_S$ with $k_L = k_S$. For realistic parameters for the width, d, and the thickness, h, of stripes and for $v_S/D$ ($v_S$ is the scanning velocity of the laser beam, D is the thermal diffusivity of the substrate) the temperature profiles are essentially unaffected by the scanning velocity of the laser beam and they are therefore very similar to the profiles shown in Fig. 2. The main difference results from the heat transport along the stripe, which yields a reduction of the center temperature with increasing cross-section of the stripe. This effect is especially significant for $k_D \gg k_L = k_S$.

## 4. Experimental Techniques

A typical experimental setup is shown schematically in Fig. 3. The reaction chamber can be operated either with a constant flow of the reacting gaseous

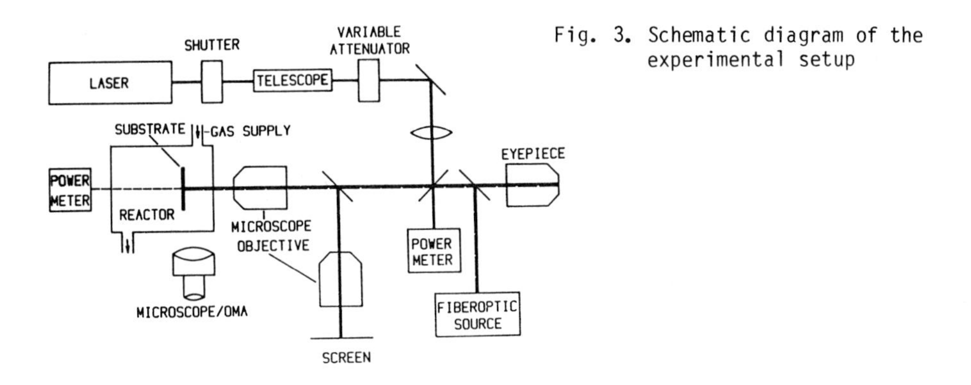


Fig. 3. Schematic diagram of the experimental setup

species with or without a buffer gas, or can be sealed off because of the small amount of gas consumed in most of the reactions.

The $TEM_{00}$ beam of a cw $Ar^+$ or $Kr^+$ laser is expanded and then focused onto the substrate by a simple lens, a microscope objective, or a combination of both. The latter arrangement was used to produce the smallest structures produced. In this case accurate positioning of the substrate can be achieved by imaging the focussed spot onto a screen using a second identical objective. For a Gaussian beam, the incident laser irradiance can be written in the form $I(w) = I(o) \exp\{-2w^2/w_o^2\}$, where $w_o$ is defined by $I(w_o) = I(o)/e^2$ and is given by $w_o = 2 f\lambda / \pi a$ where $a$ is the aperture. The length of the laser focus is defined by $L = 2\pi w_o^2/\lambda$. The diffraction-limited diameter of the laser focus is one of the essential parameters which determine the lateral resolution of patterns (see Sect. 5.2). The laser power, P, refers always to the effective laser power within the reaction chamber.

The beginning of nucleation is indicated very sensitively by the occurrence of a characteristic speckle pattern which reveals the appearance of scattering centers of submicrometer size. With the onset of speckle movement regular growth of a circular spot starts. For investigating the growth of spots (see Sect. 5.1), the time of laser beam illumination, $t_i$, could be varied continuously by means of a shutter. Deposition rates can in some cases be measured in situ from the transmission of the laser beam or a probe laser beam through the deposited film.

Further laser irradiation results in the growth of a rod (see Sect. 6). The techniques of temperature and deposition rate measurements for this case were described in detail in [1,18].

Writing of surface patterns is accomplished by translating the substrate perpendicular to the laser beam.

## 5. Flat Structures

Investigations on the growth of spots are the most simple case for which to test the adequacy of the model calculations of Sect. 3 for the description of pyrolytic LCVD. The results also allow an understanding of the initial phase of growth of rods (see sect. 6). Steady growth of stripes is relevant in direct writing of microstructures. The investigations outline the possibilities and the fundamental limitations of the technique.

Table 1: Materials deposited with visible laser light

| Solid | Gas [Carrier] | Laser λ [nm] | Deposition Rate [μm/sec] | Ref. |
|---|---|---|---|---|
| Al | $Al_2(CH_3)_6$ [$H_2$] | Kr 476-647 | 0.05-10 | [11] |
| Ni | $Ni(CO)_4$ | Kr 476-647 | 0.1-20 | [1, 7, 13,15] |
| Cu | - | Ar | - | [19] |
| Cd | $Cd(CH_3)_2$ [$H_2$] | Kr 476-647 | 0.01 | [6] |
| Sn | $Sn(CH_3)_4$ | Ar | - | [20] |
| W | $WF_6$ [$H_2$] | Kr 476-531 | | [36] |
| Pt | $Pt(CF_3COCHCOCF_3)_2$ | Ar | - | [20] |
| Au | $Au(CH_3)_2(CH_3COCHCOCH_3)$ | Ar | - | [21] |
| C | $C_2H_2$, $C_2H_4$, $CH_4$ | Ar, Kr 488-647 | 0.05-100 | [18,25] |
| Si | $SiH_4$, $Si_2H_6$ | Ar, Kr 488-647 | 0.1- 40 | [4,22, 23] |
| GaAs | $Ga(CH_3)_3$, $AsH_3$ [$H_2$] | Nd:YAG 532 (10pps) | 0.001 | [28] |
| | $Cl(CH_3)_2Ga \cdot As(C_2H_5)_3$ [$H_2$] $Cl(CH_3)_2Ga.As(CH_3)_3$ [$H_2$] | Kr 647 | < 0.01 | [27] |
| $SiO_x$ $SiO_2$ | $SiH_4 + N_2O$ | Kr 531 | 1-10 | [26] |

In the following two paragraphs the discussion concentrates on the deposition of Ni [1,7,13] from $Ni(CO)_4$ for which the most complete data are available. Similar investigations have been performed by other groups for the materials listed in Table 1. The typical range of laser irradiances used was 0.1 - 4 $kW/mm^2$; the range of partial pressures for the reactant species ranged from 0.1 to 1000 mbar. Typical deposition rates were between 0.1 to 100 μm/sec.

## 5.1 Deposition of Spots

The growth of Ni spots can be most easily investigated when using a substrate material that strongly absorbs the laser radiation and has a much smaller thermal conductivity than the deposit. These requirements are very well fulfilled for glass substrates covered with a 1000 Å a-Si layer. For such substrates, $t_n << t_i$ (see Sect. 2) and the spot grows very rapidly with $t_i$ to radii much larger than the laser focus. The large spot sizes can easily be measured by using the simple setup of Fig. 3. In addition, the high growth rates enable much data to be accumulated. Fig. 4 shows a scanning electron micrograph of Ni spots deposited with the same laser power but with different times of laser beam illumination, $t_i$. Fig. 5 shows the spot diameter as function of $t_i$ for two laser powers and a total

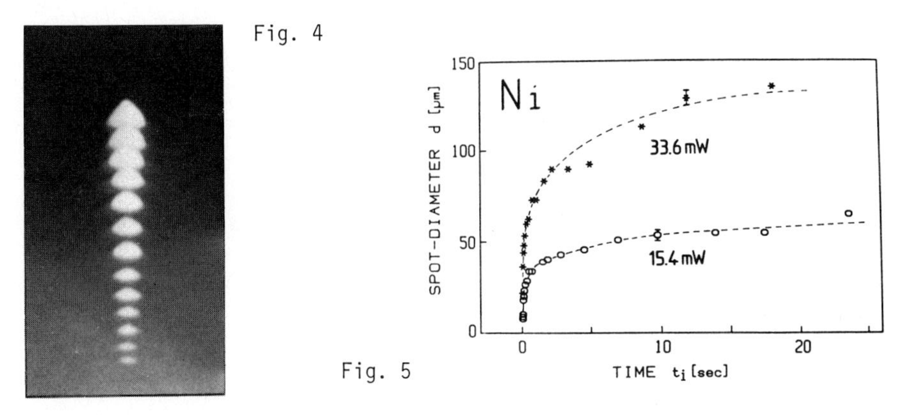


Fig. 4. Scanning electron micrograph of Ni spots deposited with the same laser power, but with different times of laser beam illumination.

Fig. 5. Diameter of Ni spots as function of laser beam illumination time for two laser powers; $2w_0$ = 6 μm. Broken lines are guides for the eyes

gas pressure $p_{tot} \equiv p\ (Ni(CO)_4) = 200$ mbar [13]. The figure shows that the condition $d >> 2w_0$ is fulfilled for all but the shortest time in the 15.4 mW curve. The spot diameter first increases very rapidly and nearly saturates for times $t_i \approx 1$ sec. Because the temperature rise $\Delta T\ (d/2)$ decreases approximately inversely with the spot diameter (see sect. 3), the saturation may indicate that the corresponding temperature at the edge, $T(d/2)$, has fallen below the threshold temperature for nucleation. However, this saturation can also be due to the exponential dependence of the deposition rate on temperature that yields an apparent threshold below which deposition is negligible (see (1)). The mechanism could be proved by depositing the same material from reactant molecules with different activation energies as, e.g., Si from $SiH_4$ or from $SiCl_4$.

The results of Fig. 5 enable the radial growth rates $v \equiv \Delta d / 2\Delta t$ of Ni spots to be calculated by numerical differentiation. It is clear from the shape of the spots that v is not parallel to the deposition rate W defined as the rate of translation of a surface element along its perpendicular (see Sect. 6). However, because spots grown with different laser powers remain similar in shape, W and v differ only by a factor which is roughly constant. In any case, the exponential dependence of the growth rate on temperature will dominate any temperature dependence of the preexponential factor. In other words, if the growth of Ni spots is thermally activated, the lateral growth velocity, v, should follow an Arrhenius type behaviour. Fig. 6 shows such an Arrhenius plot in which additional experimental data for different laser powers and laser focus diameters have been included. The plotted temperature was that at the edge of the deposit which was calculated according to Sect. 3. The values used for the thermal conductivities correspond to those in Fig. 2a. The high temperature region of very fast growth corresponds to small spot sizes, the low temperature region with much smaller growth rates to larger spot sizes. The full line represents a least squares fit to the low temperature data and shows the exponential dependence of the lateral growth rate on temperature. The apparent activation energy is $\Delta E = 22 \pm 3$ kcal/mole. The fact that this value is, within the accuracy of the measurements, independent of P and $w_0$,

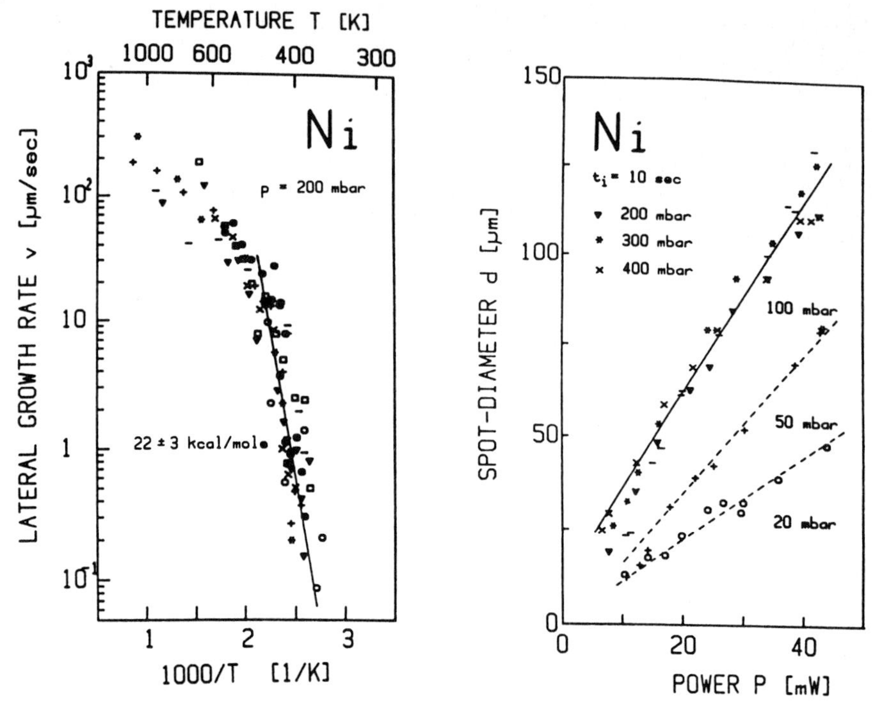


Fig. 6. Arrhenius plot for lateral growth rate v of Ni spots. The full line is a least squares fit to the low temperature data. The different symbols refer to different laser powers and focus diameters (after ⌊13⌋)

Fig. 7. Dependence of Ni spot diameters on laser power for various gas pressures and constant laser beam illumination time $t_i$ = 10 sec. The full curve was calculated correspondingly to (1). The dashed lines are guides for the eyes (after ⌊13⌋)

supports the idea that the lateral growth rate depends only on the local temperature rise, which is determined only by the total absorbed laser power. The main systematic error in the calculated temperatures, and consequently in the activation energy, arises from the uncertainty in the reflectivity $R_D$, which was measured in situ and found to be $R_D = 0.2 \pm 0.1$. For the limiting values $R_D = 0.3$ and $R_D = 0.1$ we obtain $\Delta E$ = 18 kcal/mole and $\Delta E$ = 31 kcal/mole, respectively. These values are within the range of apparent chemical activation energies reported for large area heterogeneous deposition of Ni from $Ni(CO)_4$ ⌊29-31⌋. The investigation which covered the widest temperature region (350K ≤ T ≤ 430K) gave 22 kcal/mole ⌊29⌋, which is in good agreement with our result. The marked decrease in slope above the temperature $T_b \approx 500$ K could have various origins. For example it might indicate the limits of the model calculations, which, of course, are adequate only if $d \gg 2w_0$. Another possibility, which at present seems very likely, is the change in reflectance which occurs for the very shortest times $t_i$. However, the decrease in slope could also have origins which were already discussed in connection with steady growth of rods (see Sect. 6 and ⌊1,18⌋), namely limitations in the gas phase transport of reactant molecules or reaction products, the desorption of CO, or other chemical reaction pathways which may become possible in the high temperature region.

Fig. 7 shows the diameter of Ni spots for $t_i$ = 10 sec as function of laser power and for different gas pressures. The saturation in growth observed for higher gas pressures is expected for a heterogeneous chemical reaction and is described by the pressure dependence of $k_0$ (see (1)), i.e. we find $k_0 \approx 1$ for $p > 100$ mbar. The full curve belongs to the p = 200 mbar data and was calculated by integrating the spot diameter correspondingly to (1) with the activation energies and the constant A derived from Fig. 6. The agreement is excellent and shows the consistency of the procedure. According to the calculations, the quasilinear increase in d should extend up to about 60 mW.

## 5.2 Steady Growth of Stripes

Figs. 8a-d show scanning electron micrographs of Si stripes deposited from $SiH_4$ on Si wafers with increasing powers of the $\lambda$ = 488 nm $Ar^+$ laser line. While at laser powers corresponding to center temperatures below the melting point, $T_m$, of Si, a convex cross section is observed, a dip in the middle of the stripe (Fig. 8c) occurs for center temperatures $T > T_m$ and increases with increasing laser power (Fig. 8d). The dip can be explained by the change in surface tension with temperature which pulls the liquid away from the valleys. At such laser powers polysilanes which are formed in a homogeneous reaction above the surface of the deposit condense in the region of deposition. With a further increase in laser power, the formation of polysilanes increases and the dip extends into the Si wafer. Melting of the surface of the stripe is accompanied by the occurrence of a ripple structure with grating vector k parallel to the incident electric field vector E (Fig. 9a). Formation of ripples has previously been observed after illumination on solid surfaces mainly with intense laser pulses [33]. Interesting features occur when using laser powers, which induce temperatures $T > T_m$ and increasing scanning velocities. As expected, the deposited structure becomes smaller in width and height. At some stage, a

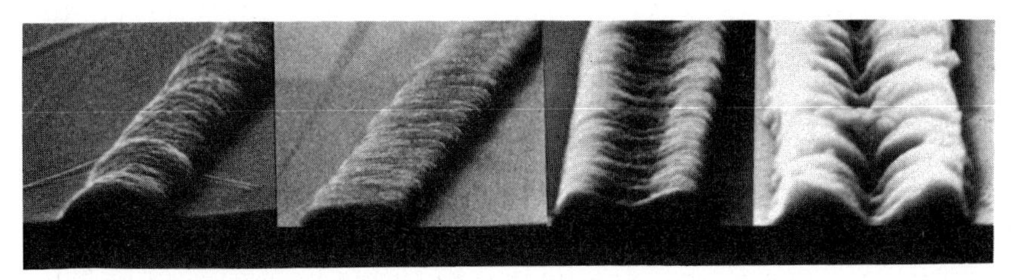

Fig. 8. Si stripes grown on Si wafers with increasing laser powers. $p(SiH_4) \approx 40$ mbar; $v_s \approx 10$ µm/sec; $\lambda$ = 488 nm (after [32])

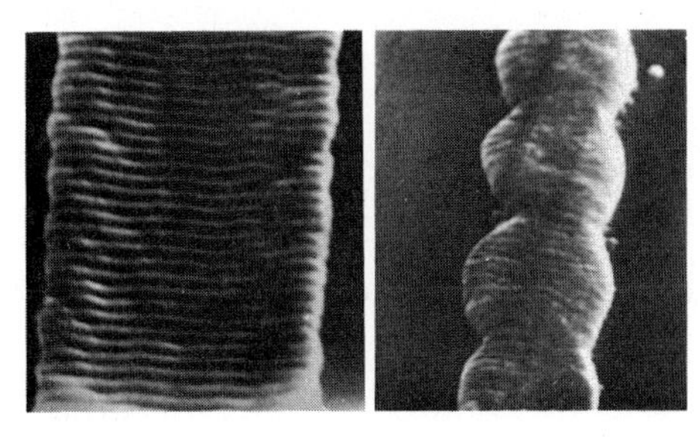

Fig. 9. Rippling and superstructure of Si grown on Si wafers

periodic superstructure occurs which still shows the rippling (see Fig. 9b). When further increasing the scanning velocity, continuous growth breaks off and nearly equidistant spots (still showing the rippling) are observed. Formation of superstructures was also observed when varying the gas pressure. The structure-forming mechanism which is probably based on the nonlinearity of the deposition process must be investigated in further detail.

The influence of melting and changes in the morphology complicate the understanding of the deposition process. The following analysis of direct writing will therefore be performed for the range of low laser powers where no appreciable changes in the shape of the cross section occur and where therefore an unequivocal definition of a width and a height of stripes is possible. The main experimental results were outlined in detail for the example of Ni stripes which were deposited on substrates of different absorbance and thermal conductivity [1,7]. Here, we will only recall some of the most essential features which are common to all systems investigated until now and compare them with the results of the model calculations of Sect. 3. Fig. 10 shows the widths of Ni stripes as function of laser power for three different substrate materials. In all cases, the cross section of stripes is similar to that shown in Fig. 8a. The height, measured in the middle of the stripe, is $h \leqslant (0.1\text{-}0.05)d$. The negligible influence of the

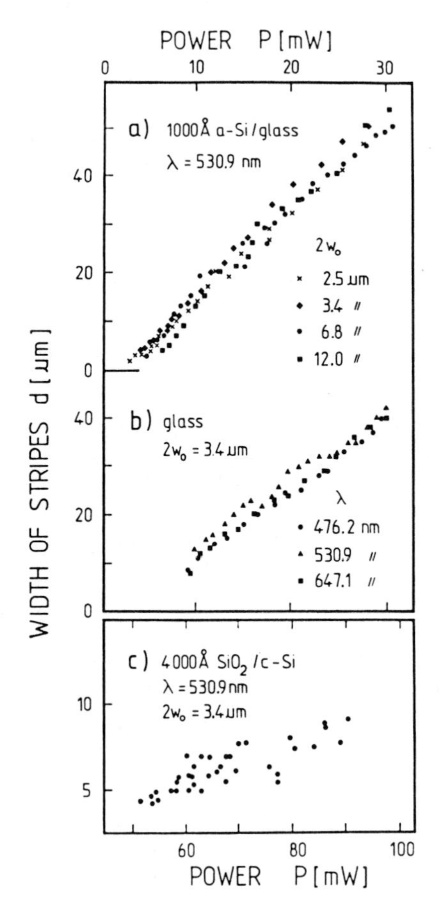


Fig. 10. Dependence of width of Ni stripes on laser power for different substrates, focus diameters and wavelengths. In all cases the total pressure was $p(Ni(CO)_4) = 400$ mbar and the scanning velocity $v = 84$ µm/s (after [7])

laser wavelength (Fig. 10b) reflects the thermal nature of the decomposition mechanism. Note that for substrates of equal thermal conductivity but absorbances differing by several orders of magnitude, the results are approximately equal (Figs. 10a,b). This strongly suggests that in steady growth of stripes the total absorbed laser power is given by $P(1-R_D)$, i.e. it depends only on the absorbance of the already deposited material. Therefore, we believe that steady growth of stripes occurs as schematically drawn in Fig. 11. During the dwell time of the laser beam lateral growth occurs. In steady growth of stripes, the lateral growth velocity in the scanning direction must be equal to the scanning velocity of the laser beam, i.e. $v = v_s$. Steady growth of the stripes tails off when the scanning velocity of the laser beam exceeds the maximum lateral growth velocity. In fact, the maximum lateral growth rates reported in Sect. 5.1 for Ni/1000 Å a-Si/glass, agree, to within a factor of about two, with the maximum scanning velocities obtained for the same system and the same parameter set [1,7]. Another feature in Fig. 10 is that in cases a) and b) the width $d \gg 2w_0$ (except for the lowest laser powers) and independent of $2w_0$ while in case c) $d \approx 2w_0$. This can be understood from the results of the model calculations presented in Fig. 2 by the following arguments. Assume we produce the same center temperature, $T_c$, for all three substrate materials (full curves in Figs. 2a-c). It is clear from Fig. 2 that in cases b) and c) the temperature falls off much faster away from the center than in case a). Because growth occurs only down to a threshold temperature, $T_t$ (see also Sect. 5.1), the stripe, in case b) or c), grows to a final width much smaller than the width in a). Fig. 2 also shows that doubling of the laser focus (chain-dotted curves) results in a stripe of equal width in a), while deposition will stop in b) or c). On the other hand, if $T_c$ approaches $T_t$, deposition in case a) will continue to lower laser powers the smaller the diameter of the laser focus becomes. This is directly reflected in the experimental results of Fig. 10a. In other words, the smallest widths of structures that can be achieved depend on $2w_0$. The fact that stripes which are narrower than the diffraction limit of the optical system can be produced (see Fig. 10a) also originates from the threshold for deposition.

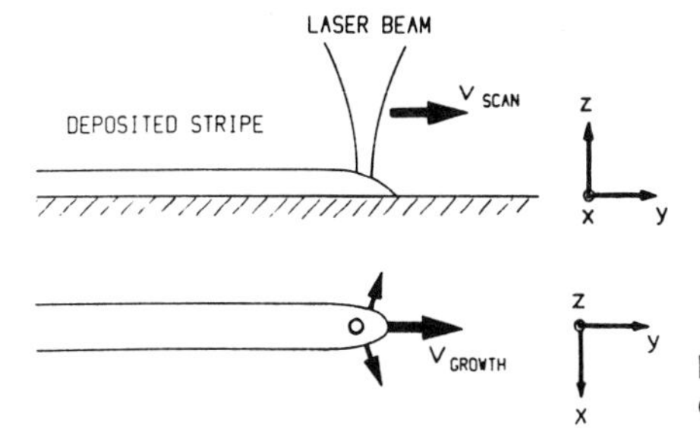


Fig. 11. Schematic for steady growth of stripes

The foregoing results are, of course, by no means specific for Ni deposits but are characteristic for pyrolytic LCVD of flat structures in general. Similar results corresponding to those in Figs. 10a,b, i.e. to the case $k_D \gg k_S$, were also obtained for the deposition of Al and Si on 1000 Å a-Si/glass [11,35], for C on $Al_2O_3$ [25] and for Cu on Si [19]. In addition to the example of Ni/4000 Å $SiO_2$/Si (Fig. 10c) the case $k_D \approx k_S \gg k_L$ (Fig. 2b) has also been demonstrated for Si/4000 Å $SiO_2$/Si [22,35]. The case $k_D = k_S = k_L$ has been verfied experimentally for Ni on Si [15] and for Si on Si [22,23,35]. As expected from Fig. 2c, in these latter cases the widths of stripes is typically $d \lesssim 2w_0$.

From the above discussion it is clear that many features in direct writing can be qualitatively understood from the calculated temperature profiles of Fig. 2. Also the decreasing width of stripes with increasing scanning velocity [1,7] can be explained from the analysis of the lateral growth of spots. Quantitative calculations, however, require consideration of the exact position of the laser focus with respect to the tip of the growing stripe (this position changes with scanning velocity) and of the heat transport along the stripe. The effect of the latter has been calculated for a simplified model in [12]. The results also show that in direct writing, the range of parameters and therefore the lateral and axial growth rates and the related maximal scanning velocities strongly depend on both the physical properties of the deposited material and of the substrate. While the possible range of variation in the width of stripes is very large for $k_D >> k_S$, it is very small for $k_D \approx k_S$. The upper limitation is essentially based on the maximum temperature rise up to which controlled deposition is possible, i.e. no dramatic changes in the geometry of the deposit (Fig. 8), no damaging of the substrate and no triggering of a homogeneous gas phase reaction above the surface of the deposit occurs. Furthermore, small changes in $2w_0$, or in the positioning of the substrate or in the laser power (due to systematic uncertainties or due to mechanical or electrical instabilities) will have a much stronger influence for systems where $k_D \approx k_S$ than for those where $k_D >> k_S$. This may also explain the larger scattering in the data of Fig. 10c with respect to those in Figs. 10a, b.

## 6. Steady Growth of Rods

A typical example of a rod grown by LCVD is shown in Fig. 12 for the case of Si which was deposited from $SiH_4$. Two phases of growth can be observed. Near the onset, the deposition rate depends strongly on the physical properties of the substrate. This phase of growth corresponds to the growth of spots and was discussed in Sect. 5.1. In steady growth, which is characterized in Fig. 12 by a constant rod diameter, the deposition rate is independent of the substrate material. Therefore, in contrast to the growth of spots, the temperature profile in the tip of the rod is independent of time, i.e. T = f(r), if the laser irradiance is held constant. The constant rod diameter is a consequence of the threshold in lateral growth - as discussed in Sect. 5.1. It is clear from the shape of the rod that in steady growth the maximum growth rate is at the center of the tip and identical with the axial growth velocity. Therefore, the deposition rate can be defined by

$$W(T) \equiv v(r = 0,T) = \Delta h(r = 0,T) / \Delta t \quad (4)$$

where h(r = 0, T) is given by (1). T is the surface temperature measured in the center of the tip of the rod [18]. The upper part of Fig. 13 shows an Arrhenius plot for the laser-induced deposition of Si from $SiH_4$. In the kinetically controlled regime, which reaches up to about 1400 K, the deposition rate increases exponentially with temperature and is characterized

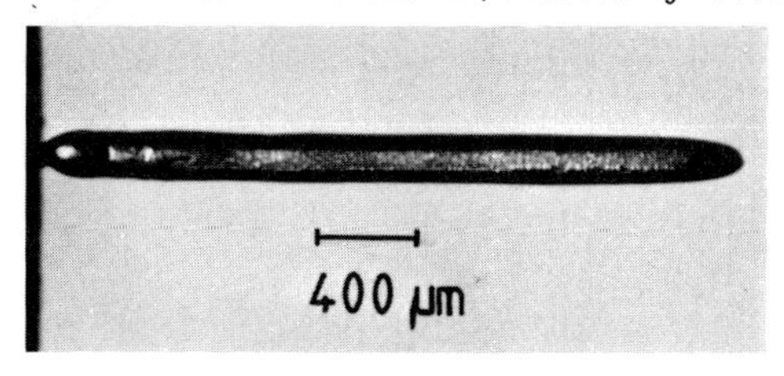


Fig. 12. Silicon rod grown from $SiH_4$ with 488 nm $Ar^+$ laser radiation. P = 400 mW, $p(SiH_4)$ = 133 mbar

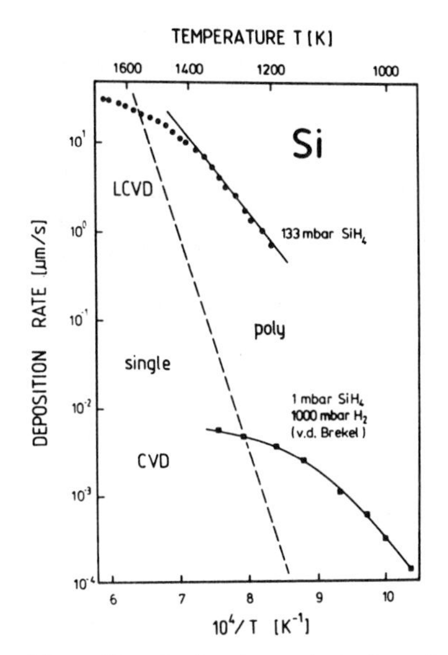


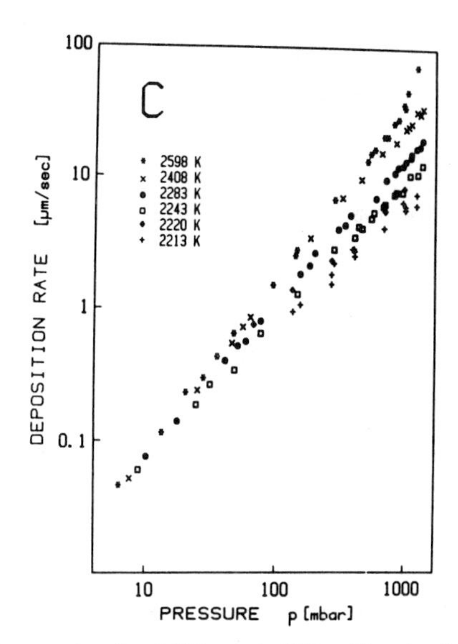


Fig. 13. Arrhenius plot for deposition rate in LCVD and CVD. The broken line separates regions of single- and polycrystalline growth

Fig. 14. Deposition rate of C as function of $C_2H_2$ pressure for various temperatures (after [34])

by an apparent chemical activation energy of $\Delta E = 46.6 \pm 4$ kcal/mol (this value is corrected by using the ansatz $k_0 \propto 1/T$). The characteristic decrease in slope observed above a certain temperature may indicate that deposition is no longer controlled by the chemical kinetics, but instead becomes limited by transport. However, alternative explanations cannot be ruled out (see Sect. 5.1 and [1]). The lower part of Fig. 13 shows the deposition rate for Si deposited from $SiH_4$ - with $H_2$ as carrier gas ($p(SiH_4)$ = 1 mbar, $p_{tot}$ = 1000 mbar) - according to standard CVD techniques. The comparison of LCVD and CVD curves shows the remarkable differences for small and large area heterogeneous chemical reactions as discussed in Sect. 2.

The diameter of Si rods could be varied between 20 µm and 380 µm for effective laser powers of 25 mW and 1.4 W of the $\lambda$ = 488 nm $Ar^+$ laser line, respectively. The lower limit was essentially determined by the mechanical stability of the apparatus, the upper limit by the available laser power. Due to the step-like increase in reflectivity at the melting point, the total absorbed laser power, $P(1-R_D)$, falls dramatically at this temperature.

Similar investigations were performed for the deposition of C from $C_2H_2$, $C_2H_4$ and $CH_4$ [18,25]. The apparent chemical activation energy derived for the deposition from $C_2H_2$ was $\Delta E = 51 \pm 2$ kcal/mol (corrected value). This activation energy was independent of the gas pressure within the investigated range 67 mbar $\leq p$ ($C_2H_2$) $\leq$ 980 mbar. Fig. 14 shows the pressure dependence of the deposition rate for various temperatures. The apparent reaction order for temperatures 2000 K $\leq T \leq$ 2350 K was found to be 0.95 $\pm$ 0.05 and this increases for higher temperatures. For pressures $p \leq 50$ mbar the deposition rate becomes independent of temperature. This indicates that deposition becomes limited by transport for all the temperatures investigated.

Rods of $SiO_x$ and of stoichiometric $SiO_2$ were deposited with $\lambda$ = 530.9 nm $Kr^+$ laser radiation from a mixture of $N_2O$ and $SiH_4$ [26]. The growth of Ni rods deposited from $Ni(CO)_4$ was investigated for laser powers ranging from about 10 mW up to about 200 mW [7]. The deposition rate did not change when using $Kr^+$ laser wavelengths between $\lambda$ = 476.2 nm and 647.1 nm - as expected for a thermally activated process (see sect. 2). The limit of growth up to which controlled deposition was possible was determined by the occurrence of spontaneous breakdowns - probably an autocatalyzed reaction - within the gas phase above the surface of the tip of the rod.

Investigations of the temperature dependence of the deposition rate during the steady growth of the rods are up to now the most accurate method which yields information on the reaction kinetics in LCVD. Furthermore, because of the extremely high deposition rates together with the possibility of in situ temperature measurements, this technique seems to be unique for rapid and accurate determination of apparent activation energies which are also relevant to CVD and gas phase epitaxial processes. The determination of such activation energies by the standard techniques is very time-consuming and problematic because a number of parameters, such as substrate temperature, gas velocity, gas mixture, etc., must be held constant over long periods of time, generally several hours, and only small numbers of data points can be generated [18].

Other interesting possibilities, such as the growth of complicated three dimensional structures by interference of laser beams, the production of materials with higher purity and the production of non-equilibrium materials or materials which form only under extreme conditions, were already mentioned in the introduction.

## 7. Microstructure and Physical Properties of Deposits

The microstructure of deposits was mainly investigated by optical microscopy, scanning electron microscopy (SEM), X-ray diffraction, and by Raman scattering techniques.

The microstructure of spots and stripes investigated until now was always polycrystalline with grain sizes increasing with increasing laser irradiance and decreasing with gas pressure [1,7]. In most cases spots and stripes adhered strongly to properly cleaned substrates, except in the case of glass substrates covered with 1000 Å a-Si and high laser powers, typically > 20 mW. The thermally induced lateral strain has been estimated for Si stripes, which were deposited on 3500 Å to 4000 Å thermally grown $SiO_2$ on Si, from the shift of the 520 $cm^{-1}$ $T_{2g}$ Raman line. The observed red shift of the line was < 2 $cm^{-1}$, corresponding to a tensile stress of < 4 kbar [1,22]. The electrical resistivities of Ni [7] and Cu [19] stripes were by about a factor of 2-3 larger than the corresponding bulk resistivities. Low resistivity stripes of Si have been produced by adding doping gases as $BCl_3$ or $B(CH_3)_3$ to the silane [22]. Carbon inclusions in Ni were ≤ 1%. Carbide formation is much more critical with the deposition of W, Mo and Al from the carbonyls and the alkyls, respectively. However, it can be strongly reduced by addition of suitable amounts of $H_2$.

The microstructure of rods also depends on the laser-induced temperature and the gas pressure. Rods have been grown in the amorphous [26], polycrystalline [7,18,23,25] and single crystalline phases [1,4]. Fig. 13 includes the border line (broken line) for single and polycrystalline growth of Si by CVD and LCVD. This border line is essentially determined by the ratio of the flux of Si atoms giving rise to the observed growth rate, and the value of the self-diffusion coefficient of Si, needed to arrange the arriving atoms on proper lattice sites.

## 8. Conclusions

Pyrolytic LCVD allows single-step production of microstructures of nearly all materials deposited by standard CVD techniques. Laser pyrolysis at visible wavelengths combines high deposition rates (typically 0.1 μm/sec to 100 μm/sec) and small lateral dimensions of deposits (down to ~ 0.5 μm) with standard laser techniques, simple optics and adjustments. At present, the highest scanning speeds are about 500 μm/sec. The growth of spots and stripes can be qualitatively - and in some cases even quantitatively - understood from temperature distributions which are calculated for combined structures and which take into account the heat transport through the deposited material itself.

Three-dimensional structures in the form of rods have been grown, even as single crystals, within the laser beam, i.e. without any crucible and in otherwise cold surroundings.

Among the advantages of laser pyrolysis with respect to photolysis are the large variety of materials which can be deposited, the high deposition rates which exceed those in photolysis by a factor $10^2$ to $10^4$, and the better morphology and higher purity (especially with respect to carbon inclusions for deposition from alkyls or carbonyls) which result in better electrical properties. Disadvantages of pyrolysis are the higher local temperatures and - in case of flat structures - the stronger influence of the physical properties of the substrate material, especially its thermal conductivity.

## Acknowledgements

I wish to thank K. Piglmayer for additional computer calculations and the Fonds zur Förderung der wissenschaftlichen Forschung in Österreich for financial support.

## References

1 For earlier reviews see, e.g.: D. Bäuerle: In Laser Diagnostics and Photochemical Processing for Semiconductor Devices, ed. by R.M. Osgood et al. (North Holland, New York 1983) Vol. 17, p. 19-28; and Springer Series in Chemical Physics 33, ed. by F. Aussenegg et al. (Springer, Heidelberg 1983) p. 178-188 and references therein
2 For an earlier review on photolytic LCVD see, e.g.: D.J. Ehrlich, R.M. Osgood, T.F. Deutsch.: J. Vac. Sci. Technol. 21, 23 (1982)
3 For a review see, e.g.: J. Bloem, L.J. Giling: In Current Topics in Materials Science, Vol. 1, ed. by E. Kaldis (North-Holland, New York 1978) p. 147-342
4 D. Bäuerle, G. Leyendecker, D. Wagner, E. Bauser, Y.C. Lu: Appl. Phys. A 30, 147 (1983)
5 see, e.g.: Handbook of Thin Film Technology, ed. by L.I. Maissel, R. Glang, (LMcGraw Hill, New York, 1970)
6 Y. Rytz-Froidevaux, R.P. Salathé, H.H. Gilgen, H.P. Weber: Appl. Phys. A 27, 133 (1982)
7 W. Kräuter, D. Bäuerle, F. Fimberger: Appl. Phys. A 31, 13 (1983)

8 A.M. Bradshaw: this volume
9 K.L. Kompa: this volume
10 D.J. Ehrlich, R.M. Osgood: Chem. Phys. Lett. 79, 381 (1981)
11 U. Kempfer, K. Piglmayer, D. Bäuerle: to be published
12 K. Piglmayer, J. Doppelbauer, D. Bäuerle: In Laser Controlled Chemical Processing of Surfaces, ed. by D.J. Ehrlich et al. (North Holland, New York, 1984)
13 F. Petzoldt, K. Piglmayer, W. Kräuter, D. Bäuerle: Appl. Phys. (1984)
14 A.J. Davies: The Finite Element Method (Clarendon Press, Oxford 1980)
15 J.P. Herman, R.A. Hyde, B.M. McWilliams, A.H. Weisberg, L.L. Wood: Ref. 1a, p. 9-18
16 H.C. Webber, A.G. Cullis, N.G. Chew: Appl. Phys. Lett. 43, 669 (1983)
17 H.S. Carslaw and T.C. Jaeger: Conduction of Heat in Solids (Oxford University Press 1959), p. 216
18 G. Leyendecker, H. Noll, D. Bäuerle, P. Geittner, H. Lydtin: J. Electrochem. Soc. 130, 157 (1983)
19 F.A. Houle and C.R. Jones: private communication
20 D. Braichotte, H. v. d. Bergh: this volume
21 C.R. Jones, C.A. Kovac, T.H. Baum, F.A. Houle: private communication
22 D.J. Ehrlich, R.M. Osgood, T.F. Deutsch: Appl. Phys. Lett. 39, 957 (1981)
23 D. Bäuerle, P. Irsigler, G. Leyendecker, H. Noll, D. Wagner: Appl. Phys. Lett. 40, 819 (1982)
24 D. Bäuerle, G. Leyendecker, D. Wagner: unpublished
25 G. Leyendecker, D. Bäuerle, P. Geittner, H. Lydtin: Appl. Phys. Lett. 39, 921 (1981)
26 S. Szikora, W. Kräuter, D. Bäuerle: Mat. Lett. 2, 263 (1984); see also reviews by I.W. Boyd and T. Tokuyama: this volume
27 D. Bäuerle, J. Doppelbauer, S. Szikora, G. Constant, F. Maury: to be published
28 H. Beneking: this volume
29 H.E. Carlton, J.H. Oxley: AICHE Journal 12, 86 (1967)
30 A.J. Goosen, J.A. Van den Berg: J.S. African Chem. Inst. 25, 370 (1972)
31 J.P. Day, R.G. Pearson, F. Basolo: J. Am. Chem. Soc. 90, 6933 (1968)
32 J. Otto, D. Bäuerle: unpublished
33 For reviews see, e.g.: Z. Guosheng, P.M. Fauchet, A.E. Siegman: Phys. Rev. B 26, 5366 (1982); and H.M. van Driel, J.E. Sipe, J.F. Young: Phys. Rev. Lett. 49, 55 (1982); Phys. Rev. B 27, 1424 (1983)
34 G. Leyendecker, H. Noll, D. Bäuerle: unpublished
35 F. Petzoldt, S. Szikora, D. Bäuerle: unpublished
36 S.D. Allen, A.B. Trigubo, R.Y. Jan: see Ref. 1a, p. 207-214

# Structure of Platinum and Tin Films Formed by Laser-Induced Chemical Vapor Deposition

D. Braichotte and H. van den Bergh

Institut de Chimie Physique, Ecole Polytechnique Fédérale,
CH-1015 Lausanne, Switzerland

## Introduction:

Working integrated circuits have recently been produced by LCVD techniques (1), and much of the laser chemistry effort at the gas-solid and liquid-solid interfaces is directed towards this goal (2-4). In the present communication we report on the LCVD of Pt and Sn by observing the deposited thin films using electron microscopy. The dependence of the structure of the metallic deposit on the following variables is measured:

A) The LCVD mechanism which can be either pyrolytic or photolytic.
B) The laser irradiation time.
C) The laser power density at the surface.

The dependence of the LCVD on the gas pressure in these experiments has been reported elsewhere (5). In a future paper we will try to correlate the observed structures of the metallic deposits with their electric conductivity (6).

## Experimental:

The experimental setup has been described in some detail previously (5), and only some of the more essential features are repeated here briefly. For electron microscopy the metallic films are deposited on a support consisting of a thin layer (about 100 Å thick) of amorphous carbon previously evaporated under vacuum and transposed onto a fine copper wire grid.

The laser used for pyrolytic LCVD is a single mode Ar ion laser operating at $\lambda$=514.5 nm. The laser beam is focussed onto the surface with a 5 cm focal length quartz lens. Following Bäuerle and coworkers (4) the power densities are calculated from the measured laser beam power and the diffraction limited diameter of the laser beam at the focal point of the lens:

$$2W_o = 1.27\lambda f/d$$

where $2W_o$ is the beam diameter at the focal point, $\lambda$ is the laser wavelength, f is the focal length of the lens, and d is the diameter of the laser beam.

For photodeposition at $\lambda$=257 nm the green light is frequency doubled in a temperature tuned KDP crystal. The green light is then removed using a Glan-Thompson prism and a reflection filter. The maximum power obtained at $\lambda$=257 nm is 0.7 mWatt.

The electron microscopes used are Philips EM300 for transmission electron microscopy (TEM) as well as diffraction electron microscopy (DEM).

The materials used are platinum-bishexafluoroacetylacetonate synthesized and purified according to (7). The tetramethyltin is from Ventron (99.5%) and is freeze-pumped before use. Hereafter these compounds are abbreviated respectively as $Pt(HFAcAc)_2$ and TMSn.

Results and Discussion:

I) The pyrolytic LCVD of Sn:

The first results presented here show several aspects of the growth of Sn particles in pyrolytic LCVD from TMSn. Figs. 1a-e show the TEM pictures of the deposited particles at constant laser intensity but at varying irradiation times between 0.01 s and 3 s. At first, at times up to about 1/60 s at the applied conditions, the metal clusters grow. Simultaneously we see that the number of metal clusters of a given size (the darker spots in Figs. 1a,b) increases. At a later stage (see for instance Figs. 1c-e) on a time scale between 1/15 s and 3 s, the size of the clusters continues to increase, but the number density of the larger clusters decreases due to the coalescence of clusters on the hot surface. DEM pictures of the pyrolitically deposited Sn show the diffraction pattern characteristic of polycrystalline material.

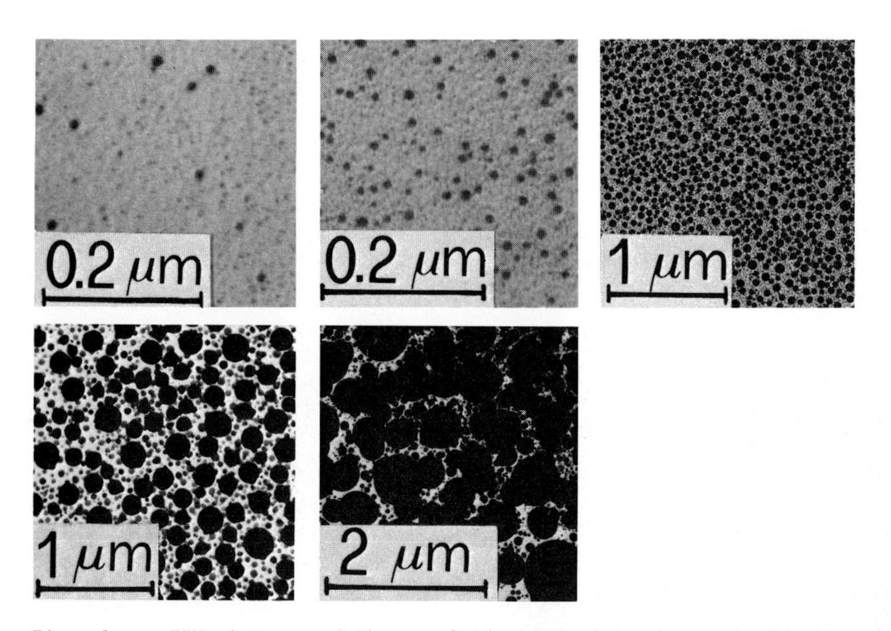


Figs. 1a-e: TEM pictures of the pyrolytic LCVD of Sn observed with increasing irradiation times. 1a=1/100 s, 1b=1/60 s, 1c=1/15 s, 1d=1/2 s, 1e=3 s. Power density at $\lambda$=514.5 nm is 50 kW/cm$^2$. The pressure of TMSn is 30 torr as in all experiments described below.

The results of many measurements such as reported in Figs. 1a-e have been summarized in Fig. 2.

Over the whole range of applied conditions the "average" particle size increases both with increasing irradiation time and increasing laser power density.

At very low power densities ($I<20$ kW cm$^{-2}$) no metallic deposit is observed. At higher power densities $20<I<100$ kW cm$^{-2}$ the Sn is deposited in a disc-like deposit, the detailed structure of which is similar to that found in Figs. 1 a-e. At even higher laser power densities the tin is deposited in the shape of an annulus. Such annular shapes have been observed previously (5,8) and are

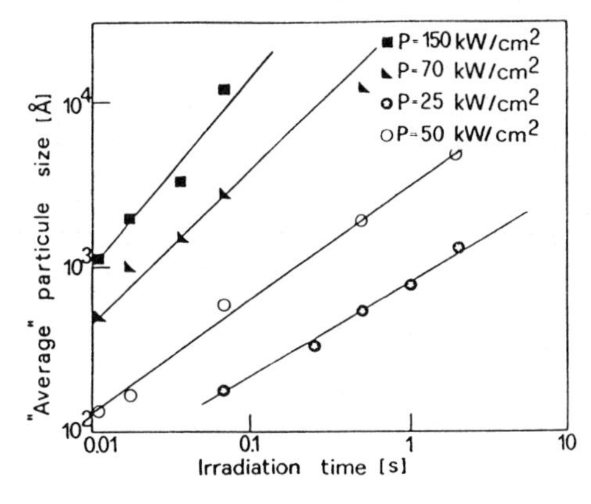


Fig. 2: The variation of the "average" particle size with the irradiation time, measured during the pyrolytic LCVD of a Sn metallic film. The measurements are made at several laser power densities at λ=514.5 nm. The tetramethyltin pressure is 30 torr. All measurements are with the LCVD cell at room temperature, and only the amorphous carbon is heated by the laser beam.

probably due to overheating at the center of the laser beam focus. The tin formed at the hottest part of the surface will not "stick", and will move to a lower temperature region away from the laser beam centroid, thus leaving an area without metallic deposit in the middle of the heated area.

II) The photolytic LCVD of Sn:
The photolytic LCVD of tin yields a metallic deposit which is apparently (even at the largest magnifications) quite homogeneously distributed in space. This is shown in Fig. 3.

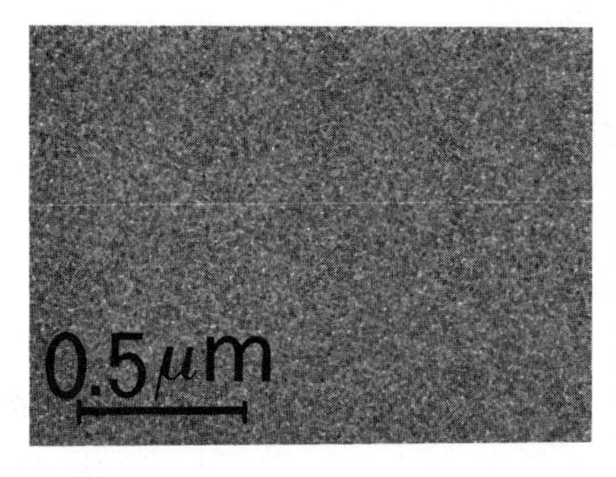


Fig. 3: TEM picture of a section of a photolytically deposited film of Sn which has been strongly enlarged. Note the homogeneity of the deposit as compared to the deposits of Fig. 1. The deposit is amorphous. The laser power density is 0.5 kW $cm^{-2}$ at λ=257 nm. The irradiation time is 10 s, and the TMSn pressure is 30 torr.

Contrary to the pyrolytic LCVD of Sn which yielded predominantly polycrystalline material, the photolytic LCVD yields amorphous tin. One possible explanation for this is that the surface temperature is too low for the tin atoms to rearrange from the positions where they settle on the surface to the positions of the crystalline matrix.

III) The pyrolytic LCVD of Pt:
A typical photodeposit is shown in Fig. 4a. The deposit appears at first from the DEM picture to be polycrystalline as evidenced by the concentric circles in the diffraction pattern. However if the electron beam is focussed so well that essentially only one of the small cubic crystals (see Fig. 4b) of which the film is made up is analysed, then the spot pattern typical of monocrys-

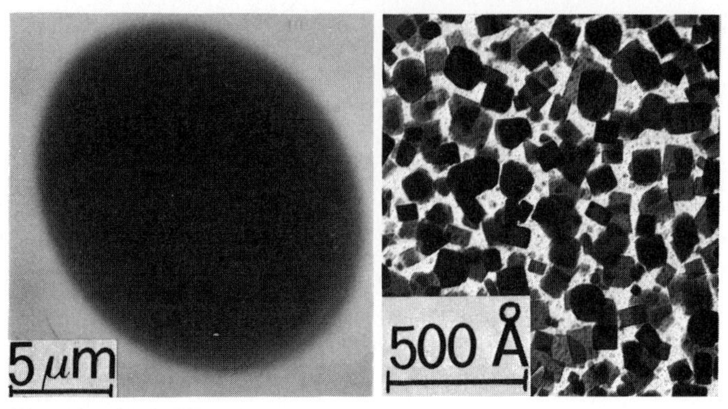

Fig. 4: (4a) TEM picture of a Pt deposit obtained by pyrolytic LCVD from $Pt(HFAcAc)_2$. The laser power density is 15 kW $cm^{-2}$ at λ=514.5 nm, the pressure of $Pt(HFAcAc)_2$ is 0.5 torr, the irradiation time is 10 s. Note that this deposit is significantly more homogeneous than the pyrolytically deposited Sn of Fig. 1. (4b) shows an enlargement of a section at the fringe of Fig. 4a which shows the microscopic monocristalline structure of the deposited Pt.

talline material appears. The deposit is much more homogeneous in overall structure and distribution of material than is the case for pyrodeposition of tin. Contrary to the case of pyrolytic LCVD of tin, in the case of pyrolytic LCVD of platinum, at all tested laser intensities, a disc of deposited metal is observed. The annular deposits observed in the pyrolytic LCVD of Sn at high laser intensities are not observed in the pyrolytic LCVD of platinum. The fact that the Pt is not as easily removed from the spot where it is deposited as in Sn, may involve the much higher melting and boiling points of Pt as compared to Sn (MP(Sn)=231 $^{o}C$, MP(Pt)=1772 $^{o}C$ and BP(Sn)=2270 $^{o}C$, BP(Pt)= 3827 $^{o}C$). Thus for a given temperature of the surface the Sn will much easier sublime and/or distil away from the laser beam centroid than the platinum.

IV) The photolytic LCVD of Pt:

The general aspect of the photolytic LCVD of Pt is the same as in the case of pyrolytic LCVD of platinum, i.e. it is quite homogeneous, as was the case for the pyrolytic LCVD of Sn. The photolytically deposited Pt is however amorphous as was the case of the photolytically deposited Sn.

The parent compound used, $Pt(HFAcAc)_2$, is very efficient as a source of photolytically deposited Pt, as has been shown recently (5). The deposition rate of Pt from $Pt(HFAcAc)_2$ was observed to be several orders of magnitude higher for photolysis at λ=257 nm than the photolytic LCVD of Sn from TMSn at the same wavelength and laser power density.

## Conclusions:

Some of the main similarities and differences in the structure and shape of the metallic deposit have been studied in the case of photolytic and pyrolytic LCVD of tin and platinum. The photolytically deposited thin metallic films appear to be more homogeneous and tend to be amorphous. The pyrolytically deposited films are polycrystalline and are more irregular, in particular in the case of Sn where the hot drop-like particles coalesce on the surface yielding a microscopic deposit of quite varied sizes and shapes.

## Aknowledgement:

The authors are grateful to J.-M. Philippoz for helping with some of the measurements, and to the Swiss Fonds National for financial support.

References:

1. Laser Focus, April 1984, p.14
2. R.M. Osgood, Ann. Rev. Phys. Chem. 34,77(1983).
3. D.J. Ehrlich and J.Y. Tsao, J. Vac. Sci. Technol. B1(4)969(1983).
4. D. Bäuerle, P. Irsigler, G. Leyendecker , H. Noll and D. Wagner, Appl. Phys. Lett. 40(9),819(1982).
5. Qiu Mingxin, R. Monot and H. van den Bergh, Scientia Sinica A, 27(5), 531 (1984).
6. D. Braichotte and H. van den Bergh, to be published.
7. S. Okeya and S. Kawaguchi, Inorg. Synth. 20,65(1980).
8. H. Schröder, private communication.

# Laser Deposition of Single Crystalline GaAs and Stimulated Sheet Doping

H. Beneking

Institute of Semiconductor Electronics, Technical University Aachen,
Sommerfeldstraße, D-5100 Aachen, Fed. Rep. of Germany

## 1. Introduction

The growing application of laser light in processing depends on several reasons. Firstly the possibility to achieve light spots down to 1 μm diameter combined with extreme high power density offers applications in mechanical engineering. Secondly the quantum energy of the light quanta emitted can be used to energize chemical reactions in a specific way leading to photolytic interactions. Thirdly the possibility to create extremely short laser pulses permits correspondingly short heating cycles in small volumes where the absorption takes place. This allows cracking thermally adsorbed species as well as diffusion into the bulk material. The first of these effects can be used as the initiator of crystal growth, the second allows to distribute dopants over a very short distance. Both effects are of high practical importance for modern semiconductor device fabrication.

## 2. The MOCVD process

In the conventional MOCVD process for GaAs growth the metalorganic compounds $(CH_3)_3$ Ga (TMG) and Arsine are used. After Schlyrer and Ring [1], both react at the substrate surface in the following way:

$$(CH_3)_3Ga + AsH_3 \rightarrow (CH_3)_2GaAsH_2 + CH_4$$

$$(CH_3)_2GaAsH_2 \rightarrow CH_3GaAsH + CH_4$$

$$CH_3GaAsH \rightarrow GaAs + CH_4 .$$

A sufficient surface mobility is afforded and the reaction decreases rapidly at lower temperatures ($T < 550^oC$). In the high temperature region ($T > 550^oC$) the process is limited by mass transport of reactant species through the gas phase towards the substrate. The reaction limited and diffusion limited regions can be seen in fig. 1 [2].

## 3. The growth system

The system used consists of a conventional gas supply unit, fig.2. The graphite susceptor is heated by a lamp spot heater as can be seen in fig. 3. An air lock is used to avoid direct contact to the atmosphere in the loading procedure. Besides the susceptor heating from the rear a hydrogen purged quartz window allows illumination of the surface of the wafer. As this additional light source a Nd-YAG laser ($\lambda$= 1064 nm ) is used where the fundamental frequency is doubled ($\lambda$= 532 nm ). This wavelength allows strong absorption at the surface of the GaAs wafer, see fig. 4. At elevated temperatures the fundamental wavelength is also absorbed due to the

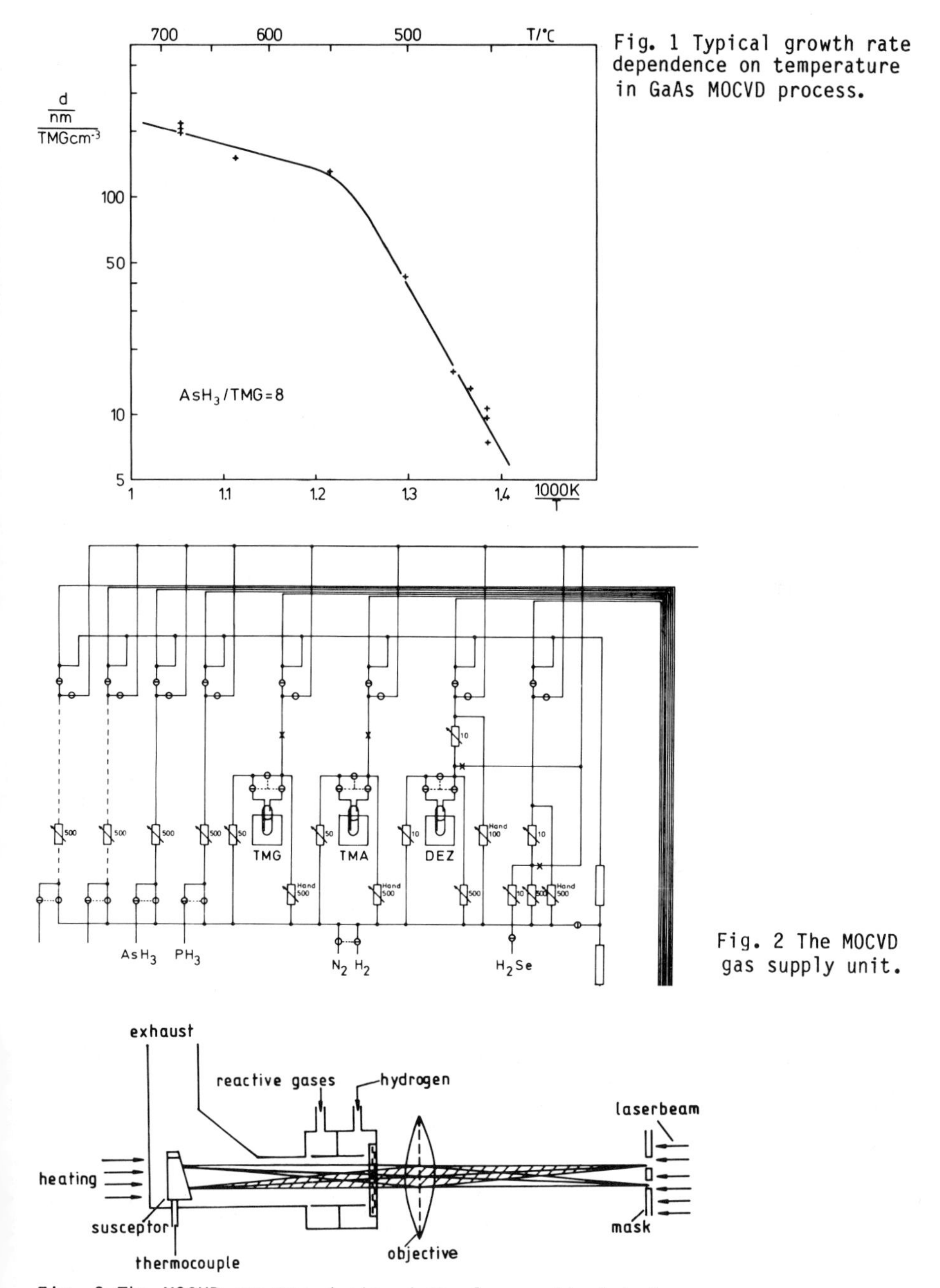


Fig. 1 Typical growth rate dependence on temperature in GaAs MOCVD process.

Fig. 2 The MOCVD gas supply unit.

Fig. 3 The MOCVD reactor designed for laser stimulated processes.

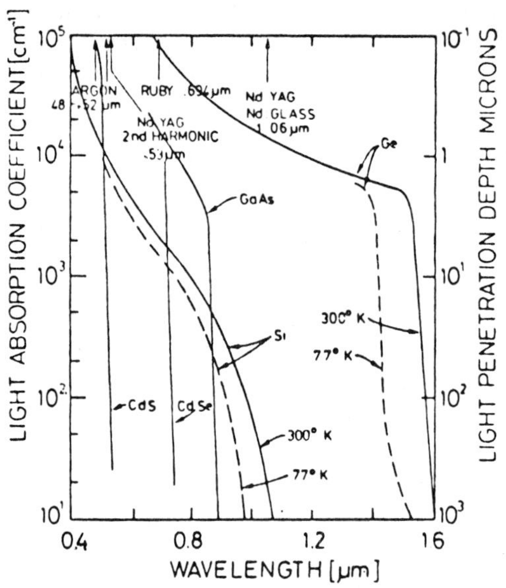


Fig. 4 Absorption coefficients for different semiconductors vs. wavelength, after [3].

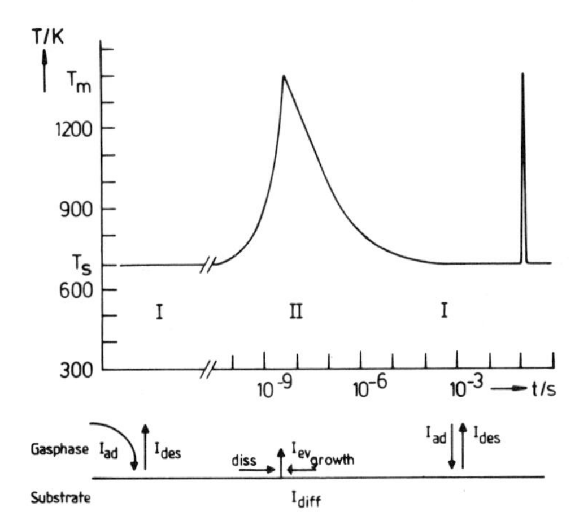


Fig. 5 Surface temperature of GaAs additionally heated to 460 °C and illuminated with 3 ns, 120 mJ/cm² laser pulses vs. time and schematic process steps.

shift of the absorption edge. This effect and additionally the free carrier absorption has to be taken into account by evaluating the temperature rise achievable.

The laser delivers 3 ns pulses with a max. repetition rate of 10 Hz. Therefore at each period a sudden temperature rise occurs followed by a slower decay. This can be seen in fig. 5 where the calculated temperature cycle is shown.

## 4. Growth procedure

Applying the system as in chapter 3 and using an ambient gas atmosphere as conventionally used for MOCVD growth, the laser assisted growth can be performed. The different processes which occur at the surface of the substrate are also indicated in fig.5. The time-dependent temperature variation can be

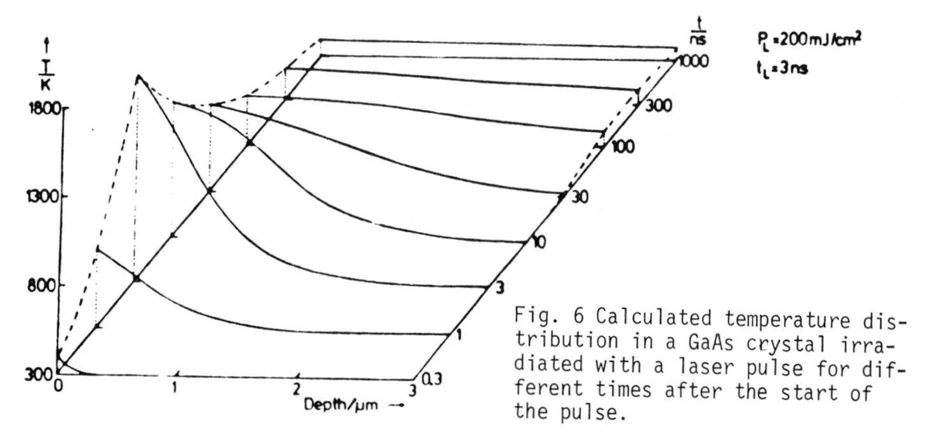


Fig. 6 Calculated temperature distribution in a GaAs crystal irradiated with a laser pulse for different times after the start of the pulse.

seen in fig. 6 which indicates that only a very narrow region of the substrate is influenced. In the recovery phase species from the gas phase are adsorbed whereas the reaction and the growth take place at the high temperature excitation. The relation $N_a(t) = N(1 - \exp(t/\tau))$ indicates that the number of adsorbed reactive species $N_a(t)$ depends exponentially on time with $\tau = (K_a+K_d)^{-1}$ and $N_a = N \cdot K_a$ ($K_a$ adsorption coeff., $K_d$ desorption coeff., N number of available places ). This results in the laser assisted growth behaviour as shown in fig. 7 [4]. Contrary to the conventional growth process, enhanced single crystalline growth of GaAs occurs in the normally reaction limited region, see fig. 8. The quality of the layers grown depends strongly on the laser fluence applied. Fig. 9 gives examples of the morphology achievable.

The growth occurs only at the laser illuminated surface regions of the wafer. Therefore by projection (or scanning) techniques island growth is possible. Fig. 10 shows the expanded side view of a mesa diode grown by this method [5]. At the edges a higher growth rate is observable which can be understood by taking into account the larger gas supply from the ambient atmosphere at corners.

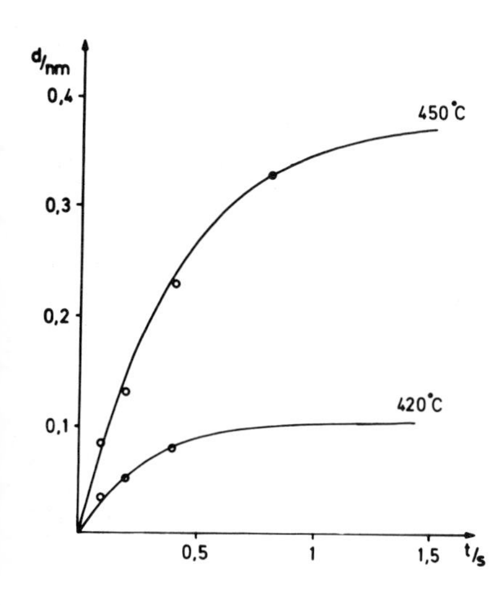


Fig. 7 Deposited layer thickness vs. time between laser pulses, drawn lines are fitted.

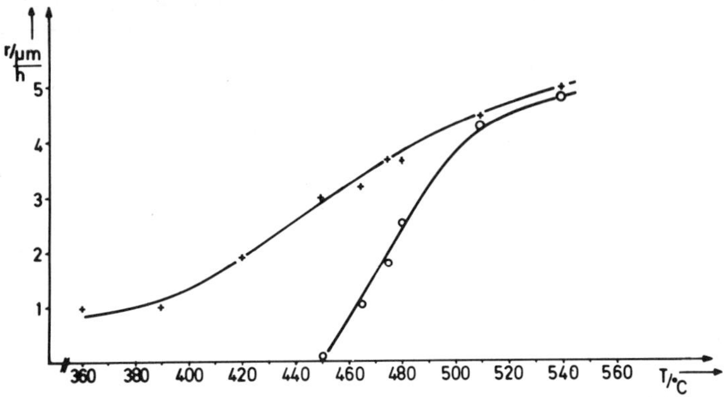


Fig. 8 Growth rate vs. temperature in conventional (o) and laser enhanced (+) MOCVD

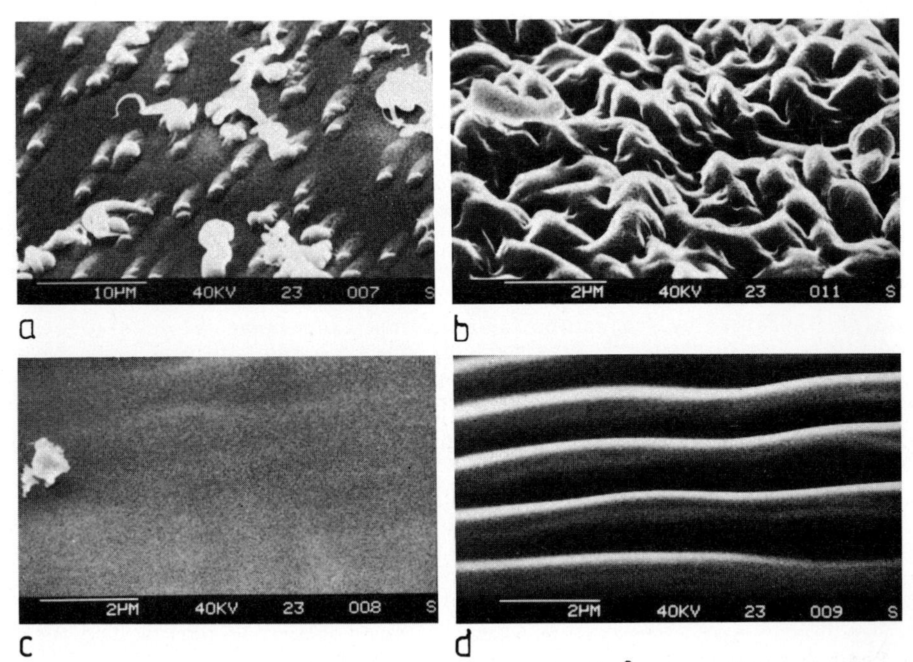


Fig. 9 Morphology of GaAs surfaces grown at 450 $^{0}$C for different laser fluences. (a) no laser, (b) 70 mJ/cm$^2$, (c) 120 mJ/cm$^2$, (d) 150 mJ/cm$^2$

## 5. Laser assisted diffusion

If the ambient atmosphere contains no species for crystal growth but those containing dopant atoms, the laser induced cracking of the adsorbed molecules allows to dope the substrate. The short temperature cycle, Figs. 5 and 6, allows to drive the dopants in over a correspondingly short distance. As a result extremely high dopant densities are achievable along some 10nm.

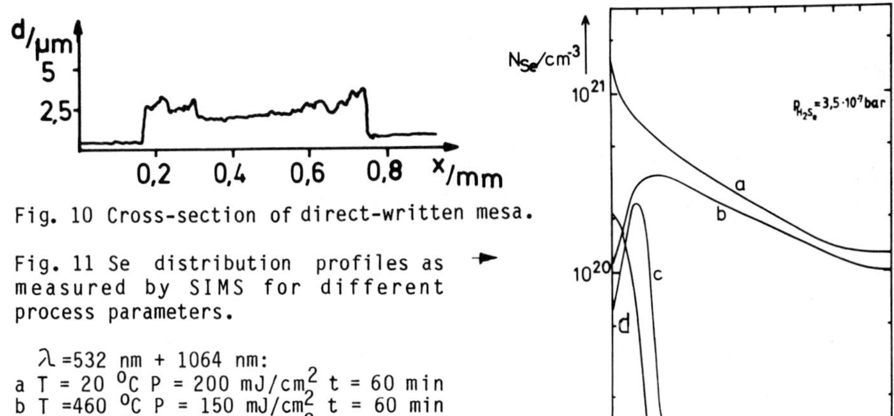


Fig. 10 Cross-section of direct-written mesa.

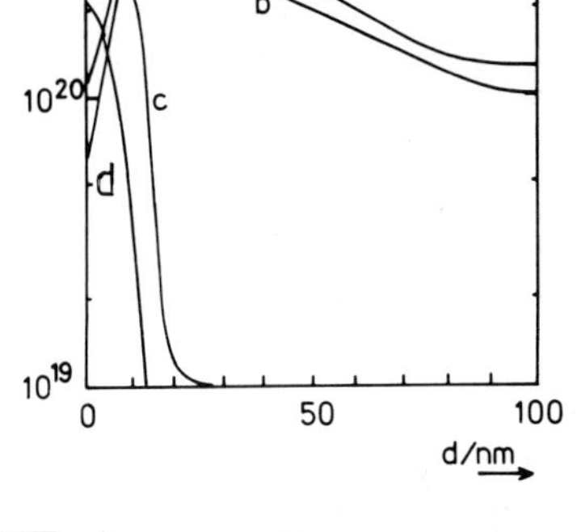


Fig. 11 Se distribution profiles as measured by SIMS for different process parameters.

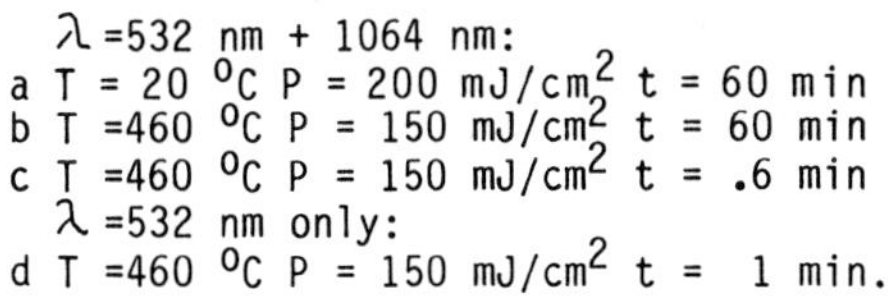

λ =532 nm + 1064 nm:
a T = 20 °C P = 200 mJ/cm² t = 60 min
b T =460 °C P = 150 mJ/cm² t = 60 min
c T =460 °C P = 150 mJ/cm² t = .6 min
λ =532 nm only:
d T =460 °C P = 150 mJ/cm² t = 1 min.

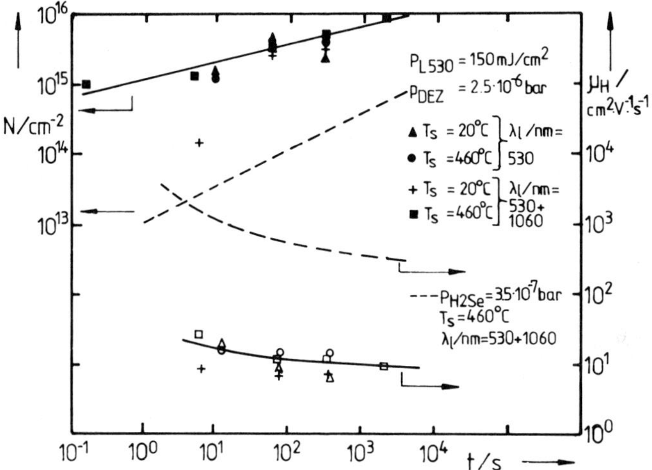


Fig. 12 Sheet carrier concentration and Hall mobility of GaAs irradiated with 3 ns laser pulses in a $H_2Se$ or DEZ gas atmosphere vs. processing time.

For n-type doping $H_2$ Se is used [6], for p-type doping $(C_2H_5)_2Zn$ (DEZ) [7]. Fig. 11 demonstrates the sheet-like doping achievable, where also the difference arising is indicated if the residual long wavelength radiation is excluded. The doping content can be seen in fig.12, where in the case of Se the $t^{1/2}$ dependence indicates a normaldiffusion behaviour.Contrarily,the Zn doped samples show a $t^{1/4}$ dependence resulting from anormal interstitial diffusion of Zn in GaAs.

## 6.Devices

Because of the short settling time the perfection of the single crystalline grown layers is not as qualified as conventionally grown material. This is

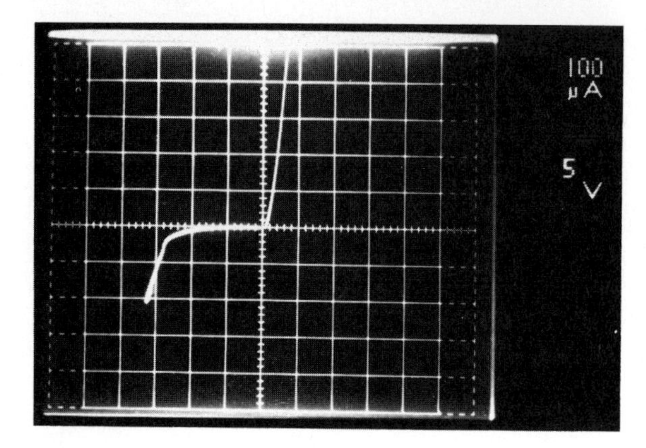


Fig. 13 I-V characteristic of a direct-written p-n mesa diode.

indicated by the reduced carrier mobility. Nevertheless device quality can be achieved. Fig. 13 shows the I-V characteristics of a laser grown pn diode [5]. The large n-factor, n = 1.75, see fig. 14, indicates the minor quality of the laser grown GaAs.

The correspondent short lifetime allows to fabricate fast optical detectors using the photoconductive effect [8]. This is demonstrated in fig. 15 where the pulse response of such a photoconductive detector is shown. The active material has been grown on s.i. GaAs, leading to a lateral detector configuration.

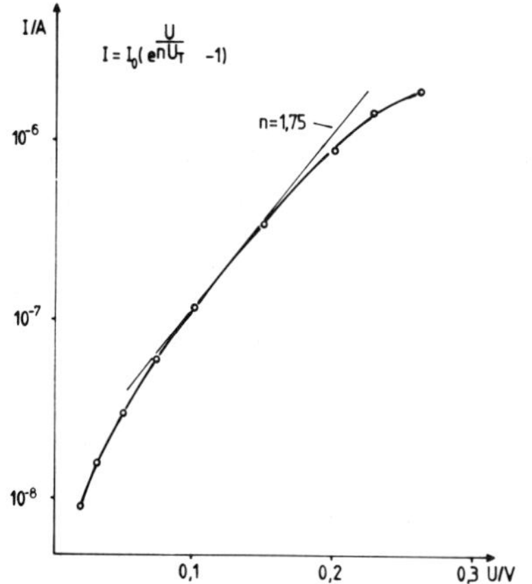


Fig. 14 (left) Semi-logarithmic I-V characteristic of the mesa diode.

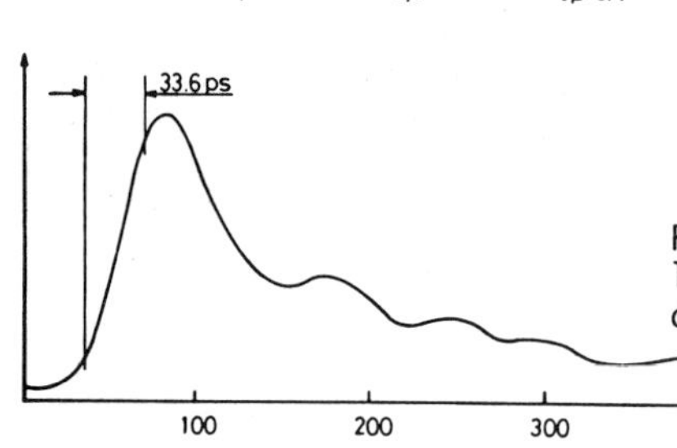


Fig. 15 (bottom) Pulse response of a laser grown GaAs photoconductive detector.

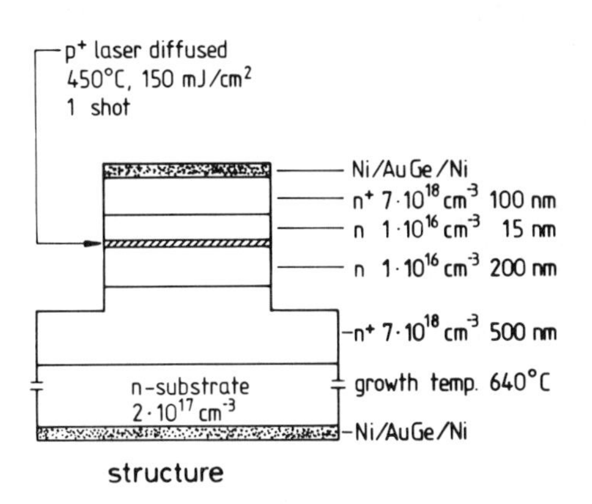


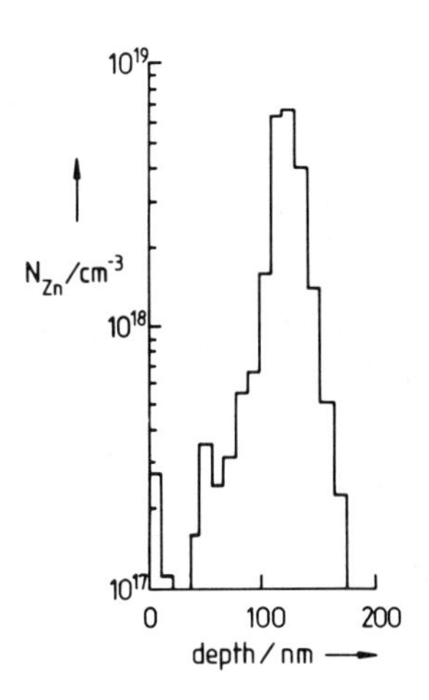


Fig. 16 Planar doped barrier structure and Zn SIMS profile.

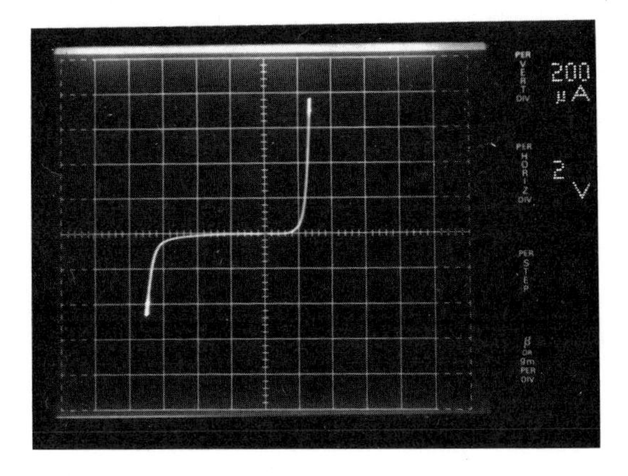


Fig. 17 I-U characteristics of the bulk barrier structure in the laser doped region.

The laser assisted doping of thin layers has been applied in fabricating bulk barrier devices. An example is shown in fig. 16. The resulting DC characteristics, fig. 17, indicate that overgrowth of these thin laser assisted sheet doped layers is possible. However, the conventional growth procedure over this narrow doped layer leads to a strong outdiffusion which changes the initial dopant profile remarkably.

A further application of this method might be the fabrication of luminescent diodes, where the carbon incorporation which occurs in the laser assisted growth procedure does not influence the device quality.

## 6. Acknowledgement

The assistance of my group at the Institute of Semiconductor Electronics has to be mentioned as well as the financial support from the State Government of Nordrhein-Westfalen and of the Volkswagen Foundation. The cooperation of P. Roentgen, H. Kräutle, W. Roth, A. Krings and M. Maier is greatly appreciated.

References

1 D. J. Schlyrer and M.A. Ring, J. Organomet. Chem. 114, 9 (1976)
2 H. Kräutle, H. Roehle, A. Escobosa, H. Beneking, J. of. Electronic Mat. 12, 215 (1983)
3 E. Rimini, Proc. of Laser Effects in Ion Implanted Semiconductors, Catania, Aug. 1978
4 W. Roth, H.Kräutle, A. Krings and H. Beneking, Mat. Res. Symp. Proc. 17, 193 (1983)
5 W. Roth, H. Beneking, A. Krings and H. Kräutle, Micrelectronics Journal 15, 26 (1984)
6 H. Kräutle, W. Roth, A. Krings and H. Beneking, to be published in Mat. Res. Symp. Proc., Boston 1983
7 P. Roentgen, H. Kräutle, W. Roth and H. Beneking, CLEO Proceedings, 222 (June 1984) Anaheim/Cal.
8 W. Roth, H. Schumacher, H. Beneking, Electronics Letters, 19, 142 (1983)

# IR Laser Photo-Assisted Deposition of Silicon Films

M. Hanabusa, H. Kikuchi*, T. Iwanaga, and K. Sugai

Department of Electrical and Electronic Engineering, Toyohashi University of Technology, Tenpaku, Toyohashi, 440, Japan

Amorphous hydrogenated silicon films can be deposited conveniently with efficient $CO_2$ lasers, using monosilane or disilane. The $CO_2$ laser beams are irradiated either normal or parallel to substrates. Although the deposition process is basically thermal, the photoassisted effects following light absorption play a role in deposition. The gas-phase conditions under laser irradiation have been studied by a CARS technique. It was shown that the gas is heated by the $CO_2$ laser and silane molecules are internally excited.

## 1 Introduction

For the so-called laser CVD various kinds of light sources have been used. Among them the $CO_2$ laser is unique, because it is highly efficient and powerful. The main drawback of $CO_2$ laser CVD is that photon does not carry enough energy to break common chemical bonds needed for photolysis of material gases. Therefore, often we make a use of pyrolysis in $CO_2$ laser CVD.

In the present paper we describe the results obtained so far with $CO_2$ laser CVD for silicon films. It is shown that silicon films can be prepared efficiently with $CO_2$ lasers using material gases such as monosilane $SiH_4$ [1-5] and disilane $Si_2H_6$ [6]. This technique is so advanced that probably a practical industrial application will be made possible in very near future. The reactional mechanism is basically thermal, as expected, but it is not limited to the pyrolysis taking place at the substrate surface. In fact, the $CO_2$ laser beam does not have to strike the surface, as long as it runs closely above the surface and the light is absorbed by gas [2-4]. This and other experimental results indicate the importance of some kind of gas-phase reactions following light absorption by material gas molecules. In an attempt to clarify the nature of the gas-phase dynamics we used the powerful laser diagnostic means of coherent anti-Stokes Raman spectroscopy (CARS).

## 2 Methods

In preparing silicon films using $CO_2$ lasers there are two basic configurations: one is the normal irradiation scheme and the other is the parallel irradiation scheme. In the former the laser beam strikes a substrate normal. The substrate opaque to the light is heated by the $CO_2$ laser beam, and the pyrolysis taking place at the heated substrate surface dominates the deposition process. Therefore, this kind of $CO_2$ laser CVD and conventional thermal CVD are alike. However, there are certain important differences. First, deposition is well-defined spatially, in particular when the

---

* Present address: Nippon Hoso Kyokai (NHK), Kobe Station, Chuoku, Kobe 650, Japan.

substrate with low thermal conductivity is used. Using a focused beam, it is possible to deposit films with a high spatial resolution. Also, deposition rates vary with $CO_2$ laser wavelengths; deposition is accelerated when the light is absorbed by material gas. This indicates that there are some photo-induced effects in $CO_2$ laser CVD of silane. This conclusion is further strengthened by the parallel irradiation experiment, where the laser beam running close to but above substrates plays an essential role in deposition.

The experimental setup we used for the normal incident scheme is shown in Fig. 1. The $CO_2$ laser generates a cw power up to 60 W. The beam size measured by deposited films is about 10 mm in diameter. It is either tuned to a particular line or used without any wavelength selection. The substrate is a quartz plate 0.38 mm thick. The gas was either monosilane or disilane. A thermocouple was placed behind the substrate. Film growth was monitored by measuring the interference of a reflected He-Ne laser beam.

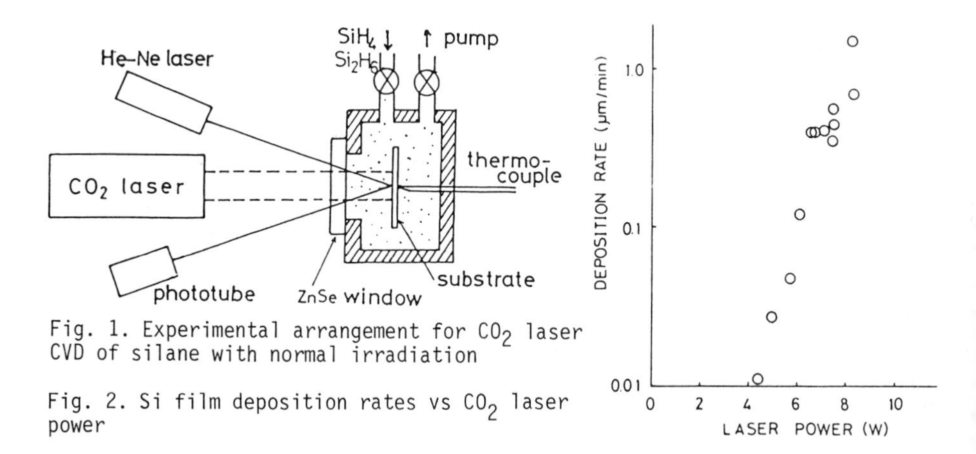


Fig. 1. Experimental arrangement for $CO_2$ laser CVD of silane with normal irradiation

Fig. 2. Si film deposition rates vs $CO_2$ laser power

As an example we show in Fig. 2 the results obtained with 3 Torr of disilane. The deposition rates are shown as a function of laser powers obtained without wavelength selection. The substrate temperatures, measured by the thermocouple and corrected for the error that was discovered through the CARS study [7], are 360, 415, and 495°C at laser powers of 4, 6, and 9 W, respectively. It is seen that silicon films are deposited fast at reasonably low laser powers and substrate temperatures. Similar results were obtained with monosilane; however, the deposition rates were slower roughly by a factor of ten than with disilane at the same substrate temperatures. Therefore, for a practical application, disilane seems a better choice. It is noted that in the case of monosilane, a distinct dependence of deposition rates on $CO_2$ laser wavelengths had been observed [5]. The rates were enhanced at the wavelength where the light was absorbed. This makes a sharp contrast with disilane, which shows little wavelength dependence even though this gas absorbed light at certain wavelengths. It is concluded that the deposition mechanism is different for these two gases.

In a completely different setup, the laser beam is sent parallel to the substrate. However, for successful deposition the substrate must be heated. The experimental setup we used is shown in Fig. 3. The main laser (1) sends the beam above a quartz substrate, while the second low-power laser

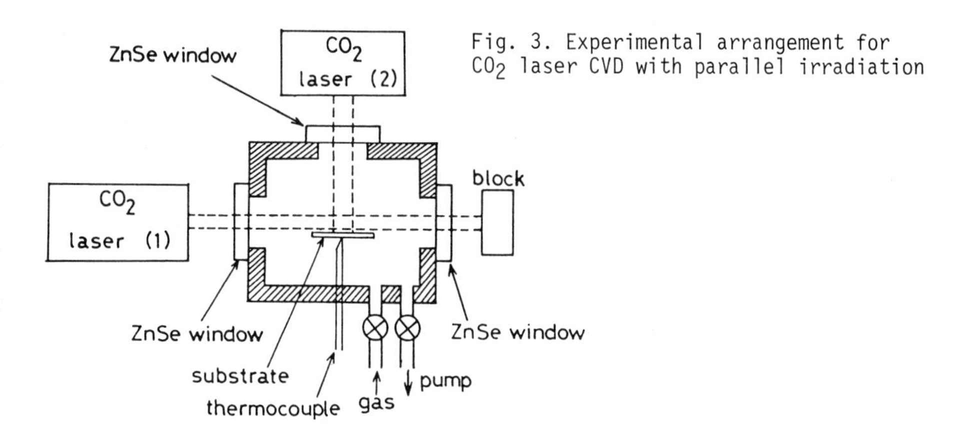


Fig. 3. Experimental arrangement for $CO_2$ laser CVD with parallel irradiation

(2) is used to heat the substrate. The parallel experiment has been done by other groups, who used an independent electronic heater [2-4]. With the present setup we can retain some of spatial resolution characteristic of the normal incident arrangement. Silicon films were deposited at a speed of 0.01 µm/min with the main laser power of 40 W and 5 Torr of $SiH_4$ at a substrate temperature of 380°C. Generally speaking, the deposition rates become slower with the parallel irradiation, compared to the normal irradiation. However, the films are more uniformly deposited, and the minimum substrate temperature required for appreciable deposition is lowered. The substrate temperature can be as low as 200°C if a higher main laser power is used [2,3]. For comparison the threshold temperature needed for the present normal incident arrangement used with disilane was 320°C. It seems that we have a choice between a high-speed deposition at low powers and medium substrate temperatures with the normal irradiation and a medium speed deposition at high powers and low substrate temperatures with the parallel irradiation.

The physical properties of the deposited films have been studied. Basically they are hydrogenated amorphous silicon. Details of the results on electrical properties, optical gap, IR absorption spectra, ESR, etc. can be found in the literature [3-6]. To control their electrical properties, doping was carried out by mixing silane with phosphene or diborane [8].

## 3 Process Analysis by CARS

Following light absorption, the molecule is vibrationally excited, and as a result several processes are induced. It is noted that the excitation to the first vibrationally excited state v=1 is not sufficient to cause molecular dissociation. When two photo-excited molecules in the state v=1 collide with each other, a molecule in the state v=2 is generated, and this molecule , after colliding with another molecule in v=1, is transformed to the state v=3. This sequence continues and gives rise to highly excited molecules. This may contribute to deposition. On the other hand, the excess energy stored in the vibrational mode following the light absorption is distributed to other degrees of freedom of molecules via collisions. Through this randomization of energy, the gas temperature is raised. The rise in gas temperature should in turn induce gas-phase decomposition. This process is known as HOMO CVD [9]. The processes which are thought to be involved in $CO_2$ laser CVD are summarized in Fig. 4.

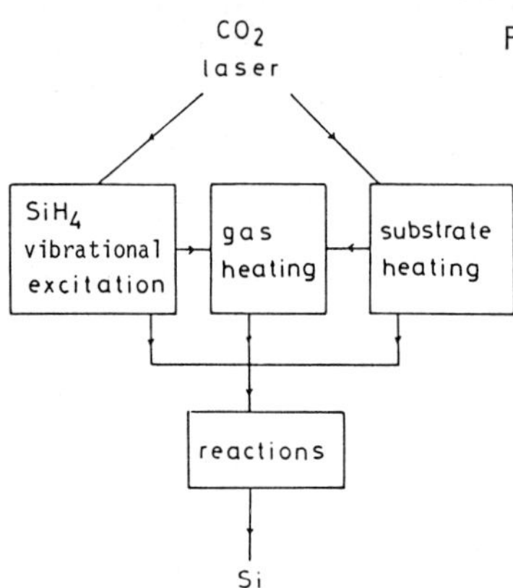


Fig. 4. Processes in $CO_2$ laser CVD of silane

We applied the CARS technique to examine the expected internal excitation of material gas molecules and measure gas temperature. CARS is ideally suited for the present purpose, because its spectral profile reflects distribution among various vibrational and rotational levels of molecules, and, in addition, it can be used as a thermometer.

We can not use silane CARS to measure gas temperature because the molecule is not in thermal equilibrium. Therefore, we mixed nitrogen with monosilane, and observed $N_2$ CARS spectra. Nitrogen is not involved in reactions directly, and the observed spectral profile agrees with a theoretical curve predicted on the basis of a Boltzmann distribution among its rotational levels.

The experimental arrangement used for $N_2$ CARS thermometry is shown in Fig. 5 [7]. Second harmonic beam at 532 nm from a Nd:YAG laser (Quanta Ray DCR-IA) was used as a pump beam for CARS and also to pump a dye laser whose output was a tunable Stokes beam for CARS. In the laser CVD experiment a

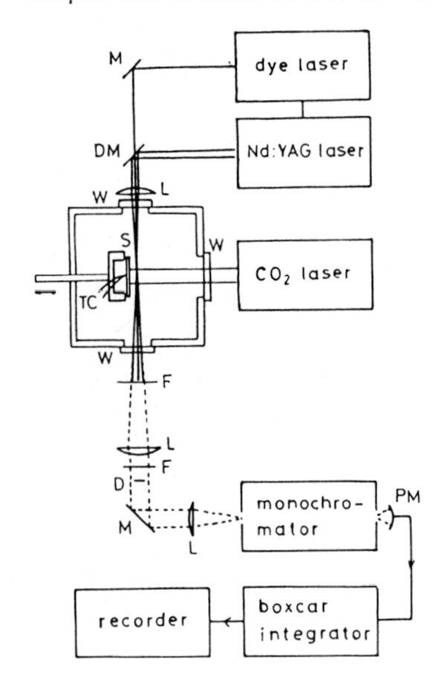


Fig. 5. Experimental arrangement used for CARS diagnosis of $CO_2$ laser CVD of silane. Code: M, mirror; DM, dichroic mirror; L, lens; W, window; S, substrate; TC, thermocouple; F, filter; D, disc; PM, photomultiplier tube

reaction zone is set precisely by the laser beam, and good spatial resolution is required. We met this requirement by overlapping a donut-shaped pump beam with a fine Stokes beam passing at its center. This is a modification of the so-called BOXCARS. Its spatial resolution depends greatly on the size of a disc placed after the collecting lens; we used a disc of 10 mm in diameter to obtain a resolution better than 10 mm. The focal lengths of the focusing and collimating lenses were 10 and 20 cm, respectively. The CARS signal was separated from the laser beams by filters, a disc, and a monochromator. It was detected by a photomultiplier and averaged by a boxcar integrator. The energy per pulse was at most 50 and 4 mJ for the pump and Stokes beams, while spectral resolution was roughly 0.8 and 1 $cm^{-1}$ (FWHM), respectively.

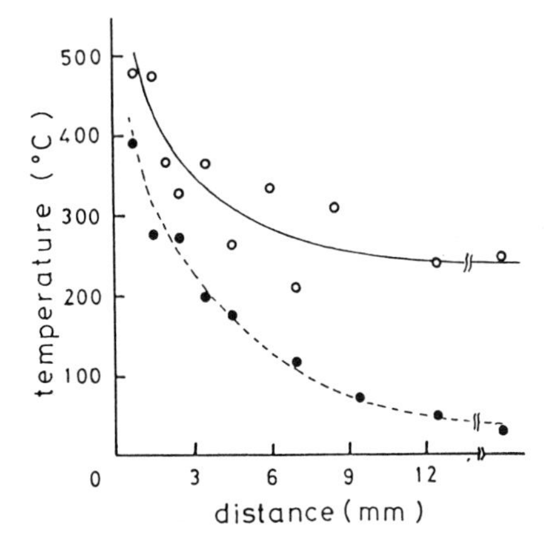


Fig. 6. Gas temperature determined by $N_2$ CARS thermometry vs distance from substrate: open circles, the P(20) line, and closed circles, the R(24) line. The points far right were taken without substrates

Gas temperature determined by $N_2$ CARS thermometry in a mixture of 5 Torr of $SiH_4$ and 25 Torr of $N_2$ is shown in Fig. 6 as a function of distance from the substrate [7]. The results were obtained with the P(20) line (944 $cm^{-1}$), where the light is absorbed strongly and thus the deposition is fast, and also with the R(24) line (978 $cm^{-1}$), where absorption is weak and deposition is slow. Note that there is a distinct difference in temperature without the substrate for the two lines, as shown at far right in Fig. 6. In the case of the R(24) line the gas remains at room temperature, while it is heated to 240°C with the P(20) line irradiation. This clearly demonstrates the gas heating effect present in $CO_2$ laser CVD of silane. Upon introducing the quartz substrate the gas temperature rises near the substrate, because the substrate is heated by $CO_2$ laser to 500°C, as indicated by the thermocouple, for both the P(20) and R(24) lines. However, there is still a clear difference in gas temperature between the P(20) and R(24) line; even at the closest point (0.75 mm) to be measured with the present setup, there is a temperature difference of about 100°C. It is emphasized again that the results shown in Fig. 6 indicate real substrate temperature roughly 20 % higher than the value obtained by the thermocouple because of the heat loss through thermocouple wires.

The thermal decomposition of $SiH_4$ in gas phase takes place with an activation energy of 51 kcal/mol, whence the monosilane gas decomposes 140 times faster at 500°C than at 400°C near the substrate. This ratio could account fully for the difference in deposition rates with the P(20) and R(24) line. A similar gas-heating process must take place when disilane is used, as evidenced by the fact that at pressures higher than 5 Torr the ZnSe window used to introduce the laser beam into the cell was covered with either film or powder. However, since it is decomposed easily at the heated surface, the gas-phase decomposition is overshadowed: hence, the deposition rates are independent of whether the molecule absorbs the light or not.

We observed CARS spectra for $SiH_4$ and $Si_2H_6$ under $CO_2$ laser irradiation. Parts of the $SiH_4$ spectra observed with the same apparatus as used for $N_2$ CARS thermometry were published already [7]. However, the observed complicated spectral shape could not be explained completely. Therefore, we used an alternative system built around two excimer-pumped dye lasers with higher spectral resolution in an attempt to find the clue for a better understanding of the spectra. The schematic diagram for the new apparatus is shown in Fig. 7. The XeCl excimer laser (Lambda Physik EMG 103 MSC) pumped two dye lasers (Lambda Physik FL 2002), one for the CARS pump beam at 480 nm and the other for the tunable Stokes beam around 536 nm for $SiH_4$ and $Si_2H_6$ (Raman shift is 2186 and 2163 $cm^{-1}$, respectively). The output power and spectral resolution for two dye lasers were 15 mJ and 0.1 $cm^{-1}$, respectively. We employed a conventional BOXCARS arrangement with the beams intersected at an angle of about $3^o$ by a lens with a focal length of 10 cm. The spatial resolution was about 3 mm.

In Fig. 8 the $SiH_4$ CARS spectra observed with this new apparatus are shown with the $CO_2$ laser off and on. The 10 W power of the P(20) line was used. The gas pressure was 5 Torr. As observed before with low spectral resolution, an additional broad peak appears on the low Raman-shift side of the main peak when the $CO_2$ laser beam is on. Here, however, we observed an extra feature in both spectra which could not be seen before; namely, there is a small peak on the higher Raman shift side of the main peak (see arrows). This peak grows in size when the laser is on. At the same time we observed $Si_2H_6$ CARS for the first time under the condition of the $CO_2$ laser irradiation, as shown in Fig. 9. The beam was 10 W of the P(20) line. The gas pressure was 3 Torr. For $Si_2H_6$, even the spectrum observed without the beam is characterized by a profile with many peaks; the spectrum under the laser irradiation exhibits a broadened and more separated satellite peak. The way the spectra change under laser irradiation is basically identical for both $SiH_4$ and $Si_2H_6$.

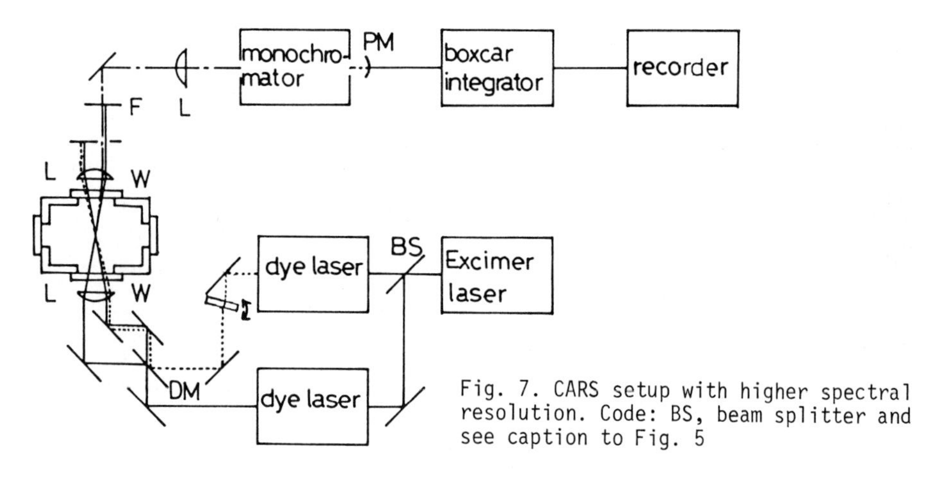


Fig. 7. CARS setup with higher spectral resolution. Code: BS, beam splitter and see caption to Fig. 5

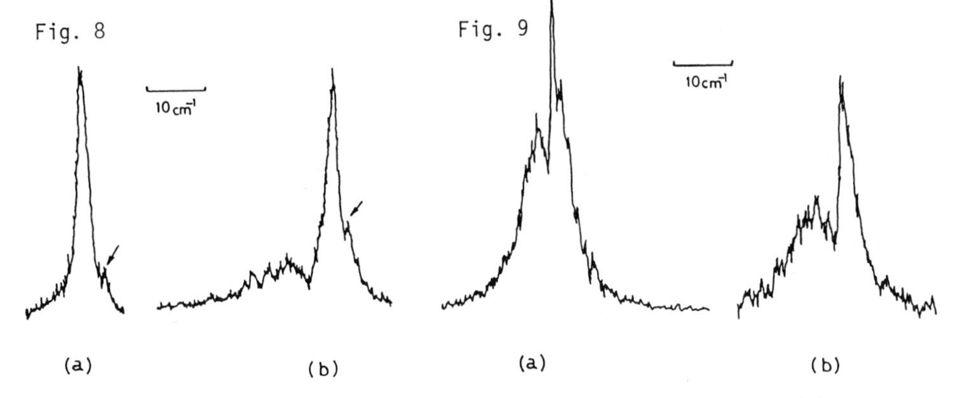


Fig. 8. $SiH_4$ CARS spectra observed with the $CO_2$ laser turned off (a) and on (b). For arrows, see the text

Fig. 9. $Si_2H_6$ CARS spectra observed with the $CO_2$ laser turned off (a) and on (b)

It is not easy to explain all the details of the observed silane CARS spectra. We note first that the $SiH_4$ spectra observed near an electrically heated substrate showed similar profile as observed with the laser irradiation. Therefore, gas temperature has an important effect on the observed profile. Then we are tempted to identify the additional peaks in $SiH_4$ spectra as hot bands in the same $\nu_1$ mode that are observed by CARS. However, this explanation is unlikely, because the hot bands should appear only on the low Raman shift side. Besides, their peak position should not change with temperature, as observed previously [7]. For this reason and others, it was assumed previously that the observed spectral profile was induced by rotationally excited silane molecules that were involved in a complicated series of chemical reactions [7]. The main difficulty with such an explanation is that the gas pressure is too high to achieve such a non-equilibrium state among rotational levels. Here, we propose an alternative explanation based on the appearance of the peak on the larger Raman shift side. We note that the present $SiH_4$ CARS is induced in its $\nu_1$ vibrational mode and its vibrational energy depends on how other vibrational modes ($\nu_2$ to $\nu_4$) are populated [10]. If other vibrational modes are populated, the $\nu_1$-mode CARS spectral peak is to be shifted, depending on the sign and magnitude of the inter-mode coupling. As temperature increases or the $CO_2$ laser induces vibrational excitation, the population increases in the modes coupled with the $\nu_1$ mode, whence the satellite peak grows in height. This can account for the appearance and growth of the arrowed peaks observed in $SiH_4$ spectra. If the peaks are caused by coupling with more than one mode and they are located close together, the central position of the overlapping signals changes with temperature, because the relative populations among the vibrational levels change. In this way, we can explain the observed growth and shift of the broad satellite peaks observed in both $SiH_4$ and $Si_2H_6$.

## 4 Conclusion

We have shown that $CO_2$ laser CVD is very promising for preparation of amorphous silicon films. Basically, the normal and parallel irradiation schemes are used with material gases such as monosilane and disilane.

Although the process is basically thermal, the photo-induced effects contribute to film deposition. An emphasis was placed in the present work on process diagnostics based on CARS. The results confirm the gas heating by $CO_2$ laser and internal excitation of silane molecules in gas phase.

## Acknowledgements

We thank Prof. M. Kawasaki for valuable discussions on interpretation of silane CARS spectra. We are indebted to Dr. R. Vehrenkamp at Lambda Physik for his cooperation in setting up the excimer-based CARS system. Disilane was kindly provided by Toa Gosei Chemical Co. and Mitsui-Toatsu Chemicals, Inc. Finally, we thank Mr. M. Danno for the help in improving the $CO_2$ laser. This work was partly supported by Special Coordination Funds for Promoting Science and Technology of the Science and Technology Agency of the Japanese Government.

## References

1. C. P. Christensen and K. M. Lakin: Appl. Phys. Lett. 32, 254 (1978)
2. R. Bilenchi, I. Gianinoni and M. Musci: J. Appl. Phys. 53, 6497 (1982)
3. T. R. Gattuso, M. Meunier, D. Adler and J. S. Haggerty: Proc. Materials Research Society, Laser Diagnostics and Photo-chemical Processing for Semiconductor Devices, Boston, 1982 (North-Holland, New York, 1983) 17, p.215
4. M. Meunier, T. R. Gattuso, D. Adler and J. S. Haggerty: Appl. Phys. Lett. 43, 273 (1983)
5. M. Hanabusa, S. Moriyama and H. Kikuchi: Thin Solid Films 107, 227 (1983)
6. T. Iwanaga and M. Hanabusa: Jpn. J. Appl. Phys. 23, L492 (1984)
7. M. Hanabusa and H. Kikuchi: Jpn. J. Appl. Phys. 22, L712 (1983)
8. R. Bilenchi, A. Ferrario and M. Musci: 1984 Conference on Lasers and Electro-Optics Proc., p.222
9. B. A. Scott, R. M. Plecenik and E. E. Simonyi: Appl. Phys. Lett. 39, 73 (1981)
10. G. Herzberg: Infrared and Raman Spectra (Van Nostrand Reinhold, New York, 1945)

# IR Laser Pyrolysis of Silane

V.V. Nosov, S.M. Repinskii, and F.N. Dulcev

Institute of Semiconductor Physics, Siberian Branch of the USSR Academy of Sciences, SU-630090 Novosibirsk-90, USSR

Synthesis of dielectric silicon films by means of chemical vapour deposition has recently come into wide practice. These methods are usually based on the interaction of silane with ammonia, oxygen or $N_2O$ [1-3]. Also chlorosilanes are often used for this purpose [1, 4]. Studies show that the reactions under discussion involve many routes and stages. To optimize the process and to obtain films of the needed chemical composition require the identification of properties of individual stages, particularly for gas-phase stages.

The aim of our work was to study gas-phase pyrolysis of silane and silane-ammonia mixtures. Laser heating of the reactive gas excludes heterogeneous processes that usually occur on the walls of a reactor [5,6].

We used a continuous-wave $CO_2$ laser. Laser power was stabilised by the system of automatic frequency control and by pumping a gas mixture. With the maximum laser power of 10 W an instability per hour was less than 2%. Pyrolysis was performed in a cavity equipped with NaCl end windows. The cavity volume was 70 ml.

The mixture composition was controlled with a manometer, the total pressure being 300 Torr. In order to provide identical thermal conditions and temperature distributions argon was added. The heating gas was $SF_6$ (5 Torr), as $SF_6$ absorbs well a laser beam and is chemically inert up to 1500 K [6]. Partial pressure of the studied gas ranged from 1 to 10 Torr. Argon served as a buffer gas. The pyrolysis products were analysed in the UR-20 spectrograph monitoring the IR absorption bands at 505, 975, and 805 $cm^{-1}$ for $SiH_4$, $NH_3$, and $CHClF_2$, respectively.

The laser power ranged from 2 to 7 W. Temperature of the laser-heated zone was determined by means of "chemical thermometer", in our case it was the following reaction

$$CHClF_2 \longrightarrow CF_2 + HCl$$

with known kinetic characteristics [8]. This reaction was held in the same conditions as the studied reaction. Kinetic parameters of the two reactions form the following equation [6]:

$$\lg K_{2eff} = \frac{E_2}{E_1} \lg K_{1eff} + B , \qquad (1)$$

where $K_{1eff}$ and $K_{2eff}$ are rate constants of the reference and the studied reactions, respectively, $E_1$ and $E_2$ are activation energies of the reference and the studied reactions, respectively, B is a constant.

Varying the laser power and thus the temperature we obtained the set of $K_{1eff}$ and $K_{2eff}$ for each value of laser power. $E_1/E_2$ was determined graphically in the $\lg K_{1eff}$ - $\lg K_{2eff}$ coordinates. Since the reactive zone is not isothermal, $K_{02}$ can be precisely determined only when $E_1$ and $E_2$ differ within 10% if

$$B = \lg K_{02} - \frac{E_2}{E_1} \lg K_{01} , \qquad (2)$$

where $K_{01}$ and $K_{02}$ are preexponential factors of the reference and the studied reactions, respectively.

Figure 1 shows a typical change of concentration with time. Experimental data processing shows that silane decomposition follows the first-order kinetics in the range 1 to 10 Torr of silane.

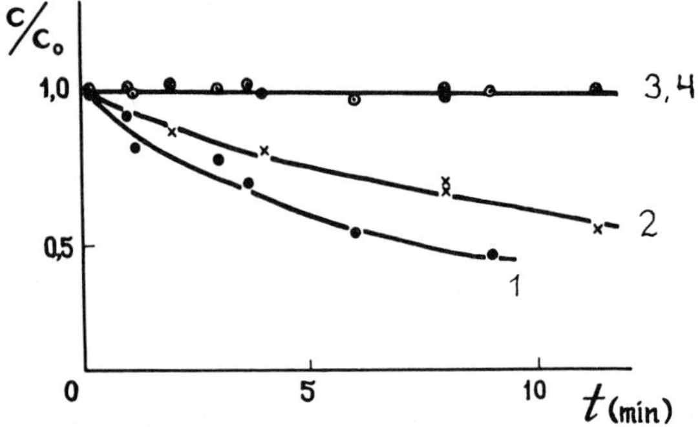


Fig.1. Concentration of silane (1,2) and ammonia (3,4) as function of time for pyrolysis of mixture $SiH_4$-$NH_3$ (1,3) and $SiH_4$-$NH_3$-$C_3H_6$ (2,4). At P=300 Torr, $p_{SiH_4}$=1.5Torr, $p_{NH_3}$= 1.5 Torr, $p_{C_3H_6}$ = 7 Torr.

In other experiments propylene was added as an inhibitor of radical processes. The results are given in Fig. 2. The presence of propylene decreases the rate constant of silane pyrolysis, the efficiency of this influence being less for silane-ammonia mixtures.

Figure 3 depicts the curves with the help of which activation energies for pyrolysis of the studied mixtures were cal-

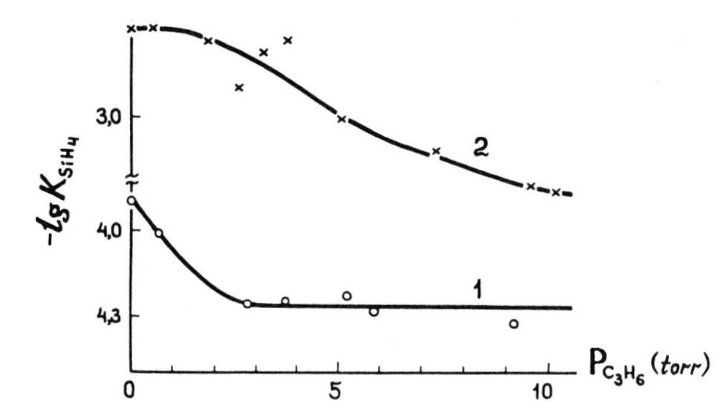


Fig.2. Rate constant for decomposition of silane as function of propylene pressure for pyrolysis of $SiH_4$ (lower curve) and mixture $SiH_4$-$NH_3$ (upper curve). At P=300Torr, $p_{SiH_4}$ =1.5Torr, $p_{NH_3}$ =1.5Torr. Radiation powers are 3.0 and 4.7W, respectively.

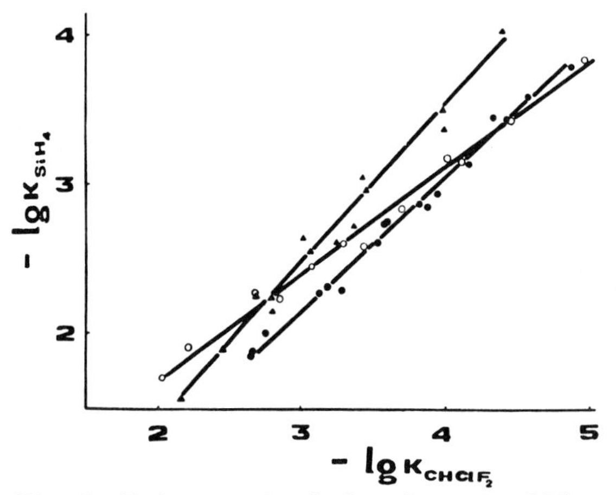


Fig.3. Rate constant for decomposition of silane as a function of rate constant for decomposition of $CHClF_2$ (chemical thermometer) for • - $SiH_4$, o - $SiH_4$-$NH_3$, ▲ - $SiH_4$-$C_3H_6$. Conditions have been given in Fig.1.

TABLE 1 Kinetic parameters for initial stages of silane pyrolysis

| Mixture composition | $K_o$ ($s^{-1}$) | E (kcal/mole) |
|---|---|---|
| $SiH_4$ + propylene | 13.5±0.8 | 59.9±2.0 |
| $SiH_4$ | 11.5±0.6 | 46.6±1.7 |
| $SiH_4$ + $NH_3$ | 9.2±0.9 | 36.9±2.0 |

culated. The results are summarized in Table 1. An activation energy for the $SiH_4$-$NH_3$ mixture pyrolysis appears to be lower than that for the pure silane pyrolysis. However the ammonia consumption is negligible: with the 35% silane decomposition ammonia loss is not more than 5-6% (see Fig. 2).

Silane pyrolysis has been studied in many works [9-13] , although its mechanism is vague. Our data confirm that silane pyrolysis follows two routes, molecular and radical. It is important that adding propylene does not decrease the silane pyrolysis rate lower than some definite value for the given temperature. This is evidence that following stages are be initial [11] :

$$SiH_4 \longrightarrow SiH_2 + H_2$$

$$SiH_2 + SiH_4 \longrightarrow Si_2H_6^*.$$

Judging by thermodynamic data, the most probable chain-initiating stage is [7] :

$$Si_2H_6^* \longrightarrow 2SiH_3 .$$

In the presence of inhibiting species the process follows a molecular route and has an activation energy of 59.9 kcal/mole [11, 12]. With no inhibitors,radical stages become important and the effective activation energy decreases down to 46.2 kcal/mole [10, 18]. Thus, using common type reactors one should take into account both possible routes. In particular, these peculiarities of silane pyrolysis are responsible for the change of external morphology of polysilicon layers formed by vapour deposition [14].

Note that our kinetic data coincide with the kinetics of silicon nitride film formation from the $SiH_4$-$NH_3$ mixture [1]. Thus, our experiments give the activation energy of $37.0 \pm 2.0$ kcal/mole and the silicon nitride synthesis experiments give 38.4 kcal/mole. Our measurements, while being extrapolated to 800°C, give the rate constant $0.25 \times 10^{-3}\ s^{-1}$ which is close to the value of $1.0 \times 10^{-3}\ s^{-1}$ determined from the silicon nitride film synthesis experiments [17]. This evidences that the limiting stages of both processes are identical.

Our results show that silane pyrolysis in the presence of ammonia is not accompanied by the formation of stable gaseous products with Si-N bonds. But an intermediate is likely to be formed causing a decrease of the effective activation energy of silane pyrolysis.

References

1. Silicon Nitride in Electronics, ed. by A.V.Rzhanov (Izd. Nauka, Novosibirsk 1982)
2. L.L.Vasilyeva, V.N.Drozdov: In Problems of Physical Chemistry of Semiconductor Surfaces, ed. by A.V.Rzhanov (Izd. Nauka, Novosibirsk 1978) p. 155

3. L.L.Vasilyeva, L.I.Rabinovich: Izv. SO AN SSSR, Ser.Khim. 4, No. 9, 65 (1981)
4. O.I.Semyonova, L.A.Nenasheva, S.M.Repinskii: Izv.AN SSSR, Neorgan.Materialy 17, No. 7, 1223 (1981)
5. W.M.Shaub, S.H.Bauer: Int.J.Chem.Kinet. 7, No. 4, 509 (1975)
6. Yu.N.Samsonov, A.K.Petrov, Yu.N.Molin: Kinetika i Kataliz 20, 17 (1979)
7. M.Bowrey, J.H.Purnell: Proc.Roy.Soc., Ser. A 321, 341 (1971)
8. V.I.Vedeneyev, A.A.Kibalko: Rate Constants of Gas-Phase Monomolecular Reactions (Izd. Nauka, Moscow 1972) p. 100
9. J.H.Purnell, R.Walsh: Proc.Roy.Soc., Ser. A 293, 543 (1966)
10. G.Cochet, H.Mellotee, R.Delbourgo: J.Chem.Phys. 71, No. 10, 1363 (1974)
11. C.G.Newman, H.E.O'Neal, M.A.Ring, F.Leska, N.Shipley: Int. J.Chem.Kinet. 11, No. 11, 1167 (1979)
12. P.Neudorfl, A.Jodhan, O.P.Strausz: J.Phys.Chem. 84, No. 3, 338 (1980)
13. V.N.Panfilov: Thermal Decomposition and Other Reactions of Monosilane in Gas Phase (Preprint of Institute of Chemical Kinetics and Combustion, Sib.Branch, USSR Ac. of Sci., Novosibirsk 1981)
14. M.S.Sukhov: Physical Chemistry of Monocrystalline Semiconductor Surfaces, IV Seminar, Abstracts (Novosibirsk 1981) p. 33
15. N.M.Emmanuel, D.G.Knorre: Course of Chemical Kinetics (Izd. Vysshaya Shkola, Moscow 1969) p. 288
16. Lin Sin Shong: J.Electroch.Soc. 125, No. 11, 1877 (1978)
17. L.L.Vasilyeva, A.S.Ginovker, V.P.Popov, S.M.Repinskii: Izv. SO AN SSSR, Ser.Khim.Nauk 5, 54 (1979)
18. D.Bäuerle, P.Irsigler, G.Leyendecker. H.Noll, D.Wagner: Appl.Phys.Letts. 40, No. 9, 819

# Multiphoton Excitation and Dissociation of $SiH_4$ Exposed to $CO_2$ Laser Radiation

M. Snels*, E. Borsella, R. Fantoni, and A. Giardini-Guidoni

ENEA, Dip. TIB, Divisione Fisica Applicata, C.R.E. Frascati,
C.P. 65 - 00044 Frascati, Rome, Italy

The mechanism of $SiH_4$ laser excitation has been investigated in the 10 μm region using a continuously tunable pulsed $CO_2$ laser. At variance with previous results, multiphoton resonances have been observed by photoacoustic detection.

## 1. Introduction

In the past silanes have been widely used for thin silicon film production via conventional plasma enhanced CVD deposition [1]. More recent methods utilize IR laser photolysis mainly to control thickness, area and doping of deposits [2,3]. Effective excitation of silane molecules up to their decomposition threshold (the main channel $SiH_4$+nhv → $SiH_2$+$H_2$) has been achieved [4,5] by irradiating the gaseous sample with $CO_2$ laser radiation tuned to the (100 ← 001) emission lines. Due to the rather low $SiH_4$ pressure (1 - 100 Torr) during the laser induced photodissociation [2,3], and due to the peculiarity of this light molecule with respect to the heavier and widely studied highly symmetric species [6], much interest arose in the mechanism of laser absorption. In particular, since collisions are effective in increasing both the absorption probability and the dissociation yield [4,5], up to now it was not clear whether the process could be considered as an IR multiple-photon absorption occurring also in the collision-less regime, in contrast to laser heating with full thermodynamical redistribution of the absorbed energy through the V-T relaxation. Some remarks in Ref. [4] seem to rule out the last simple hypothesis, since a more than linear pressure dependence in the absorption is observed. However the requirement of pressure broadening in order to match absorption of $SiH_4$ lines to the $CO_2$ line tunable emission (in combination with the power broadening) can be more important than the need of fast V-T relaxation for the thermal redistribution and could lead to a non-linear pressure dependence of the absorption probability. This fact pushed us to carry out an investigation of $SiH_4$ absorption under the high power ($10^5$ - $10^7$ W/cm$^2$) pulsed radiation supplied by a continuously tunable $CO_2$ laser (sect. 3).

Before discussing the results (sect. 3), it is worthwhile to recall some features of the well studied [7,8] IR absorption of $SiH_4$ molecule in the frequency range 850-1100 cm$^{-1}$, which is partially overlapping the $CO_2$ laser emission. Two vibrational modes of $SiH_4$ ($\nu_4$ at 913.3 cm$^{-1}$ and $\nu_2$ at 972.1 cm$^{-1}$) fall into this wavelength region; the Q branch of the $\nu_4$ IR active mode is red shifted with respect to the $CO_2$ emission so that only R branch of vibrorotational transitions can be observed by laser radiation. Since a red shift of vibrationally excited levels due to the anharmonic shift has been generally observed in multiphoton excitation of

* Guest from Nijmegen University

polyatomic molecules [6], $SiH_4$ is expected to hardly show multiphoton excitation. Moreover the dipole moment of the $\nu_4$ mode of $SiH_4$ ($\mu^{\nu_4}_{0\to1}$ = 0.21D) [9] is considerably lower than for vibrational modes of heavier fluorinated compounds which have shown the occurrence of multiphoton resonances [11,12]. Furthermore to counteract the multiphoton process also the low density of vibrorotational levels in the spectrum of this light molecule should be mentioned (the high rotational contant B = 2.85941 $cm^{-1}$ [10] for $^{28}SiH_4$ yields a narrow J distribution even at room temperature, $J_{max}$ ~ 23 at T = 300 K).

On the other hand, of primary importance for the onset of the multiphoton process could be the occurrence of Coriolis coupling between the $\nu_4$ and the close lying $\nu_2$ mode [7,8]. In fact, this last mode, being IR forbidden, scarcely contributes to linear absorption, but should affect the absorption bands of the excited levels involved in multiphoton excitation. In this respect another relevant effect arises from the second-order anharmonic splitting of degenerate levels in the tetrahedral symmetry of the molecule. In fact, within the allowed selection rules [13], it can furnish different pathways for multiphoton resonance occurring through the same vibrorotational transition.

## 2. Experimental

The infrared radiation was provided by a pulsed multimode continuously tunable $CO_2$ laser (Lumonics model TE 281). Continuously tunable emission with a pulse energy up to 500 mJ, over a 0.38 $cm^2$ area, a pulse width of less than 100 nsec (FWHM) and a short tail of 400 nsec was obtained by operating the laser at 9 atm with an 8:8:84 = $CO_2$:$N_2$:He gas mixture. Under these conditions the output energy varied less than 50% when moving from a $CO_2$ line center to a neighboring line both in the P and R branches of the 10 μm band [10P32-10P10, 10R34-10R8]. With a 135 lines/mm Cu grating the resolution was found to be 0.12±0.02 $cm^{-1}$ as measured using a Fabry-Perot interferometer. The well-known linear absorption spectrum of $NH_3$ [14] was used for absolute calibration of the grating. The laser energy was monitored throughout the course of the experiment by collecting 40% of the laser beam which was reflected by a CdTe beam splitter onto the surface of a calibrated pyroelectric joulemeter (Lumonics mod. 20D).

Multiphoton absorption was measured by using a previously described optoacoustic cell [15]. A capacitance microphone detects the acoustic pulse due to V-T relaxation of the vibrationally excited molecules. The maximum of the integrated optoacoustic signal is proportional to the average energy deposited in the molecules [15]. A 1 m long absorption cell filled with 20 Torr of $NH_3$ with a second pyroelectric detector at its exit was used to monitor "on line" the frequency calibration on a fraction of the laser beam.

A TMS 9900 based microcomputer controls the experiment. The laser is triggered by the computer; the signals from the two pyroelectrics and from the optoacoutic cell are digitized, stored and processed. A synchronous motor moves the grating in prefixed steps in order to obtain the frequency spectrum. Any long term changes of fluence from the selected value are detected and automatically corrected by adjusting the high voltage in the laser discharge. Careful screening of the experiment has been achieved by means of copper mesh cages in order to minimize the effect of the electromagnetic noise created by the laser discharge.

## 3. Results and Discussion

All the measurements here reported were performed on commercial $SiH_4$ (purity 99.999%) at p = 1 Torr and room temperature.

Preliminary measurements performed by using a line-tunable pulsed $CO_2$ laser have shown several peaks in agreement with the results of Ref. [4] both on P and R branch of the $CO_2$ 10 μm emission. Spectra taken at $\phi$ = = 0.3 J/cm² and different pressures (1-10 Torr) have shown an increase with pressure of some peaks, namely the one excited with the 10P24 laser line, thus indicating a better frequency matching due to pressure broadening.

A large portion of the absorption spectrum of $SiH_4$ measured with the continuously tunable laser at $\phi$ = 0.07 J/cm² is shown in Fig. 1. Numbers mark one frequency resonances (linear absorption) assigned on the basis of positions and intensities given in Ref. [8], while the expected width (0.15 cm⁻¹) takes into account both the laser resolution and the power broadening. Some peaks appear broader than expected, thus indicating

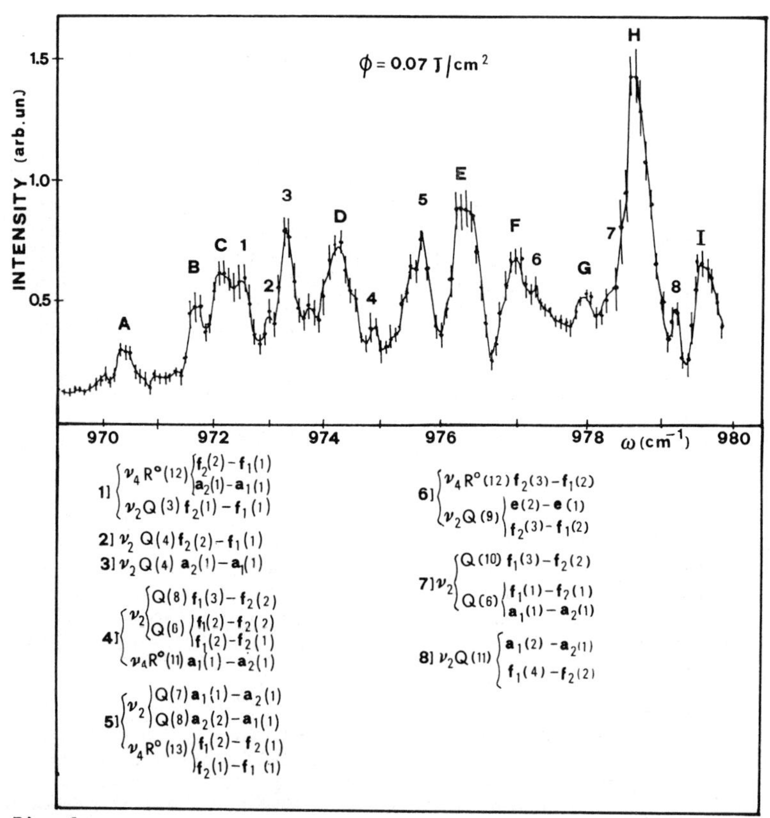


Fig. 1
Multiphoton excitation spectrum of 1 Torr $SiH_4$ taken at $\phi$ = 0.07 J/cm² in the wavelength range 969-980 cm⁻¹. Assignement of linear absorption peaks is shown. Capital letters indicate multiphoton resonances not already assigned.

unresolved high order contributions, and some new features appear clearly overimposed to the linear spectrum.

In order to ascertain the non-linearity of the process which gives rise to the new structures (labelled in the figures with capital letters) several regions of the spectrum have been measured at different laser fluences. As an example, the region between 10P24 and 10P20 laser lines, measured at $\phi$ = 0.07 J/cm and $\phi$ = 0.16 J/cm² is reported in Fig. 2. Some linear absorption peaks are identified in the figure, while the capital letters label multiphoton resonances at 941.1 cm⁻¹, 941.9 cm⁻¹, 942.2 cm⁻¹, 943.5 cm⁻¹, 944.0 cm⁻¹, 944.4 cm⁻¹ and 944.6 cm¹ which become dominating in the high fluence spectrum.

In order to fully assign $SiH_4$ multiphoton resonances a better knowledge of its excited state spectroscopy is required. Namely the $\chi_{44}$ and $\chi_{24}$ anharmonicity constants, the $\zeta_{24}$ Coriolis contant and the anharmonic splittings in the v = 1 and v = 2 levels are needed.

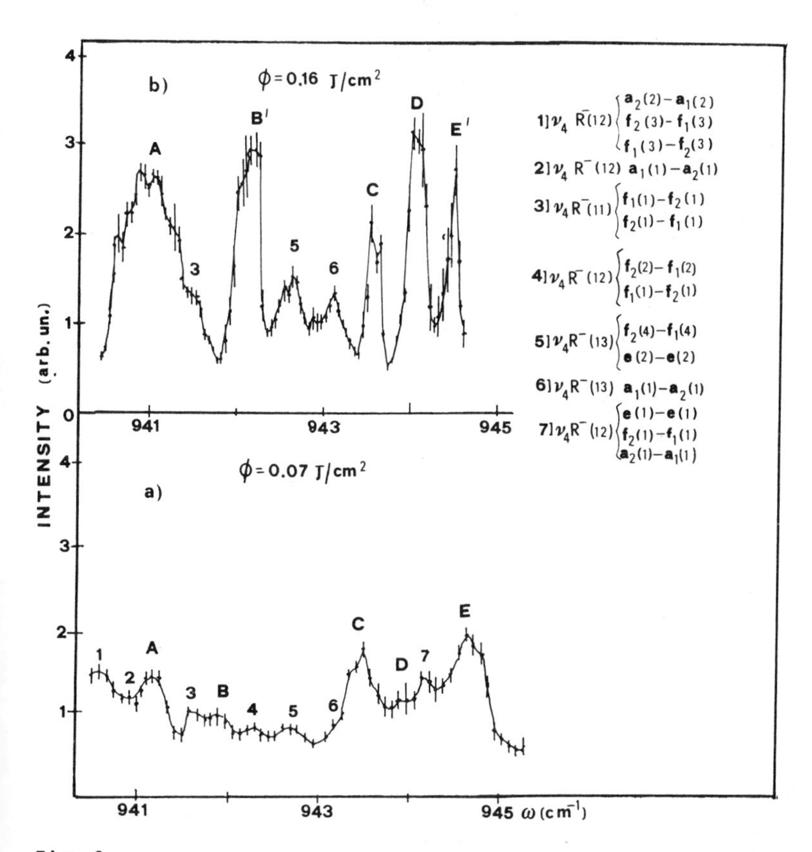


Fig. 2
Multiphoton excitation spectra of 1 Torr $SiH_4$ taken at $\phi$ = 0.07 J/cm² (a) and $\phi$ = 0.16 J/cm² (b) in the wavelength range 940-945 cm⁻¹. Assignement of linear absorption peaks is shown. Capital letters indicate multiphoton resonances not already assigned.

As far as $SiH_4$ multiphoton dissociatior is concerned, the molecule has been dissociated by using pulsed radiation at fluence $\phi$ = 2.5 J/cm$^2$ tuned on the 10P20, which is almost degenerate with a multiphoton resonance (see Fig. 2). By irradiating a 1:1 mixture of $SiH_4$ and Ar at 20 Torr total pressure, almost complete dissociation has been achieved after 100 laser pulses. Eye monitoring of the dissociation was allowed by the strong red fluorescence of the $SiH_x$ (x = 1,2,3) radical involved in the process. In this condition a homogeneous deposition of hydrogenerated silicon was formed on a glass substrate heated at ~ 120 °C.


Acknowledgements

Author gratefully acknowledge helpful discussion with Prof. J. Reuss. Thanks are due to Mr. R. Belardinelli, R. Larciprete and G. Schina for assistance during the experiment.


References


[1] H. Dun, P.Pan; F.R. White, R.W. Douse: J. Electrochem. Soc. 128, 7 (1981)
[2] T.J. Chuang: J. Chem. Phys. 74. 1453 (1981)
[3] R. Bilenchi, I. Gianninoni, M. Musci: J. Appl. Phys. 53, 6479 (1982)
[4] T.F. Deutsh: J. Chem. Phys. 70, 1187 (1979)
[5] P.A. Longeway, F.W. Lampe: J. Am. Chem. Soc. 103, 6813 (1981)
[6] R. Fantoni, E. Borsella, A. Giardini-Guidoni: Laser Applications in Chemistry , K.L. Kompa and J. Wanner Eds. (Plenum Press, Oxford, 1984), p. 151
[7] J.W.C. Johns. W.A. Kreisner, J. Susskind: J. Mol. Spectr. 60, 400 (1976)
[8] D.L. Gray, A.G. Robiette, J.W.C. Johns: Mol. Phys. 34, 1437 (1977)
[9] L.A. Pugh, K.N. Rao in "Molecular Spectroscopy in Modern Research" Vol. 2 (K.N. Rao Ed. Acad. Press N.Y. 1976)
[10] M. Dang-Nhu, G. Pierre, R. Saint-Loup: Mol. Phys. 28, 447 (1974)
[11] S.S. Alimpiev, N.V. Karlov. S.M. Nikiforov. A.M. Prokhorov. B.G. Sartakov, E.M. Khokhlov and A. Shtarkov: Opt. Commun. 31, 309 (1979)
[12] E. Borsella, R. Fantoni, A. Giardini-Guidoni, D.R. Adams, C.D. Cantrell: Chem. Phys. Lett. 101, 86 (1983)
[13] A.G. Robiette, D.L. Gray, F.W. Birss: Mol. Phys. 32, 1591 (1976)
[14] A.R.H. Cole: "Table of Wavenumbers for the Calibration of Infrared Spectrometers" (Pergamon Press, London 1976)
[15] G. Sanna, M. Nardi, M. Bernardini: Proceedings of the Int. Conf. on Laser '81, ed. C.B. Collins (STS Press, McLean VA, 1982) p. 83

# Deposition of Silicon Films by Photodissociation of Silane Under IR Laser Irradiation

Y. Pauleau, D. Tonneau, and G. Auvert

Centre National d'Etudes des Télécommunications, BP : 98
F-38243 Meylan Cedex, France

## 1. Introduction

In the field of semiconductor processing, a considerable amount of interest has been devoted to laser-induced deposition of silicon films [1]. For example, hydrogenated amorphous silicon (a-Si) films can be successfully deposited on quartz or glass substrates at temperatures below 400 °C [2-4]. The technique involves vibrational excitation of silane molecules by absorption of the P(20) $CO_2$ laser line at 10.59 μm. Since the absorption of $SiH_4$ molecules is known to be enhanced by buffer gases such as hydrogen and nitrogen, the deposition rate of a-Si films formed by irradiating $SiH_4$-$N_2$ mixtures is likely to be altered.

The purpose of this study is to measure and compare the deposition rate of a-Si films produced from pure silane and $SiH_4$-$N_2$ mixtures under $CO_2$ laser irradiation. The optical absorption of silane is determined and the homogeneous decomposition threshold of molecules is investigated as a function of laser fluence and gas pressures. The experimental procedure and results are reported in this paper.

## 2. Experimental Techniques

Silane molecules are irradiated using a pulsed $CO_2$ laser tuned to 10.59 μm and at a pulse repetition frequency of 1 Hz. The maximum output energy of the laser and the pulse duration are 2.2 J and 100 nsec, respectively. The beam is about 22 mm in diameter. The photon beam is made to pass through both a telescope and a variable attenuator in order to reduce the beam diameter by half and allow adjustment of the laser fluence. The beam is introduced into the stainless steel reaction chamber through a NaCl window (Fig. 1). Quartz substrates (25 x 25 mm) are mounted on a heating stage and placed parallel to the laser beam. The optical path length between the substrate and the NaCl window is 15 mm. Before laser irradiation, the reaction chamber is first evacuated to a $10^{-5}$ Torr vacuum

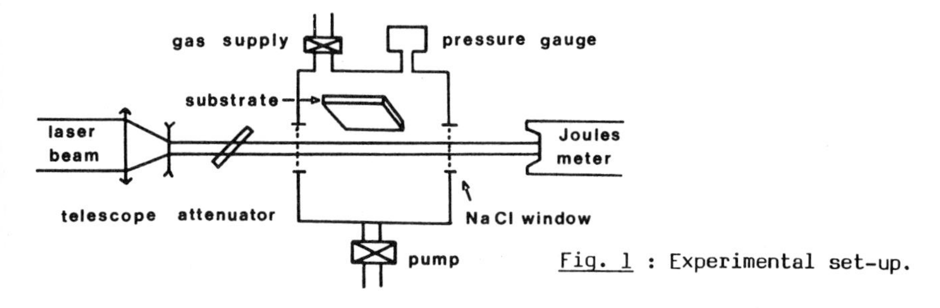


Fig. 1 : Experimental set-up.

by a turbomolecular pump, followed by introduction of the reactive gas into the cell. During irradiation, the cell is sealed off ; the change in pressure due to the chemical reaction is negligible.

The optical absorption of silane molecules is determined by measuring the laser fluence transmitted through the gas cell. The homogeneous decomposition threshold of silane is reached when powdery silicon forms on the NaCl window [4]. Laser fluence versus silane pressure has been determined for pure silane and $SiH_4$-$N_2$ mixtures at the decomposition threshold. a-Si films were deposited on quartz substrates using minimum 2700 laser pulses (45 min.). Film thickness is determined by $\alpha$-step measurements carried out after partial submersion of samples in a 4N KOH etching solution.

## 3. Optical Absorption of Pure Silane and Silane-Nitrogen Mixtures

The IR absorption of silane molecules has been investigated as a function of silane and nitrogen pressures. Under a laser fluence of 0.8 $J/cm^2$ and a pressure of about 20 Torr, the absorption of pure silane is 100 % at room temperature (Fig. 2). Deposition of powdery silicon on the NaCl window occurs at a silane pressure of 15 Torr. This in no way hinders gas absorption measurements, for silicon does not absorb the P(20) laser line.

The absorption of photons by silane molecules is enhanced in the presence of nitrogen. The silane partial pressure in the gas cell was fixed at 5 and 10 Torr. In each case, the pressure of nitrogen was progressively increased until a constant absorption of gas was reached. A maximum absorption of about 80 % is reached at a nitrogen pressure of 200 Torr for a silane partial pressure of 5 Torr. Under 10 Torr of silane, the maximum absorption is between 95 and 100 % for a nitrogen pressure of 80 Torr (Fig. 2) indicating that $SiH_4$-$N_2$ mixtures have a larger absorption coefficient than pure silane. The optical absorption of silane molecules reaches a limit value solely dependent on silane partial pressure in the mixture.

## 4. Homogeneous Decomposition Threshold of Silane

Irradiation of silane with the P(20) laser line causes $SiH_2$ and $SiH_3$ radicals to form ; a visible luminescence due to molecular and atomic hydrogen

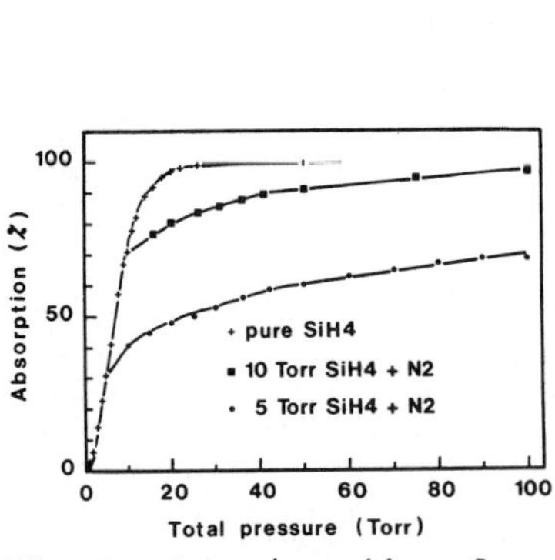


Fig. 2 : I.R. absorption of pure $SiH_4$ and $SiH_4$-$N_2$ mixtures.

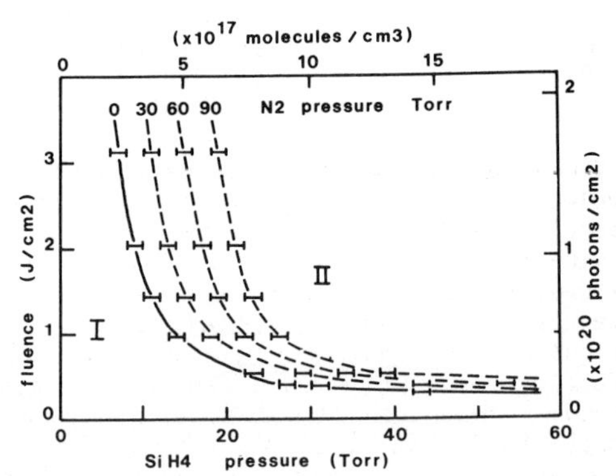


Fig. 3 : Homogeneous decomposition threshold of $SiH_4$ : pure $SiH_4$ (solid line) ; $SiH_4$-$N_2$ mixtures (dashed lines).

accompanies the molecule dissociation [5, 6]. A further increase in laser fluence or gas pressure will result in the formation of powdery silicon on the NaCl window. The onset of powdery silicon deposition is taken as the threshold of homogeneous decomposition of the gas. The powder has been determined to be polycrystalline silicon by X-ray diffraction.

Laser fluence versus silane pressure for the homogeneous decomposition threshold of gas is represented in Fig. 3. When fluence and silane pressure values are chosen from zone I, molecules will be vibrationally excited without any formation of silicon and radicals may be produced. When values are chosen from zone II, silane molecules or radicals are decomposed and powdery silicon is formed by volume reactions in the homogeneous phase. On a microscopic scale, the most important parameters are the flux of photons at the window and the density of silane molecules. At room temperature, the ratio of photon flux to molecule density required to reach the homogeneous decomposition threshold is about 100.

Nitrogen molecules prevent the decomposition of silane. The silane partial pressure needed to attain the decomposition threshold increases with increasing nitrogen pressure in the gas mixture (Fig. 3). At a given nitrogen pressure, the difference between silane pressure in the $SiH_4$-$N_2$ mixture and pure silane pressure at the homogenenous decomposition threshold decreases with increasing laser fluence (fig. 4). In other words, the ability of nitrogen to prevent the decomposition of silane molecules is greater at low fluence.

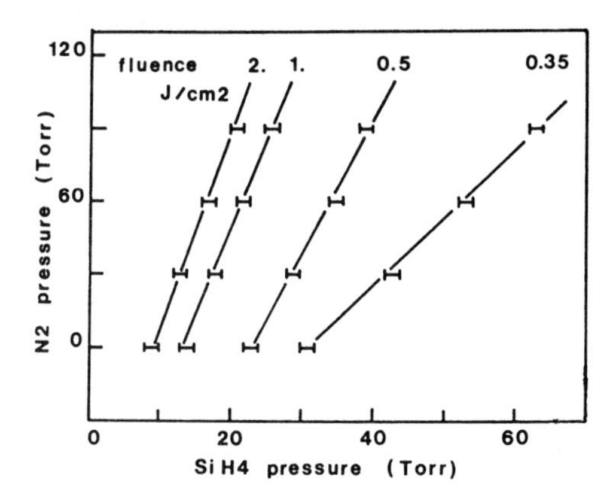


Fig. 4 : Nitrogen effect on the homogeneous decomposition threshold of silane.

The effect of nitrogen can be interpreted on the basis of a mechanism involving collisional processes. During a molecular collision, a nitrogen molecule can deenergize an excited silane molecule by removing an amount of vibrational energy sufficient to prevent its decomposition. In $SiH_4$-$N_2$ mixtures for a given fluence, the number of IR photons absorbed by silane molecules increases with increasing nitrogen molecule density since molecular collisions cause the absorption line width to broaden (Lorentz effect). Thereby, at a fixed silane pressure, the density of excited molecules in a $SiH_4$-$N_2$ mixture is higher than in pure silane, but the vibrational and translational energies of these excited species are lower. In a gas mixture, a part of the excitation energy is transferred to the nitrogen molecules under the form of translational energy and the temperature of the gas increases. At the decomposition threshold, it must be at least 600 °C, since the powdery silicon deposited on the window is polycrystalline.

## 5. Deposition of Silicon Films from Pure Silane

Silicon films deposited using the laser beam perpendicular to quartz substrates have been found to be non-adherent [4]. For the present study, the parallel and tangential direction of the laser beam has been adopted and silicon films tightly adherent to substrates have been produced under various experimental conditions. The films have been determined to be amorphous by the electron diffraction technique. The width of a-Si films is equal to the beam diameter (10 mm). The thickness of deposits is fairly constant all across the substrates.

At a fluence of 1 $J/cm^2$ and under a silane pressure of 20 Torr, 2700 laser pulses yield negligible deposits below 300 °C (Fig. 5). The effect of substrate temperature on film thickness appears greater here than in the case of cw $CO_2$ laser-induced deposition [2, 5]. The activation energy cannot be directly derived from the dependence of the deposition rate on substrate temperature. Indeed, according to MEUNIER et al. [7], the deposition rate of films actually depends on gas temperature which is in turn a function of laser intensity, gas pressure, gas composition and substrate temperature. The activation energy is reported to be $(46 \pm 5)$ kcal/mole. Owing to the considerable effect of temperature on deposition rate, all our experiments have been carried out at the base substrate temperature of 350 °C.

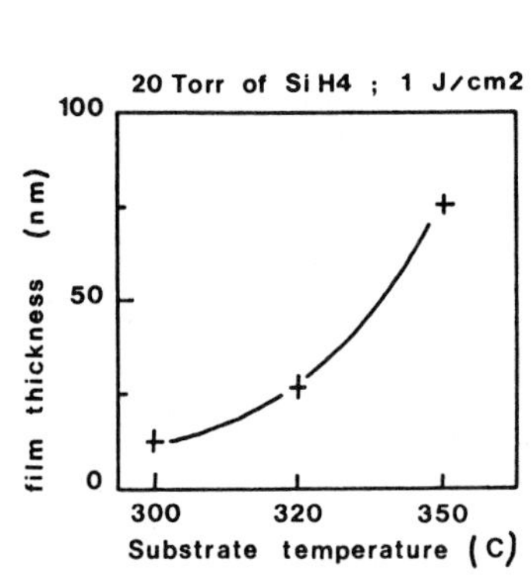


Fig. 5 : Temperature effect on deposition of a-Si films from pure silane.

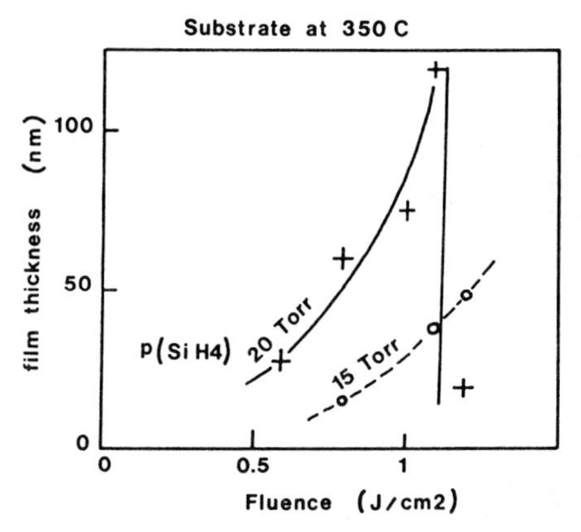


Fig. 6 : Fluence effect on deposition of a-Si films from pure silane.

The depositon rate of films deposited at 350 °C is dependent on laser fluence (Fig. 6). At a silane pressure of 20 Torr, the deposition rate decreases very rapidly for laser fluences higher than 1.1 $J/cm^2$. In this fluence range, the formation of powdery silicon by volume reactions takes place in the homogeneous gas phase. A large depletion of reactive gas occurs close to the substrate surface and then the deposition rate drops off sharply. The growth rate of films increases with increasing silane pressure, i. e., when the photon absorption by gas molecules is greater. Since the homogeneous decomposition threshold of silane molecules is not reached at a fluence of 1.2 $J/cm^2$ at a silane pressure of 15 Torr, these silicon films are thicker than those deposited at 20 Torr. With the gas at room temperature and at a laser fluence of 1 $J/cm^2$ (Fig. 3), the homogeneous decomposition threshold is reached at a silane pressure

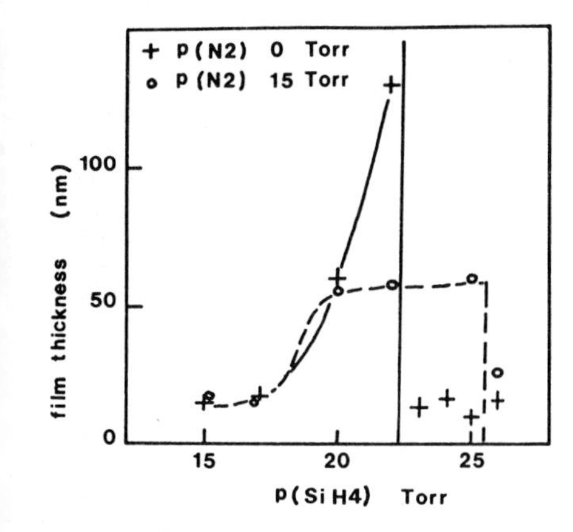


Fig. 7 : Silane pressure effect on deposition of a-Si films from pure silane and silane-nitrogen mixtures.

of 13 Torr. Actually, by heating the substrate to 350 °C, the threshold is attained at a higher silane pressure, but for an identical value of molecular density in the deposition zone.

The deposition rate of films from pure silane is strongly dependent on the gas pressure (Fig. 7). At 350 °C and at a laser fluence of 0.8 $J/cm^2$ the thickness of films begins to increase for a gas pressure of 18 Torr and drops off rapidly at silane pressures higher than 22 Torr. The a-Si films start to build up for a gas pressure in the neighbourhood of a silane pressure corresponding to the homogeneous decomposition threshold. Above 22 Torr, silane molecules are converted into powdery silicon and molecular hydrogen by volume reactions. Consequently, the gas pressure range in which a-Si films are produced at a satisfactory rate is very narrow and the deposition process is difficult to control.

## 6. Deposition of Silicon Films from Silane-Nitrogen Mixtures

The silane pressure range for deposition of a-Si films can be expanded by irradiating $SiH_4$-$N_2$ mixtures. For a nitrogen partial pressure of 15 Torr in $SiH_4$-$N_2$ mixtures, the thickness of films is dependent on silane pressure (Fig. 7). Below a silane pressure of 20 Torr, films of identical thickness are deposited from either pure silane or gas mixtures. Above this partial pressure, the thickness is independent of silane pressure up to the homogeneous decomposition threshold, which is attained at a silane pressure higher than 25 Torr. Between 20 and 25 Torr of silane, the wide plateau makes the deposition process easy to control. With a nitrogen partial pressure of 20 Torr in the gas mixture, the plateau can be extended beyond 27 Torr of silane ; the films, however, are only about 10 nm thick for 2700 laser pulses.

## 7. Reaction Mechanism

MEUNIER et al. [7] suggest that the reaction mechanism for laser-induced pyrolysis of silane consists of two elementary steps :

$$SiH_4(g) \longrightarrow SiH_2(g) + H_2(g) \qquad (1)$$

$$SiH_2(g) \longrightarrow SiH_y(s) + \frac{2-y}{2} H_2(g). \qquad (2)$$

In the first step, $SiH_2$ radicals and molecular hydrogen are produced by decomposition of vibrationally excited $SiH_4$ molecules. Under a relatively high pressure of silane, $SiH_2$ radicals react together during collisions to produce powdery silicon by volume reactions. At lower pressures, hydrogenated amorphous silicon films can grow by pyrolysis of $SiH_2$ radicals on the surface of the substrate. Step (1) is considered to be the rate-limiting process.

Since $SiH_2$ species are vibrationally excited by photon absorption, the pyrolysis of these radicals and the growth of a-Si films occur at much lower temperatures than in the conventional pyrolysis of silane. Nitrogen molecules screen the vibrationally excited $SiH_4$ molecules and $SiH_2$ radicals. Therefore, collisions between excited species and the formation of particles by homogeneous reactions are hampered. Photon absorption by silane molecules is likewise more intense in $SiH_4$-$N_2$ mixtures. Consequently, the concentration of excited silane molecules is higher in gas mixtures than in pure silane, but a lower level of excitation energy is reached by gaseous species. Nitrogen molecules act as a buffer agent making the deposition rate of a-Si films more regular.

## 8. Conclusion

Amorphous silicon films can be deposited at 350 °C from pure silane or $SiH_4$-$N_2$ mixtures under P(20) $CO_2$ laser line irradiation. The optical absorption of gas mixtures is greater than that of pure silane. The homogeneous decomposition of silane into powdery polycrystalline silicon can be hindered by adding nitrogen to silane. The deposition rate of films deposited from gas mixtures is lower than that of films produced from pure silane. However, by using $SiH_4$-$N_2$ mixtures, adherent a-Si films can be deposited under a wider range of silane pressures and the deposition process is easier to control.

## References


1 M. Hanabusa, S. Moriyama, H. Kikuchi, Thin Solid Films, 107, 227 (1983)

2 R. Bilenchi, I. Gianinoni, M. Musci, J. Appl. Phys., 53, 6479 (1982)

3 M. Meunier, T. R. Gattuso, D. Adler, J. S. Haggerty, Appl. Phys. Lett., 43, 273 (1983)

4 Y. Pauleau, R. Stawski, P. Lami, G. Auvert, in "Laser-Controlled Chemical Processing of Surfaces", Mat. Res. Soc. Symp. Proc., Vol. 29, ed. by A. Wayne Johnson and D. J. Ehrlich, (North-Holland, New York, 1984) (to be published)

5 R. Bilenchi, M. Musci, in "Proceedings of the 8th International Conference on Chemical Vapor Deposition", ed. by J. M. Blocher, G. A. Vuillard and G. Wahl, (The Electrochemical Society Softbound Proceeding Series, Pennington, 1981) p. 275

6 T. F. Deutsch, J. Chem. Phys., 70, 1187 (1979)

7 M. Meunier, J. H. Flint, D. Adler, J. S. Haggerty, in "Laser-Controlled Chemical Processing of Surfaces", Mat. Res. Soc. Symp. Proc., Vol. 29, ed. by A. Wayne Johnson and D. J. Ehrlich, (North Holland, New York, 1984) (to be published)

# Characterization of Reactive Intermediates in Silicon Etching and Deposition Using Laser Techniques

S.A. Joyce, B. Roop, J.C. Schultz, K. Suzuki, J. Thoman, and J.I. Steinfeld

Department of Chemistry, Massachusetts Institute of Technology, Cambridge, MA 02139, USA

## 1. Introduction

Plasma reactive etching and chemical vapor deposition (CVD) are widely used techniques in the fabrication of semiconductor microelectronic devices. Both processes are complex and difficult to characterize because of the large number of reactive components which may be present; in addition, the field gradients present in plasmas and the temperature gradients present in CVD reactors must be considered in any general model of these processes. The use of optical probes for plasma [1,2] and CVD [1,3] processes has begun to provide important information on the elementary reactions taking place in these systems. The high sensitivity and time and energy resolution afforded by laser spectroscopic techniques, in particular, have been extremely valuable for this purpose.

Lasers have also started to find application for photoinitiation of etching and CVD processes, in which reactive species can be generated in isothermal, field-free environments [4]. There are numerous examples of reactions initiated by irradiation of a surface in the presence of reactive vapor-phase species. EHRLICH, OSGOOD and co-workers at the M.I.T. Lincoln Laboratory have used ultraviolet irradiation to create microstructures on semiconductor surfaces [5]. CHUANG [6] has studied the influence of infrared excitation on the reactions between silicon and $XeF_2$ or $SF_6$, while HOULE [7,8] has investigated visible-wavelength photostimulation of the $XeF_2$/Si reaction. In these studies, the laser radiation was partially absorbed by the surface, producing local thermochemical as well as photochemical effects. In our own work [4], we have been using laser-induced chemical reactions such as infrared multiple-photon dissociation (IRMPD) to generate reactive fragments in the gas phase in close proximity to a well-characterized surface, thereby elucidating the details of the interaction of these species with the surface. We make use of several standard surface analysis techniques, such as photoelectron spectroscopy (XPS, UPS) [9,10] and thermal desorption spectrometry (TDS) [11,12], for characterization of surface binding sites and product identification. Scanning electron microscopy (SEM) is also used to observe the overall morphology of surface modifications.

## 2. Interaction of Fluorine Atoms with Si(111)7x7

Xenon difluoride has been proposed as an emulant system for fluorine etching, since this species spontaneously etches silicon with a rate of (2-5) x $10^5$ Å $min^{-1}$ $Torr^{-1}$ [13-15]. The initial step is presumed to be dissociative chemisorption of the $XeF_2$,

$$XeF_2(g) + Si(S) \rightarrow Si{:}F(ads) + Xe(g).$$

A full understanding of the binding in this system is particularly apropos, since it has been suggested [13] that the initial step in the reactive etching of silicon by fluorocarbons proceeds in a similar way,

$$CF_3(g) + Si(S) \rightarrow Si{:}C(ads) + Si{:}F(ads).$$

Following controlled exposure of Si(111)7x7 to $XeF_2$ and evacuation to a base pressure below $10^{-9}$ Torr, we have used XPS to characterize the species found at the surface and TDS to detect reaction products. We observe a peak at m/e = 85($SiF_3^+$) at T = 220-350 °C, and peaks at m/e = 66($SiF_2^+$) and

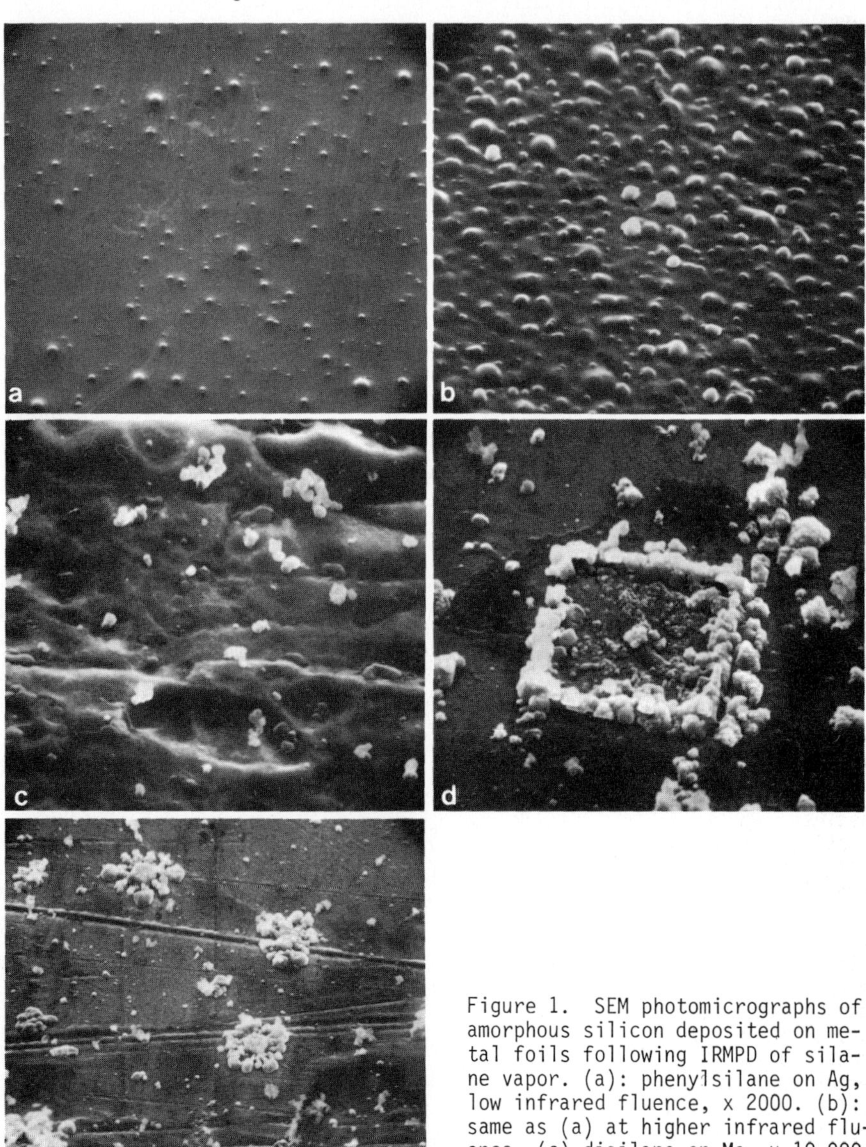

Figure 1. SEM photomicrographs of amorphous silicon deposited on metal foils following IRMPD of silane vapor. (a): phenylsilane on Ag, low infrared fluence, x 2000. (b): same as (a) at higher infrared fluence. (c) disilane on Mo, x 10,000. (d) and (e): disilane on Ag, x 10,000.

47($SiF^+$), both arising from $SiF_2$ at higher temperatures (>450°C), indicating at least two distinct reactive sites. However, the F(1s) peak in XPS shows only a single feature with fwhm = (2.0±0.1)eV. Interstitial F (*i.e.*, fluorine diffused into the silicon lattice) may play an important rôle, as suggested by HOULE [7,8]. This may be especially important for the Si(111)7x7 face, which contains several open channels penetrating down 3 or 4 atomic layers in the lattice [16].

## 3. Deposition of Amorphous Silicon on Metallic Surfaces

IRMPD of $RSiH_3$ (R = $C_2H_5$, $C_4H_9$, phenyl, or $SiH_3$) leads to deposition of amorphous silicon (a:Si-H) on proximal surfaces [17]. The presumed active intermediate is $SiH_2$ resulting from secondary IRMPD of "hot" silane eliminated in the initial dissociation. The form of these deposits depends on both the precursor molecule and the substrate.

Figures 1a and 1b show deposits on a silver foil substrate resulting from IRMPD of phenylsilane at low and high infrared fluence, respectively [18]. In both cases, Si-rich nodules are deposited on a carbonaceous overlayer which results from breakup of the phenyl ring [19]. (It is actually more of a matrix than an overlayer, since depth profiling with XPS shows a nearly constant C/Si ratio.) There is no evidence of clustering or aggregation of these nodules. Figure 1c shows the deposit resulting from IRMPD of disilane ($Si_2H_6$) on molybdenum foil. In this case, the silicic nodules are locally aggregated, but there is no evidence of long-range order in the deposits. On silver foil, however, similar nodules are formed but now form striking patterns, typically possessing fourfold symmetry; examples are shown in Figs. 1d and 1e.

Comparison of Figs. 1a and 1b with Figs. 1d and 1e shows that the presence of the carbon overlayer completely inhibits aggregation of the a:Si-H nodules, even at high coverage. In the absence of this overlayer, in material derived from IRMPD of disilane, individual nodules tend to aggregate locally, but in the rough Mo surface (Fig. 1c) there is no gross ordering on the surface. On a Ag surface, which is smooth but contains many defect sites corresponding to grain boundaries of microcrystallites, preferential nucleation appears to occur at these sites, with the resulting patterns reflecting the cubic close-packed (face-centered cubic) structure of the silver lattice.

A possible interpretation of these observations is that initial small cluster formation may be occurring in the gas phase prior to deposition, as in the formation of $Si_2$ dimers in silane CVD [3]. The adsorption and possible subsequent migration of these clusters on the surface will depend on sticking coefficients at specific sites or defects. Aggregation or preferential deposition may occur if there are large site-to-site differences in surface chemical potential.

## 4. Discussion

Both processes described here - silicon removal by chemical etching and amorphous silicon deposition from the vapor phase - are controlled by chemical transport processes taking place between the gas and the solid surface [20]. These processes are, in turn, driven by chemical potential gradients in the system which depend on local values of concentration, temperature, and (in the case of plasmas) electric field, as well as on the surface free energies at various binding sites. Although some elementary treatments of chemical transport processes have appeared in the literature [21], detailed theoretical analysis remains to be done. The real-time, *in situ* concentration profiles afforded by laser diagnostics will be of great importance in testing the predictions of these models.

Acknowledgments
This work was supported by the National Science Foundation and the Air Force Office of Scientific Research.

References

1. J. Wormhoudt, A.C. Stanton, and J. Silver: Proc. SPIE 452 (1983), Spectroscopic Characterization Techniques for Semiconductor Technology.
2. R.A. Gottscho, R.H. Burton, D.L. Flamm, V.M. Donnelly, and G.P. Davis: J. Appl. Phys. 55, 2707 (1984).
3. W.G. Breiland and P. Ho: Electrochemical Soc. Vol. 84-6 (1984), Proc. Ninth Intl. Conf. on Chemical Vapor Deposition (McD. Robinson, C.H.J. van den Brekel, G.W. Cullen, J.M. Blocher, Jr., and P. Rai-Choudhury, eds.), pp. 44-59.
4. D. Harradine, F.R. McFeely, B. Roop, J.I. Steinfeld, D. Denison, L. Hartsough, and J.R. Hollahan: Proc. SPIE 270 (1981), High Power Lasers and Applications, pp. 52-60.
5. R. Osgood: Ann. Rev. Phys. Chem. 34, 77 (1983).
6. T.J. Chuang: J. Chem. Phys. 74, 1453, 1461 (1981).
7. F.A. Houle: J. Chem. Phys. 79, 4237 (1983).
8. F.A. Houle: J. Chem. Phys. 80, 4851 (1984).
9. B. Feuerbacher and R.F. Willis: J. Phys. C: Solid State Phys. 9, 169 (1976).
10. M. Cardona and L. Ley (eds.): Photoemission in Solids. I. General Principles, Topics in Applied Physics Vol. 26, Springer-Verlag, Berlin (1978).
11. P.A. Redhead: Vacuum 12, 203 (1962).
12. D. Menzel: in Interactions on Metal Surfaces (R. Gomes, ed.) Topics in Applied Physics Vol. 4, Springer-Verlag, Berlin (1975), pp.101-142.
13. H.F. Winters and J.W. Coburn: Appl. Phys. Letts. 34, 70 (1979).
14. H.F. Winters and F.A. Houle: J. Appl. Phys. 54, 1218 (1983).
15. D.L. Flamm, D.E. Ibbotson, J.A. Mucha, and V.M. Donnelly: Solid State Technology 117 (April, 1983).
16. F.J. Himpsel and I.P. Batra: J. Vac. Sci. Tech. A2, 952 (1984).
17. J.S. Francisco, S.A. Joyce, J.I. Steinfeld, and F. Walsh: J. Phys. Chem. (in press).
18. The yield of dissociation products is, in general, a logarithmically increasing function of infrared fluence; see for example H.W. Galbraith and J.R. Ackerhalt: in Laser-Induced Chemical Processes (J.I. Steinfeld, ed.), Plenum Press, New York (1981), pp. 1-44.
19. Such nodules are also observed in the formation of polycrystalline Si from $SiCl_4$ in laser-heated substrates: see V. Baranauskas, C.I.Z. Mammana, R.E. Klinger, and J.E. Greene: Appl. Phys. Letts. 36, 930 (1980).
20. C.B. Zarowin: Thin Solid Films 85, 33 (1981).
21. H. Schäfer: Chemical Transport Reactions, Academic Press, New York (1964).

# The Physics of Ultraviolet Photodeposition*

H.H. Gilgen, C.J. Chen, R. Krchnavek, and R.M. Osgood, Jr.

Columbia Microelectronics Sciences Laboratories, Columbia University,
New York, NY 10027, USA

Ultraviolet photodeposition is a technique for direct laser writing of submicrometer metal patterns on solid substrates. The process involves a wealth of unexplored physical phenomena including micrometer-scale ultraviolet photochemistry and surface and interface chemical dynamics. This paper briefly reviews the current developments in understanding the process physics. In addition, the applications of the technique to microelectronics fabrication are briefly discussed.

## I. INTRODUCTION

In photodeposition, selected molecular species decompose by direct absorption of light. One of the photofragments then condenses on a nearby solid-substrate surface to form a thin-solid film. There are many variations on this simple process. For example, it is possible to decompose the parent molecule as the result of multiple- or single-photon absorption; the former generally involving infrared radiation, the latter almost exclusively uses ultraviolet radiation. Photodeposition may also occur from gas, adsorbed-, or liquid-phase molecular species. The "dry " gas and adsorbed phases are more convenient from a practical point of view since they are convenient to handle and mix. However, the liquid phase is a well established chemical medium in which even relatively inert materials can be readily solvated. Finally, it is possible to use subseqent reactions in conjunction with photodecomposition to enable the deposition of useful materials such as $SiO_2$ and $Si_3N_4$ [1].

In this paper, we will review the simplest form of photodeposition; namely the deposition of metal from organometallic compounds using ultraviolet light. We will discuss the materials and molecules used in photodeposition, the process phenomena, the microstructure of the deposits, and recent measurements of the electrical properties of the deposit. We will also include a comparison of photodeposition with other laser writing techniques as well as a brief summary of demonstrated applications involving photodeposition.

Historically photodeposition was one of the first laser-chemical processing techniques to be extensively investigated. The initial result with focused laser light was obtained with photodeposition of iodine from $CH_3I$ using a frequency-doubled $Ar^+$ laser [2]. The appearance of blurred, but distinct interference fringes in the resulting deposit showed that high spatial resolution could be obtained from such a process. In subsequent work with metallorganics, submicrometer-wide metal lines with low

* This work was supported by the Defense Advanced Research Projects Agency and the Air Force Office of Scientific Research, the Department of Army (ARO), and the Joint Services Electronics Program.

resistivity were written. In these experiments differences in the sticking coefficients between the illuminated and unilluminated regions of the surface gave rise to well defined depositions even from gas-phase reagents. The use of a computer-controlled x-y table in conjunction with a UV microscope allowed one to metallize a substrate in a predetermined pattern, thus opening up a variety of practical applications in microelectronics [3].

In addition to the practical results, research in photodeposition has generated interest in many basic areas of photochemistry. For example, recent progress in understanding the photochemistry of metal alkyls and other metal-bearing organic molecules can be directly linked to work in photodeposition. Similarly new research in UV and IR spectroscopy at gas-solid interfaces has also been motivated in part by photodeposition.

## II. LASER WRITING

Laser writing involves using a focused, scanning laser beam to deposit patterns on a solid substrate. Table 1 summarizes the various chemical techniques which have been used for laser writing.

TABLE I.

| MEDIUM | | |
|---|---|---|
| GAS | LIQUID | SOLID (Film) |
| Photolysis<br>$Cd/Cd(CH_3)_2$<br>Cu/Cu(AcAc) | Au, Cu<br>from corresponding metal salt solution | |
| Pyrolysis<br>$Si/SiH_4$<br>$Ni/Ni(CO)_4$ | Au, Cu<br>from corresponding metal salt solution | Spin-on organo silicates and organo metallics |

The two techniques, which use gas phase-reagents, are commonly classed as either photochemical [4] or thermochemical deposition [5,6]. This classification is based on the somewhat simplified idea that reactions in a focused laser beam can depend exclusively on photodissociative processes or light beam initiated thermal chemistry, respectively. In fact, with high intensity, deep UV light, it is easy to initiate thermal chemistry as well; or alternatively, if the "pyrolytic" light source is in the near UV or blue, photodissociation of weakly bound complexes may also occur.

Nonetheless, it is useful to compare briefly pyrolytic and photolytic deposition. In the former, one uses the heating of the substrate to decompose the gases above it. In the latter, one dissociates the gas or at least a weakly bound film on the substrate directly by relying on a bound-free electronic transition in the parent molecule. As a result it is clear that pyrolytic deposition cannot be used in cases where the substrate melts before the gas decomposes. Photolytic deposition can be used for depositing on fragile substrates such as organic materials or on thin film layers of complex III-V compounds, see Fig. 1a. It is, however, possible that the presence of even low intensity UV light may alter some of the electrical or chemical properties of the underlying substrate; further studies are needed before the importance of such effects can be gauged.

Another advantage of photolytic deposition is that it appears to be more surface insensitive than pyrolytic deposition, since in the former the light acts directly on the parent molecules whereas in the latter it acts through the substrate. Thus, in pyrolytic-writing as one writes over a surface containing $SiO_2$, Si, and metal, each with different thermal conductivities, the laser power must be readjusted at each interface or the deposition-rate and width will vary. In fact, in cases where even the pyrolytic deposit and substrate have different conductivities, e.g. metal on $SiO_2$, the deposit width may be controlled by the deposit itself [7]. Such substrate dependent effects are greatly reduced in photolytic deposition (See Fig. 1b).

Photolytic deposition does face two serious drawbacks. First, it requires a cw, deep-UV laser source, since most practical parent molecules

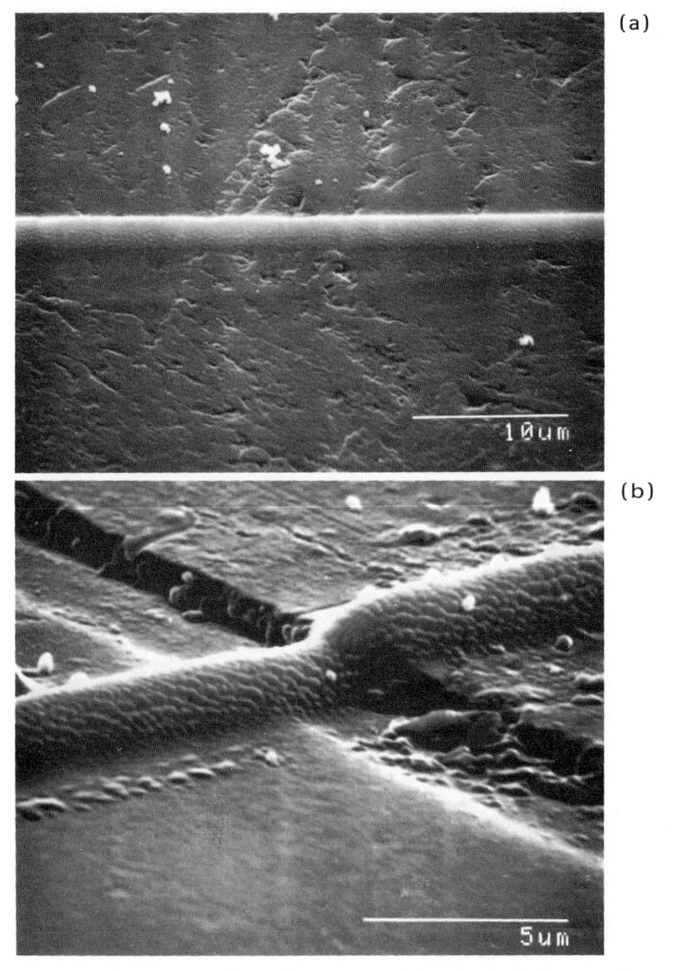


Fig. 1(a) Cd-line deposited from dimethylcadmium on low melting plastic material. (b) Cd-line deposited over a step of $SiO_2$ on Si.

use wavelengths of 250 - 300 nm or shorter to initiate a dissociative process.

Thus far the only available laser has been the frequency doubled $Ar^+$ at 257 nm, with a typical power of 10 mW. This low power limits the rate of deposition. In addition, this wavelength is not short enough to permit deposition from many important molecules such as $SiH_4$, which are compatible with pyrolytic deposition. The second drawback is the fact that good electrical properties are not readily obtained because of the low deposition temperature in photolytic deposition. Low substrate temperature can allow impurity incorporation and cause a loose microstructure. Nonetheless, recent results have shown that by paying careful attention to specific deposition parameters, it is possible to obtain workably low electrical resistivities (see below).

In summary, both pyrolytic and photolytic deposition are capable of directly writing submicrometer conductors. However, both appear to have significant drawbacks which must be solved before generalized applications in microelectronics can be envisioned.

## III. THE PROCESS OF PHOTOLYTIC DEPOSITION

### A. General

In photolytic deposition, a UV laser beam illuminates a gas-solid interface. Generally the beam impinges on the substrate and the deposit as it is formed. As a result photodissociation occurs in both the gas and surface phases. The deposit, then, consists of atoms which have been produced in both phases. The details of these processes depends sensitively on the specific parent-molecule substrate combination used. For the purposes of our discussion here, we will emphasize the processes encountered with the Group-II-metal alkyls since the physics of this group is comparatively well studied.

### B. The Photochemistry of Group II Metal Alkyls.

The precursor metal alkyls for the Group II are typically the dimethyl or diethyl species such as $(CH_3)_2Cd$ or $(C_2H_5)_2Cd$. The absorption spectrum of dimethylcadmium, from 330 to 175 nm is shown in Fig. 2. It consits of two

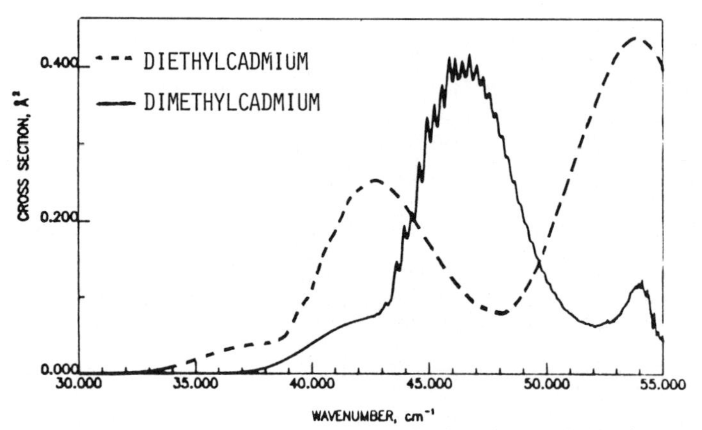


Fig. 2. The absorption spectra of dimethyl-and diethyl-cadmium.

electronic transitions with distinguishable features. At lower photon energy (37,000 $cm^{-1}$ to 43,000 $cm^{-1}$), the absorption is weak and structureless. For higher photon energies (43,000 $cm^{-1}$ to 52,000 $cm^{-1}$), a strong absorption with clear vibrational structure appears. Analysis shows that the vibrational structure consists of a double series with two characteristic frequencies.

The photodissociation processes of the two transition are as follows. The first electronic transition, ($X^1\Sigma_g^+ \rightarrow A^1A_1$) results in a bent dissociative excited state which dissociates into a cadmium atom and two methyl radicals. The second electronic transition, ($X^1\Sigma_g^+ \rightarrow B^1\Pi_u$), results in a linear dissociative excited state which separates into a methyl radical and an excited cadmium monomethyl. The later radiatively decays or dissociates afterwards. The observed two-frequency vibrational structure is due to the excitations of the out-of-plane mode of $CH_3$ ligand and cadmium-carbon stretching mode of cadmium-monomethyl fragment [8].

The absorption spectrum of diethylcadmium (Fig. 2.) has a basically similar overall structure with two specific differences: An overall shift of the spectrum to the red by 5,000 $cm^{-1}$, and a broadening of the vibrational peaks in second electronic transitions. Note that for these compounds a third, very strong transition is visible at 53,000 $cm^{-1}$, perhaps corresponding to a molecular state correlated to the Cd $^1P_1$ state. For the first two transistions an almost identical photodissociation mechanism and excited-state assignment are applicable. Note that the redshift in spectrum compared to the corresponding methyl-alkyl increases the dissociative cross section at 257 nm.

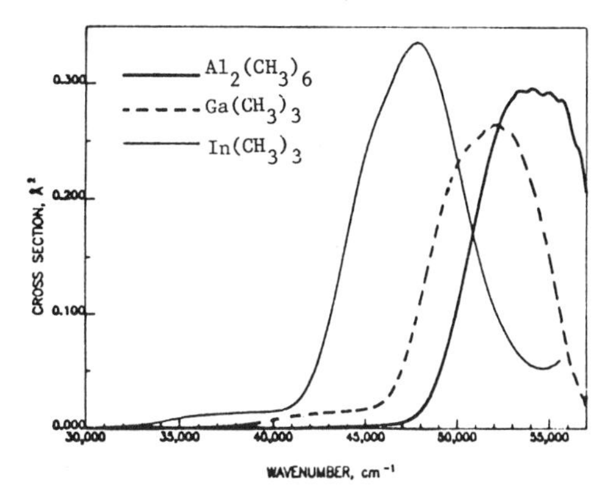


Fig. 3. Absorption spectra of the three metal-(Al,Ga,In) trimethyl molecules.

The measured absorption spectra of three metal-trimethyl molecules ($Al_2(CH_3)_6$, $Ga(CH_3)_3$, and $In(CH_3)_3$) are shown in Fig. 3. Similar features to those in the dimethyl precursors are found except that three electronic transitions are distinguishable. The first transiton is very weak, for the gallium and indium compounds and extremely weak for trimethylaluminum. The second and third transitions are strong, somewhat overlapping. A systemtic red shift was found from $Al_2(CH_3)_6$ to $In(CH_3)_3$.

Almost all of these metal-alkyls form chemisorbed layers on fused silica surfaces with the absorption spectra substantially smoothed and substantially more absorbing in the long-wavelength tail compared to gas-phase spectra. On top of the chemisorbed layer, physisorbed layers form, with coverage increasing as the pressure of the metal-alkyl gas increases. When the pressure of the gas is about one-half of its vapor pressure at the ambient temperature, the thickness of physisorbed layer is about one complete monolayer. The spectra of physisorbed layers are also broadened and red-shifted from gas spectra of the same material [9].

### C. Deposition Model

In order to describe the deposition process we have to consider the growth from the adlayer, the contribution from the gas phase and the diffusion of the reactants and products towards the activated zone. Formula (1) results from a simplified model which takes care of the different contributions to the metal growth and is correct only for low laser intensities:

$$\text{growth rate} \propto p \cdot I \cdot (A + Br). \qquad (1)$$

In this formula p is the partial gas pressure of the reactive gas, I is the laser power density. A and B are the cross sections of the reactants on the surface and in the gas-phase respectively and r is the spot radius [10]. At high laser intensities and/or high total gas pressure the growth rate can be limited by the diffusion (D) of the reactions or the products towards or from the active zone. At extremely high intensities ($> 100$ kW/cm$^2$), the diffusion would dominate the process and the growth rate would be given by formula (2):

$$\text{growth rate} \propto p \cdot D. \qquad (2)$$

An effect not included in this simple model is the interaction of the deposited material with the incident laser light. As described in Ref.[11], the statistical roughness of the deposited metal give rises to light scattering. The roughness can be introduced by the inhomogeneous adlayer, nucleation in the gas phase with subsequent formation of small balls on the surface or by local fluctuations in the laser beam. The resulting scattered light has components which travel parallel to the surface. This surface electromagnetic field drastically influences the growth rate of the material on the surface and results in a ripple pattern with a ripple spacing close to the wavelength. Similar patterns are observed in the field of laser annealing and etching of different semiconductors [12]. In some applications this ripple formation and field enhanced reactions can be very useful [12]. However, in many cases this phenomena is undesirable, and further work is needed to develop techniques to avoid growth [13].

### D. Resolution

As has been pointed out previously, the submicrometer resolution in laser direct writing is a result of process nonlinearities. In the case of writing with UV photodissociation, the nonlinearity arises from nucleation by photolysis of the adsorbed layer of gas. The physics of this process has been discussed in detail elsewhere. Basically, however, metal atoms from gas-phase photolysis condenses much more efficiently in regions of a substrate where metal nuclei already exist. As a result the metal films form only where the UV intensity is sufficient to dissociate completely the adlayer and form metal nuclei.

The existence of such a threshold flux is shown clearly in the data of Fig. 4. In this experiment a scanned laser beam was slowly increased in power, while at the same time keeping the spot size fixed. The experiment

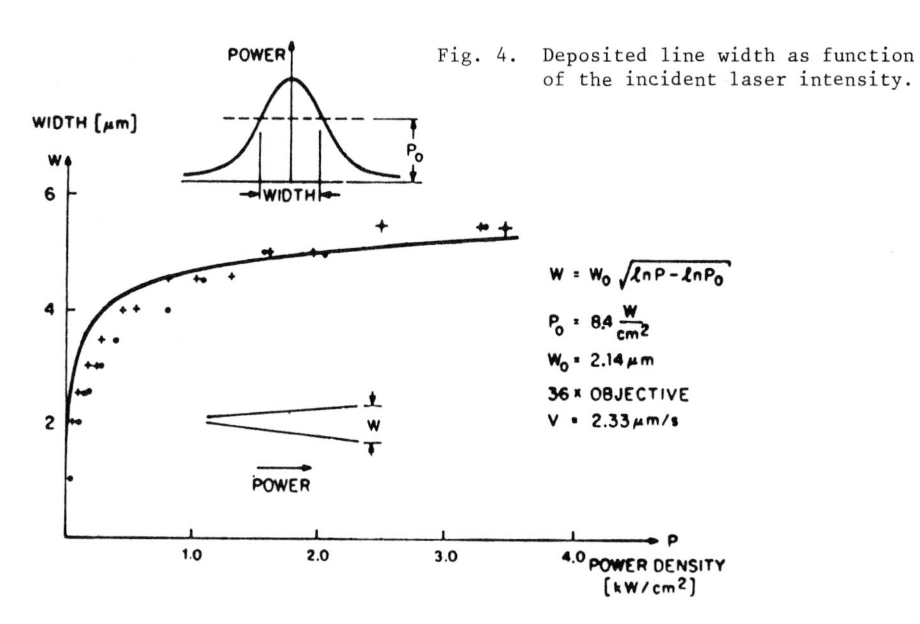


Fig. 4. Deposited line width as function of the incident laser intensity.

was done in a cell filled with 3 Torr of dimethylcadmium using a 257-nm laser beam. As seen in Fig. 4, the width of the line broadened monotonically with the laser beam power. The broadening occurs because as the laser power increases the portion of the Gaussian beam which was above threshold also increases. The data could be fit with a simple theory based on the existence of a sharp threshold for nucleation to occur. The measured threshold for this materials system was $3 - 10\ W/cm^2$.

## IV. DEPOSITION CHARACTERISTICS

### A. Electrical Properties

Clearly for most applications of laser direct writing, the electrical and optical properties of the deposited material must be well characterized and adequate for the application at hand. Therefore, we have concentrated our efforts on measurements of the electrical resistance of cadmium and indium lines. The experiments were done with lines which had a typical width of $2\mu m$ and connected on two gold islands separated by $100\mu m$. The resistance between the two gold patterns was normalized with the corresponding bulk resistance of the line. The bulk resistance value of the line was found by optically measuring their length and width and by determination of the thickness by a mechanical profilometer.

The normalized resistivity (or resistivity ratio) is plotted in Fig. 5 for cadmium as function of the dimethyl cadmium gas pressure. We found that for deposition without buffer gas a distinct minimum occurred at seven times the bulk resistivity. At the low pressure end equation (1) holds. With a spot size of $2\mu m$ and using the results of the absorption spectra, we find the growth rate is dominanted by the adlayer growth. Under these conditions the light interaction with the deposition is strong and results in a pronounced ripple formation. The resistivity is increased by the regions of thin metal thickness in the ripple and is therefore very high. Raising the pressure decreases the diffusion coefficient and the growth rate becomes diffusion limited. At high gas-pressure atoms away from the surface can nucleate homogeneously and a heavy "rain" of cadmium particles occur. Under these

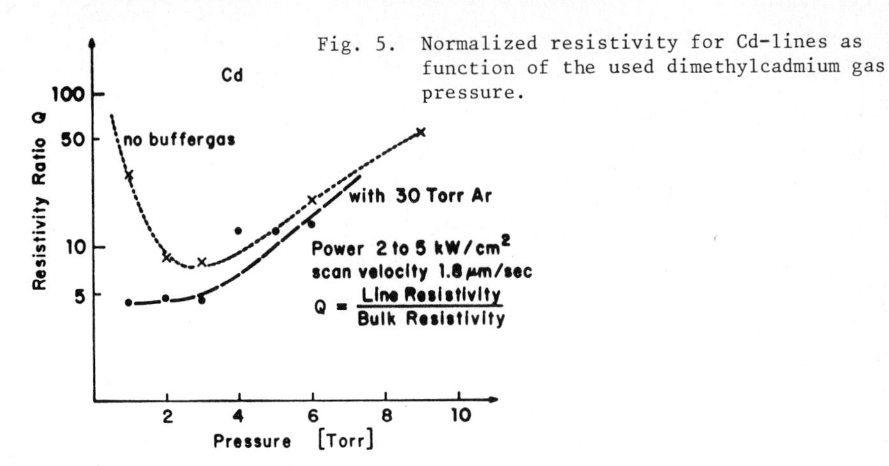


Fig. 5. Normalized resistivity for Cd-lines as function of the used dimethylcadmium gas pressure.

conditions fairly well-resolved structures occur, but the deposited material is less dense and therefore has higher resistivity. Adding 30 Torr or argon buffer gas also increases the diffusion time to the surface. Under these conditions the growth is diffusion limited and the best values of four times the bulk resistivity are obtained. This value compares favorably with values obtained by vacuum evaporation of metal lines which are in the order of three times the bulk.

B. Deposit Structure - Step Coverage

Metal or insulator patterns produced by photoresist and subsequent lift-off techniques possess very well-defined steps. It is important to be able to write good conducting metal lines over such vertical steps. We have recently shown that using photodeposition of a line thickness equal to the step height we can write with constant velocity over such a step without a drastic increase in the line resistivity. For example, we have found good conducting lines with no change in width or thickness (0.7 μm) over a step of 0.5 μm. In addition the large optical depth of field with UV light makes a deposition with constant line parameters in deep U-shaped grooves possible. Coverage of steps larger than the thickness of the lines can be achieved by a speed reduction in the step region.

## V. APPLICATIONS

Despite the fact that the majority of experiments with UV photolytic direct writing have involved the Group-II-metal alkyls, it has still been possible to demonstrate a number of important new applications of laser direct writing. The first practical demonstration used laser deposition of metals to repair defects in a chrome-quartz photolithographic mask [14]. In this case the descretionary requirement of repairing necessitates direct, one-step processing. Recently we have applied this same philosophy to the repair of simple integrated circuits. Fig. 6. shows a low magnification SEM of such a circuit. The circled areas from left to right show a broken circuit element which was repaired with the addition of a directly written conducting link and by the shorting out of a defective transistor. Other applications of laser photolytic writing are described in a companion paper by Ehrlich and Tsao in this volume.

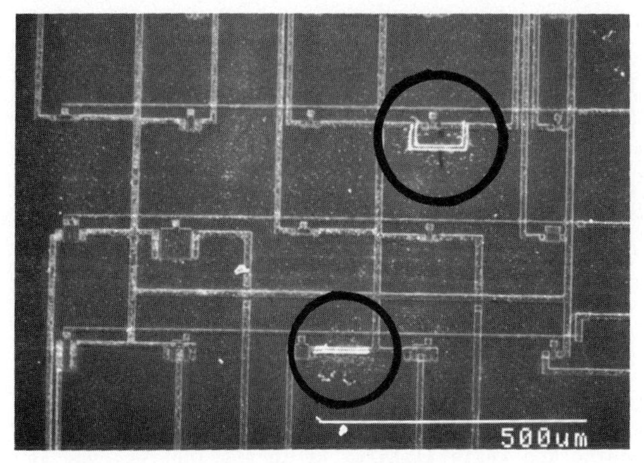


Fig. 6. Low magnification SEM of a repaired integrated circuit.

## Acknowledgments

The authors would like to thank other members of the Columbia Microelectronics Sciences Laboratories for many helpful comments during the preparation of this work. We thank I.P. Herman for several helpful comments.

## References

1. P.K. Boyer, G.A. Roche, W.H. Ritchie, and G.J. Collins, Appl. Phys. Lett. 40, 716 (1982).
2. T.F. Deutsch, D.J. Ehrlich and R.M. Osgood, Appl. Phys. Lett. 35, 175 (1979).
3. D.J. Ehrlich, R.M. Osgood, and T.F. Deutsch, IEEE Journal of Quantum Electronics, 16, 11 (1980).
4 R.M. Osgood, Ann. Rev. Phys. Chem. 34, 77 (1983).
5. S.D. Allen and M. Bass, J. Vac. Sci. Technol. 16, 431 (1979).
6. D. Bäuerle, Proc. Int. Conf. on "Surface Studies with Lasers," 1983, ed. by F. Aussenegg, et al., Springer, Chem. Phys. 33 178 (1983)
7. I.P. Herman, R.H. Hyde, B.M. McWilliams, A.H. Weisberg, and L.L. Wood Mat. Res. Soc. Symp. Proc. 17, 9 (1983).
8. C.J. Chen and R.M. Osgood, J. Chem. Phys. 81, 318; 327 (1984).
9. C.J. Chen and R.M. Osgood, Chem. Phys. Lett. 98, 363 (1983).
10. T.H. Wood, J.C. White and B.A. Thacker, Appl. Phys. Lett. 42, 408 (1983).
11. S.R.J. Brueck and D.J. Ehrlich, Phys. Rev. Lett. 48, 1678 (1982).
12. H.H. Gilgen, D.V. Podlesnik, C.J. Chen and R.M. Osgood, Mat. Res. Soc. Symp. Proc. 29, (in press), (1984).
13. Zhou Guosheng, P.M. Fauchet and A.E. Siegmann, Phys. Rev. B. 26, 5366 (1982).
14. D.J. Ehrlich, R.M. Osgood, D.J. Silversmith, and T.F. Deutsch, IEEE Electron Device Lett. EDL-1 (1980).

# Low Temperature Growth of HgTe by a UV Photosensitisation Method

S.J.C. Irvine, J.B. Mullin, and J. Tunnicliffe

Royal Signals and Radar Establishment, St. Andrews Road, Great Malvern, Worcestershire. WR14 3PS, U.K.

## 1. Introduction

The binary semi-metal HgTe is an end member of the important infrared detector alloy $Cd_xHg_{1-x}Te$. As the requirement for low temperature epitaxial growth of this alloy is due to the instability of Hg in the lattice, the compound, HgTe, is an important material to investigate with new, low temperature growth techniques. Previous publications have considered the limitation on low temperature growth of $Cd_xHg_{1-x}Te$ by Metal-Organic Vapour Phase Epitaxy (MOVPE) to be related to the thermal stability of the Te metal-organic; the preferred source being diethyltelluride ($Et_2Te$) [1-5]. Significant growth rates are not achieved by pyrolysis below 400°C but control during growth of the electrically active Hg vacancy requires growth temperatures below 300°C. A further attraction of low temperature growth is the potential ability to grow abrupt HgTe/CdTe interfaces and hence superlattice structures [6].

The thermal stability of $Et_2Te$ at low temperatures can be circumvented by photolytic decomposition. A study of the deposition of Te from $Et_2Te$ using a Hg arc lamp has been described elsewhere [7]. $Et_2Te$ will photodissociate but tellurium deposition will not occur onto a silica reaction tube in the region where it is illuminated with high UV intensity. In a previous report on epitaxial growth of HgTe using a Hg arc lamp to bring about the reaction between Hg vapour and $Et_2Te$ in a $H_2$ carrier gas, deposition on the substrates and on the reactor wall would only occur with a Hg pressure greater than $10^{-2}$ [atm] [8]. These pressures are close to the Hg rich solidus for HgTe in the temperature range 200-300°C. The growth process was interpreted as a surface selective photosensitisation reaction which relied on absorption of UV radiation by surface adsorbed Hg atoms which could decay to the ground state by dissociating the $Et_2Te$ molecules.

This paper is concerned with the surface and crystalline quality of HgTe epitaxial layers grown onto InSb substrates over the temperature range 200-310°C. It is particularly important at these low temperatures to establish the structural quality of epitaxy because of the lower surface mobility of the reactants.

## 2. Experimental

A description of the growth method has been given in a previous paper [8]. A horizontal, open flow reactor, operated at an atmosphere total pressure is used to flow a predetermined mixture of $Et_2Te$, Hg and $H_2$ into the reaction zone. Substrates of polished InSb {100} etched in 25:4:1, lactic acid, nitric acid, HF, prior to loading are situated on a graphite substrate holder which is heated by an infrared lamp. A Hg arc lamp (3[kW] total power dissipation) is situated above the reactor and can be focussed onto the substrate. Typical growth conditions for these experiments are Hg partial pressure 2-8x10$^{-2}$ [atm], $Et_2Te$ partial pressure 1.3-9.2x10$^{-3}$ [atm] and growth temperatures 230-310°C.

Epitaxial layers were examined after growth using a Philips 500 Scanning Electron Microscope (SEM), a Nomarski contrast microscope and a Philips single crystal diffractometer. The x-ray diffractometer used a Cu $k_\alpha$ source and diffraction traces of the HgTe and InSb (400) reflection were examined.

## 3. Results and Discussion

The surface selective photosensitisation reaction, previously described [8], relies on the Hg partial pressure being maintained above 2x10$^{-2}$ [atm]. Under this condition, epitaxial HgTe layers have been grown over the temperature range 200-310°C. Figure 1 shows a plot of growth rate versus substrate temperature where $Et_2Te$ partial pressure was maintained at 5.9x10$^{-3}$ [atm] and Hg partial pressure 3x10$^{-2}$ [atm]. From 230°C to 310°C the growth rate does not depend on temperature which indicates that surface kinetics are not a limiting factor. Hence under these growth conditions it should be possible to achieve higher growth rates either with higher $Et_2Te$ partial pressure or with higher photon fluences. At temperatures below 230°C a decrease in growth rate is observed which is consistent with surface kinetics limiting the growth at these low temperatures.

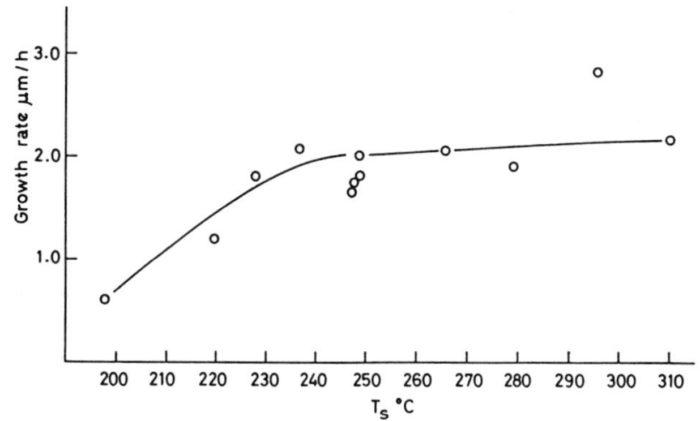


Fig. 1. Growth rate versus substrate temperatures $T_s$ for $P_{Hg} > 3x10^{-2}$ [atm] and $P_{Et_2Te} = 5.9x10^{-3}$ [atm] on {100} InSb substrates.

In a previous report [8] it was suggested that a thin HgTe layer (0.3 [µm]) had tetragonally distorted to accommodate the larger lattice of InSb (6.4798 [Å]). The HgTe (400) reflections were shifted to larger 2θ angles than expected from an unstrained lattice parameter of 6.4605 [Å], resulting in the InSb $k_{\alpha_2}$ and HgTe $k_{\alpha_1}$ peaks being resolved. By contrast, the present results are on thicker HgTe layers (~ 1 [µm]) and a tetragonal distortion is not observed, resulting in the complete overlap of InSb $k_{\alpha_2}$ and HgTe $k_{\alpha_1}$, as can be seen in Fig 2. This result is not surprising as calculations on the formation of misfit dislocations in the system $Cd_xHg_{1-x}Te$/CdTe by Basson and Booyens [9] have shown that for HgTe rich compositions the critical thickness to avoid misfit dislocations is below 0.2 [µm].

The crystalline quality of these layers were studied for different growth temperatures by measuring the HgTe $k_{\alpha_1}$ and $k_{\alpha_2}$ separation. Due to the

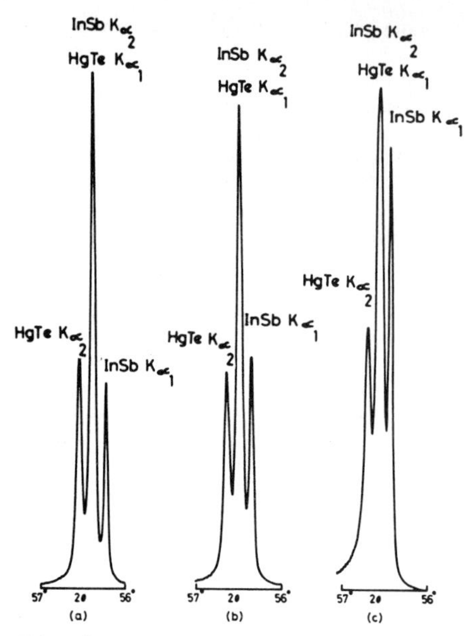


Fig. 2. X-ray diffractometer traces of the (400) reflections using Cu $k_\alpha$ radiation for ~ 1[μm] HgTe layers on InSb substrates at different growth temperatures (a) 230°C, (b) 266°C, (c) 310°C.

similar thicknesses of the HgTe layers, the overlapping InSb $k_{\alpha 2}$ peak would make the same contribution in each case; see examples in Fig 2. Another measure of lattice strain is the Full Width Half Maximum (FWHM) measurement but in each case the InSb FWHM is limited by diffractometer resolution of 0.06° and the HgTe peaks are only displaying slight broadening on this figure to a maximum of 0.1°. The $k_{\alpha 1}/k_{\alpha 2}$ separation was measured as the ratio of the HgTe $k_{\alpha 2}$ peak height to the minimum between the $k_{\alpha 1}$ and $k_{\alpha 2}$ peaks. This ratio, called $\gamma$, is plotted for a range of growth temperatures in Fig 3. The higher $\gamma$ values indicate greater $k_{\alpha 1}/k_{\alpha 2}$ separation and hence less strain in the lattice, surface kinetics would make this more favourable at higher temperatures. However, Fig 3 shows a trend of decreasing $\gamma$ at the higher temperatures, being 3 at 230°C and 1.6 at 310°C.

It has been shown by Rutherford Back Scattering (RBS) [10] that considerable Te sublattice disorder occurs near the HgTe/InSb interface. Channeling yields improve away from this interface and can be as low as 12% of the random signal near the surface. The order on the Hg sublattice is clearly sufficient to maintain the epitaxial structure near the interface but the Te sublattice disorder decreases during growth and is therefore not a fundamental problem of the growth method. Indeed, thicker HgTe layers give improved $k_{\alpha 1}/k_{\alpha 2}$ separation with a $\gamma$ of 5.5 at 3[μm]. Poor interface structure may occur from preferential etching of Sb from the substrate prior to growth. It has been observed that after thermal cleaning at temperatures above 310°C surface roughening occurs. The loss of Sb on the monolayer scale at temperatures lower than 310°C could have a disruptive effect on the initial stages of growth, resulting in more lattice strain at higher growth temperatures. This is consistent with the plot of $\gamma$ versus growth temperature in Fig 3 and would indicate that over this temperature range, the surface mobility of the reactants is not a major problem.

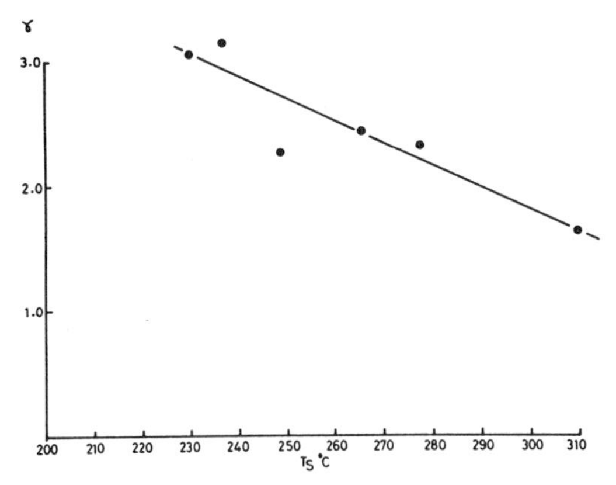


Fig. 3. Plot of γ (see text) versus HgTe growth temperatures over the range 230°C to 310°C.

The surface morphology of the layer grown at 310°C is shown in Fig 4(a) and reveals a large density of pyramid features. Some large facets have developed which is an indication of good surface mobility but much of the structure is irregular and this is consistent with the poor crystalline quality of this layer. At lower temperatures, the surface becomes much flatter but regions of poor growth can still be observed. Fig 4(b) is a typical example of poor nucleation due to contamination being left on the substrate after the cleaning procedure. Inside the oval region no growth has occurred; this has been confirmed on similar examples by Energy Dispersive X-ray microanalysis (EDX) which has also shown that the central feature contains silicon, possibly a remnant from siton polishing. Clearly, substrate preparation is very critical as is the thermal treatment prior to growth, however, improvements in this procedure have resulted in almost featureless surfaces at growth temperatures below 260°C. It can be seen in Fig 4(b) in the region where growth has occurred that the pyramid features observed in Fig 4(a) are smaller and lower in density. At lower growth temperatures these pyramids are not present. The pyramids may form by a VLS mechanism where Sb depletion leaves an In rich surface which would be liquid at these growth temperatures.

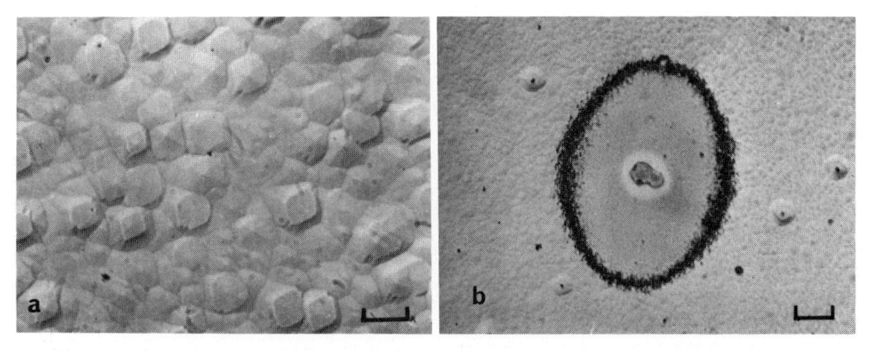


Fig. 4. Optical micrographs with Nomarski contrast of HgTe layers grown at (a) 310°C and (b) 266°C (showing region of poor growth). The scale markers are 20 [μm] wide.

## 4. Conclusions

A new low temperature growth technique using UV photosensitisation has been used to grow epitaxial layers of HgTe over the temperature range 200°C - 300°C. These layers, grown onto InSb substrates, have been assessed for crystalline and surface quality. The major limitation to the quality of the thin films ~ 1[μm] in thickness is the quality of the InSb surface. It is suggested that loss of Sb prior to growth even at temperatures less than 300°C results in greater lattice strain. Regions of poor surface preparation can result in no nucleation of HgTe, this is associated with contamination in these regions with Si containing material or could be due to hydrolysis products from the etching. On substrates free from accidental contamination, where a careful final rinse in deionised water was used, the surface morphology is smooth at temperatures below 250°C but becomes structured at higher temperatures.

Further work will be carried out on substrate preparation procedures and on the assessment of thicker HgTe layers to establish the inherent quality of epitaxy by this technique.

## Acknowledgements

The authors wish to thank Mrs J Clements for technical assistance and Mr P Hagger for SEM studies.



## References

1. S.J.C. Irvine and J.B. Mullin: J.Crystal Growth 55 (1981) 107.
2. J.B. Mullin and S.J.C. Irvine: J. Vac. Sci. Technol., 21 (1982)178.
3. S.J.C. Irvine, J.B. Mullin and A. Royle: J. Crystal Growth 57 (1982) 15.
4. S.J.C. Irvine, J. Tunnicliffe and J.B. Mullin: J. Crystal Growth 65 (1983) 479.
5. I. Bhat and S.K. Ghandhi: J. Electrochem. Soc., in press.
6. J.P. Faurie, A. Million, R. Boch and J.L. Tissot: J. Vac. Sci. Technol., A1(3) (1983) 1593.
7. S.J.C. Irvine, D.J. Robbins, J.B. Mullin and J.L. Glasper: Proc. MRS Symp. Laser-Controlled Chemical Processing of Surfaces, Elsevier, 1984.
8. S.J.C. Irvine, J.B. Mullin and J. Tunnicliffe: J. Crystal Growth proceedings ICMOVPE II in press.
9. J.H. Basson and H. Booyens, Phys. Stat. Sol.(a) 80 (1983) 663.
10. J.A. Grimshaw: to be published.

# Applications of Excimer Lasers to Semiconductor Processing

T.F. Deutsch[2]

Lincoln Laboratory, Massachusetts Institute of Technology
Lexington, MA 02173-0073, USA

## I. Introduction

The basic processes involved in making an integrated circuit are the production of patterns by photolithography, the deposition of thin films of insulators and conductors, doping of semiconductors, and patterning of material by etching. Excimer lasers are being used to perform each of these operations in the laboratory and, in some cases, are being considered for use in a production environment. This paper will review the developments in each of these areas. Two conference proceedings contain a number of articles dealing with excimer laser processing [1,2].

Excimer lasers have a number of unique properties that make them of special interest for semiconductor processing. The wavelengths emitted by excimers correspond to photon energies ranging from 6.4 eV for ArF radiation to 3.5 eV for XeF radiation; these photon energies are adequate to break molecular bonds in a variety of compounds and allow the excimer laser to initiate photochemical reactions. Silicon and the III-V semiconductors have absorption coefficients of the order of $10^6$ $cm^{-1}$ at the excimer wavelengths, resulting in absorption lengths of ~ 10 nm. This, combined with the short output pulse length of excimer lasers, allows the surface of a semiconductor to be heated rapidly while the bulk of the material remains cool. Hence excimer radiation may be used to obtain effects due to rapid thermal heating, as well as to initiate photochemistry. Finally, the high average powers that can be obtained from excimer lasers today, in excess of 100 W at 248 nm, allow the high throughputs necessary for production environments.

## II. Doping

Excimer lasers have been used to dope Si, GaAs and InP using gas-phase donor molecules [3]. Figure 1 shows a schematic diagram of the system used for pulsed excimer laser doping of semiconductors. The laser serves both to release dopant atoms from an appropriate parent molecule and to melt a thin layer on the semiconductor surface, allowing dopant incorporation by liquid state diffusion.

In a typical experiment the sample is enclosed in a 1-cm-long stainless-steel cell which is translated normal to the beam axis. Scan rates

---

[1]This work was sponsored by the Department of the Air Force, in part under a specific program sponsored by the Air Force Office of Scientific Research, by the Defense Advanced Research Projects Agency, and by the Army Research Office.
[2]Present address: Department of Dermatology, Massachusetts General Hospital, Boston, Massachusetts 02114.

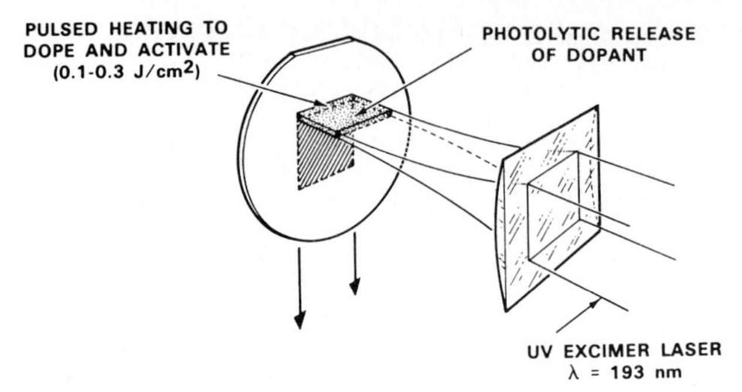


Fig. 1. Schematic diagram of pulsed excimer laser doping of semiconductors.

range from 0.25-10 mm/min and laser pulse repetition rates range from 2-10 Hz. Typical fluences at the substrate range from 0.1-1 J/cm$^2$. In the case of compound semiconductors such as GaAs the energy density at the surface is limited by the occurrence of damage at the surface.

A variety of doping gases including $BCl_3$, $PCl_3$, $H_2S$ and $Cd(CH_3)_2$ were used. Gas pressures were chosen to give 193 nm absorptions of 10-50% in a 1-cm path. In addition, B doping was also demonstrated using commercial spin-on dopants.

The electrical properties of UV excimer laser doped Si have been examined for B and P doping [4]. Figure 2 shows the profile of B concentration vs depth obtained by secondary ion mass spectroscopy (SIMS) for an n-type (100) Si wafer (2-5 Ω-cm) doped using ArF radiation. The estimated junction depth, obtained by extrapolating the linear portion of the B depth profile to the substrate doping level of $2 \times 10^{15}$ cm$^{-3}$, is about 0.35 μm. The sheet resistance of the B-doped layer was about 50 Ω/□. The curve indicates that high dopant concentrations, up to the solid solubility limit, and shallow profiles can be obtained by laser doping.

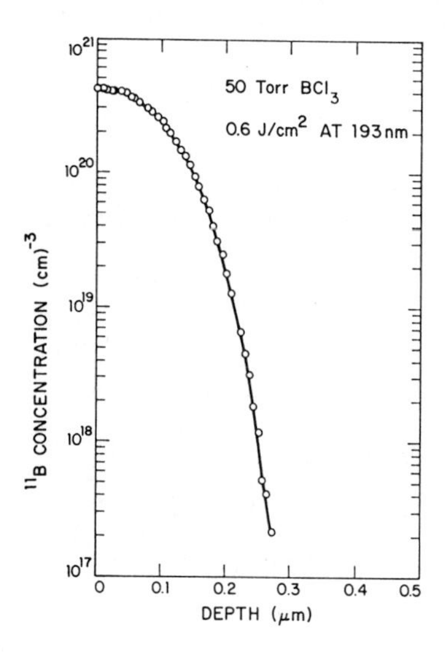


Fig. 2. $^{11}B$ concentration vs depth for Si sample doped using 50-Torr $BCl_3$ and a 193 nm fluence of 0.6 J/cm$^2$ at the sample.

Doping can also be obtained using wavelengths that are not absorbed by the doping gas; this was demonstrated using 351 nm XeF radiation and $BCl_3$ gas. In this case pyrolysis of the gas on the laser-heated Si surface is the most likely mechanism. Similar doping effects have been seen by other workers using much longer wavelengths (0.73 μm) [5]. The sheet resistivities obtained using XeF radiation are about three times those obtained using ArF radiation, indicating that the photolytic mechanism enhances the doping substantially.

Adlayers can also serve as a source of doping atoms. This was demonstrated by exposing a Si sample to $BCl_3$, evacuating the cell, and then irradiating it with 351 nm radiation. Doping was observed, indicating that pyrolysis of the adlayer served as a source of dopant atoms. The use of adlayers as doping sources may have applications in the production of flat doping profiles; the adlayer serves as a finite source of doping atoms, in contrast to the gas phase case, where the doping gas constitutes an infinite reservoir. With multiple laser pulses the doping atoms should become distributed uniformly up to the depth of the solid-liquid interface during irradiation. The production of such profiles by laser annealing of ion implanted samples has been discussed by HILL [6].

ArF and KrF radiation have been used to dope Si with B by heating and ablating a spun-on dopant film. Both Borofilm (Emulsitone) and XB-100 (Allied Chemical) were used. Sheet resistances as low as 50 Ω/□ were obtained, but damage to the substrate may occur.

The laser doping technique was used to form junctions which could be fabricated into solar cells. ArF radiation was used to B dope n-type wafers which were then fabricated into solar cells up to 0.5 x 1.0 cm in size. The best 0.5 $cm^2$ cell had a measured efficiency of 10.3% without an antireflection coating [7]; such a coating would be expected to increase the efficiency significantly.

The laser doping technique has also been applied to fabrication of metal-gate Si MOSFETs. Metal gate electrodes and interconnects have the advantage of having lower resistivity than the more conventional polysilicon gate technology allows and are desirable for high speed circuits. Conventional self-aligned technology, in which the gate serves as a mask during ion-implantation, cannot be used with Al gates because the low melting point of Al is not compatible with thermal annealing of the implant. A number of laser annealing schemes have been used to allow the fabrication of self-aligned aluminum gate MOSFETs [8,9].

We have used a combination Mo-Al gate metallization (80 nm Mo, 500 nm Al) to serve as a mask during ArF laser doping of n-Si substrates (10-20 Ω-cm) using $BCl_3$ doping gas. The substrates were scanned through the focus of the ArF laser as shown schematically in Fig. 1. The Mo layer was used to minimize laser ablation of the Al film by enhancing the adhesion of the Al. Such ablation limits the fluences that can be used for doping. Figure 3 shows the I-V characteristics of a MOSFET made by laser doping. The process allows self-aligned doping of MOSFETs in single step.

Laser doping has also been applied to GaAs [10] and InP [11]. For laser doping, as well as for laser or electron beam annealing, decomposition at the surface of a III-V semiconductor can occur by evaporation of the more volatile component. In addition, beam heating can introduce slip planes and other defects which degrade the electrical properties of GaAs. The greater vulnerability of GaAs and InP to damage by the laser beam re-

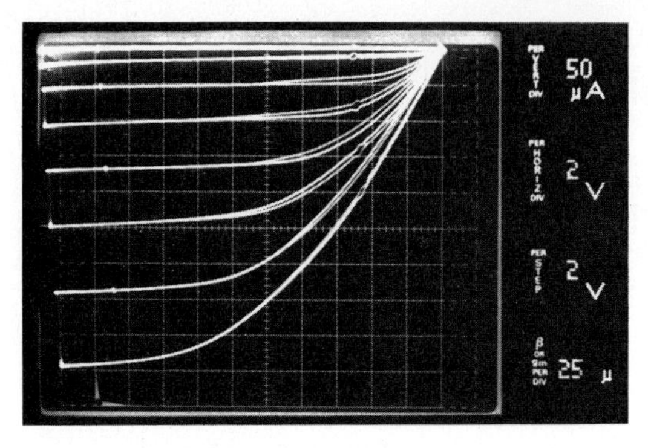


Fig. 3. I-V characteristics of a metal gate MOSFET made using laser doping.

sults in a more limited range of laser operating parameters than in the case of Si. Nevertheless, GaAs has been doped with S using $H_2S$ as the doping gas. S concentrations of $10^{19}$ were obtained and solar cells were fabricated from laser-doped junctions. Antireflection coated, 3 x 3 mm square, cells gave AM1 efficiencies of 10.8%.

## III. Deposition

The use of UV radiation to initiate photolytic reactions which deposit conducting and insulating thin films at lower substrate temperatures than those used with conventional chemical vapor deposition (CVD) has been investigated by several groups. Initially, UV lamps were used to deposit $SiO_2$, $Si_3N_4$ and other compounds on a variety of substrates [12,13]. More recently, excimer laser radiation, generally ArF or KrF, has been used to deposit $SiO_2$, $Si_3N_4$, $Al_2O_3$, and other insulators [14,15, 16], as well as a number of metals [17] on Si and other substrates. The high average powers available from excimer lasers make possible higher growth rates than are possible with lamp sources.

Low-temperature processing has a number of advantages for semiconductor processing. It reduces or eliminates unwanted diffusion or chemical reactions on a semiconductor wafer. It also reduces wafer warpage in processing, an increasingly important issue as larger wafer diameters are used in production. Furthermore, it makes it possible to deposit films on compound semiconductors, such as GaAs and InP, that would dissociate at the temperatures required for conventional CVD.

Since the reagents used in conventional CVD can generally be dissociated by excimer laser radiation, photolytic initiation of film deposition appears to be generally applicable to most CVD systems. A possible advantage of photolytic initiation of the deposition reaction is that the laser may give a more controlled chemistry than pyrolysis, since a specific dissociation channel is accessed by the laser.

Figure 4 shows a schematic diagram of the deposition system. The deposition chamber is a stainless-steel cross capable of accepting 2" diameter wafers. The substrates were mounted on a stainless-steel pedestal, which contained a heater element capable of producing substrate temperatures of 500°C. The 193-nm ArF laser was operated at 50 Hz and produced average powers of 4-7 W. A beam reducing telescope was used to produce a colli-

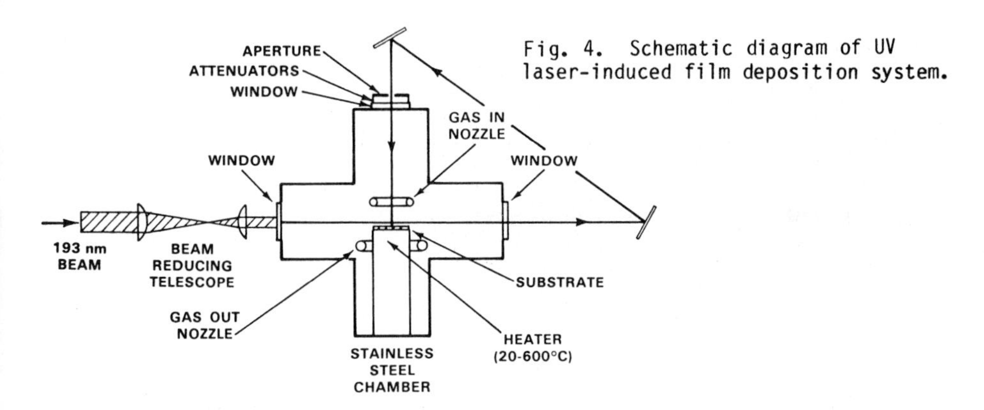


Fig. 4. Schematic diagram of UV laser-induced film deposition system.

mated beam having a cross section ~ 2 cm wide and ~ 1 mm high; the beam passed about 1 mm above the substrate; in some cases the emerging beam was then directed onto the top surface of the substrate. The gases used as deposition reagents were either premixed in a reservoir and then flowed through the chamber, or, in some cases, electronic mass flow controllers were used.

The physical, and to a lesser extent the electrical, properties of laser-deposited insulator films have been discussed in the literature cited. One relatively poorly understood phenomenon is the effect of surface UV radiation on the properties of the deposited material. This was investigated for the deposition of $Al_2O_3$ using 193 and 248 nm radiation [18]. A rectangular aperture was used to produce a defined irradiated region on the substrate. Measurements of refractive index and film thickness as a function of position were made using an automatic ellipsometer. Figure 5 shows the positional dependence of the refractive index for two different levels of 248 nm surface irradiation. The refractive index of single crystal $Al_2O_3$ is 1.76 and values of 1.64 are typical of films deposited by other techniques. Surface fluences as low as 1 $mJ/cm^2$ produce readily measurable changes in refractive index. At 193 nm larger effects are found for similar energy levels. UV irradiation was also found to decrease the etch rate of the deposited material in $H_3PO_4$ at 67°C; such a decrease is characteristic of the densification that is achieved by annealing conventionally deposited material.

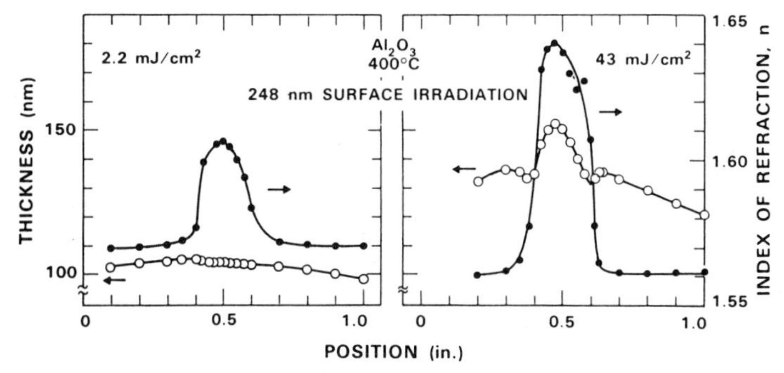


Fig. 5. Thickness and refractive index versus position for $Al_2O_3$ deposited at 400°C for two different levels of localized 248 nm fluence at the surface.

The effects described in more detail in Ref. [18] indicate that UV radiation can be used to alter the growth conditions of $Al_2O_3$ films on Si. The energy fluences involved, as low as 1 $mJ/cm^2$, are insufficient to cause transient heating that is significant compared to the substrate temperatures; a simple thermal calculation indicates that 1 $mJ/cm^2$ will raise the temperature of the Si surface by less than 10°C. A number of possible photochemical effects may be induced by the surface radiation. They include enhancement of the mobility of surface species, nucleation of the surface by photolysis of adlayers, and dissociation of clusters formed in the region above the substrate where there is normally no UV beam. At the highest fluences used, ~ 40 $mJ/cm^2$, photolysis in the volume directly above the substrate, as well as transient heating of the substrate, may come into play.

These possible mechanisms may be discussed in terms of the desired conditions for compound deposition. In order to minimize the formation of clusters which would not form a continuous film on the substrate, compound formation should occur on the substrate rather than in the volume. Surface reactions can be enhanced by having high sticking coefficients for at least one of the reacting atoms. Finally, adsorbed atoms and molecules need high surface mobilities in order to form surface clusters which serve as nucleation sites; this requires a hot substrate even when photolysis occurs in the gas phase. Previous studies have demonstrated that trimethyl aluminum (TMA) forms adsorbed layers which can be photolyzed by ArF radiation to produce Al adatoms which serve as nucleation sites for subsequent Al deposition [19]. Because the absorption coefficient of TMA is more than a decade higher at 193 nm than at 248 nm, ArF radiation will be more effective than KrF radiation in photolyzing such adlayers. While the activation energy for surface diffusion of Al on $Al_2O_3$ is not known, activation energies for systems that have been investigated typically range from 0.2-0.6 eV [20]. Thus, provided the UV radiation can be coupled into the surface-adatom system, the available photon energy, 6.4 eV at 193 nm, should be ample to increase the surface mobility.

We have observed improved physical and electrical properties for $Al_2O_3$ films subjected to surface UV radiation during deposition. Similar effects have been observed in experiments involving the effect of ion and neutral particle bombardment on film growth; a recent review summarizes the observed effects [21]. In a number of experiments involving the growth of both metal and semiconductor films on a variety of substrates, ion bombardment during film growth was shown to lead to a reduction in the "epitaxial temperature" required for film growth. Even in these experiments, where purely photochemical effects are absent, a variety of possible mechanisms for enhanced nucleation have been suggested; they include enhanced adatom diffusion as well as effects such as the production of defects which can serve as adsorption sites.

Insulating films deposited by laser-initiated CVD have potential application as encapsulants, passivating layers, and as dielectrics in active devices. The latter application is quite demanding since low levels of impurities can affect the dielectric properties of films. For example, high quality $SiO_2$ films used as dielectrics in metal-oxide-semiconductor devices typically have surface concentrations of electrically active impurities of $10^{11}$ $cm^{-2}$ or less, corresponding to volumetric concentrations of $10^{16}$ $cm^{-3}$ for a typical thickness of 100 nm. On the other hand, the purity requirements for high quality metal films are less stringent, since impurity scattering is not a significant factor in the room temperature resistivity of metals. Refractory metal films, for example, are of interest for the fabrication of low-resistance interconnects and contacts for semiconductor devices. Films of Mo, W, and Cr have been deposited over large areas (> 5 $cm^2$) by excimer laser photolysis of their respective hexacarbonyls [17]. Irradiation using the normal geometry produced metallic films while the parallel configuration led to black, particulate films. Good step coverage was obtained and resistivities of the order of 20 times the bulk values were obtained.

W films having higher purity and lower resistivity than those obtained using carbonyls as a reagent have been deposited by photodissociation of $WF_6$ [22]. Thermal CVD of W over $SiO_2$ by the reaction of $WF_6$ with $H_2$ requires temperatures in excess of 700°C; at lower temperatures deposition is difficult and films, when obtained, generally have poor adhesion. We have used ArF excimer laser radiation to initiate low-temperature (< 500°C) CVD deposition of W films on $SiO_2$ and have obtained adherent, low-resistivity films under conditions where films could not be produced without laser initiation.

The substrates were Si wafers and Si covered with 460 nm of thermal $SiO_2$. In some cases the $SiO_2$ films were patterned with gratings in order to examine conformal coverage.

Without laser irradiation W deposition did not occur on $SiO_2$ at temperatures up to 400°C; similar results have been observed by others [23]. With laser irradiation shiny metallic films were obtained at temperatures as low as 240°C; however, only films deposited at 440°C passed the adhesive tape test for adherence. Figure 6 shows two scanning electron microscope (SEM) micrographs illustrating the excellent conformal coverage and the surface morphology of W films deposited at 285°C over $SiO_2$ steps on Si.

Figure 7 shows the temperature dependence of the W deposition rate on Si or $SiO_2$ using ArF laser radiation, as well as the thermal deposition rate on Si substrates. The activation energy obtained for the thermal reaction, ~ 18 kcal/mole, is in reasonable agreement with the value of 16 kcal/mole found by others [24,25]. The effect of laser irradiation is to reduce the activation energy for the reaction to about 9.7 kcal/mole,

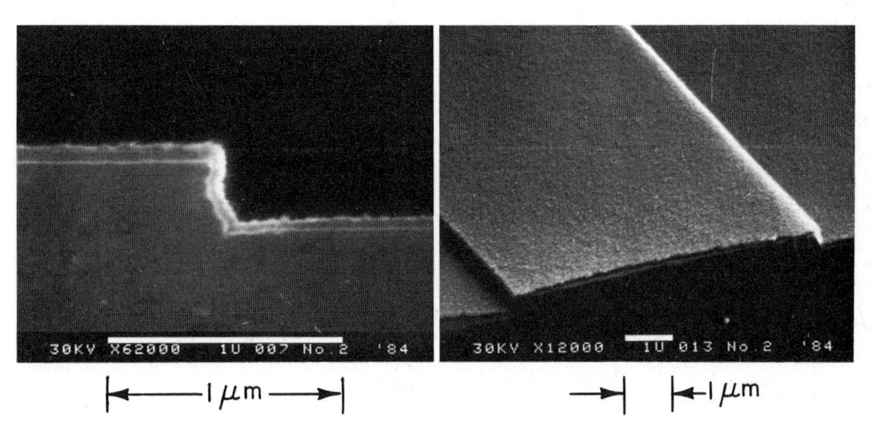


Fig. 6. SEM micrographs showing a side and top view of a W film over $SiO_2$ steps on a Si substrate. Conditions: ArF laser irradiation, $WF_6$-$H_2$ mix, 285°C.

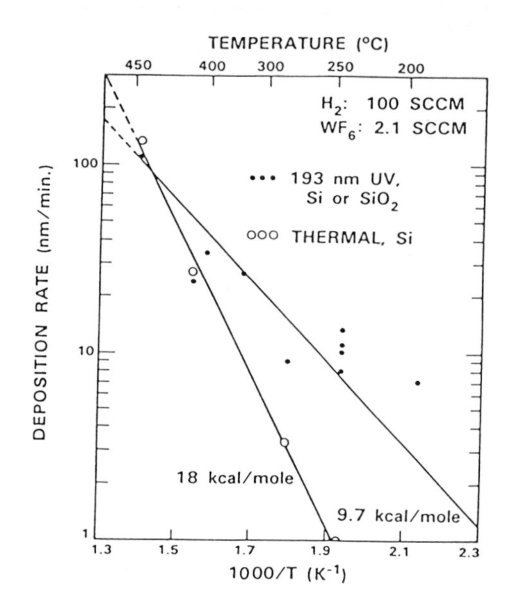


Fig. 7. Temperature dependence of the deposition rate for laser-initiated W film deposition. Conditions: 100 sccm $H_2$, 2.1 sccm $WF_6$.

increasing the deposition rate on Si for temperatures in the 200-300°C range significantly, and allowing deposition on $SiO_2$.

Sheet resistivity measurements were performed using a four-point probe and film thickness was determined by Dektak profilometer measurements of etched films. The film resistivity was found to be a strong function of deposition temperature. At 440°C a resistivity of 17 μΩ-cm, about three times the bulk value of 5.3 μΩ-cm, was obtained for a laser-deposited film on $SiO_2$; a thermally deposited film on Si had a resistivity of 8-μΩ-cm.

The dependence of film resistivity on both deposition temperature and subsequent thermal annealing can be understood in terms of the film microstructure produced. Tungsten can exist both in the stable α-W phase and in a metastable phase, the β-W phase. Studies on sputtered and evaporated [26] films have shown that β-W phase films consist of small crystallites, 5-10 nm in diameter, with a high density of stacking faults and twins, while α-W films consist of large crystallites, 150-250 nm in diameter, free of structural defects. The high resistivity (100-300 μΩ-cm) of β-W films has been attributed to diffuse scattering of electrons by grain boundaries. X-ray diffraction measurements on W films laser-deposited on $SiO_2$ substrates at three different substrate temperatures showed that the structure changes from β-W to α-W as the temperature is increased from 330°C to 440°C. This change of crystal structure, with the accompanying change in crystallite dimension discussed above, is responsible for the sharp decrease in resistivity with deposition temperature.

The chemistry of the conventional CVD of W films may be summarized by the overall reaction,

$$WF_6 + 3\,H_2 \rightarrow W + 6\,HF \quad . \qquad (1)$$

The activation energy for the deposition reaction, 16 kcal/mole, has been identified with the dissociation of adsorbed $H_2$ molecules on the surface under conditions where the reaction is not mass transport limited. In the case of laser initiation the initial step is probably dissociation of $WF_6$ by the 193 nm radiation to release one or more F atoms and produce radicals of the form $WF_n$ (n = 1-5). The reaction

$$H_2 + F \rightarrow HF + H \quad , \tag{2}$$

which is 31.9 kcal/mole exothermic, can then occur. The hydrogen atoms can react with $WF_6$ and $WF_n$ radicals via a complex series of reactions to deposit W and produce HF. Thus ArF laser radiation can serve to change the reactions involved.

A different approach to large-area film deposition involves the photolysis of adsorbed layers. The technique has been used to deposit Fe films from $Fe(CO)_5$ condensed on substrates that were either at room temperature or 77 K [27]. Both 193 nm and 248 nm radiation was used at power densities of $10^6$ to $10^7$ W/cm$^2$. Typical deposition rates were 1 nm/min and the deposited films were less than 50 nm thick. Oxygen and carbon impurities, probably from CO from the photolyzed carbonyl, were found at the level of 4-13 at.%. The technique has several potential advantages; window deposits are avoided and it may be applicable to the formation of films having a controlled, spatially varying, composition such as semiconductor quantum well structures. The low pressures involved in photolysis of adlayers lead to conditions approaching those of molecular beam epitaxy. At present several problems must be investigated, including the control of laser power so that the deposited film is not ablated but the condensed adlayers are completely photolyzed. Another potential problem is condensation of reaction products and gas impurities on the surface.

Laser-enhanced growth of single-crystal semiconductor films has been demonstrated using the excimer laser photolysis of $GeH_4$ [28].

## IV. Lithography

The use of excimer lasers as sources for photolithography is receiving increasing attention. The high resolution that UV wavelengths can provide, the increased throughput possible using high average power excimer lasers rather than lamps to expose relatively insensitive UV resists, and the absence of speckle are among the features of excimer lasers that make them attractive sources for lithography. JAIN [29] has reviewed recent developments. Both contact and proximity printing have been used to demonstrate submicrometer resolution. More recently, projection lithography has been demonstrated using a commercial projection printer [30]. Inorganic resists have also been patterned using excimer radiation [31] and the use of wavelengths as short as 157 nm ($F_2$ laser) has been explored [32].

The use of excimer laser to pattern organic polymers by ablation has been explored by several groups [33-35]. The absorption depths of most polymers at 193 nm are of the order of 100 nm, leading to deposition of absorbed energy in a very thin layer of the resist. Ablation is found to occur at a threshold energy of the order of 20 mJ/cm$^2$ for a variety of materials. Figure 8 shows the etch rate of nitrocellulose, a polymer we have studied, as a function of fluence; the threshold and the energy-dependent etch rate can lead to high contrast if the exposure is at a fluence near threshold [35]. Figure 9 shows a grating pattern in nitrocellulose produced using a 3.8-μm-period mask contacted to the substrate;

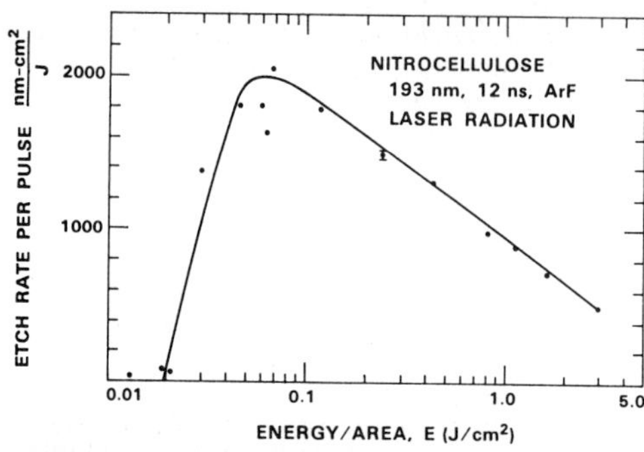


Fig. 8. Development rate per pulse for nitrocellulose vs incident 193-nm energy per unit area.

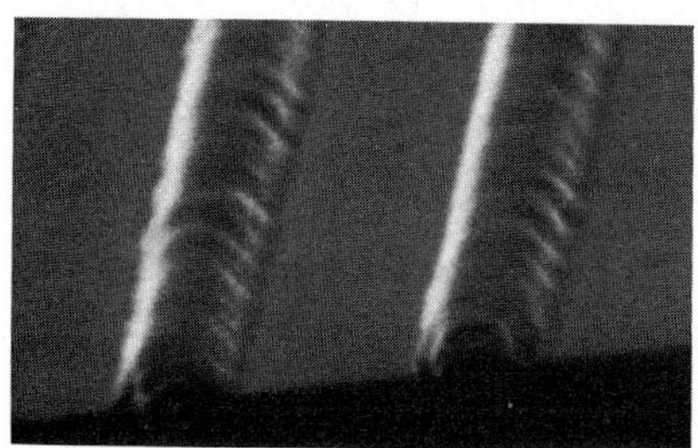

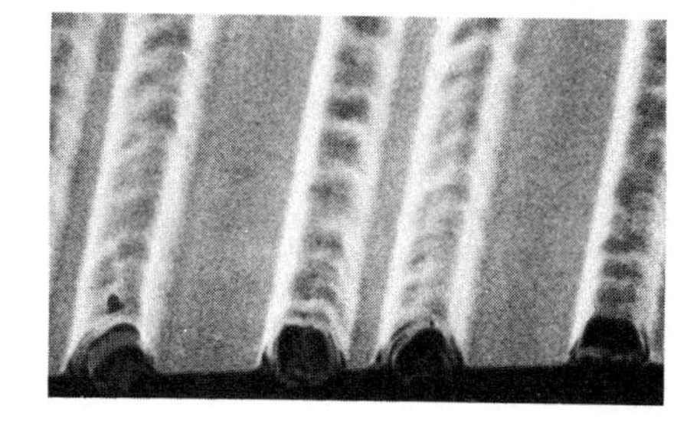

2 μm

Fig. 9. (Left) Optical micrograph of a grating pattern in nitrocellulose obtained using 193-nm ArF laser radiation and a 3.8-μm-period chrome-on-quartz mask contacted to the Si substrate. (Right) Grating pattern obtained when the mask is spaced away from the substrate in order to obtain spatial period division effects.

the pattern at the right was produced by spacing the mask about 40 μm from the substrate. The pattern is due to the phenomenon of spatial period division [36] and serves to illustrate that the resolution of the resist is about 0.3 μm.

## V. Etching

The use of excimer lasers for etching electronic materials has been studied by several groups. Both radiation parallel to the surface of the sample and perpendicular to it has been employed. In the former case, laser-induced photolysis serves to produce the species capable of etching and has the potential advantage over plasma etching that the photolysis reaction may be more species specific and that possible damage by ion bombardment is reduced. In the case of the perpendicular configuration additional processes come into play. Laser-induced desorption of reaction products can occur, photolysis of adlayers may contribute to etching, and electron-hole pair generation in semiconductor substrates may affect the interaction with etching medium. At sufficiently high energy fluences, ablation of the sample may occur.

The use of XeCl radiation to etch Si has been discussed by ARIKADO et al. [37]. Chlorine was used as the etching gas and both parallel and perpendicular illumination was used. The etch rate was found to increase rapidly with n-type doping level and to decrease slowly with p-type doping level. The dependence of etch rate on doping level was attributed to a mechanism in which electrons attach to Cl atoms formed by photolysis. Higher etch rates were found for the perpendicular configuration in which the laser generates electron-hole pairs in the Si. The maximum etch rate was about 1 $nm\text{-}cm^2/J$. Features as small as 3 µm were generated using an Al mask on the Si wafer.

The use of ArF radiation to etch GaAs using a variety of halogen containing etching gases has been reported by BREWER et al. [38]. $CF_3Br$, $CF_3Cl$, $CH_3Br$ and $CF_3Cl$ were used at pressures from 0.1 to 10 Torr, substrate temperatures up to 120°C were employed, and both the parallel and perpendicular geometries were studied. Laser-induced fluorescence was used to monitor the concentrations of Ga and As atoms produced and an activation energy of ~ 11 kcal/mole was deduced from the temperature dependence of the fluorescence in the parallel geometry. The activation energy was identified with the thermal desorption of nonvolatile etching products. The use of the perpendicular geometry led to higher etch rates than obtained with parallel illumination, up to 1 µm/min at 2 $W/cm^2$ intensity. The higher etch rates were attributed to laser-induced desorption of reaction products from the surface. At sufficiently high fluences, > 35 $mJ/cm^2$, ablation of the GaAs increases the etch rate even further. Patterned etching was demonstrated using both a substrate masked with patterned $SiO_2$ and by projecting a pinhole onto the substrate. The direct masking technique gave a resolution of better than 200 nm.

ArF etching of a number of electronic materials, including Si, $SiO_2$, W and Mo, has been studied by LOPER et al. [39]. $COF_2$, $NF_3$ and $CCl_2F_2$ were used as etch gases; room temperature substrates were irradiated in a perpendicular geometry. The relatively modest etch rates obtained, of the order of 0.05 nm/pulse at 85 $mJ/cm^2$, correspond to about 1 atom removed per 300 incident photons and are comparable to those obtained with Si [37]. The possible formation of nonvolatile reaction products has been suggested as a rate limiting step for the etch process.

The ablative processes that occur at significantly higher energies have been used by ANDREW et al. [40] to remove and pattern films of Al, Cr, and Ni on dielectric substrates. The thresholds for ablating 100 nm films range from 0.03 to 0.24 $J/cm^2$. These fluences correspond to the threshold for melting, rather than vaporization, of the metals and pressure buildup at the interface has been suggested as a possible mechanism for ablation. Projection techniques were used to examine the resolution of technique, which was found to be in the micron to submicron range despite relatively low-resolution optics. The high resolution is at least in part due to the fact that for a threshold process, extremely high contrast in the pattern produced can be obtained by operating near threshold [35]. The actual resolution of the process may be limited by the possible production of debris.

At present many of the etch rates obtained are relatively low. Using the value of 1 nm of Si removed per $J/cm^2$ [37] one can estimate the power required to remove 100 nm from a 5 inch dia Si wafer (A = 127 $cm^2$) in 1 min, a typical etch rate obtainable with conventional technology. The required power is 220 W, about twice what currently available commercial excimer lasers produce. The excimer process may be commercially attractive if it can lead to higher resolution features than are currently possible. This may be the case for perpendicular illumination, which would be expected to produce highly anisotropic etching, allowing the fabrication of features with vertical walls, if such surface processes as desorption, adlayer photolysis, and carrier generation are significant contributors to the etch process. However, such direct illumination may not be suitable for devices made of relatively fragile materials, such as GaAs, whose electrical properties may be degraded by irradiation [10]. The appropriate patterning technique for each application needs to be investigated. Projection techniques eliminate the need for masks, but, because of optical considerations, limit patterning to a single small area at a time. Large areas can be patterned using photoresist masks if low temperatures (<~ 100°C) are used; at higher temperatures the use of metal masks may be required.

## VI. Conclusions

We have reviewed some of the applications of excimer lasers to semiconductor processing. Many new techniques are evolving. Significant, but not discussed here, are applications of excimers to rapid thermal processing such as laser annealing and the formation of metastable alloys.

## VII. Acknowledgments

The work performed at Lincoln Laboratory involved the participation, at various times, of R. Chapman, D. J. Ehrlich, J. C. C. Fan, M. W. Geis, R. W. Mountain, R. M. Osgood, D. D. Rathman, D. J. Silversmith and G. W. Turner. Valuable technical assistance was provided by J. Burke, M. Finn, and P. Nitishin. Technical discussions with S. R. J. Brueck and P. L. Kelley are gratefully acknowledged.

## References

1. Laser Diagnostics and Photochemical Processing for Semiconductor Devices, edited by R. M. Osgood, Jr., S. R. J. Brueck and H. R. Schlossberg, (North-Holland, New York, 1983).
2. Laser-Controlled Chemical Processing of Surfaces, edited by A. W. Johnson and D. J. Ehrlich (North-Holland, New York, 1984).
3. T. F. Deutsch in Ref. 1, p.225.
4. T. F. Deutsch, D. J. Ehrlich, D. D. Rathman, D. J. Silversmith and R. M. Osgood, Jr., Appl. Phys. Lett. 39, 825 (1981).
5. G. B. Turner, D. Tarrant, G. Pollack, R. Pressley and R. Press, Appl. Phys. Lett. 39, 967 (1981).
6. C. Hill, A. L. Butler and J. A. Daly in Laser and Electron-Beam Interactions with Solids, edited by B. R. Appleton and G. K. Celler, (North-Holland, New York, 1982), p. 579.
7. J. C. C. Fan, T. F. Deutsch, G. W. Turner, D. J. Ehrlich, R. L. Chapman and R. M. Osgood, Jr., Proceedings of Fifteenth IEEE Photovoltaics Specialists Conference, (June, 1981), p. 432.
8. S. Iwamatsu and M. Ogawa, Electron. Lett. 15, 827 (1979).
9. S. Iwamatsu and M. Ogawa, J. Electrochem. Soc. 128, 384 (1981).
10. T. F. Deutsch, J. C. C. Fan, G. W. Turner, R. L. Chapman, D. J. Ehrlich and R. M. Osgood, Jr., Appl. Phys. Lett. 38, 144 (1981).
11. T. F. Deutsch, D. J. Ehrlich, R. M. Osgood, Jr. and Z. L. Liau, Appl. Phys. Lett. 36, 847 (1980).
12. H. M. Kim, S. S. Tai, S. L. Groves and K. L. Schuegraf, in Proceedings of the Eighth International Conference on Chemical Vapor Deposition, (Electrochemical Society, Pennington, New Jersey, 1981), Vol. 81-7, p. 258.

13. J. W. Peters, in Technical Digest of the International Electron Devices Meeting 1981, (Institute of Electrical and Electronics Engineers, New York, 1981), p. 240.
14. P. K. Boyer, G. A. Roche, W. H. Ritchie and G. J. Collins, Appl. Phys. Lett. 40, 716 (1982).
15. R. Solanki, W. H. Ritchie and G. J. Collins, Appl. Phys. Lett. 43, 454 (1983).
16. T. F. Deutsch, D. J. Silversmith and R. W. Mountain in Ref. 1, p. 129.
17. M. R. Solanki, P. K. Boyer and G. J. Collins, Appl. Phys. Lett. 41, 1048 (1982).
18. T. F. Deutsch, D. J. Silversmith and R. W. Mountain in Ref. 2.
19. D. J. Ehrlich, R. M. Osgood, Jr. and T. F. Deutsch, Appl. Phys. Lett. 38, 946 (1981).
20. G. Ehrlich, CRC Crit. Rev. Solid-State Mat. Sci. 10, 391 (1982).
21. J. E. Greene, CRC Crit. Rev. Solid-State Mat. Sci. 11, 47 (1983).
22. T. F. Deutsch and D. D. Rathman, to be published in Appl. Phys. Lett.
23. T. Moriya, S. Shima, Y. Hazuki, M. Chiba and M. Kashiwagi, 1983 International Electron Device Meeting (IEDM) Technical Digest 550 (1983).
24. E. K. Broadbent and C. L. Ramiller, 163rd Meeting of the Electrochemical Society Extended Abstracts 83-1, 657 (1983), Abstract No. 420.
25. W. A. Bryant, J. Electrochem. Soc. 125, 1534 (1978).
26. A. K. Sinha, T. E. Smith, T. T. Sheng and N. N. Axelrod, J. Vac. Sci. Technol. 10, 436 (1973).
27. P. J. Love, R. T. Loda, P. R. LaRoe, A. K. Green and V. Rehn in Ref. 2.
28. J. G. Eden, J. E. Greene, J. F. Osmunsen, D. Lubben, C. C. Abele, S. Gorbatkin and H. D. Desai in Ref. 1, p. 185.
29. K. Jain, Proceedings International Conference Microcircuit Engineering, (Cambridge, United Kingdom, September, 1983), p. 181.
30. K. Jain and R. T. Kerth, Appl. Opt. 23, 648 (1984).
31. D. J. Ehrlich and J. Y. Tsao in Ref. 2.
32. J. C. White, H. G. Craighead, R. E. Howard, L. D. Jackel, R. E. Behringer, R. W. Epworth, D. Henderson and J. E. Sweeney, Appl. Phys. Lett. 44, 22 (1984).
33. R. Srinavasan and V. Mayne-Banton, Appl. Phys. Lett. 41, 576 (1982).
34. J. E. Andrew, P. E. Dyer, D. Forster and P. H. Key, Appl. Phys. Lett. 43, 717 (1983).
35. T. F. Deutsch and M. W. Geis, J. Appl. Phys. 54, 1201 (1983).
36. D. C. Flanders, A. M. Hawryluk and H. I. Smith, J. Vac. Soc. Technol. 16, 1949 (1979).
37. T. Arikado, H. Okano, M. Sekine and Y. Horiike in Ref. 2.
38. P. Brewer, S. Halle and R. M. Osgood in Ref. 2 and to be published.
39. G. L. Loper and M. D. Tabat in Laser-Assisted Deposition, Etching, and Doping, edited by S. D. Allen, Proceedings SPIE 459, 1217 (1984).
40. J. E. Andrew, P. E. Dyer, R. D. Greenough and P. H. Key, Appl. Phys. Lett. 43, 1076 (1983).

# Linear-Focused ArF Excimer Laser Beam for Depositing Hydrogenated Silicon Films

M. Murahara

Faculty of Engineering, Tokai University, Kitakaname 1117, Hiratsuka
Kanagawa 259-12, Japan

K. Toyoda

Riken, the Institute of Physical and Chemical Research, Hirosawa 2-1
Wako, Saitama 351-01, Japan

## 1 INTRODUCTION

Excimer lasers provide high intensity beams in the ultraviolet wavelength region. Using these photons, it is possible to cut the molecular bonds in materials such as PMMA by photochemical reactions [1]. As the results of the photochemical reactions, the deposition of metals [2], semiconductors [3] and other compound materials [4-5] has been realized. In uv laser-induced chemical vapor deposition (uv CVD) of thin films the excitation of gas phase has been studied extensively in recent years. These methods are expected to be applied to a low temperature technique in new production processes. However, these methods involve some difficulties: the attachment of the photochemical product to the incident window of the laser beam might be an unavoidable problem in many cases. However, use of this process has led to some successful results.

In this report, it will be shown how the photochemical decomposition of monosilane and disilane assisted by uv excimer lasers is used for large area deposition of silicon film. Using an apparatus for observing the scattered visible laser light in the gas cell with spatial resolution, the spatial distribution of cluster formation and the difference between single photon and two-photon decomposition were specified. As the result of these experimental observations, it was concluded that the silicon films are deposited on the incident quartz window of laser beam due to the single photon absorption of disilane. Linear-focused ArF beam satisfies requirement for large area deposition of thin film on the incident window plate. On the contrary, it is also suggested that the two-photon absorption of monosilane can cause the silicon deposition on the substrate placed in the gas without any attachment to the incident window.

## 2 OBSERVATION of SCATTERED VISIBLE LASER LIGHT

For the photochemical deposition of silicon films, monosilane ($SiH_4$) and disilane ($Si_2H_6$) were used. Absorption of $SiH_4$ starts at the wavelength of 170nm and the bonding energy of Si-H is 94kcal/mol. Absorption of $Si_2H_6$ starts at 200nm and the bonding energy of $SiH_3$-$SiH_3$ is 71kcal/mol. The photon energy of ArF excimer laser (193nm) is 6.4eV which corresponds to 114kcal/einstein. Therefore, it is considered that the $Si_2H_6$ is easily decomposed with single-photon excitation of ArF excimer laser. However, $SiH_4$ may not be decomposed by single-photon excitation because the significant absorption does not occur at the wavelength in spite of the fact that the photon energy is higher than the bonding energy of molecular bond.

However, when the excimer laser beam was focused in the cell, decomposition due to two photon excitation might occur. The two photon decomposition could also occur in the case of KrF excimer laser irradiation.

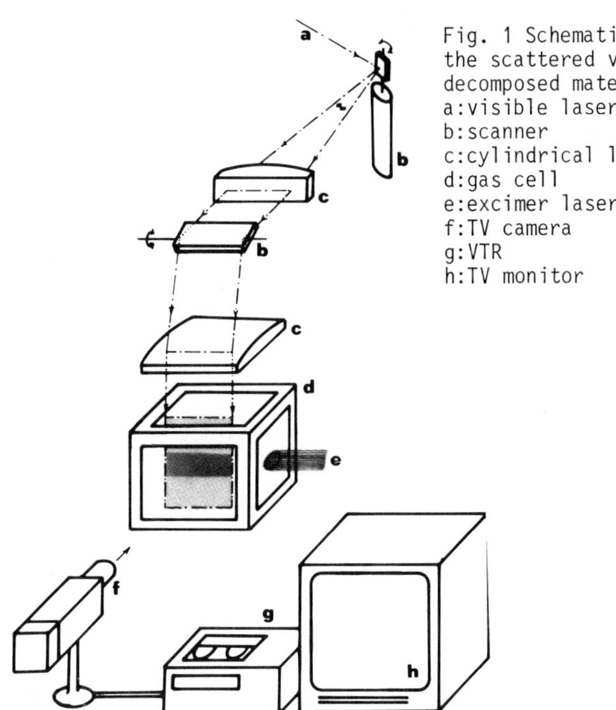


Fig. 1 Schematic diagram for observing the scattered visible laser light from decomposed materials
a:visible laser light
b:scanner
c:cylindrical lens
d:gas cell
e:excimer laser beam
f:TV camera
g:VTR
h:TV monitor

In order to observe the spatial distribution of the fine particles comprising the clusters of decomposed material, an apparatus for observing the scattered visible laser light was constructed as is illustrated in Fig. 1.

The experiments were carried out as follows: 20 Torr of $Si_2H_6$ gas was sealed in a reaction cell and the ArF excimer laser beam entered the cell through the quartz window. The decomposed materials of $Si_2H_6$ along the laser beam combine to produce small clusters. When the visible laser light is scanned over the irradiated region, the spatial distribution of clusters is visible by scattering observations. In case of repetitive irradiations of ArF laser pulses, the two-dimensional structure of scattered light reveals the dynamic flow inside the cell.

When $SiH_4$ gas was irradiated by the unfocused beam, no clusters due to decomposition were observed. To examine the two photon decomposition, the laser beam was focused in the reaction cell. When the laser power increased, scattering light from the cluster was observed around the focal point, which is believed due to two photon excitation since it has a strong power dependence.

## 3 HIGH SPEED GROWTH of SILICON THIN FILMS

The disilane ($Si_2H_6$) has become of major interest as the gas material of high speed growth of thin Si films because the bonding energy is lower than that of $SiH_4$ and because the absorption spectra covers the ArF laser wavelength. However, the decomposition due to single photon excitation causes the attachment of the decomposed materials to the incident window, which usually must be avoided. However, use of the attachment of the decomposed material onto the incident window is a solution to realize the high speed deposition process.

In order to evaluate the deposition on the incident window, the film thickness was monitored by He-Ne laser transmission as shown in Fig 2. The excimer laser energy of $70mJ/cm^2$ per pulse was incident at the rate of 50pps on the gas cell containing 20 Torr $Si_2H_6$ gas. In Fig. 3, the transmittances are recorded as the functions of laser pulse number. It is clear that effective photochemical deposition occurs by the irradiation of ArF excimer laser. For comparison, KrF laser is not effective for deposition.

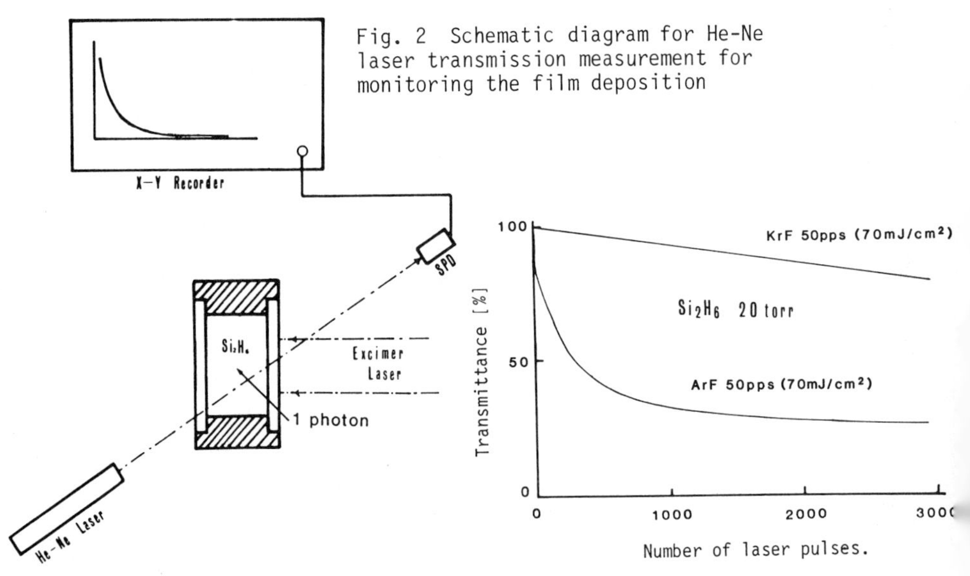


Fig. 2 Schematic diagram for He-Ne laser transmission measurement for monitoring the film deposition

Fig. 3 Transmittances of deposited films by ArF and KrF excimer lasers as the function of number of shots

The transmittance becomes constant above about 1000 shots of ArF laser pulse which means the decrease of the laser energy incident on the cell because the surface reflection at uv wavelength becomes dominant. However, during first several hundred shots, rapid deposition might occur. Therefore it was suggested that the large area deposition may be possible by moving the cell. Speed of the irradiation cell was 1mm/sec. As the beam pattern of the usual excimer laser is rectangular, the linear-focused laser beam which is of importance for large area deposition is easily obtained by using a double-cylindrical lens as is shown in Fig. 4.

In the experiment, the gas pressure was varied from 1 to 760Torr and the laser repetition rate from 1 to 50pps. In Fig. 5, the absorbance of deposited film at two wavelengths of 193nm and 633nm is plotted as a function of the gas pressure. The increase of absorbance is due to both increase of absorption coefficient and film thickness. Absorbance increases strongly above 200Torr and becomes almost constant above 400Torr.

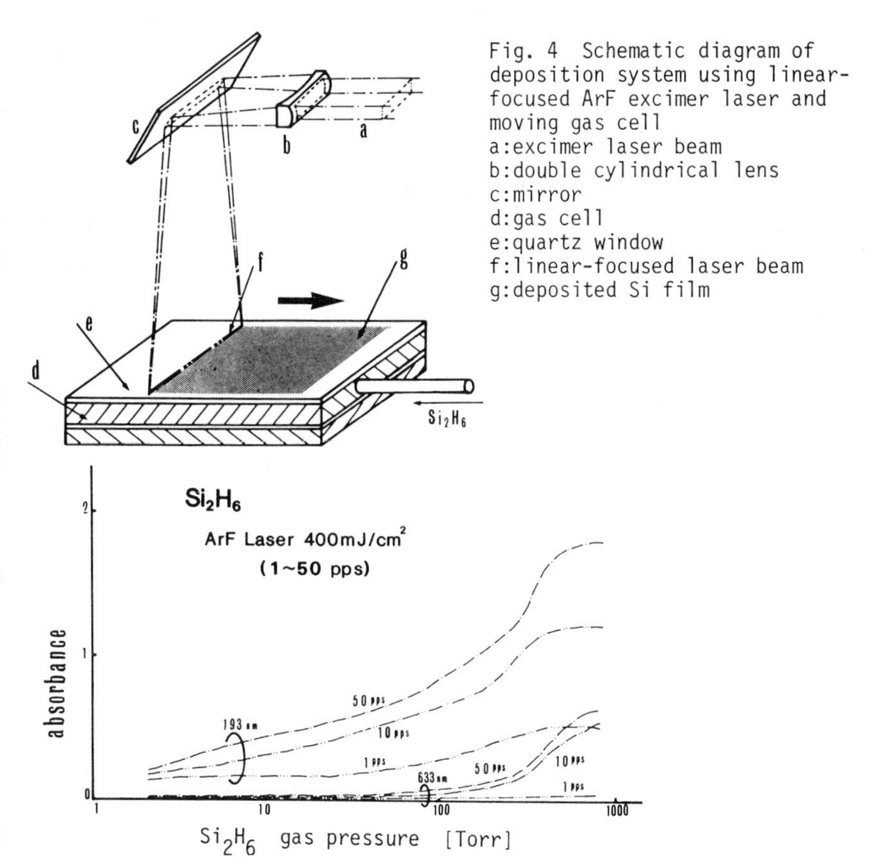


Fig. 4 Schematic diagram of deposition system using linear-focused ArF excimer laser and moving gas cell
a:excimer laser beam
b:double cylindrical lens
c:mirror
d:gas cell
e:quartz window
f:linear-focused laser beam
g:deposited Si film

Fig. 5 Absorbance of Si film vs. $Si_2H_6$ pressure at 193nm and 633nm for laser repetition rate of 1, 10 and 50pps

In Fig. 6, the absorption curves used to obtain the optical band gap of the films are shown for three different repetition rates of excimer laser. In the case of 1pps, optical band gap, $E_{opt}$ = 1.7eV was obtained. Whereas $E_{opt}$ = 1.2eV for 10 and 50pps.

## 4 DISCUSSION

In the scattering observations of visible laser light, it is shown that the ArF excimer laser effectively decomposes the $Si_2H_6$ gas even in unfocused condition. The attachment of the decomposed materials to the incident window is monitored by the He-Ne laser transmission measurement. The results suggest again that the deposition by ArF excimer laser is very effective and that the high speed growth of thin film is possible as compared with KrF excimer laser. The result means that purely photochemical reaction is responsible for the deposition of thin film. In the case of focused beam condition, the two-photon excitation effect becomes dominant.

In order to apply the photochemical decomposition by ArF excimer laser to the thin film deposition, the moving gas cell scheme with linear-focused

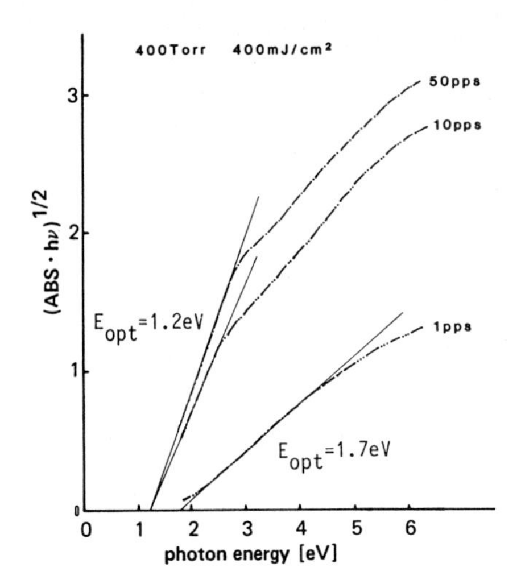


Fig. 6 Absorption curves of various Si films to obtain the optical band gap
Pressure of $Si_2H_6$: 400 Torr
ArF laser energy: 400mJ/cm$^2$ (per pulse)

laser beam has been developed. The linear-focused laser beam is easily obtained from conventional excimer laser beam with the simple double-cylindrical lens. Furthermore, the operating pressure of $Si_2H_6$ gas can be high enough to obtain very short photon mean free path. Therefore, in the high pressure operation, the distance between the location of decomposition and the solid surface to be deposited becomes short. In fact, high speed deposition is realized at the high pressure of 750Torr. The growth rate is 1mm/sec with the width of 1cm.

From the optical band gap measurements, $E_{opt}$=1.7eV is obtained by the low repetition of 1pps and $E_{opt}$=1.2eV by 10-50pps of laser pulse repetition rate. The high optical band gap corresponds to amorphous system of Si. The decrease is due to the heating effect of uv excimer laser in which the deposited Si is changed into polycrystal due to the repetitive heating of high repetition laser.

## 5 CONCLUSION

High speed deposition of Si films was demonstrated using a linear-focused ArF excimer laser which irradiated a moving gas cell containing high pressure disilane gas. The scheme would be effective for the large area deposition of thin films on transparent substrates.

## REFERENCE

1 Y. Kawamura, K. Toyoda, and S. Namba: Appl. Phys. Lett., 40, 374 (1982)
2 T.F. Deutsch, D. J. Ehrlich, and R. M. Osgood, Jr.: Appl. Phys. Lett., 35, 175 (1979)
3 R. Solanki and G. J. Collins: Appl. Phys. Lett., 42, 662 (1983)
4 P. K. Boyer, G. A. Roche, W. H. Ritchie, and G. J. Collins: Appl. Phys. lett., 40, 716 (1982)
5 R. Solanki, W. H. Ritchie, and G.J. Collins: Appl. Phys. Lett., 43, 454 (1983)

# Analysis of UV Laser-Induced Heterogeneous Deposition: Platinum

H. Schröder, I. Gianinoni, D. Masci, and K.L. Kompa
Max-Planck-Institut für Quantenoptik, D-8046 Garching, Fed. Rep. of Germany

In this communication we wish to discuss some aspects of UV-laser induced metal deposition, with special emphasis on the structure and the composition of the deposit. Our starting molecule is tetrakis trifluorophosphine platinum(0), $Pt(PF_3)_4$. This class of complexes has extensively been studied by Kruck and co-workers [1], their chemistry has been reviewed by Ugo [2]. As these molecules have no measurable dipole moment and because of the large charge concentration at the outer F atoms they are, despite their mass, remarkably volatile and do not tend to be adsorbed. On the other hand they are thermally quite unstable. $Pt(PF_3)_4$ decomposes at 130° C and $Pd(PF_3)_4$ at only -20°C. Therefore, Rand [3] studied $Pt(PF_3)_4$ for the CVD of Pt. The origin of this mean stability has some consequence for the later discussion, since decomposition is not a homogeneous process but starts heterogeneously, preferably at metal films on the walls which act as a catalyst for further decomposition [4]. The reader who is interested in the electronic structure should refer to Ref. [5], wherein the similarity between the Me-$PF_3$ bond on the surface and in the molecule is discussed in particular.

It is a novel observation that linear excitation in the electronic absorption band of $Pt(PF_3)_4$ at 248 nm ($\sigma = 2\times10^{-19}$ $cm^2$) with a KrF laser induces an intensive orange luminescence with no pronounced peak in the visible range. Two-photon excitation results in a blue emission with a weak maximum around 450 nm. The emission spectra are completely continuous and resemble in this respect those of $CrO_2Cl_2$ and $OsO_4$ [6]. Equally outstanding is the long emission lifetime of 60 µs at 0.6 mbar in the case of one-photon excitation.

Thus, the above outlined attributes suggest consideration of $Pt(PF_3)_4$ as an ideal test system to explain some of the problems concerning the dominant mechanisms in CVD with pulsed lasers; for example, to discriminate photolytic processes in the gas phase from laser-heating on the surface and to determine the role of photo-electrons [7]. Furthermore, there should be a difference between pulsed and continuous surface irradiation. This means, that for cw heating [8] an equilibrium temperature is established, according to which deposited particles can move on the surface to yield the thermodynamically favored morphology. On the contrary, with pulsed laser irradiation (15 ns) the diffusion length is only a few Å. Hence, interaction of neighboring atoms is rather restricted; as a consequence, "they stick where they hit" and a new structrue of the deposition might result. In this case, concepts of nucleation theory are only of limited usefulness. The pure photolytic CVD-process, i.e. the case when the metal containing molecule is completely photo-decomposed in the isolated gas phase, has been intensively studied in the past for organometallics and especially for the case of $Me(CH_3)_2$ (Me=Hg, Cd, Zn) [9]. The anisotropic photodissociation of $Cd(CH_3)_2$ [10] with polarized light merits special interest. For elements with large heats of formation in the gas phase like Pt, C, W and for those compounds with strongly bound ligands (eg. $SiH_4$) photolytic decomposition becomes increasingly difficult because of the increasing energy demand. In this case one can often observe that single atoms are released only due to secondary chemical reactions between photo-fragments and, in addition, the formation of cluster-molecules at higher pressures [11]. $Pt(PF_3)_4$ also seems to follow this scheme.

Taking a pressure increase as indicative for irreversible dissociation in our reaction chamber and a perceptible film for a positive Me-deposition, we observe the following: At p = 0.6 mbar there is no dissociation with the unfocussed KrF-laser beam, although the energy in the molecules is, even after the emission of a 2 eV photon, still 3 eV, which should be enough to break at least one of the $Pt-PF_3$ bonds. We interpret this as a result of a recombination process analogous to the adsorption of $PF_3$ on a Pt-surface which has a sticking coefficient of 0.14 [5]. If we focus the laser beam (E ~ 60 mJ) with a spherical lens (f = 150 mm) we excite the blue-luminescing fragments. By means of light scattering, at pressures above some 100 µbar, one also readily observes the development of a radially expanding cloud of dust particles, which later form a particulate layer. Presumably, fragments like $Pt(PF_3)_2$ which recombine to large clusters could explain this phenomenon. Since the film quality from this photo-chemical deposition was poor we did not further investigate this process. From the point of view of reaction kinetics and photo-catalysis [12] it still deserves some mentioning.

We will discuss the experiments, for which the laser beam is directed perpendicular to the substrate in somewhat more detail. For guidance the following simple picture will be used which also elucidates the difference between homogeneous and heterogeneous metal deposition. First of all, similar to the gas phase one has to remove one of the $PF_3$ ligands in order to generate a coordinate unsaturated intermediate. This can be done by photolysis, thermally or by harpooning of a surface photo-electron. The $Pt(PF_3)_x$ can then react with the Pt surface - only a few atoms are needed - during which process a certain amount of sublimation energy is released, roughly inversely proportional to the number of ligands. This excess energy could be dissipated in the substrate, but it is likewise possible that it serves to separate the ligands further. Anyhow, for the remaining ligands it should be energetically and, for reasons of entropy, more favorable to be finally adsorbed at different Pt sites. Therefore, at least in the case of $Pt(PF_3)_4$ the process of metal deposition seems to be intimately related to the mechanism of ligand desorption. Analysis of our deposits with respect to their composition and morphology underline this model.

It has already been mentioned above that electronically excited fragments are produced by the KrF laser. Therefore it is seductive to make these particles responsible for the Pt-deposition. Experiments, however, did not support this idea. With a graphite substrate we achieved comparable depositions with KrF - and XeCl - laser irradiation at comparable fluences, although 308 nm was not absorbed by the $Pt(PF_3)_4$ molecules and hence no luminescence could be excited. Following a suggestion in Ref. [13], we compared the initial deposition rates in our quartz-cell at the inner side of the front and rear windows, respectively, and observed no striking difference. This occurs despite the fact that the rear window was always in contact with the column of electronically excited gas whereas electronic excitation was reduced at the front window due to the increasing absorption.

A discussion of the absolute number of deposited Pt atoms should also be instructive. According to Rutherford backscattering and scanning Auger measurements we deposit $7x10^{14}$ Pt atoms/($cm^2$ x shot), in the case of an Al substrate, 0.6 mbar $Pt(PF_3)_4$ and 200 $mJ/cm^2$ KrF laser fluence; roughly half a monolayer. If this amount of deposition would be only due to the excited fragments ($\sigma = 2x10^{-19}$ $cm^2$) a 2.3 cm long luminescing column would be required, to approach the surface at a diffusion limited velocity without being deactivated. This seems to be rather unlikely. It is interesting to mention that similar simple appraisals also exclude laser heating of the surface as a dominant process, because a deposition time of the order of 100 μs would be necessary; and, during this long time interval, thermal conductivity would have caused a complete surface cooling.

Comparing the number of photons hitting the surface and the number of deposited Pt-atoms, we can evaluate the deposition quantum yield to be about $10^{-3}$. This value, on the other hand, is typical for the yield of photoelectron emission at 5 eV. Therefore, it is not unreasonable to presume that photoelectrons from the surface play an essential role in initiation of the deposition process. This means, that thermal electrons are captured by the $Pt(PF_3)_4$ molecules, the excess charge gives rise to a dissociation step, and negatively charged fragments finally fall back into the positive holes on the surface where they are further decomposed in the way described before. If the surface mobility is low enough the model could also explain why deposition occurs exclusively within the laser irradiated area.

We shall now discuss the composition and morphology of our Pt deposits. We shall concentrate on quartz and grahite substrates and keep the KrF laser fluence low enough to avoid photochemical gas phase processes from dominating.

Deposition on quartz is possible only above a fluence threshold of about 50 $mJ/cm^2$. The layer grows outwards from the center of irradiation. At a certain thickness a new process comes into play, forming a distinct padded halo around the original deposit, see Fig. 1. This ring, in contrast to the central area, is strongly adhesive. The deposits exhibit a measurable electrical conductivity. After removal of the central deposit no damage on the quartz surface is discernible. It should be mentioned that the size of the halo coincides with the visible size of the laser beam diameter. This observation shows that laser CVD is not a continuous growth of a particle layer, but also involves kinetic processes like desorption and

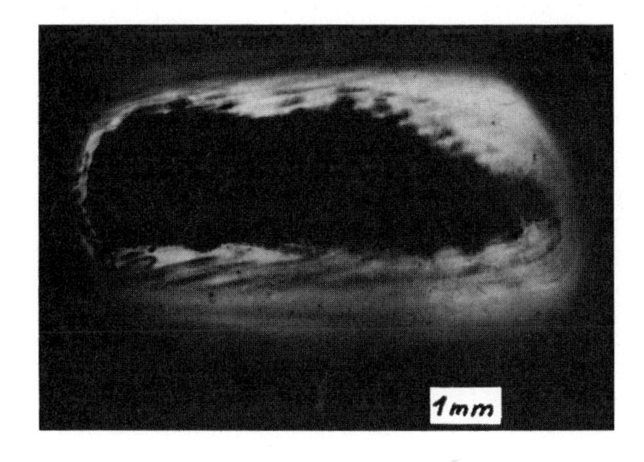


Fig. 1.
KrF-laser induced Pt-deposition on a quartz substrate. 4000 laser shots, 35 mJ input energy. A halo is clearly observable

segregation. For a better analysis of these processes graphite is much more suitable.

The deposition rate on graphite is somewhat slower than on aluminum. The amount of deposit increases linearly with respect to pressure, fluence and the number of shots. No fluence threshold was apparent down to 10 mJ/cm$^2$ and single laser shot. This is in contrast to quartz and might be interpreted as a difference in the anchoring ability, since the adhesive power on graphite is also distinctively higher than on quartz. The adhesive power on graphite, in turn, correlates with the local laser fluence, and the outer deposited ring can easily be peeled off.

Platinum does not grow as a uniform layer but it is composed of microcrystallites, see Fig. 2. Their final size reflects the total amount of deposited platinum, which is proportional to the laser fluence. This means, we can look at the deposition process as a continuous increase of cluster size. Because of the low surface mobility no enslaving processes are being observed. The globular shape may be connected to the fact that platinum is preferably deposited at platinum surfaces. At any rate, a definite interpretation is possible only if a detailed model of the deposition process is available. Surface and profile analysis of the deposits are certainly quite informative in this respect. They show that surface - catalyzed reactions proceed during the deposition. This shall be discussed for only one example.

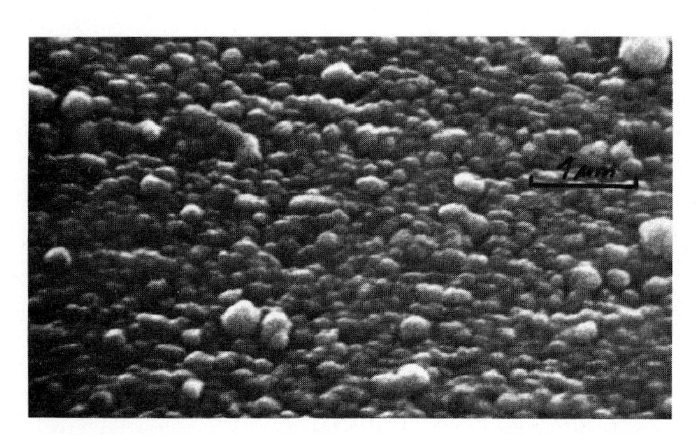


Fig. 2.
KrF laser induced Pt deposition on graphite.
10000 laser shots, 20 mJ/cm$^2$

The SEM micrograph in Fig. 3 shows, on the left hand side a dark border, ramifications in the middle and a relatively smooth structure on the right. The whole picture is a section of a platinum deposition at 0.58 mbar $Pt(PF_3)_4$ ($p_0$ = $4 \times 10^{-6}$ Torr), 50 mJ/cm$^2$ and 10000 laser shots. The left border is part of a 400 μm wide groove that is the result of 100 additional exposures at the same vapor pressure but with the laser fluence doubled. By means of scanning Auger spectroscopy we have measured distribution patterns of all observable elements (Pt, S, P, N, O). Part of the results is shown in Fig. 4. The ramifications appear to be due to phosphorus and oxygen in non - stoichiometric compositions. Platinum is exactly anticorrelated to the P,O-distribution. We interpret this result as being due to the fact that phosphorus, which is always a contamination on the Pt-deposit is preferably desorbed from areas of higher laser fluences. This means that it should be possible to purify the deposited ma-

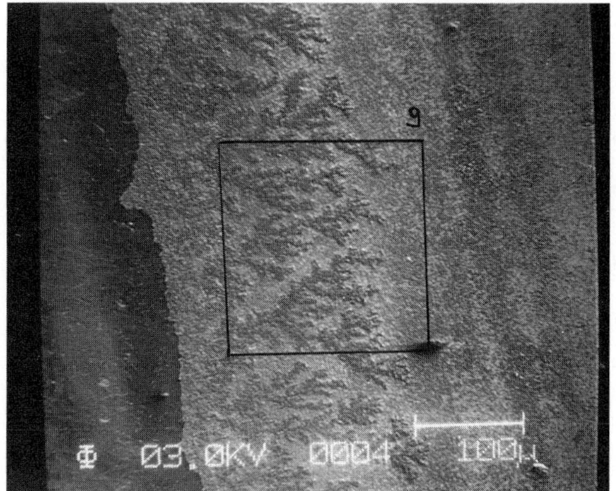


Fig. 3.
KrF laser induced Pt-deposition on graphite, similar to Fig. 2. Subsequent 100 shot deposition at higher laser fluence causes a remarkable desorption pattern

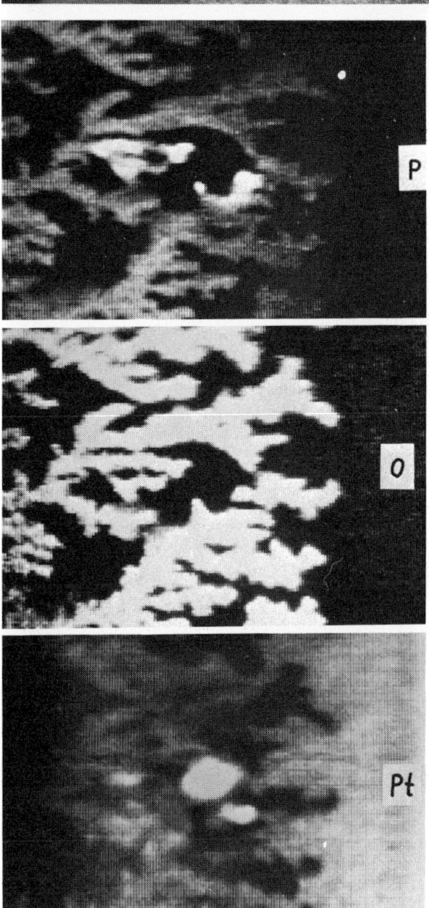


Fig. 4.
Spatial distribution of the elements according to Fig. 3

terial within certain limits. Fluorine is not observed on the platinum, but it becomes dominant on remote areas and presumably right at the graphite-platinum boundary.

Irrespective of the deposition mechanism it is interesting to compare purely thermal and UV-laser induced Pt deposits. Figure 5 shows the case when graphite was heated with a lamp. There is a distinct difference in the morphologies with respect to smoothness and thermal stress. Moreover, the elements are distributed in a different way. In the thermal case we find: Pt (69%), P (11%). C (0%), O (20%), and for laser deposition: Pt (38%), P (3%), C (52%), O (4%). As already suspected, there is more phosphorus and oxygen on the thermal deposit, whereas carbon is dominant in the laser case. This amount of carbon does not result from the holes between the Pt crystallites and is rather due to adsorbed hydrocarbons on this sample because the carbon disappears after ion sputtering, and platinum increases to 82 %.

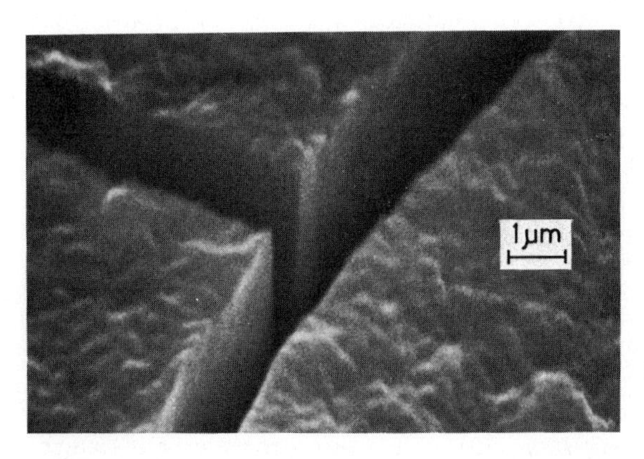


Fig. 5. Thermal deposition of platinum on graphite

These results show that a more detailed understanding of laser surface chemistry is still needed before laser CVD can be developed to practical applications.

References:


1 Th. Kruck: Angew. Chem. 79, 27 (1967)
2 R. Ugo: Coordin. Chem. Rev. 3, 319 (1968)
3 M.J. Rand: J. Eletrochem. Soc. 120, 686 (1973)
4 H.G.M. Edwards, L.A. Woodward: Spectrochimica Acta 26A, 897 (1970)
5 F. Nitschke: Thesis, Ludwig-Maximilians-Universität München (1980)
6 H. Schröder: MPQ Jahresbericht (1981)
7 J.L. Beauchamp, P.M. George: US patent, 4324854 (1982)
8 D. Bäuerle: this issue
9 S.J.W. Price: "The Decomposition of Metal Alkyls, Aryls, Carbonyls and Nitrosyls" in Chemical Kinetics, Vol. 4 ed. C.H. Bamford, C.F.H. Tipper, Elsevier (1972)
10 C. Jonah, P. Chandra, and R. Bersohn: J. Chem. Phys. 55, 1903 (1971)
11 H. Schröder, H. Lamprecht, K.L. Kompa: J. Appl. Phys. 1328, 180 (1982)
12 K.-I. Fu, R.L. Whetten, and E.R. Grant: Ind. Eng. Chem. Prod. Res. Dev. 23, 33 (1984)
13 S.D. Allen: J. Appl. Phys. 52, 6501 (1981)

# Laser Photolytic Deposition of Metals on Indium Phosphide

M. R. Aylett and J. Haigh

British Telecom Research Laboratories,
Martlesham Heath,
Ipswich IP5 7RE,
UK.

## 1 INTRODUCTION

Current interests at British Telecom Research Laboratories include advanced optoelectronic and integrated optics device structures in III-V semiconducting materials. To improve device yields, alternative methods for preparation and fabrication of these structures are evaluated. For example, contact metallisations for III-V optoelectronic devices are conventionally defined by photolithography, a multi-stage process. It has been shown that focused laser beams can be used to pyrolytically or photolytically deposit localised regions of many materials on various substrates, and also for localised etching; a recent review is given in [1].

We are currently investigating the possibility of using a laser photolysis system to deposit metals on indium phosphide substrates in localised areas to act as electrical contacts. Such contacts typically have their smallest dimensions constrained by the dimensions of the optoelectronic devices to be in the 0.2 - 10 μm region, so that a laser 'writing' process should be suitable for their preparation. Such an approach is attractive since it is a single-stage process which can easily be integrated with metallo-organic chemical vapour deposition (MOCVD), one of the techniques used for the growth of epitaxial III-V optoelectronic device heterostructures. This compatibility with MOCVD arises because the metallo-organic precursors used for the two techniques are similar, as are the requirements therefore of the gas-handling systems and reactor cells.

Other workers have generally used continuous wave (cw) lasers (such as frequency-doubled argon ion lasers) for localised photolytic deposition [2], reserving pulsed excimer lasers for applications where broad-area deposition [3] or thermal diffusion of species into the substrate is required [4]. This situation has been due to both the pulsed nature of the excimer laser emission, and also its higher available average power and generally poorer beam quality. A system for localised laser photolytic deposition of metals onto indium phosphide substrates using a pulsed excimer laser has been developed. The system has been designed to be suitable for deposition of contact metallisations for III-V optoelectronic devices.

For the production of ohmic contacts to n- and p-type indium phosphide, metallisations of tin and zinc may be used, these being n- and p-type dopants respectively in this material. Deposition of tin from the metallo-organic precursor tetramethyl tin [5], and zinc from diethyl zinc [6] have been reported by others using a frequency-doubled argon ion laser; with the excimer laser operating at a wavelength of either 193 or 249 nm, localised regions of tin and zinc have been deposited by us from tetraethyl tin and diethyl zinc. Etching of indium phosphide and gallium arsenide using methyl bromide and a cw UV laser was also reported by EHRLICH *et al.* [7]. We have achieved localised etching of indium phosphide using methyl bromide with a pulsed excimer laser. In this paper the excimer laser photolytic deposition system is described, and examples are given of the deposits and etch patterns obtained. The use of an excimer laser rather than a cw laser (such as a frequency-doubled argon ion laser) for localised metal deposition is discussed.

## 2 EXCIMER LASER LOCALISED DEPOSITION SYSTEM

Figure 1 is a schematic diagram of the apparatus that has been developed. The excimer laser used as the source of UV radiation is a Lambda Physik model EMG 102E. Because the laser medium has a high gain, with the normal resonator optics installed the beam from an excimer laser has rather a high divergence (2x4

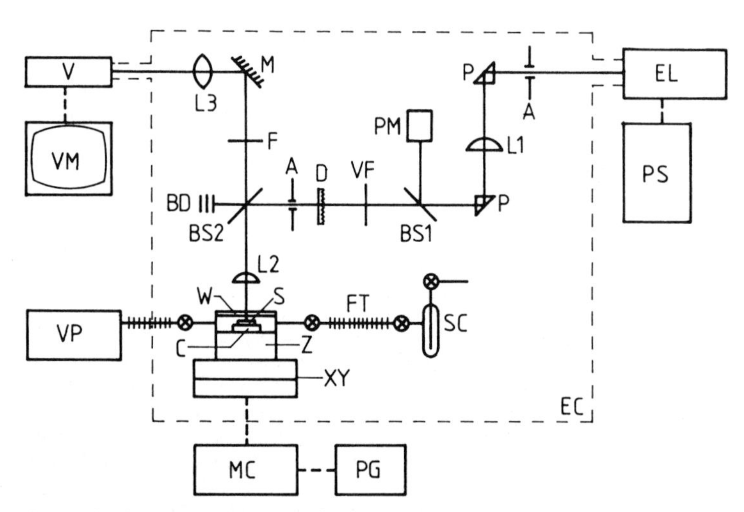


Figure 1 Schematic diagram of laser deposition apparatus

Key to abbreviations:

| | |
|---|---|
| A | Aperture stop |
| BD | Beam dump |
| BS1 | Beam splitter for power meter |
| BS2 | Beam splitter for viewing with vidicon |
| C | Peltier cooler |
| D | Removable ground silica diffuser plate |
| EC | Fume-extracted light-tight cabinet |
| EL | Excimer laser |
| F | Neutral density filter |
| FT | Flexible stainless steel tubing |
| L1 | Fine focusing lens (1" diameter, 350 mm f.l.) |
| L2 | Lens focusing beam onto substrate (0.5" diameter, 25 mm f.l.) |
| L3 | Transfer lens for imaging onto vidicon (1.5" diameter, 50 mm f.l.) |
| M | Front-aluminised mirror |
| MC | Stepper-motor control electronics |
| P | Fused silica 90° prism |
| PG | Pulse generator |
| PM | Power meter |
| PS | Excimer laser power supply |
| S | Substrate |
| SC | Metallo-organic precursor sample container |
| V | UV sensitive vidicon in CCTV camera |
| VF | Variable circular linear-wedge neutral density filter (motorised) |
| VM | Video monitor |
| VP | Hermetically sealed two-stage rotary vacuum pump |
| W | UV grade fused silica rotatable window |
| XY | Stepper motor controlled x-y translation stage |
| Z | Manual z translation stage. |

mrad) and would not be suitable for micron-scale localised deposition as the focused spot would be too large. With unstable resonator cavity optics fitted, however, the divergence is reduced to 0.5 mrad, which allows the beam to be focused to a near-diffraction-limited spot size. The excimer laser is accordingly fitted with positive branch confocal unstable resonator optics. Operation at 193 and 249 nm output wavelengths is achieved using ArF and KrF excimer gas mixtures respectively. The maximum repetition rate attainable is 150 Hz; in most experiments a repetition rate of 22.5 Hz has been used. With both ArF and KrF excimer gas mixtures the pulse length of the laser is about 15 ns.

The indium phosphide substrate is placed in a stainless steel vacuum-tight cell which is equipped with a UV grade fused silica window and gas inlet and outlet ports. The silica window is rotatable in order to allow a clean window area to be used should deposition take place on it, and is sealed to the cell with a viton o-ring. Also inside the cell, underneath the substrate, is a thermoelectric (Peltier) cooling device, which can be used to cool the substrate. This has the effect of increasing the amount of precursor on the substrate surface. The substrate is limited by the size of the cooler to a maximum of 9.2 mm square. The laser beam is focused perpendicularly down onto the substrate surface by a 0.5" diameter UV grade fused silica plano-convex lens of 25 mm focal length. The lens is stopped down to about f/4.5 to reduce the effects of spherical aberration.

The cell is fixed to an x-y-z translation stage assembly, with the z motion being manually controlled with 10 $\mu m$ resolution for focusing of the beam onto the substrate surface, and the x-y motion provided by two 0.1 $\mu m$ per step stepper motor translation stages. Lines of deposit can thus be formed by moving the substrate under the focused beam during deposition, and areas can be built up by scanning the substrate in a raster pattern. The stepper motor controller allows movement at between 4 and 200 $\mu m\ s^{-1}$. A pulse generator has been added which allows slower speeds; for deposition of lines and areas of metal speeds in the range 0.1 to 2 $\mu m\ s^{-1}$ have been used. The cell is pumped out using a two-stage rotary pump to $10^{-2}$ Torr and the metallo-organic precursor admitted to a pressure of typically a few torr.

The laser beam is directed onto the substrate by an uncoated 10 mm thick fused silica beamsplitter, through which the substrate surface or laser spot can be imaged onto a UV-sensitive vidicon in a closed-circuit TV camera (Hamamatsu N983 vidicon). The UV laser is used to illuminate the substrate since this allows the laser spot and substrate surface to be viewed without refocusing or use of achromatic optics. Neutrai density filters are inserted into the beam paths to provide the correct power densities for deposition and viewing. For imaging the substrate surface, a diffuser is placed in the laser beam to give diffuse illumination. The diffuser is spun to eliminate speckle patterns. For imaging the laser spot at the substrate surface, the diffuser is removed. Magnification at the monitor is about 650x, although this can be varied by changing the positions of the transfer lens and vidicon faceplate.

Steering of the beam into the apparatus is accomplished using either UV grade fused silica prisms for the 249 nm wavelength or dielectric coated mirrors for 193 nm. Average power is monitored with a 1" diameter volume absorbing disc calorimeter with a spectral range of 190 to 250 nm. The laser beam path and deposition apparatus are completely enclosed [8] in a light-tight cabinet equipped with filtered air inlets and fume extraction to provide a safe operating environment.

## 3 EXPERIMENTAL RESULTS

Initial results obtained before the stepper-motor controlled x-y stage was installed [9] indicated that with tetraethyl tin or diethyl zinc vapour in the cell, operating the laser at a wavelength of 193 nm resulted primarily in gas-phase photolysis of the precursor giving poorly defined, diffuse deposits of metal on the substrate. At

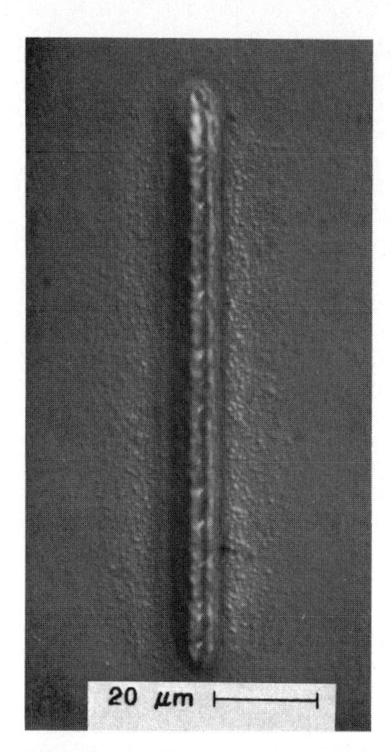


Fig. 2 Deposit of tin produced using tetraethyl tin as the metallo-organic precursor, at a laser wavelength of 249 nm.

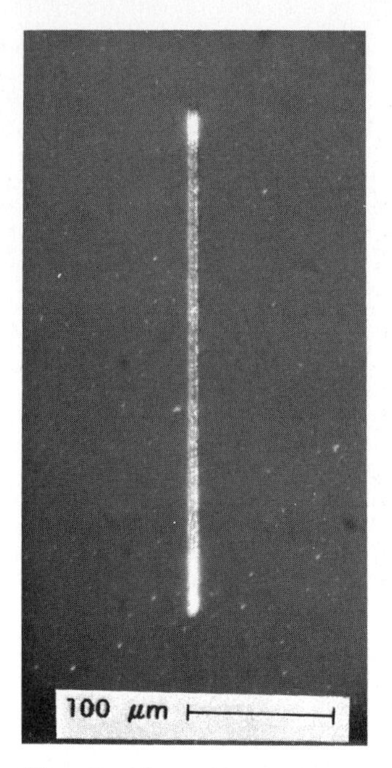


Fig. 3 Line of zinc deposited from diethyl zinc, varying the rate of translation of the substrate along the line.

249 nm however, there was a significant contribution to the deposition from photolysis of precursor adsorbed on the surface of the substrate, and the definition of the deposit was sharper. The minimum spot diameter achieved for the deposition of zinc was about 2 μm (although this could presumably be improved upon if necessary by using aberration-free optics for focusing the beam onto the substrate rather than the currently used simple plano-convex lenses). The deposition rate was found to be increased by a factor of 2-3 by using the Peltier cooler to cool the substrate some 10-20 °C below ambient; this is due to an increase in the amount of the precursor at the surface of the substrate.

The deposits shown in Figs. 2-4 were all obtained using the excimer laser at a wavelength of 249 nm with a KrF excimer gas mixture. A detailed examination of these deposits is currently in progress; the results will be published elsewhere. Figure 2 shows a line of tin deposited from tetraethyl tin. The substrate was moved at a rate of 0.4 $\mu m\ s^{-1}$ and the deposit shown resulted from a single pass. The ridged structure on the deposit may have been the result of multiple reflections at slightly different angles produced in the laser beam by passage through slightly non-parallel neutral density filters or beamsplitters. The amount of deposit observed depended on the pressure of the precursor in the cell; upon cooling the substrate the precursor will condense out onto it until the vapour is again in equilibrium with the cooler surface. Lack of accurate control over the pressure in the cell made the deposition rate rather unreproducible. The energy density at the substrate was about 0.6 $J\ cm^{-2}$ for all the deposits shown.

Figure 3 shows a longer line of deposited zinc; here the rate of movement was varied at different points along the line from 0.5 to 2.0 $\mu m\ s^{-1}$. More deposit can

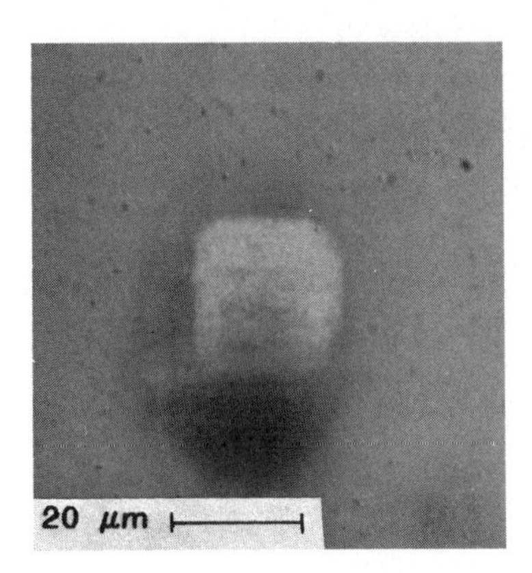


Fig. 4 Area of zinc deposited from diethyl zinc (laser beam somewhat defocused).

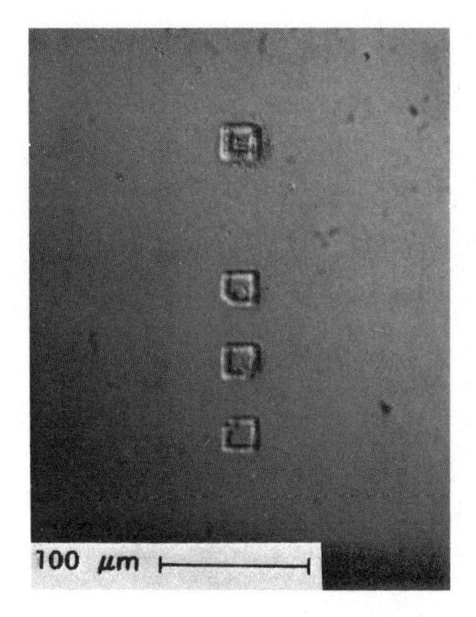


Fig. 5 Patterns etched in indium phosphide by photolysis of methyl bromide.

be observed where the movement was slower. The zinc deposit shown in Fig. 4 was built up by scanning the substrate under the (slightly defocused) laser beam in a series of 20 μm long lines to form a deposit nominally 20 μm square. Because the laser beam was not optimally focused the definition of this deposit does not represent the capability of the system. The dark region at the bottom of the photograph appears to be a thin non-metallic deposit caused by a less intense part of the laser spot.

Etching of the indium phosphide substrate material as shown in Fig. 5 was observed wher. methyl bromide vapour was introduced to the cell at a pressure of 500 Torr or less (down to about 10 Torr). The energy density at the substrate in this case was again about 0.6 J $cm^{-2}$. The 20 μm squares were etched by moving the substrate at 0.4 μm $s^{-1}$.

## 4 LOCALISED DEPOSITION AND ETCHING USING AN EXCIMER LASER

The experiments reported here have been mainly concerned with determining the suitability of the excimer laser-based deposition system for production of localised metallic regions on indium phosphide substrates; this is still at an early stage and the deposits obtained have not been fully characterised. The results suggest however that it is possible to deposit lines and areas of metal with this system which are reasonably well localised. Similarly the etching of indium phosphide using methyl bromide has given well-localised etched regions. It thus appears that an excimer laser can be used to initiate localised reactions at indium phosphide substrate surfaces; the possibility of having a choice of ultra-violet wavelengths available should provide insight into their mechanisms.

## ACKNOWLEDGEMENT

Acknowledgement is made to the Director of Research of British Telecom for permission to publish this paper.

## REFERENCES


1 D.J. Ehrlich and J.Y. Tsao, J. Vac. Sci. Technol. **B1**(4), Oct.-Dec. 1983, 969.

2 For example, D.J. Ehrlich, R.M. Osgood, Jr. and T.F. Deutsch, J. Electrochem. Soc. **128**(9), 1981, 2041.

3 For example, R. Solanki and G.J. Collins, Appl. Phys. Lett. **42**(8), 1983, 662.

4 T.F. Deutsch, D.J. Ehrlich, R.M. Osgood, Jr. and Z.L. Liau, Appl. Phys. Lett. **36**(10), 1980, 847.

5 T.F. Deutsch, D.J. Ehrlich and R.M. Osgood, Jr., Appl. Phys. Lett. **35**(2), 1979, 175.

6 D.J. Ehrlich, R.M. Osgood, Jr. and T.F. Deutsch, IEEE J. Quantum Electronics **QE-16**(11), Nov. 1980, 1233.

7 D.J. Ehrlich , R.M. Osgood, Jr. and T.F. Deutsch, Appl. Phys. Lett. **36**(8), 1980, 698.

8 BS 4803, 'Radiation safety of laser products and systems.' British Standards Institution, 1983.

9 Reported at 2nd. International Conference on Metallo-Organic Vapour Phase Epitaxy, Sheffield, UK, April 1984.

# Laser Photochemical Deposition of Metals

A.E. Adams, M.L. Lloyd, S.L. Morgan, and N.G. Davis
GEC Research Laboratories, Hirst Research Centre
Wembley, HA9 7PP, England

## Introduction

The trend towards finer device geometries and increased packing density places severe requirements on the materials and techniques used to form interconnects, ohmic contacts, and low resistivity gates. As device dimensions approach 1 μm, the sheet resistance contribution of polysilicon gates (20 Ω/square) to RC delay times becomes significant and the advantages of such fine device geometries cannot be fully realised. Further, as lateral dimensions are decreased there is also a concomitant reduction in the depths of the junctions which form the device structure, for example the source and drain regions of an MOS transistor. Shallow junctions ultimately limit the use of aluminium and its alloys for ohmic contacting because of its known penetration into silicon. In order to overcome these limitations, the use of refractory metals, in particular tungsten, is being widely considered. Its bulk resistivity of 6 μΩ/cm, high resistance to electromigration, and its ability to form a stable low resistivity silicide $WSi_2$ makes it an ideal choice for use as a VLSI metallisation material. Currently, the preferred method of obtaining good quality tungsten layers is by low pressure chemical vapour deposition, this however, is only one of a series of multistep sequences which for complex fine geometry structures are becoming less reliable.

An alternative approach is to form patterned metal films directly by laser deposition techniques, either Laser Chemical Vapour Deposition (LCVD), or Laser Photochemical Deposition (LPD). LCVD is analogous to conventional CVD but offers the advantage of being able to produce delineated deposits. LPD can also be used to pattern films directly but has further advantages including the capability to form high resolution features, and the freedom to select substrate deposition temperature. These properties make LPD a potentially important technique for the fabrication of microelectronic structures [1].

In previous studies the LCVD of aluminium and tin from their trimethyl species has been examined by us using a $CO_2$ laser [2]. We have also investigated the photolysis of iron from $Fe(CO)_5$ [3], and elsewhere the photodissociation of tungsten from $W(CO)_6$ [4] has been described. Here we examine the deposition of tungsten from $WF_6$ selected because of its conveniently high vapour pressure, and discuss attempts to directly deposit $WSi_2$.

## Experimental

The experimental configuration used for these studies has been described in detail previously [3]. Essentially the system consists of a stainless steel reaction chamber together with auxiliary gas handling facilities which control the pressure and flow of the reaction vapours permitting a wide variety of operating conditions. A quartz input window allows the substrate to be illuminated; fogging of the inside face is inhibited by jetting nitrogen across it. The substrate to be coated, which is usually sapphire, silicon, or quartz, is mounted on a ceramic sample holder and may be heated to 500°C. The laser employed is a Lambda Physik EMG101E operated at the argon fluoride wavelength, 193 nm, and provides typical output energies of 10 mJ per pulse up to a maximum pulse repetition rate of 40 Hz.

The formation of deposits is monitored in real-time by measuring the change in sample reflectivity with a helium neon laser. Sheet resistivity measurements, scanning electron microscopy, X-ray fluorescence and Auger analyis have been used to characterise the deposited layers.

## Results

Initial attempts to obtain deposits on silicon and quartz substrates by the photolysis of $WF_6$ were not totally successful; the deposition rates were extremely slow and the resultant deposits were soft, easily removed, and highly insulating. The reason for this is a strong bidirectional reaction between the dissociated tungsten and fluorine, which causes a rapid recombination of the photolysed products to reform $WF_6$. To prevent this from occurring hydrogen is introduced in to the reaction system to act as a fluorine scavenger by forming HF thus:

$$WF_6 + 3H_2 + nh\nu \underset{193\ nm}{\rightarrow} W\downarrow + 6\ HF\uparrow.$$

This reaction was first studied in a statically filled cell to a pressure of 50 Torr with a $WF_6$ partial pressure of between 5 and 15 Torr. The best quality deposits were obtained when the silicon substrate was heated to a temperature in excess of 200°C. Under these conditions there was a prenucleation time of ~20 s after which the deposition rate was 3.2 nm/min Figure 1. The film's adhesion was determined as good by sticky tape tests and four point probe measurements gave a minimum value for sheet resistance

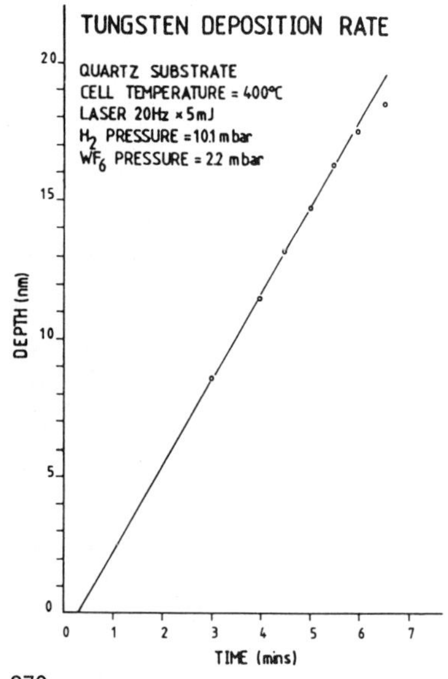


FIGURE 1 : Depth evolution by real time reflectivity.

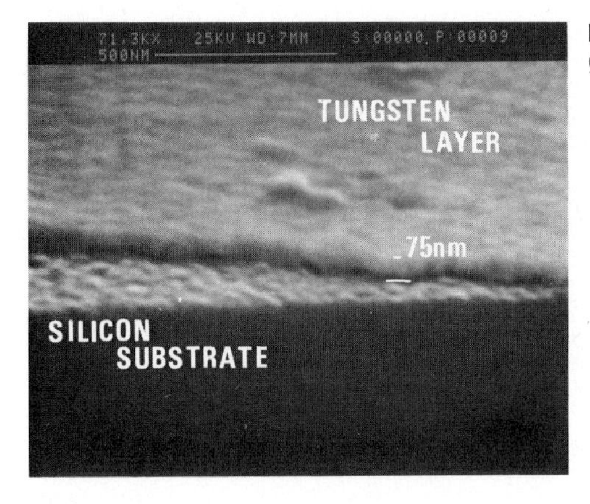


FIGURE 2 : Scanning electron micrograph showing tungsten on silicon.

of 30 Ω/square. Sheet resistance was found to be a function of deposition temperature with the lowest values obtained at 400°C. The reason for this temperature dependent resistivity has not yet been positively identified but it is likely to be related to either crystal structure or impurity incorporation. Auger analysis has shown the films to consist mainly of tungsten, with traces of oxygen and this may be responsible for the higher than expected bulk resistivities obtained [5]. The morphology of the films was examined in a scanning electron microscope, Figure 2. The layers are largely flat and featureless with typical thicknesses in the range 70 to 100 nm. At the highest magnification, the layers appear to be constructed from columnar growths. However, further studies at higher magnification, e.g. cross-sectional TEM, are required to identify more fully the nucleation and subsequent growth evolution of the tungsten layers.

In order to examine the effect of a heterogeneous substrate surface, layers were deposited onto patterned silicon on sapphire. Once again flat, featureless low resistivity layers were obtained with no observable deposition selectivity between the surface of the silicon islands or the sapphire substrate, Figures 3 and 4.

The attempts to deposit tungsten silicide directly were undertaken using tungsten hexafluoride and silane (10% in helium) as the precursor vapours.

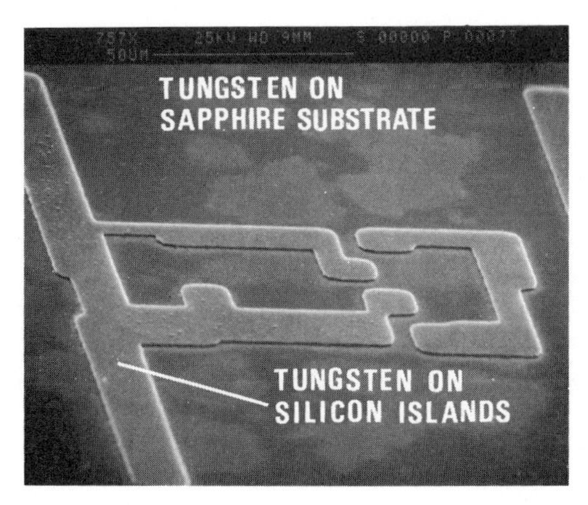


FIGURE 3 : Scanning electron micrograph showing tungsten on silicon-on-sapphire structure.

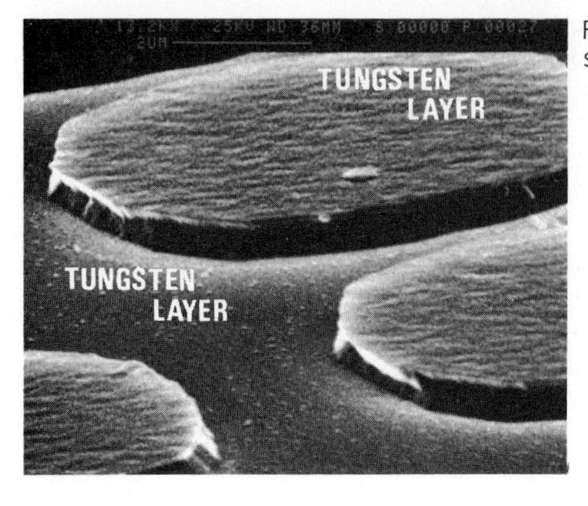


FIGURE 4 : Surface detail of tungsten on patterned SOS.

The experiments involved flowing the two gases at nominally equal flow rates (~10 cc/min). Above 150°C the gases decomposed spontaneously to form a metallic like deposit. At 150°C pyrolysis did not occur at these flow rates. Illuminating the substrate with the excimer laser initiated the reaction and again a metallic like deposit was formed. However extinguishing the beam did not affect the deposition rate. Reducing both the $WF_6$ and $SiH_4$ flow rates and decreasing the total cell pressure to 2 mbar caused the reaction to become more beam dependent although ceasing illumination did not prevent the reaction completely. Monitoring the deposition process using real time reflectivity indicated that the reaction was initially slow then increases to higher rate, suggesting a heterogeneous gas phase reaction, with the high rate reaction process being totally beam dependent.

Analysis of the pyrolysed and photolysed deposits by Auger depth profiling showed the films to be compositionally different, Figure 5. The pyrolysed films, Figure 5a, consisted of both tungsten and silicon, with

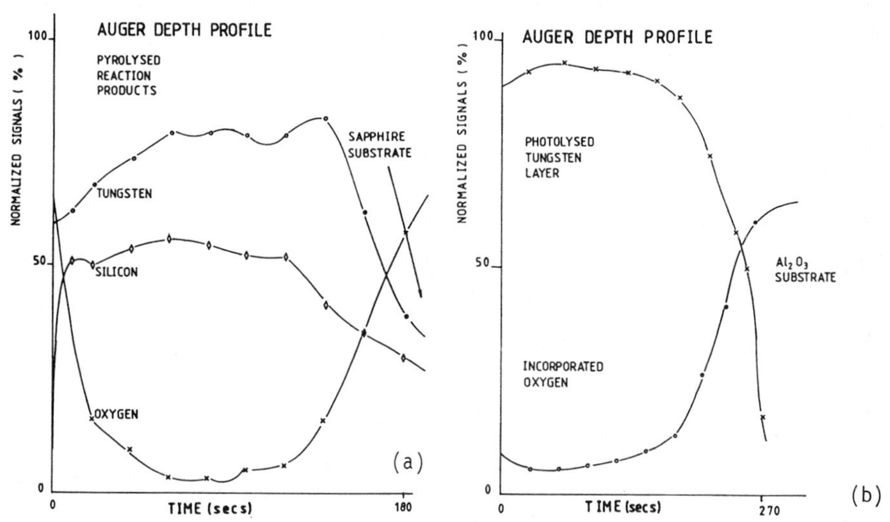


FIGURE 5a : Auger depth profile of pyrolysed layer.
FIGURE 5b : Auger depth profile of photolysed layer.

XPS indicating some bonding between the two. The photolysed films, Figure 5b, on the other hand, contained no detectable amounts of silicon, suggesting the reaction pathways leading to film formation are different. From bond enthalpy considerations, it can be shown that the preferable pyrolytic reaction pathway is:

$$2\,(WF_6 + SiH_4) \rightarrow 2\,(4\,HF + W + Si + F_2)$$

$$Si + 2F_2 \rightarrow SiF_4$$

which is exothermic with an excess energy of 2337 KJ/mol. The photolytic reaction is more complicated and less certain. A likely scenario is that first the $WF_6$ molecule absorbs one or more of the incident ultraviolet photons causing it to dissociate photolytically. The free tungsten atoms then condense onto the substrate and the fluorine abstracts hydrogen from the silane to form HF and $SiF_4$, thus:

$$WF_6 + SiH_4 + \underset{193\ nm}{nh\nu} \rightarrow WF^*_2 + 4F^* + SiH_4$$

$$WF^*_2 + 4F^* + SiH_4 \rightarrow SiF_4 + WF^*_2 + 2H_2$$

$$SiF_4 + WF^*_2 + H_2 \rightarrow SiF_4 + W\downarrow + 2HF\uparrow + H_2\uparrow.$$

The exact form of the reaction intermediates is unknown and so this reaction is stated by way of example only. However, abstraction of hydrogen from the silane by free fluorine does provide an explanation for the continued reaction after the laser has been turned off as some will inevitably still be present within the reaction volume.

In conclusion, we have shown that it is possible to deposit good quality tungsten layers by the photolytic reduction of $WF_6$. This technique will be developed further to improve the conductivity of the tungsten layers. Effort will also be directed towards obtaining $WSi_2$ layers and to understand, in greater detail, the processes leading to nucleation and subsequent growth evolution of atomic and molecular films.

## References


1 D. Ehrlich, R. Osgood and T. Deutsch: J. Quant. Elect., Vol 16 (11), 1233 (1980)

2 K.G. Ibbs: Nat. Quant. Elect., Conference, September 1981

3 M.L. Lloyd and K.G. Ibbs: Laser controlled chemical processing of surfaces, MRS Meeting, Boston, November 1983

4 R. Solanki, P. Boyer, J. Mahan and G Collins: Appl. Phys. Lett., 38(7), 572 (1981)

5 F. Blatt: Physics of Electronic Conduction in Solids, (McGraw-Hill, New York, 1980) p 155

## 3.2 Oxide Formation

# Laser Assisted Pyrolytic Growth and Photochemical Deposition of Thin Oxide Films

Ian W. Boyd

Center for Applied Quantum Electronics, Department of Physics,
North Texas State University, Denton, TX 76203, USA

Lasers offer a diverse approach to fabricating oxide films for a wide variety of applications. This paper will review the field of laser oxidation in general but particular attention will be focused on oxide formation on silicon. Two main areas will be detailed, namely Laser Chemical Vapor Deposition (LCVD) and Laser Pyrolytic Growth (LPG). The kinetics involved with film preparation will be discussed while the various structural, optical and electrical properties of the films will be compared.

## 1. Introduction

The successful application of silicon toward large scale device integration is due not only to the tailorability of its semiconducting properties, but also to the ease with which it can be effectively passivated by its natural oxide. Although various forms of silicon oxide exist, the most technologically important is silicon dioxide ($SiO_2$). It is an excellent insulator (resistivity $>10^{16}$ Ωcm), can withstand very large electric fields (dielectric breakdown strength ~$10^7$ V $cm^{-1}$) and passivate the silicon surface (surface states reduced to $<10^{11}$ $cm^{-2}$), and is chemically very stable. Many methods of $SiO_2$ preparation are commonly available [1] and the physical and chemical properties of the differently prepared films can be varied considerably. Direct thermal oxidation of the Si surface at elevated temperatures (~1000°C) in an oxygen rich environment is the most commonly followed preparation technique. From the point of view of device performance, it has been found that such thermally grown layers are reproducibly quite stable and contain a very low level of interface state charge, mobile ionic charge and fixed charge [2]. However, there is an anticipated need for smaller geometry integrated circuits in particular for very large scale integration (VLSI) applications, and an essential requirement for the fabrication of such devices is the minimization of high temperature processing techniques. It is known,for example, that high temperatures can induce some degree of wafer warpage, and promote the generation of stacking faults and other defects, as well as encourage significant redistribution of dopants. Therefore, it has become increasingly desirable in recent years to form good quality $SiO_2$ films at lower substrate temperatures, or with a sizeable reduction in high temperature processing times.

Low temperature preparation techniques are already quite widely used to deposit thin films of $SiO_2$. For example, Chemical Vapor Deposited (CVD) $SiO_2$ is employed as a dielectric on top of various narrow bandgap semiconductors such as InP in high speed electronic devices [3] and InSb in advanced infrared sensor arrays [4]. In fact, since the mid 1960s [5] CVD methods consisting of pyrolytic decomposition of silane ($SiH_4$) in $O_2$ have been successfully introduced into the Si Integrated Circuit industry. Although these films in general can be grown at much faster rates than thermal oxides, their slightly poorer electrical properties have restricted applications mainly to the role of masking or protective overlayers. It has been found that an increase in electrical performance can usually only be obtained by increasing the deposition temperature. Reactive sputtering, in which Si atoms are ejected from a high purity source by energetic ion bombardment and consequently react with an oxygen rich atmosphere to form a thin layer of insulating $SiO_2$, has all but been replaced by rf sputtering from a silica target [6]. Under ideal conditions, rf sputtered $SiO_2$ films can be prepared that more closely resemble those grown thermally than other types of deposited films formed at the same temperature [7]. However close similarity has only been achieved by raising the substrate temperature, as with CVD films. Furthermore, layers prepared in this manner are usually subject to uniformity problems, while the substrate is prone to radiation damage, although these particular difficulties are continually being minimized [8]. Microwave plasma technology has also been investigated as a means of oxide formation in VLSI production [9,10]. In this case oxygen forms a reactive species that must be transported to the substrate to oxidize the Si. However similar damage formation and impurity incorporation also threatens to restrict potential applications. Progress in this direction, which includes the use of photon enhancement techniques, will be discussed elsewhere in these proceedings [11]. Interest continues to develop in the area of high pressure oxidation which surprisingly was first demonstrated around 1960 [12]. More recently these high pressure techniques have yielded oxides whose dielectric strength and fixed charge content are as good as or better than those grown at one atmosphere [13].

Lasers offer a variety of alternative methods of oxide preparation. Although many of these techniques often result in more novel than useful structures, it is very important to realize that the laser can dramatically confine high temperature processing to only the near surface regions, and for much shortened time periods, through the fine directionality inherent in beam technologies and also the extreme heating and cooling rates intrinsic to beam heating. Additionally, lasers offer a most unique processing procedure, so desirable in the future VLSI production line--that of locallized microchemistry. As has been already pointed out in these proceedings [14],lasers allow the possibility of direct writing, sometimes with submicron resolution, and therefore offer a step towards non-photolithographic processing and discretionary restructuring of devices. Here, the various methods involving the use of lasers to produce oxide layers on the crystalline Si surface will be reviewed. Particular emphasis will be directed towards the areas in this field which have attracted most attention--those of laser photolytic deposition (LPD) and laser pyrolytic growth (LPG). The kinetics of these processes will be described while their physical properties and potential applications will be discussed.

## 2. The Applications of Silicon Oxide

Figure 1 schemes the layered structure typical of a non-volatile floating gate MOS memory device. Clearly the dominating features are the oxides and oxide based layers. The highest quality $SiO_2$ films, i.e., the tunnel and gate oxides, are grown thermally after elaborate surface preparation, and must exhibit high dielectric integrity and low interface and fixed charge content. Thermal oxides are also used for isoplanarisation which helps maintain the step coverage of, for example, metallization patterns. Field oxides provide electrical isolation between neighboring devices and since thick layers (> 0.5 μm) are required, are usually deposited to minimize processing time. The PSG overlayer protects the circuitry from physical abuse during subsequent mounting and packaging stages, and must also be rapidly deposited at low temperatures in order to minimize further diffusion of impurities within the carefully arranged lower layers. Excellent microalloyed metal contacts can be formed by heating a thin $SiO_2$ layer sandwiched between Al and Si, while thicker PSG films can be used as insulating layers between metal interconnections. The oxide layer also serves as a dielectric in MOS capacitors, and of course as a mask which provides surface protection by absorbing energetic ions during implantation, and by restraining impurity diffusion. In contrast, doped oxide layers can be used as diffusion sources in self-aligning schemes [15] which allow complementary transistors to be fabricated in a single operation. Additionally, localized oxidation techniques can form the basis of a technology where device geometries can be significantly reduced while oxide isolation techniques provide near perfect isolation between pockets of crystalline Si on an insulating substrate. The latter application has been widely adopted for the fabrication of microcircuits which must be radiation hardened, and also in special high voltage applications.

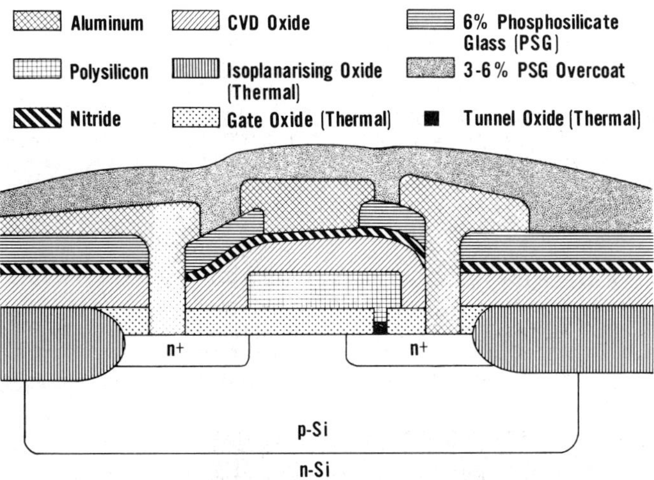


Fig. 1 Schematic representation of an MOS non-volatile memory device

As previously mentioned, oxidation can be spatially confined using lasers by reactively exciting only extremely small volumes on or near the material surface in such a way that the required patterns can be obtained directly. In contrast, it may be more desirable to achieve total coverage of particularly large areas by VLSI standards, such as complete chips or wafers, in which case much larger beam dimensions would generally be required. Laser induced etching techniques can also be combined with these oxide-forming methods as a secondary, or intermediate step toward direct pattern formation. The next section will review the various novel laser-based methods of preparing thin oxide films.

## 3. Formation of Novel Oxide Layers Using Lasers

### 3.1 Non-Silicon Oxides

It has already been extensively shown that lasers can be used to prepare a wide variety of elemental thin films and compound layers [16,17]. However, as table 1 shows, many of these laser initiated reactions involve oxidation. Extremely fine control over the temporal resolution of the laser radiation enables accurately defined film thicknesses to be grown, thereby allowing the oxidation reaction to be essentially frozen at any stage. This has become useful in studying the fundamental properties of the initial oxide formation. However, as evidenced in table 1 most of the studies are application driven. For example, semiconducting ZnO [22,23] exhibits favorable piezoelectric properties and serves as a window for visible and near IR radiation, while niobium oxides [18,19] have important applications for Josephson junction devices. $Al_2O_3$ [21] has been shown to be a better barrier against $Na^+$ contamination than $SiO_2$ in microelectronic devices, and is also used in optical waveguides. Pattern generation of $Cr_2O_3$ [24] on chromium has applications in mask-making for microelectronic circuits. Binary semiconducting compounds have suffered a restricted application in microelectronics due to problems in forming satisfactory passivating layers. Lasers now offer new approaches to growing oxides on GaAs [26,27].

The two main modes of laser oxidation are apparent from table 1. The first, and conceptionally most simple, is laser heating (LH). This can be initiated by either continuous (cw) or pulsed lasers, although in general the heating cycle is most controllable with cw beams, while melting can be most easily achieved with pulsed radiation [28]. The laser wavelength must be chosen such that sufficient absorption takes place. Heating occurs when

Table 1 A Summary of Laser Applications Toward Oxide Formation

| COMPOUND | SUBSTRATE/ SOURCE, GAS | METHOD | LASER | POSSIBLE APPLICATION | REF. |
|---|---|---|---|---|---|
| $Nb_2O_5$ $NbO_2$, NbO | Nb/$O_2$ | PLH | XeCl | Josephson Junction | [19] |
| $Nb_2O_{5-\delta}$ | Nb/$O_2$ | LPPT | $CO_2$ | " | [18] |
| CdO | Cd/Air | LH | $Kr^+$ | - | [20] |
| $CuO_2$ | Cu/Air | | | - | |
| $Al_2O_3$ | Si/TMA+$N_2O$ | LCVD | KrF, ArF | replace $SiO_2$ | [21] |
| ZnO | Si, Quartz/ DMZ+$N_2O$,$NO_2$ | LCVD | ArF, KrF | piezoelectric | [22] |
| ZnO | Si,$Al_2O_3$,Au,Ti Glass,GaAs/ZnO | LE | $CO_2$ | Solar Cell windows | [23] |
| $Cr_2O_3$ | Cr/Air | PLH | Nd:glass | microelectronics | [24] |
| $Cu_2O$ | Cu/Air | LH | $CO_2$ | - | [25] |
| $Ga_2O_3$/ $As_2O_3$ | GaAs/$O_2$ | PLM | Ruby | passivation | [26] |
| " | GaAs/$O_2$ | PLH | $Ar^+$ | passivation | [27] |
| CuO | Cu/Air | LH | $Kr^+$ | - | [65] |
| $TeO_2$ | Te/Air | | | - | |
| $In_2O_3$ InO | Quartz,InP GaAs/$O_2$ + $(CH_3)_3InP(CH_3)_3$ | LCVD | ArF | dielectric | [69] |

the absorbed energy is transferred to collective atomic vibrations, and in the presence of oxygen the reaction generally proceeds as would furnace oxidation. In this case however, the chemistry is confined to those areas of the substrate elevated to sufficiently high temperature. With a knowledge of the activation energy of the process, the heating and cycle times can be adjusted to activate the reaction on the scale of microns.

The second class of laser induced oxidation reactions involve Laser Chemical Vapour Deposition (LCVD) where all the components of the deposited layer are created in the gas phase and diffuse to a nearby substrate where they react. The reactants can be obtained from the gas-phase donor molecules in a number of ways using lasers. The technique most analogous to conventional CVD is laser pyrolysis, where the substrate is locally heated by the laser beam and the reactant atoms are liberated when the parent molecules decompose by collisional excitation with the surface. It is also possible by carefully choosing the donor molecules and the appropriate wavelength to encourage the gas to absorb resonantly the photonic energy and subsequently dissociate. Sometimes the photons are directly absorbed by an intermediate species which then de-excites by collisional transfer of the appropriate energy to the donor molecules. Such photosensitized reactions are common in photochemical studies, but are not favored for localized microchemistry due to the reaction-spreading properties intrinsic to the process. Direct photolytic techniques have been used to deposit oxide films via the following reactions (see table 1):

$$Al\,(CH_3)_3 + NO_2 + h\nu \rightarrow Al_2O_3 + \text{products} \quad (1)$$

$$Zn\,(CH_3)_2 + NO_2 + h\nu \rightarrow ZnO + \text{products} \quad (2)$$

$$Zn\,(CH_3)_2 + N_2O + h\nu \rightarrow ZnO + \text{products} \quad (3)$$

$$(CH_3)_3InP(CH_3)_3 + O_2 + h\nu \rightarrow In_2O_3 + \text{products.} \quad (4)$$

Efficient and direct energy coupling in this process have enabled growth rates greater than 2000 - 3000 A/min to be attained [21,22]. Thin films of ZnO have also been grown by laser evaporation (LE) of ZnO powder [23], while another novel technique of laser induced electrical breakdown (LPPT) promises to allow self-limiting growth of particular metallic oxide films [18]. Laser evaporated ZnO films have been shown to exhibit crystalline, optical, and electrical properties comparable to films grown by other techniques with little optimizing effort [23]. Since the power source is external to the vacuum environment and the response time for this method is essentially instantaneous, leading to flash evaporation conditions, laser evaporation in general appears to merit significant investigation as a potentially useful technique for compound film formation.

### 3.2 Silicon Oxides

Various methods involving the use of lasers as the primary energy source have been followed in recent years to prepare different oxide layers on Si (see table 2). These films have been made by, for example, implanting $O^+$ atoms into the Si lattice, and then pulse laser annealing the oxygen-enriched amorphous layer [29], or simply by annealing with either pulsed [30] or cw laser [31] any previously damaged or amorphous layer in an oxygen-rich environment. Even by deliberately melting [32] amorphizing [34] or heating [37-38] a crystalline silicon sample in air or $O_2$, such layers can readily be formed. Blum et al. [39] have recently prepared $SiO_2$ films by photo-oxidation of SiO, while deposition from the gas phase by photolytic [40,41] or pyrolytic [42] methods has also been reported. Here,

Table 2 Formation of $SiO_x$ With the Laser as the Primary Energy Source

| MATERIAL/ OXYGEN SOURCE | METHOD | WAVELENGTH | REFERENCE |
|---|---|---|---|
| $O^+$ Implanted Si | Pulse Laser Anneal | 1.06 μm | Chiang et al. [29] |
| a-Si/Air or $O_2$ | Pulse Laser Anneal | 694 nm | Garulli et al. [30] |
| a-Si/$O_2$ | cw Laser Anneal | 10.6 μm | Boyd [31] |
| c-Si/Air or $O_2$ | Pulse Laser Melting | 1.06 μm<br>530 nm | Hoh et al. [32] |
| c-Si/$O_2$ | Pulse Laser Melting | 308 nm | Orlowski et al. [33] |
| c-Si/$O_2$ | Pulse Laser Amorphization | 266 nm | Liu et al. [34] |
| c-Si/$O_2$ | cw Laser Heating | 500 nm | Gibbons [35] |
| c-Si/$O_2$ or Air | cw Laser Heating | 10.6 μm<br>500 nm | Boyd et al. [36,37,49] |
| c-Si/$O_2$ | Pulse Laser Heating | 694 nm | Cros et al. [38] |
| SiO/Air | Photo-oxidation | 193 nm | Blum et al. [39] |
| c-Si/$SiH_4$ & $N_2O$ | Pulse Laser Photodeposition | 193 nm | Boyer et al. [40,41] |
| c-Si/$SiH_4$ & $N_2O$ | cw Laser Pyrolysis | 531 nm | Szikora et al. [42] |

we will discuss the two most prolific areas of research in laser-$SiO_2$ formation, where the properties of these layers have already been studied, namely, the areas of controlled laser heating of c-Si in $O_2$, and of thin film deposition.

## A. Laser Deposited Silicon Oxides

Traditionally, silica films are grown by the pyrolytic oxidation of various alkoxysilanes, for example,tetraethylorthosilane (TEOS), or simply silane itself,via the following reactions:

$$Si\ (C_2H_5O)_4 + 12O_2 \rightarrow SiO_2 + 8CO_2 + 10H_2O \tag{5}$$

in a cold wall CVD system around 800°C, and

$$SiH_4 + 2O_2 \rightarrow SiO_2 + 2H_2O \text{ at } 600\text{-}1000°C \tag{6}$$

$$SiH_4 + O_2 \rightarrow SiO_2 + 2H_2 \text{ at } 300\text{-}500°C. \tag{7}$$

However, secondary reactions often occur during the oxidation of alkoxysilanes, and the presence of carbon, silicon monoxide, and various organic radicals, as well as water, significantly degrades the quality of the oxide layers. $SiO_2$ formation from silane is preferred at reduced temperatures for similar reasons, and has become the most commonly followed route to obtaining high quality deposited films. The reaction proceeds by the strong adsorption of oxygen on to the silicon surface where it subsequently reacts with silane to form silicon dioxide. Typical growth rates around 500-1000A/min are achieved, while the $O_2$:$SiH_4$ mole ratio should not exceed 10:1 [43]. It is also most usual to use diluted silane, commonly 5-10% by volume in argon or nitrogen. More recently, photochemical decomposition using mercury photosensitization has developed as an alternative low temperature technology for preparing similarly large area silica films using the following scheme:

$$Hg + h\nu \rightarrow Hg^* \tag{8a}$$

$$Hg^* + N_2O \rightarrow N_2 + O\ (^3P) + Hg \tag{8b}$$

$$2O + SiH_4 \rightarrow SiO_2 + 2H_2 \tag{8c}$$

and a low pressure mercury lamp as a source of incoherent UV radiation [44]. Direct photodeposition of $SiO_2$ using conventional radiation sources but eliminating the requirement for sensitization has been reported for this reaction [44], and also for the system:

$$Si_2H_6 + O_2 \rightarrow SiO_2 + \text{products.} \tag{9}$$

For the latter, enhanced growth rates (approaching 1000A/min), and an observable stability increase over thermal CVD films grown using the same gaseous system, together with a complete absence of Hg contamination [45], indicate that a promising low temperature alternative to thermochemical deposition of silica may be on hand.

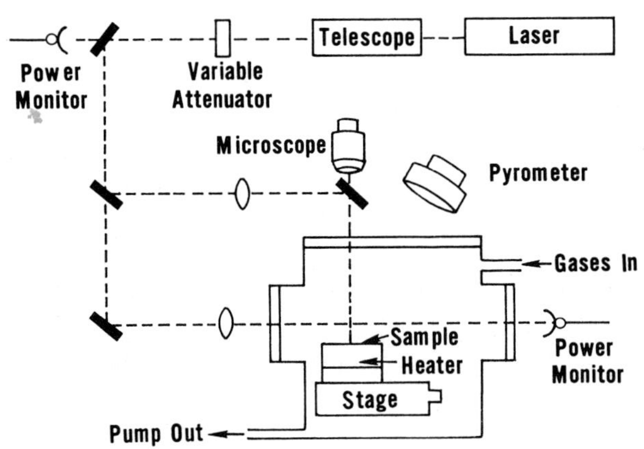


Fig. 2 Experimental configuration representing the two main modes employed for laser assisted growth of silicon oxides.

The capability of confining the reaction to a predetermined region in the reaction chamber using lasers allows much greater efficiencies and growth rates to be achieved. Fig. 2 shows a typical scheme used for laser deposition of thin oxide layers, using either a directly incident or a parallel passing beam [42,40]. Nearly stoichiometric $SiO_2$ films have been successfully grown by laser photolytic deposition at low substrate temperatures, with growth rates up to 3000A/min, using a cylindrically focused ArF laser beam parallel to and at a controlled distance above the substrate surface [42]. In this system, $SiH_4$ diluted in He or $N_2$, and $N_2O$ provided the reactant species with a $N_2O/SiH_4$ ratio >90, and an operating pressure of 8 Torr. Oxide stripes uniform to within 100A could be grown, and these were reported to be most adherent and scratch resistant when deposited at $T > 250°C$. Moreover, nitrogen contamination was low while pinhole densities, dielectric breakdown strengths and step-coverage abilities were comparable to thermally grown native oxides [41]. The localized nature of the photofragment creation just above the substrate surface provides an enormous advantage over alternative deposition methods, and furthermore, beam power, wavelength and spatial location can be varied independently of other processing parameters. The film stoichiometry and refractive index can be reproducibly maintained to essentially $SiO_2$, and 1.48 respectively (see table 3), while conformal step coverage can be achieved over a wide range of deposition conditions [41]. The dielectric strength of 1000 A thick LCVD layers has also been measured to be in the range 6.5 - 8 MV/cm; this is only slightly inferior to films deposited by conventional methods. Details of the photolytic reaction have yet to be fully explored, as have alternative variations of the operating parameters and their effects on the film properties, but this technique already appears to offer some desirable operating conditions.

Table 3 Comparison of Laser-formed Silicon Oxides

| | LASER PHOTOLYTIC DEPOSITION | LASER PYROLYTIC DEPOSITION | LASER PYROLYTIC GROWTH |
|---|---|---|---|
| Stoichiometry | $SiO_2$ | $SiO_2$ | $SiO_2$ |
| Impurities | H,N | H,N | K,Na? |
| Refractive Index | 1.48 | $1.461 \pm 0.002$ | $1.465 \pm 0.01$ |
| Breakdown Voltage [MV/cm] | 6.5 - 8 [1000A] | - | 8.3 [89A,$7\times10^{-6}$cm$^2$]<br>6.5 [>350A,$2\times10^{-3}$cm$^2$] |

Localized heating induced by an impinging cw $Kr^+$ laser beam has been shown to initiate pyrolytic decomposition of $N_2O$ and $SiH_4$ [42], with deposition rates of a-$SiO_2$ up to 2 μm/sec being achieved. These rates are three orders of magnitude faster than are currently available with those conventional oxide preparation techniques described previously. Initial studies reveal no observable inhomogeneities across the center of the silica which was typically grown in rods with diameters 50 - 100 μm, and that the films were essentially stoichiometric $SiO_2$ with a refractive index of 1.46.

## B. Laser Pyrolytic Growth

Thermal oxidation of Si has traditionally been performed under thermal equilibrium conditions provided by precisely controlled quartz tube furnaces. More recently it has been shown that cw lasers can be used as the primary heating sources for the reaction [35-37]. Additionally, when used as a secondary or auxilliary heat source lasers can locally induce an increased oxidation rate [46-48]. As will be discussed later, there is strong evidence for a non-thermal enhancement of the reaction when laser radiation of photon energy $E = h\nu$ is greater than the Si bandgap (1.12 eV). Laser oxidation basically involves the Si sample, preheated to several hundred degrees, being irradiated to a predetermined lattice temperature. In the presence of an oxygen-rich environment, the $Si(s) + O_2(g) \rightarrow SiO_2(s)$ reaction proceeds at a rate determined primarily by the surface temperature. Pyrolytic oxidation of Si by $CO_2$ and argon lasers will be discussed in this section.

Absorption of $CO_2$ laser radiation ($h\nu$= 11.7 meV) in Si is dominated by free-carrier absorption, and preheating to 400°C provides a sufficient carrier density to initiate the absorption process [49]. The lattice heats up when the excited carriers relax by phonon scattering interactions, and often the sample surface can be seen to glow dull red, orange, yellow and

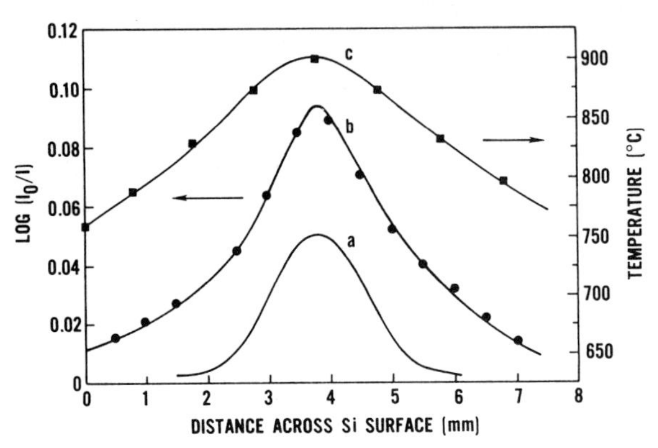


Fig. 3 Spatial profile of an oxide layer (b) grown in 90 min using a $CO_2$ laser beam (a). The calculated temperature profile is also shown (b).

brilliant yellow as the temperature increases above 700°C to the melting point at 1412°C. Fig. 3 shows a typical profile of a $CO_2$ laser grown oxide. Films up to 1800 A thick have been grown at a rate of 20 A/min. By assuming the growth rate to be totally thermally dominated, the thermal gradient induced by the laser beam can be calculated. The refractive index of these films has been measured to be 1.465 ± 0.01 for the thickness range 320-1400 A, while the spectral width of the Si-O stretching mode at 1075 $cm^{-1}$ is found to be consistently narrower than for furnace grown layers; the latter observation has been interpreted in terms of structural disorder, and that the laser grown films do not contain the more extreme bonding configurations present in furnace grown layers. It is suggested that the degree of electronic excitation during the free-carrier absorption is important in determining the specific bonding configuration of the O atoms with the Si.

Devices incorporating $CO_2$ laser grown oxide layers have been fabricated by conventional photolithographic methods [50]. An array of 10 x 10 capacitors, each 3 μm in diameter, was defined on each chip across the entire 3" wafer. Laser grown oxides were incorporated in a group of 12 neighboring arrays. Electrical breakdown measurements showed that the average dielectric strength of the first capacitor in each bank of 100 to break down was 8.3 MV $cm^{-1}$. The true dielectric strength of these films is by implication slightly higher than this value. However, it is useful to know this lower limit since devices which incorporate 100 such structures per chip will break down if only one capacitor fails. The average area under test for these measurements was $7 \times 10^{-6}$ $cm^2$. Breakdown measurements were also performed on larger area devices incorporating $2 \times 10^{-3}$ $cm^2$ of $CO_2$ laser grown oxide in the thickness range 200-1300 A. These exhibit an average dielectric breakdown, $E_{bd}$, of 6.5 MV $cm^{-1}$ for films > 350 A, revealing an areal dependence of the dielectric integrity of the films similar to thermally prepared layers.

Fig. 4 compares the known values for $E_{bd}$ for laser grown layers with the known dielectric strength of conventionally prepared films. Clearly the $SiO_2$ obtained by LCVD or LPG exhibits quite a favorable dielectric integrity, $E_{bd}$ being in general only slightly inferior to that obtained by layers produced under class 100 clean room conditions. The successful continuation of wafer-mask alignment subsequent to the laser oxidation

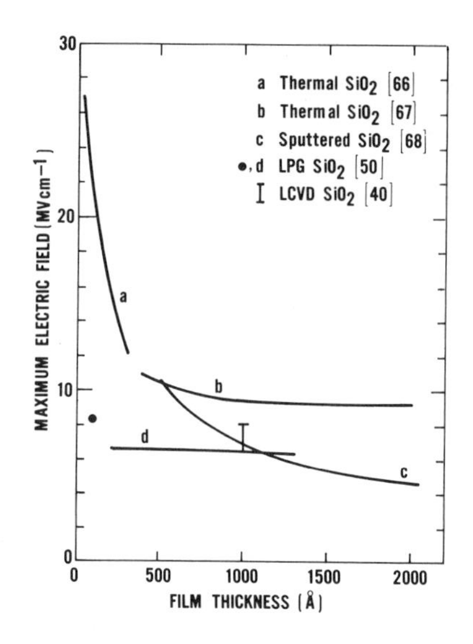


Fig. 4 Comparison of the dielectric strength of variously prepared silicon oxide layers.

process can be achieved only for a particular range of laser beam power densities [50]. It has been previously shown that processing above this operating window results in undesirable slip dislocation formation and wafer warpage, even below the melting point of the Si. However, under ideal conditions $CO_2$ laser oxidation can become an integral processing step in the manufacture of non-volatile random access memory devices, incorporating ultrathin 50 - 150 A thick oxide films [50].

Oxide growth can also be thermally activated by using shorter wavelength radiation, where the individual quanta are sufficiently energetic to promote bound carriers from the valence band across the bandgap well into the conduction band. For Si, uv (excimer laser) and visible (argon laser) radiation is strongly absorbed in this way. Again lattice heating is initiated by electron-phonon scattering. The temperature induced by a slowly scanned, strongly absorbed laser beam can be quite reasonably determined using various well established theories [51,52]. A comparison of the reported $Ar^+$ laser oxidation rates with those obtained by furnace heating (see table 4) reveals an enhancement in the former, which has been attributed to various nonthermal mechanisms [35,36,46,47,53]. Young and Tiller [48] have also confirmed the photonic effect on the oxidation rate of Si, by observing a linear dependence of the enhancement of the photon flux density and a greater enhancement for <100> than for <111> oriented crystals.

The main difficulties of isolating and interpreting the kinetics controlling the photonic role in Si oxidation are twofold. Firstly, the rise in lattice temperature associated with the redistribution of energy in the material cannot be accurately measured. Although several theoretical studies of the expected temperature rise in Si irradiated with cw argon laser radiation have been published, there lacks an absolute agreement between each set of data. In order to determine the degree of photon enhancement, one is required to know the lattice temperature very accurately, certainly well within 10%. For example, a 5% change in temperature, from 1000 to 1050°C, results in an increase of some 75% in the oxidation rate. Nevertheless, within the framework of the laser heating

Table 4 Summary of cw argon laser induced oxidation rates for Si. The increased lattice temperatures and associated thermal oxidation rates were determined using previously published theory [52] and oxidation data in the given references. The oxidation rates (A), (B), and (C) are those rates attributed to the original lattice temperature, the laser induced increase in lattice temperature, and the observed oxidation rate, respectively.

| LATTICE TEMPERATURE Original/Increased [°C] | LASER BEAM PARAMETERS [W/mm] | OXIDATION RATE (A)/(B)/(C) [A/min] | PHOTON ENHANCEMENT [%] | REF. |
|---|---|---|---|---|
| 900/910 | 1.1 | 2.5/2.9/3.2 | 10 | [48] |
| 900/923 | 2.4 | 2.25/3.1/3.3 | 7 | [47] |
| 880/902 | | 1.85/2.4/2.8 | 17 | |
| 810/831 | | 0.75/0.95/1.05 | 11 | |
| 770/790 | | 0.36/0.49/0.56 | 14 | |
| 820/841 | 2.4 | 0.65/1.06/1.29 | 22 | [46] |
| 400/866 | 6.4 | $10^{-5}$/2.3/11 | x4.8 | [53] |
| 400/977 | 7.8 | $10^{-5}$/9.8/22 | x2.2 | |

theories it has been established that cw argon laser oxidation is thermally dominated. It also seems that once the thermal contribution has been accounted for, the photon enhancement is only a secondary process within the reaction (see table 4). Nevertheless, it can be seen that using these particular laser techniques, oxidation can be encouraged to proceed at rates more typical of higher lattice temperatures.

A further complication in determining the kinetics controlling the photon-enhanced oxidation process lies in the basic lack of understanding and general controversy regarding the mechanism of conventional thermal oxidation. Traditionally, the Deal-Grove model, based on Fickian diffusion of neutral oxygen through the growing oxide to the $Si/SiO_2$ interface, followed by a first-order chemical reaction [54], has been satisfactorily used for steam oxidation, and for the latter stages of dry oxidation. This linear-parabolic rate law, however, is inadequate in its original form for describing the faster initial stages of the Si + $O_2$ interaction. Several modifications and alternatives to this model have recently been proposed. Revesz and Evans [55] and later Irene [56] postulated that normal diffusion may be short-circuited by fast diffusion through microchannels close to the $Si/SiO_2$ interface, while Grove [57] and Tiller [58] believed that an electric field in the layer could promote the diffusion of an ionic oxidizing species, perhaps $O_2^-$. In contrast, Fargeix et al. [59] proposed that diffusion through the first few hundreds of A of the oxide layer is much slower than in the rest of the film because of the compressive stress near the interface. Lora-Tamayo et al. [60] have specifically considered the influence of both $O_2^-$ and $O^-$ on the overall reaction. Ghez and Van der Meulen [61] introduced the idea of dual process of direct oxidation by oxygen molecules as well as indirect oxidation by oxygen atoms, while Blanc [62] suggested that molecular oxygen dissociates into atomic oxygen and maintains a local equilibrium at the reacting interface before bonding to the silicon. Hu [63] has recently extended the Deal-Grove and Blanc models to a more generalized form incorporating the pressure dependence of the chemisorption of molecular oxygen, and has proposed yet another ionic species, $O^-$, as a parallel oxidant to $O_2$.

The laser now presents a set of processing parameters never previously achievable in the field of oxidation of Si. The presence of a large photon flux has already been shown to modify the reaction rate of the process but the precise mechanism of photonic oxidation is not yet fully formulated. For example, the importance of the increased density of conduction band electrons in the absorbing Si has been discussed by several groups [36,46,53]. It has also been suggested that electronic transfer from the conduction band of the Si via the $SiO_2$ conduction band to an $O_2$ molecule diffusing from the gas phase creates an $O_2^-$ species which may become important, or more important in the overall reaction [64,47]. It must be noted however that this should become important only for photon energies $h\nu>3.2$ eV, the barrier height between the Si and $SiO_2$ conduction bands. At present, therefore, the photonic effect on the silicon oxidation reaction has not yet been satisfactorily incorporated within the context of a generally accepted model for the $Si+O_2$ reaction. Since this reaction is presently one of the most widely studied in the scientific field, it may not be long before such a system is adequately modelled. In addition to the aforementioned cw laser applications toward oxide growth enhancement, a 30x enhancement in Si oxidation has been found using pulsed uv laser heating [33]. Although the bulk of this increased rate may be due to localized melting of the surface, this presents a new regime of oxidation clearly not yet fully explored. Interestingly, optically enhanced oxidation of other semiconductors has also been reported recently [26,27,46]. Other novel developments, including twin-beam oxidation [49], where an argon laser promotes an excess of free carriers in the conduction band such that $CO_2$ laser radiation can be absorbed with an effective absorption coefficient greater than $10^4$ $cm^{-1}$, offer the possibility for improved localization and greater control of the heating process.

## 4. Conclusions

Clearly this field has highlighted several important processing conditions potentially useful for semiconductor manufacturing. Indeed, laser activated local micro-fabrication presently allows a wide range of high quality oxide layers to be prepared more efficiently and usually at a faster rate than previously available. These new areas of rapid melting and solidification, flash evaporation, and pulsed-plasma chemistry seem certain to bring about whole new fields of thin film formation in general, rather than remaining only oxide preparation techniques. In the field of Si oxidation, lasers now enable deposition rates of 2 $\mu$m/sec to be achieved, while cw laser heating with visible radiation allows increased oxidation rates to be obtained for lower lattice temperatures. Initial studies on the structural, optical and electronic characteristics for the laser grown layers reveal properties quite comparable to those of conventionally prepared layers. A continuing effort in these areas is bound to provide most fruitful gains in the understanding of gas/surface interactions, and for future applications toward VLSI devices.

## 5. Acknowledgements

I would like to thank my colleagues at Heriot-Watt University, Hughes Microelectronics Ltd., and North Texas State University for their invaluable assistance. In particular, I acknowledge rewarding collaboration with Prof. S. D. Smith, J. I. B. Wilson, M. J. Colles, T. D. Binnie, and J. L. West.

## 6. References

1. S. T. Pantelides, "The Physics of $SiO_2$ and Its Interfaces" (Pergamon, New York 1978) and references therein.

2. B. E. Deal in "Semiconductor Silicon",eds. H. R. Huff, E. Sirtl (Electrochem. Soc., Princeton, 1977), p. 276.
3. P.A. Bertrand, P.D. Fleischauer, J. Vac. Sci. Tech., B1, 832 (1983).
4. G. W. Anderson, W. A. Schmidt, J. Comas, see ref. 1, p. 200.
5. N. Goldsmith, W. Kern, RCA Rev., 28, 153 (1967).
6. L. I. Maissel, in "Handbook of Thin Film Technology," eds. L. I. Maissel, R. Glang (McGraw-Hill, NY 1970) Ch. 4; J. L. Vossen, 1971, J. Vac. Sci. Technol., 8, 512 (1971).
7. W. A. Pliskin, R. A. Gdula, in "Handbook on Semiconductors," ed. T. S. Moss, 3, Ch. 11 (1982).
8. K. Urbanek, Solid State Tech. 20 (4), 87 (1977).
9. See for example S. Dzioba, G. Este, H. M. Naguib, J. Electrochem. Soc., 129, 2537 (1982), and references therein.
10. V. Q. Ho, Jpn. J. Appl. Phys. Suppl., 1, 19, 103 (1983).
11. T. Tokuyama, these proceedings.
12. J. R. Ligenza, W. G. Spicer, J. Phys. Chem. Solids, 14, 132 (1960).
13. R. J. Zeto, N. O. Korolkoff, S. Marshall, Solid State Technology, 22 (7), 62 (1979).
14. H. Gilgen, C. J. Chen, R. Krchnavek, R. M. Osgood, these proceedings.
15. W.M. Cosney, L.H. Hall, IEEE Trans. Electron. Dev., ED-20, 469 (1973).
16. "Laser Diagnostics and Photochemical Processing for Semiconductor Devices", eds. R. M. Osgood, S. R. J. Brueck, H. R. Schlossberg, (North-Holland, New York, 1983), and references therein.
17. D. J. Ehrlich, J. Y. Tsao, J. Vac. Sci. Technol., B1, 969, (1983).
18. R. F. Marks, R. A. Pollak, Ph. Avouris, in ref. 16, p. 257.
19. R. F. Marks, R. A. Pollak (unpublished), see ref. 18.
20. M. Wautelet, L. Baufay, Thin Solid Films, 100, L9 (1983).
21. R. Solanki, W.Ritchie, G.J. Collins, Appl. Phys. Lett. 43, 454 (1983).
22. R. Solanki, G. J. Collins, Appl. Phys. Lett., 42, 662 (1983).
23. H. Sankur, J. T. Cheung, J. Vac. Sci. Technol., A1, 1806 (1983).
24. S. M. Metev, S. K. Savtchenko, K. Stamenov, J. Phys. D13, L75 (1980).
25. I. Ursu, L. C. Nistor, V. S. Teodorescu, I. N. Mihailescu, I. Apostol, L. Nanu, A. M. Prokhorov, N. I. Chapliev, V. I. Konov, V. N. Tokarev, V. G. Ralchenko, SPIE Ind. Appl. of Lasers, V398, paper 398-69 (1983).
26. M. Matsuura, M. Ishida, A. Suzuki, K. Hara, Japan J. Appl. Phys., 20, L726, (1981).
27. W. G. Petro, I. Hino, S. Eglash, I. Lindau, C. Y. Su, W. E. Spicer, J. Vac. Sci. Technol., 21, 405 (1982).
28. Ian W. Boyd, Contemporary Physics, 24, 461 (1983).
29. S.W. Chiang, Y.S. Liu, R.F. Reihl, Appl. Phys. Lett., 39, 752 (1981).
30. A. Garulli, M. Servidori, I. Vecchi, J. Phys. D, 13, L199 (1981).
31. I. W. Boyd, Appl. Phys., A31, 71 (1983).
32. K. Hoh, H.Koyama, K.Uda, Y. Miura, Japan J.Appl.Phys, 19, L375 (1980).
33. T. E. Orlowski and H. Richter, in "Laser-Controlled Chemical Processing of Surfaces," eds. A. W. Johnson, D. J. Ehrlich (North-Holland, New York, 1984).
34. Y. S. Liu S. W. Chiang, F. Bacon, Appl. Phys. Lett., 38, 1005, (1981).
35. J. F. Gibbons, Japan. J. Appl. Phys. Suppl. 19, 121, (1981).
36. I.W. Boyd, J.I.B. Wilson, J.L. West, Thin Solid Films, 83 L173 (1981).
37. I. W. Boyd, J. I. B. Wilson, Appl. Phys. Letts. 41, 162, (1982).
38. A. Cros, F. Salvan, J. Derrien, Appl. Phys., A28, 241 (1982).
39. S.E. Blum, K. Brown, R. Srinivasan, Appl.Phys.Lett., 43, 1026 (1983).
40. P. K. Boyer, G. A. Roche, W. H. Ritchie, G. J. Collins, Appl. Phys. Lett., 40, 716 (1982).
41. P.K. Boyer, W. H. Ritchie, G. J. Collins, J. Electrochem. Soc., 129, 2155 (1982).
42. S. Szikora, W. Kräuter, D. Bäuerle, Materials Letters, 2,263 (1984).
43. B. J. Baliga, S. K. Ghandi, J. Appl. Phys., 44, 990 (1973).

44. J. W. Peters, Technical Digest of the International Electron Devices Meeting, (1981), p. 240.
45. Y. Mishima, M.Hirose, Y.Osaka, Y.Ashida, J.Appl.Phys. 55, 1234 (1984).
46. S. A. Schafer and S. A. Lyon, J. Vac. Sci. Technol., 19, 494 (1981).
47. S. A. Schafer and S. A. Lyon, J. Vac. Sci. Technol., 21, 422 (1982).
48. E. M. Young and W. A. Tiller, Appl. Phys. Lett., 42, 63 (1983).
49. I. W. Boyd, T. D. Binnie, J. I. B. Wilson, M. J. Colles, J. Appl. Phys., 55, 3061 (1984), and references therein.
50. I. W. Boyd, J. Appl. Phys. 54, 3561 (1983).
51. F. Ferrieu, G. Auvert, J. Appl. Phys., 54, 2646 (1983), and references therein.
52. I. W. Boyd, in "Surface Studies with Lasers," eds. F. R. Aussenegg, A. Leitner, M. E. Lippitsch (Springer Berlin, 1983).
53. I. W. Boyd, Appl. Phys. Lett., 42, 728 (1983).
54. B. E. Deal, A. S. Grove, J. Appl. Phys. 36, 3770 (1965).
55. A. G. Revesz, R. J. Evans, J. Phys. Chem. Solids, 30, 551 (1969).
56. E. A. Irene, J. Appl. Phys. 54, 5416 (1983).
57. A. S. Grove, "Physics and Technology of Semiconductor Devices," (Wiley, New York, 1967).
58. W. A. Tiller, J. Electrochem. Soc., 127, 625 (1980).
59. A. Fargeix, G. Ghibaudo, G. Kamarinos, J. Appl. Phys. 54, 2878 (1983).
60. A. Lora-Tamayo, E. Dominguez, E. Lora-Tamayo, J. LLabres, Appl. Phys. 17, 79 (1978).
61. R. Ghez, Y. J. van der Meulen, J. Electrochem. Soc., 119, 1100 (1972).
62. J. Blanc, Appl. Phys. Lett., 33, 424 (1978).
63. S. M. Hu, Appl. Phys. Lett., 42, 872 (1983).
64. A. Goodman, Phys. Rev., 152, 785 (1966).
65. M. Wautelet, Materials Letters, 2, 20 (1984).
66. E. Harari, J. Appl. Phys. 49, 2478 (1978).
67. C. M. Osburn, D. W. Ormond, J. Electrochem. Soc., 119, 591 (1972).
68. I. H. Pratt, S. S. Technol, 12 (12), 49 (1969).
69. V. M. Donnelly, M. Geva, J. Long, R. F. Karlicek, Appl. Phys. Lett., 44, 951 (1984).

# Laser-Induced Oxidation of Silicon Surfaces

T. Tokuyama, S. Kimura, T. Warabisako, E. Murakami, and K. Miyake
Central Research Laboratory, Hitachi Ltd.
Kokubunji-shi, Tokyo 185, Japan

The difference between reaction mechanisms in laser and plasma assisted silicon oxidation is discussed. Photonic rather than thermal aspects of laser irradiation are seen to be important when lasers are used as a means to lower oxidation temperature. Although laser photonic oxidation enhancement occurs with an increase in the supply of free Si atoms to the $Si-SiO_2$ interface, it is difficult to utilize this phenomenon in practical processes because the oxidation reaction is limited in the case of thick oxide structures by the supply of the oxidizing species rather than silicon atoms. Enhanced oxidation in the plasma ambient is caused by the existence of oxidizing species which are excited in the plasma though not involved in the thermal oxidation ambient.

An attempt to combine both plasma and laser assistance features is described, and experimental results are discussed. An at most 60% $SiO_2$ thickness increase was observed when a $CO_2$ laser was irradiated on to the surface of the silicon in a newly developed microwave-excited oxygen plasma ambient. Properties of the $SiO_2$ and $Si-SiO_2$ interface prepared by this method are also discussed.

## 1. Introduction

Thin insulator films, especially silicon dioxide ($SiO_2$) films, are now recognized as one of the key material components of silicon VLSI devices. Such thin films are used as device isolation and metallization insulators and surface passivation coatings (passive structure element), as well as MOSFET gate insulators or memory-cell charge storage capacitor insulators (active device element). These films are also utilized during device fabrication as masks for impurity doping, materials deposition and etching.

The technology of $SiO_2$ film formation is now well established, whether it be by means of direct thermal oxidation of silicon surfaces, or through physical or chemical vapor deposition. However, when development of future high-density and high-speed VLSI devices is considered, these technologies will no longer play an important role. Instead, the relative weight of certain novel $SiO_2$ formation methods now beginning to be seriously exploited will increase. The aims of these novel techniques are: (1) a lowering of $SiO_2$ formation temperature; (2) improvement of low temperature processed $Si-SiO_2$ interface properties; and (3) formation of very thin, perfect $SiO_2$ films.

Lowering of the processing temperature is a natural consequence when one considers precise control of impurity profiles and minimization of process-induced defects, which are vital to the development of sub-micrometer VLSIs. In the fabrication of three-dimensional LSIs, this trend becomes particularly important since fabrication of upper layer devices must be carried out without causing any effect upon the properties of the already-processed lower layer devices.

Through use of physical or chemical vapor deposition procedures or photochemical reactions, $SiO_2$ films are now being formed at reasonably low process temperatures. However, Si-$SiO_2$ interface properties with preparation using these processes are usually not sufficient for application to active device layer fabrication. Neither the physical nor chemical properties of films thus prepared are comparable to those for high-temperature oxidized films. Existence of defects which lower the breakdown voltage, and inclusion of impurities at the film-substrate interface are typical problems associated with these low-temperature-deposited films.

A high-pressure oxygen atmosphere is known to be effective in lowering the oxidation temperature[1]. However, considering the operational safety of an oxidizing furnace, the practical limit to this oxygen pressure is on the order of 10 atm. In this range, the lower limit for obtaining reasonably thick $SiO_2$ film is thus thought to be around 800°C.

Another possible way to lower the oxidizing temperature is to use an oxygen plasma atmosphere[2]-[4]. An increase in the concentration of the oxidizing species and enhancement of the flow of these species with the application of an electric field to the substrate surface have made it possible with low temperature oxidation in a plasma atmosphere to obtain an $\approx 10^2$ times faster reaction speed than with conventional high-temperature dry oxygen oxidation. The difference in the oxidation reaction mechanisms between these two oxidizing processes is another reason for expecting realization of low temperature processes. On the contrary, the electrical properties of plasma-oxidized Si-$SiO_2$ structures are not good enough for active device layer applications. This is mainly due to in-process generation of damage layers by the incidence of energetic charged particles onto the surface.

Laser assisted oxidation[5]-[9] is another new process which has recently attracted much interest. However, oxidation reaction enhancement is not to be expected when a laser is used only as a means to heat the localized substrate surface. However, visible or shorter wavelength irradiations at much lower intensities can cause direct enhancement of the oxidation reaction [10]. The mechanism is thought to involve increase in the supply of free silicon atoms at Si-$SiO_2$ interface through the breaking of Si-Si bonds with absorption of irradiation[9]. However, in the Deal-Grove oxidation model[11], as well as from experimental results with conventional oxygen atmosphere reactions, the reaction rate is limited by the supply of oxidizing species flow through the $SiO_2$ layer. Thus, a simple combination of an oxygen atmosphere and laser irradiation would probably not be effective.

The present paper describes the equipment and process results for combination of a newly developed plasma oxidation [12] with a $CO_2$-laser irradiation method.

## 2. Effects of Laser Irradiation upon Oxidation Reactions

Oren and Ghandhi[10] first reported enhancement of silicon oxidation with irradiation of UV light onto a silicon surface in high-temperature oxygen atmosphere in 1971. In this report, nearly a 10% reaction rate enhancement at 955 - 1215°C temperatures was observed. They attributed this to a photonic effect, although the detailed description of the irradiation light intensity of the UV source was missing. In addition, some improvements in Si-$SiO_2$

interface properties, and similarities of oxidation reaction mechanisms to the conventional process were also reported.

During the course of laser annealing studies in the early 80's, formation of thin $SiO_2$ films or inclusion of oxygen atoms in surface layers were noticed when the silicon surface was irradiated by a high power pulse laser in oxygen or air ambients[13][14]. Depending on the laser irradiation conditions, surface amorphization or oxygen segregation phenomena associated with the rapid cooling period were also reported.

A 10nm $SiO_2$ layer can be formed in an order of a second if the conventional dry oxygen oxidation rate is extrapolated to the melting temperature of silicon. Accordingly, under one pulse irradiation of a laser (1 - 100 ns order pulse length), it would be almost impossible to grow a practical thickness oxide, even though considerable photonic enhancement can exist.

Studies of oxidation reaction enhancement were accelerated after longer time irradiation using CW or free running pulse lasers became possible. Long time laser irradiation effects can now be considered to have both thermal and photonic aspects. The thermal effect is naturally dominant when laser irradiation power density is high. When irradiation conditions are similar to the laser annealing conditions, the silicon substrate surface can be heated and oxidized in the oxygen atmosphere using an Ar CW laser[15][16]. Some specific applications such as localized oxidation may be expected when a laser beam is focused on to a small spot. None the less, oxidation enhancement is usually difficult to observe in this type of experiment.

Infrared $CO_2$ laser irradiation was also used to heat silicon substrates by means of a free carrier absorption mechanism, and oxidation experiments have been reported[7][8]. In infrared absorption measurements of a $CO_2$ laser oxidized $SiO_2$ layer, it was reported that a more defect-less structure was obtained than with a conventional thermal (furnace) oxidation process.

In these experiments in which thermal aspects of the laser irradiation effect was stressed, there is also the possibility of photonic oxidation enhancement such as with a breaking of the Si-Si bond through the absorption of a Ar CW laser irradiation. Moreover, in the case of $CO_2$ laser irradiation, the Si-O streching vibration frequency of the grown $SiO_2$ layer is close to the incident laser wavelength. Thus, the existence of some specific effects besides merely thermal ones may be expected. No detailed studies have yet been reported, though.

Definite separation of a photonic and thermal effect was first reported by Schafer and Lyon in 1981[6]. In their experiments, Si wafers were set in a 820°C heated furnace in oxygen ambients, and Ar CW laser light with an intensity of 60 W/cm$^2$ was irradiated onto the wafer surface. Growth of oxide was investigated, and the difference of oxide thickness between cases with and without laser light incidence was observed. The intensity of laser light was low enough, and the temperature rise due to the incidence of laser was estimated to be 25°C at most. Enhancement of the oxidation rate was 60%, where 40% was estimated to be due to pure photonic non-thermal effect.

In 1983, Young and Tiller [5] reported similar results though in more detail. They pointed out that oxidation rate enhancement changed with wafer orientation ( (100) > (111) ), and was proportional to the incident laser intensity. They also found that the enhancement ratio was proportional to the incident photon flux at a 460 - 514 nm wavelength range.

Using an Ar CW laser, Boyd discussed also in 1983[9] oxide growth rate as a function of growth temperature, after temperature rise due to laser irradiation was corrected. The enhancement ratio was found to be large at a low growth temperature. This was interpreted by the equation;

$$g_{LP} = g_{th} \left[\frac{n_i + n_L}{n_i}\right]^2 \equiv f_e \, g_{th}. \quad (1)$$

Here, $g_{th}$ and $g_{LP}$ show the oxidation rate due to purely thermal and laser photonic conditions, $n_i$ is the intrinsic carrier density at the oxidation temperature, and $n_L$ is the laser generated carrier density at the silicon surface. Experimental points were found between the $g_{th}$ and $g_{LP}$ curves.

This model is based on the assumption that a supply of free silicon atoms at the Si-$SiO_2$ interface determines the rate of oxidation (Blanc, 1978[17]), and thus $f_e$ becomes large in the $n_i < n_L$ range (that is, at lower growth temperatures). However, the model is considered not to be effective when a thick $SiO_2$ layer covers the surface of silicon, since in that case, it is already known that oxidizing species supplied through the $SiO_2$ layer to the Si-$SiO_2$ interface limit the oxidation reaction rate. Therefore, Eq.(1) is valid only for a thin $SiO_2$ case, i.e. in early stages of the oxidation reaction.

The other possibility for enhancement of the oxidation reaction in a thick $SiO_2$ structure is to select the oxidizing species, and to control supply through the $SiO_2$ layer to the silicon surface. In an oxygen plasma ambient, for example, new kinds of oxidizing species other than those species effective in conventional dry oxygen thermal oxidation cases are considered to be generated. As a result, a fast enough oxidation rate at low growth temperature is commonly seen. It is thus important to consider whether laser irradiation is effective in generating new oxidizing species, or in modifying the transport mechanism through the $SiO_2$.

The possibility of ionization of oxygen molecules by UV light irradiation was eliminated by Oren and Ghandi[10]. Dissociation of oxygen molecules to atoms (requiring more than 5eV energy) is generally difficult with infrared to visible wavelength laser irradiation. Thus, the next step is naturally to implement laser irradiation simultaneously with a plasma ambient. When modulation of the oxidizing species transport mechanism through the $SiO_2$, or when enhancement of reaction rate between silicon and those oxidizing species occurs during laser and plasma ambients, a higher oxidation rate can be expected than in the plasma or laser single process case. At the same time, a new concept regarding plasma formation is necessary to ensure excluding of damage at the silicon surface before such a complex process can be used for a practical low temperature oxide formation.

## 3. Oxidation of Silicon in Oxygen Plasma, and Laser Irradiation Effect

### 3.1 Plasma oxidation and related problems

A so-called oxygen plasma atmosphere is generated with application of an external electric field to low-pressure oxygen gas. Here, various excitation processes resulting from the collision of accelerated electrons with oxygen molecules are involved. Excitation reactions include: (1) dissociation of oxygen molecules into atomic states via various excitation states; (2) positive ion species generation (ionization); (3) negative ion species generation (low energy electron attachment); and (4) interactions between these species. Plasma oxidation utilizes these excited species as oxidizing species. Considerable oxidation rate acceleration compared with the thermal process case can be observed.

In early stages of investigation, species acting as oxidizers were considered to be negative oxygen ions[18]. Experimental results regarding oxidation reaction acceleration obtained as a result of applying a positive electric field to the silicon surface (plasma anodization) gave rise to this idea [3] [19]. Recently, however, through experiments that separate the effects of electrons from negative ions, it is clarified that oxidation enhancement occurs only when electrons with some sort of oxidizing species arrive at the silicon surface. In one experimental arrangement whereby among negative charged particles only electrons arrive at the surface (Olive et al. 1972 [20]) oxidation enhancement does not decrease too much. On the contrary, when only negative ions are incident upon the surface, the oxidation rate becomes very small (Gourrier et al. (1981)[21].

In the case of Al (aluminium) anodic plasma oxidation, the oxidation rate increased where total electron current to the surface was maximum[22]. This was interpreted to mean that rather than because of high-energy ( >5eV) electrons which may generate $O^-$ ions from surface absorbed oxygen molecules, instead, slow speed electrons which may generate $O^-$ ions through attachment to surface absorbed oxygen atoms contributed to the oxidation reaction.

This type of mechanism has not yet been seen in the silicon case, however. Thus, efforts to find really effective oxidizing species should be expended in the future. At the same time, development of a plasma apparatus which efficiently generates effective species or clarification of the optimum operating conditions for achieving abundant quantities for such species are also important.

Since the oxidizing species and their quantities are very much dependent upon the experimental apparatus, oxide growth speeds reported so far using plasma oxidation tend to differ from each other. In Fig. 1, various $SiO_2$ growth speeds in plasma oxidation arrangements are replotted from the literature. Data from Ho et al. [2], and Ligenza [3] were obtained using a bias-applied anodization system, while those from Ray and Reisman [4] were obtained using a non-bias system (plasma was introduced into a quartz tube in a furnace).

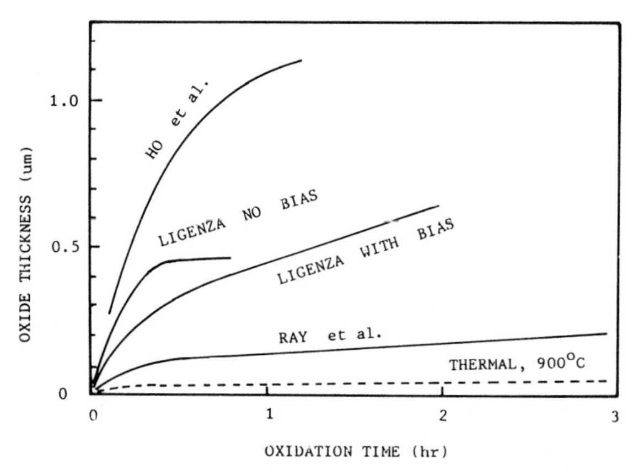


Fig.1. $SiO_2$ growth curve for various plasma oxidation systems. Data from Ho et al.[2], Ligenza[3], and Ray et al.[4]. Thermal oxidation curve estimated from data of Burger et al.[25]

Because of the difference in discharge method, oxygen pressure and discharge power are characteristic for each experiment. Futhermore, small amounts of impurity gas species such as nitrogen are known to affect greatly the in-plasma excitation processes. Therefore, variations in the growth speed can be thought as being reasonable. Nevertheless, if 900°C thermal oxidation growth speed data shown in the graph are compared, a large enhancement in the growth thickness is noticed among all plasma case data. It was also noted that in non-bias schemes, $SiO_2$ thickness shows saturation with processing time.

### 3.2 Plasma oxidation with a microwave-plasma stream system

The electrical qualities of $SiO_2$ film as well as Si-$SiO_2$ interfaces prepared by the plasma oxidation processes discussed in the preceding section are not good enough for recent MOS device gate insulator applications. The principal reasons for this are insufficiency in contamination control, and radiation damage of the silicon surface resulting during oxide formation. Charge density value at the Si-$SiO_2$ interface,for example, need sufficient annealing before actual device component use becomes possible.

We have developed a new plasma oxidation system which is characterized by a high density plasma source involving a microwave field with ECR (Electron Cyclotron Resonance) scheme, and a contamination-free reaction chamber [12]. The purpose of this design is to realize a clean ambient and sufficiently ample oxidizing species without use of an electric field. A non-bias scheme was selected in order to eliminate damage introduction to the surface. The plasma source and oxidation chamber were separated, and oxygen plasma was transported between them by means of magnetic confinement so as to prevent plasma from touching the chamber wall.

Figure 2 is a schematic view of the system. 2.45 GHz microwave power is introduced into a 100 mm diameter quartz tube through use of an isolator and a power monitor. A set of three magnetic coils for the ECR field and a fourth

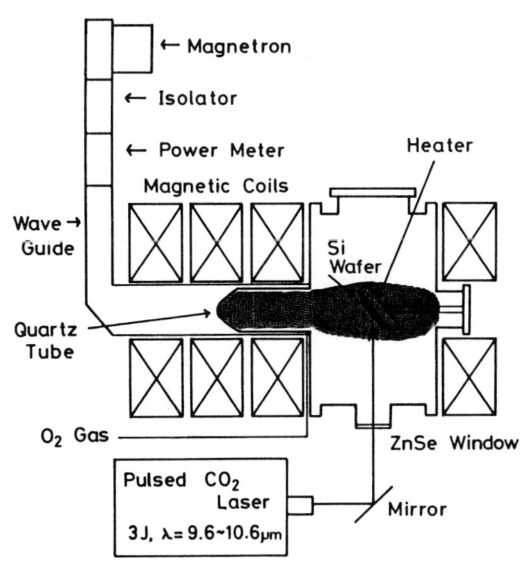


Fig.2. Schematic diagram of microwave excited oxygen plasma system with $CO_2$-laser irradiation arrangement

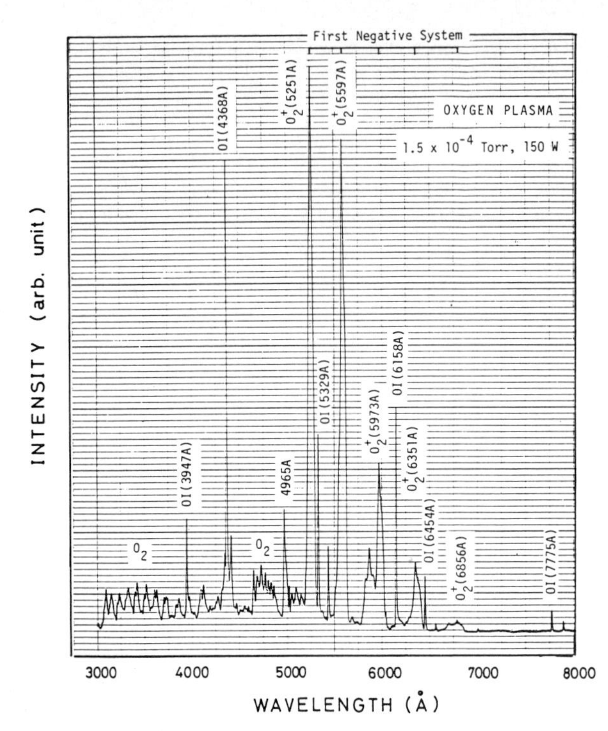


Fig.3. Optical emission spectrum from oxygen plasma

coil for confinement of plasma flow are positioned as shown in the figure. A silicon wafer is mounted on the quartz jig (electrically floated) and is heated from the back by halogen lamps. A tunable pulsed $CO_2$ laser is installed to irradiate silicon surface. Maximum power output is 3 J per pulse (0.05 - 5 μs duration), and maximum pulse repetition is 10 pps. Beam spot size is roughly 15 mm x 10 mm. Reaction chamber back pressure is $1 \times 10^{-8}$ Torr.

The optical emission spectrum in the visible range from the oxygen plasma is shown in Fig. 3. The peaks of OI shown in the figure indicate existence of excited atomic oxygen. Existence of $O_2$ molecule ions was also confirmed. Atomic ion species, however, were not found. Both OI and $O_2^+$ related emission reached maximum value at an oxygen pressure of $2 \times 10^{-4}$ Torr. In the lower pressure range, emission from $O_2^+$ (related to higher energy electrons in the plasma) increased, while in the higher oxygen pressure range an increase of emission from atomic oxygen (related to lower energy electrons) could be seen.

The $SiO_2$ growth curve is shown in Fig. 4. Compared with the extrapolated $SiO_2$ thickness to be obtained with 700°C thermal oxidation, 30 times thicker film is obtained at 640°C with the present plasma oxidation.

According to the Deal-Grove model[11] for silicon oxidation, the relation between oxide thickness, x, and oxidation time, t, can be expressed as the linear-parabolic law:

$$t - \tau = \frac{B}{A} x + \frac{1}{B} x^2 \quad . \qquad (2)$$

Here, A, B and τ are the constants. When data from Fig. 4 are fitted to eq.

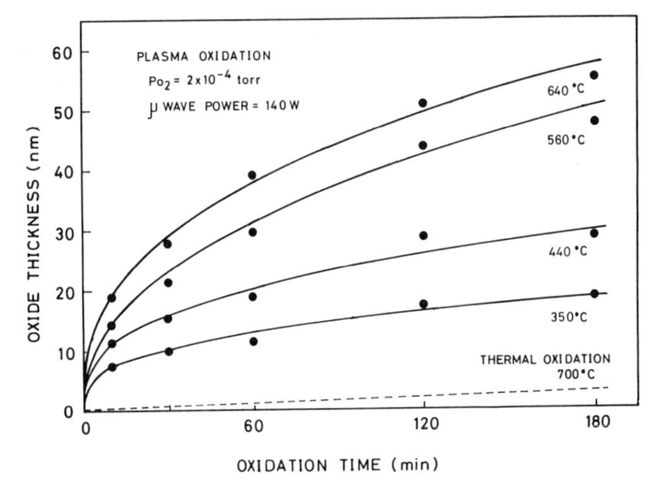


Fig.4. $SiO_2$ growth curve for microwave-excited plasma system

(2), B/A becomes negative for all curves. Furthermore, the slope of the log t - log x plot for Fig. 4 exceeds 2 in all cases. These facts imply that it is difficult to explain the reaction mechanism for the present plasma oxidation using the D-G model. Even with conventional dry oxygen thermal oxidation, some results have been reported that do not follow D-G model especially during early stages of oxidation reaction[23].

On the other hand, Cabrera and Mott[24] explained the oxidation reaction by means of the flow of silicon ions through $SiO_2$ film. They pointed out that this is accelerated by the electric field developed across $SiO_2$, which is in turn caused by the electron flow from silicon to $SiO_2$ surface absorbed oxygen. According to the C-M model, the relation between x and t can be expressed as

$$\frac{dx}{dt} = 2u\sinh\left(\frac{x_1}{x}\right), \tag{3}$$

with u and $x_1$ as constants. Using values of $x_1$ = 20 - 38 nm and u = (1.6 - 15.6) x $10^{-2}$ nm/s, the data shown in Fig. 4 fit Eq. (3) with good accuracy. The activation energy of u is determined as 0.4 eV, which is very small compared with 1.2 eV for dry oxygen thermal oxidation, where oxidizing species diffusion through the $SiO_2$ layer limits the oxidation rate.

Radioactive tracer experiment was carried out in order to clarify the plasma oxidation mechanism. The depth distribution for $O^{16}$ and $O^{18}$ in the $SiO_2$ layer was measured for samples prepared by switching the plasma ambient from $O^{16}$ to $O^{16}$ + $O^{18}$ (20%) during oxide formation. The $O^{18}/O^{16}$ concentration ratio is nearly constant from the surface to the Si-$SiO_2$ interface. Accordingly, oxidizing species flowing through the $SiO_2$ layer is more likely as the reaction mechanism than silicon atom (ions) flowing.

Considering these experimental results, moving species in the $SiO_2$ in the present plasma oxidation are thought to be $O^-$ ions. In the plasma ambient compared with the dry oxygen thermal reaction ambient, the concentration of atomic oxygen or $O^-$ ions is very high. Generation of $O^-$ ions at the surface of the $SiO_2$ layer by the low energy electron attachment to the absorbed oxygen atoms is also considered.

### 3.3 Laser irradiation effects

Effects of $CO_2$-laser irradiation on $SiO_2$ growth during plasma oxidation are shown in Fig. 5. At most, a 60% $SiO_2$ thickness increase was observed at 450°C after 1.5 hr. $SiO_2$ thickness increases with an increase of laser pulse repetition at the same irradiation power. When this 60% increase is estimated as merely originating from the temperature rise caused by laser irradiation, 140°C is obtained. Since, however, measured laser power density is on the order of 1 $J/cm^2$·pulse, (and pulse repetition of max. 10 pps) it is rather difficult to attribute this growth enhancement directly to the heating of Si substrate by irradiation.

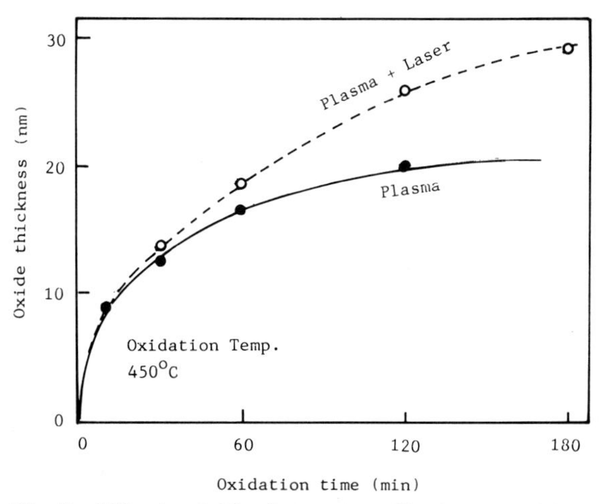


Fig.5. Effect of $CO_2$-laser irradiation on $SiO_2$ growth curve during plasma oxidation

The results of the following experiment also support the existence of a non-thermal effect. A sample with thermally grown oxide film (100 nm thick) was further oxidized in a plasma chamber for 2 hr at 450°C, and the increase in oxide thickness was measured. The same experiment was carried out with addition of laser irradiation. Two samples with irradiation wavelengths of 10.6 μm and 9.6 μm were compared. Because of a laser tuning problem, the irradiation power of the 9.6 μm wavelength sample was much smaller than the 10.6 μm wavelength sample, however. The increase in oxide thickness was 0.5 nm for the sample where laser irradiation was not employed. This should be compared with the extrapolated thickness increase of less than 0.1 nm when the sample was supposed to have been kept in dry oxygen atmosphere at the same temperature over the same processing period. For the laser-irradiated samples, the increase in the $SiO_2$ thickness was 2.5 nm and 1.5 nm for 9.6 μm and 10.6 μm irradiated samples. A laser effect was definitely clear, and what is more, the 9.6 μm irradiated sample shows a further increase even though the irradiation power was smaller.

These results imply that flow modulation of oxidizing species through the $SiO_2$ layer really take place as a result of laser light absorption. Since the 9.6 μm wavelength light is closer to the Si-O stretching mode vibration frequency of the $SiO_2$ film, it is natural to conclude that oxidizing species (supposed to be $O^-$ ions, following the description in 3.2) are subject to diffusion enhancement with this sort of absorbed energy.

### 3.4 Oxide properties

The effect of laser irradiation was also investigated from the viewpoint of both oxide and interface properties. In Fig. 6, infrared absorption spectra are shown for plasma and plasma + laser treated samples. Depending on the substrate temperature, shifts in absorption peak were observed. However, no laser irradiation effect was seen.

Etching speed of the oxide layer was also not affected by the laser irradiation. Breakdown properties were measured for MOS type samples, and no particular laser irradiation effect was observed. Breakdown field strength was on the order of 5 MV/cm, which is somewhat lower value than that for thermally grown oxide. However, with increase of substrate temperature, the number of lower breakdown voltage samples has decreased.

Clear evidence of laser irradiation was seen in the interface properties. As can be seen in Fig. 7, laser irradiated samples showed lower interface state densities than only plasma treated samples. Moreover, this difference

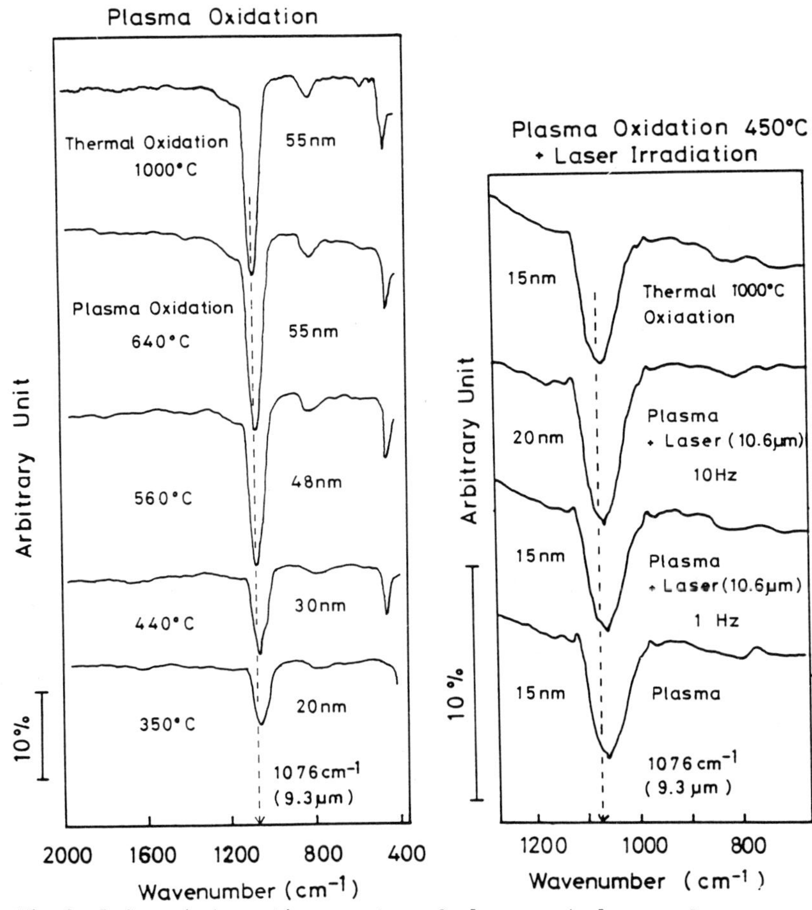


Fig.6. Infrared absorption spectra of plasma and plasma + laser grown $SiO_2$ films

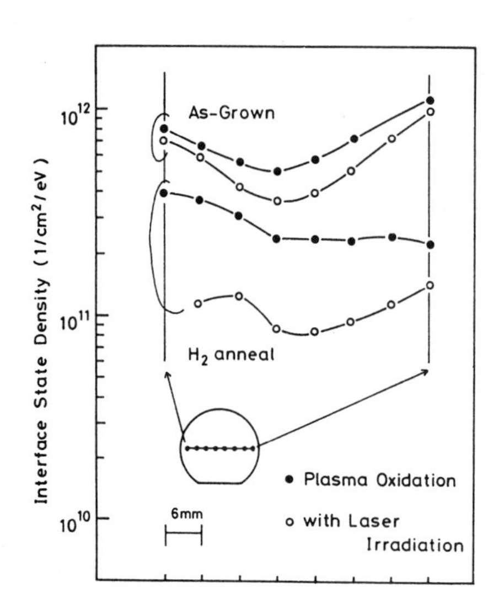


Fig.7. Interface state densities of plasma and plasma + laser grown $Si-SiO_2$ structures

became further evident after annealing in hydrogen at 395°C for 30 min. The $8 \times 10^{10}$ $cm^{-2}/eV^{-1}$ shown in the figure for laser irradiated samples is a reasonable value for utilization as a MOSFET gate insulator. This value has been hard to attain by conventional plasma oxidation methods reported up to now.

## 4. Conclusion

Laser assisted oxidation and plasma oxidation are compared as means to form oxide layers on silicon surfaces at low processing temperatures. A non-thermal photonic irradiation effect is reported for $Si-SiO_2$ interface oxidation reaction enhancement, due to breaking of Si-Si bonds through absorption of visible to UV light. In plasma oxidation, on the other hand, reaction enhancement originates from the existence of various oxidizing species excited in the plasma ambient. In addition, the existence of an electric field at the surface enhances the flow of negatively charged oxidizing species to the $Si-SiO_2$ interface.

A combination of laser and plasma methods was attempted for the purpose of developing a new low temperature oxidation. For the plasma source, a newly developed microwave-excited system was utilized, and pulse $CO_2$ laser irradiation was simultaneously applied at a low irradiation power so as to exclude thermal effects. The $SiO_2$ growth curve showed that laser enhancement of oxidation reaction really does take place, and could be tentatively interpreted as enhancement of oxidizing species flow to the $Si-SiO_2$ interface. This has been deduced from the fact that laser light at a 9.6 μm wavelength was much more effective than that at a 10.6 μm wavelength.

## References

1. N.Tsubouchi, H.Miyoshi and H.Abe : Japan. J. Appl. Phys. 17, suppl. 17-1, 223 (1978)
2. V.Q.Ho and T.Sugano : Thin Soild Films 95, 315 (1982)
3. J.R.Ligenza : J. Appl. Phys. 36, 2703 (1965)
4. A.K.Ray and A.Reisman : J. Electrochem. Soc. 128, 2460 (1981)

5. E.M.Young and W.A.Tiller : Appl. Phys. Lett. 42, 63 (1983)
6. S.A.Schafer and S.A.Lyon : J. Vac. Sci. Technol. 19, 494 (1981)
7. I.W.Boyd and J.I.B.Wilson : Appl. Phys. Lett. 41, 162 (1982)
8. I.W.Boyd : J. Appl. Phys. 54, 3561 (1983); see also this volume
9. I.W.Boyd : Appl. Phys. Lett. 42, 728 (1983)
10. R.Oren and S.Ghandhi : J. Appl. Phys. 42, 752 (1971)
11. B.E.Deal and A.S.Grove : J. Appl. Phys. 36, 3770 (1965)
12. K.Miyake, S.Kimura, T.Warabisako, H.Sunami and T.Tokuyama : J. Vac. Sci. Tech. A2, 496 (1984)
13. Y.S.Liu, S.W.Chiang and F.Bacon : Appl. Phys. Lett. 38, 1005 (1981)
14. K.Hoh, H.Koyama, K.Uda and Y.Miura : Japan. J. Appl. Phys. 19, L375 (1980)
15. J.F.Gibbons : Japan. J. Appl. Phys. 19, suppl. 19-1, 121 (1980)
16. I.W.Boyd, J.I.B.Wilson and J.L.West : Thin Solid Films 83, L173 (1981)
17. J.Blanc : Appl. Phys. Lett. 33, 424 (1978)
18. P.J.Jorgensen : J. Chem. Phys. 37, 874 (1962)
19. J.Kraitchman : J. Appl. Phys. 38, 4323 (1967)
20. G.Olive, D.L.Pufrey and L.Young : Thin Solid Films 12, 427 (1972)
21. S.Gourrier et al. : Plasma Chem. Plasma Processing 1, 217 (1981)
22. K.Ando and K.Matsumura : Thin Solid Films 52, 153 (1978)
23. Y.Kamigaki and Y.Itoh : J. Appl. Phys. 48, 2891 (1977)
24. N.Cabrera and N.F.Mott : Rept. Prog. Phys. 12, 163 (1948)
25. R.M.Burger and R.P.Donovan : *Fundamentals of Silicon Integrated Device Technology* (Prentice-Hall, Englewood Cliffs, New Jersey, 1967) vol.1, P.44

## 3.3 Etching

# Laser-Assisted Chemical Etching of Inorganic Materials: Mechanistic Studies

T.J. Chuang, Ingo Hussla, and W. Sesselmann
IBM Research Laboratory, 5600 Cottle Road, San Jose, CA 95193, USA

### I. Introduction

Recent advances in applications of lasers to induce chemical etching and vapor deposition have raised the firm expectation that the laser chemical techniques may have significant impact on processing materials for microelectronics. In laser-induced chemical etching, it has been shown in various laboratories that a rather wide range of solid materials can be potentially processed by lasers [1,2]. These include the etching of semiconductors such as Si [3-9], Ge [10], GaAs [11-13] and InP [11], metals such as Ta [14], Te [15,16], Ni and Fe [1b], insulators such as $SiO_2$ [15,17,18], and magnetic and ceramic materials such as MnZn ferrites [1a,9a] and $TiC-Al_2O_3$ [1b,16], by various halogen-containing gases excited by ultraviolet, visible and infrared lasers. The laser-enhanced etch rates can be greater than 50 $\mu$m/sec and submicron spatial resolution has also been demonstrated.

In comparison with plasma-assisted etching which is presently the most important dry processing technique, the laser chemical method offers certain advantages in some cases. The method requires no lithographic resist masks. This direct-writing capability can be particularly powerful for personalized applications such as three-dimensional fabrications and circuit repairs. Most importantly, because of the fundamental differences in etching mechanisms, laser radiation in many instances can induce efficient chemical etching of solids that are difficult to process by plasma or reactive ion etching (RIE) techniques. Plasma processing involving reactive radicals and charged particles depends basically on gas-surface chemical interactions at or near ambient temperatures. In contrast, the laser beams incident on a solid surface, particularly if they are tightly focussed, can excite the solid and activate surface reactions at relatively high surface temperatures. In addition, as the electronic devices get smaller in dimension, the radiation damage induced by charged particles may become difficult to overcome. The problem can be particularly serious in RIE processing, whereas the radiation damage to the solid is expected to be relatively minor with the laser technique. While the promises of the laser technique appear to be great, there are clearly major difficulties that need to be overcome. Perhaps the most serious limitation of the method at the present time is the total process rates and throughputs. It is readily recognized that although the localized etch rate or the etch rate per unit area can be very high, *e.g.*, greater than 50 $\mu$m/sec in etching Si wafers [9], the total surface area that can be processed per unit time is still quite small for device applications. In most practical cases, the laser beams are focussed to produce high intensities and therefore scanning or step-and-repeat is necessary to cover an area of interest on a wafer. In contrast, many wafers can be simultaneously processed in a plasma reactor. To resolve this problem, we obviously need more powerful laser systems than those currently available and need to develop optical schemes that can enable us to move efficiently utilize the laser energy.

Fundamentally, we still have to understand the factors that determine the surface reaction rates and the basic photon-induced etching mechanisms. Such understanding will undoubtedly provide important guidance for the process control and optimization in practical applications.

At present, perhaps with the exception of silicon-halogen systems, the available kinetic information and our understanding of the reaction mechanisms for other materials, in particular metals and insulators, are indeed very limited. For this reason, we have continued to investigate basic laser-enhanced surface processes relevant to etching reactions. Specifically, we have continued to study silicon-halogen etching reactions as a model system for semiconductors and a metal alloy system, *i.e.*, nickel-iron. In addition, we have examined a new metal system, namely, silver. In fact, these three systems represent three different classes of surface etching reactions. For Si-$XeF_2$, chemisorption and spontaneous etching (dark reaction) can occur. For Ni, Fe, and their alloys exposed to $Cl_2$, chemisorption is followed by the formation of passivated surface layers. And, for Ag-$Cl_2$, chlorine can diffuse into the bulk of the solid. Thus, it is interesting to study and compare the laser etching behavior of these three systems. Experimentally, we have used XPS, Auger spectroscopy, thermal desorption, time-resolved mass spectrometry and quartz-crystal-microbalance methods to analyze the surface species, the etching products, and the adsorption and desorption kinetics in conjunction with three pulsed laser systems. These new experimental results are also presented and discussed here. In the consideration of laser-induced etching mechanisms, it seems conceptually useful to divide the radiation-enhanced surface processes into two parts, namely, the enhanced chemisorption followed by reaction and the enhanced desorption which is often necessary for etching to take place. The general concepts and specific examples to illustrate the basic photon-stimulated processes have been given in a recent review by Chuang [2]. In the following section, we will briefly outline the major reaction steps and mechanisms that are directly relevant to surface etching reactions.

## II. Laser-Enhanced Surface Etching Processes

### 2.1 Enhanced Chemisorption and Reactions

For an etching reaction to take place, the very first step involves surface adsorption and for a molecular adsorbate, the step is often followed by dissociative chemisorption. Since halogen-containing gases are found to be most effective and frequently used in etching reactions, surface chemisorption usually leads to halogenation to form halogen compounds or a halogen-containing layer on the surface. In some cases, halogen atoms can penetrate rather deeply into the bulk and thereby greatly weaken the chemical bonds in the solid. Photon radiation at the gas-solid interface can affect these initial chemisorption steps and subsequent diffusion process in two major ways. First, photoexcitation of gaseous species can render the species to become more reactive and thereby enhance the sticking probability. This can be accomplished by photodissociation to produce radicals via single-photon or multi-photon absorption. In elementary surface reactions, it is well established that radicals frequently can chemisorb on surfaces which are inert to parent molecules. As elucidated by Winters *et al.* [19], there are possibly two mechanisms allowing a radical to be more reactive than its parent molecule. Namely, the reaction between a parent molecule and a surface may be exothermic but require a large activation energy to proceed. When the need for activation energy is avoided by dissociating the molecule in the gas phase, the resulting fragments can spontaneously react with the surface. The multiple photon dissociated $SF_6$ interaction with Si [4b] and $CF_3$ Br reaction with $SiO_2$ [18a] very likely occur by this mechanism. The single-photon photolyzed $Cl_2$ reaction with $SiO_2$ [15] and $Br_2$ reaction with Ge [10] may also belong to this category. Another possible mechanism involving radicals is related to adsorbed states which are endothermic. In this case, the parent molecule is inert to the solid in the absence of radiation and photo-fragmentation can provide the necessary energy for the reaction to take place. In addition to direct photodissociation, surface reactivity can also be enhanced by vibrational activation of gaseous molecules with infrared lasers. For example, $SF_6$ molecules which are inert to Si at ambient temperatures can be excited by absorption of multiple $CO_2$ laser photons to react with the solid [4b].

The second major way to influence surface reaction is by photoexcitation of the solid. This can be achieved by band gap excitation of semiconductors and insulators, interband transitions and excitation of free electrons in metals, and direct excitation of lattice phonons. Enhanced chemisorption and etching reactions on semiconductor surfaces due to photo-generation of electron-hole pairs have been clearly demonstrated in Si-$XeF_2$ [7] and Si-$Cl_2$ systems [8,20]. On metal surfaces, differentiation of electronic and thermal effects are more difficult to accomplish and more experiments are needed to clearly demonstrate the nonthermal radiation effects (further discussed in Section IV).

Another important effect of laser radiation to consider is the electromagnetic field enhancement on metal and semiconductor surfaces. The effect can be particularly important in etching reactions because in most practical cases high power laser beams are directly irradiated on solid surfaces to obtain useful etch rates. It is conceivable that strong surface electric fields may influence surface adsorption. As proposed by Winters *et al.* [19], surface halogenation reaction should be quite similar to surface oxidation reactions which could be largely described by field-assisted mechanisms. According to Cabrera-Mott theory [21], oxidation could proceed via electron migration through the oxide layer and the formation of oxygen anions on the surface. The resultant electric field across the oxide layer could pull the ions through for further growth of the oxide until the oxide layer was so thick that the surface field was greatly reduced. Likewise, a surface electric field could promote the growth of surface halides. The formation of halide or halogen-containing species in the surface region has been found to be necessary for etching reactions to occur for many systems. It is also possible that strong electric fields produced by the laser beam on the surface could modify optical absorption cross sections, and enhance nonlinear absorption and multi-photon excitation processes. On rough metal surfaces, the probability of surface excitation can greatly increase if a molecular resonance overlaps significantly with excitable surface resonances, such as surface plasmons [22]. As numerically illustrated by Gerstein and Nitzan [22], the iodine photodissociation yield on a silver sphere could be greatly enhanced by visible photons incident on the metal surface. The presence of surface plasmons has been found to influence the surface structure in the photochemically deposited metal films [23]. Similar surface electric field effect is expected to be present in etching reactions. Clearly further experiments are needed to assess its importance in influencing etching behavior and surface structures.

## 2.2 Stimulated Desorption

Photon-stimulated desorption (PSD) is a very important process in surface etching reactions. With a few exception such as silicon-fluorine system, in which the reaction products are volatile, most surface reactions of interest produce nonvolatile products and therefore the most important effect of laser radiation is to induce the product species to desorb so that new solid surfaces can be exposed to the etchant gas and the etching reaction can proceed. Laser-stimulated desorption also plays a crucial role in determining the spatial resolution of etched features.

The general concepts of PSD have been outlined and quite extensively discussed in the review given by Chuang [2]. Briefly, for chemisorption systems excited by uv-visible photons, as critically examined by Lichtman, Koel and their coworkers [24], the general conclusion was that on metal surfaces, such as CO on Ni and W, the observed photodesorption could be attributed mainly to the thermal effect. The quantum effect, *i.e.*, electronic contribution, was very small with the quantum efficiency possible less than $10^{-8}$ molecules desorbed per absorbed photon. On oxide and sulfide semiconductors, on the other hand, desorption could be readily induced by band-gap excitation with uv or visible light. The quantum yields, particularly in the presence of carbon impurity, could be quite high [24a]. In the infrared region, recent experiments by Heidberg *et al.* [25] showed that $CH_3F$ molecules adsorbed on a NaCl crystal could be desorbed by resonant vibrational excitation of the adsorbed species with a $CO_2$ laser. Similar $CO_2$ laser stimulated desorption has been observed for pyridine molecules adsorbed on KCl and Ag surfaces by Chuang and Seki [2,26]. The measured photodesorption yield depends not only on the laser wavelength and intensity but also, in the case of metal surfaces, on the polarization of the incident light [27]. For instance, at near grazing angle of incidence, p-polarized IR photons are more effective than s-polarized light in inducing molecular desorption. This is because the IR absorption factor for an oscillating dipole on a metal surface is much greater for radiation polarized parallel (p-) to the plane of incidence [28]. We have recently further investigated the vibrationally activated photodesorption phenomenon using time-resolved mass spectrometry with a pulsed tunable IR laser in the 2-4 $\mu$m region. For relatively simple molecules, such as $NH_3$ adsorbed on a Cu(100) crystal, resonant excitation of N-H stretching modes can promote the molecules to desorb [29]. By studying the photodesorption yields as a function of laser wavelength at different surface coverages, we can even differentiate chemisorbed and physisorbed surface species. From the extensive investigation of $NH_3$ and pyridine desorption from different solid surfaces under various exposure conditions, we have concluded [30] that in infrared laser photodesorption, thermally assisted processes such as the direct laser substrate heating and the indirect [2,26c] or "resonant" [31] heating due to rapid energy transfer of the absorbed IR energy to surrounding molecules and solid substrate also play a crucial role in determining the desorption yields. Thus, it seems clear that from uv, visible to IR, thermal effects are very important in PSD for many chemisorption systems and for systems with relatively thin adsorbate overlayers.

In chemical etching systems induced by lasers, the distinction between thermal and electronic excitation effects on photon-stimulated desorption of etching products is less clear. This is a subject of our continuing studies. For etching reactions involving relatively thick halogen-containing surface layers as in the Ag-$Cl_2$ system in which chlorine can diffuse quite deeply into the bulk (further discussed below), the photon radiation effect is not readily predictable. In the extreme case, one could consider the heavily halogenated Ag surface to behave like a solid AgCl which is sensitive to photodecomposition. Optical absorption by exciton bands (bound electron-hole pairs) of the solid might result in photodissociation of the halide and promote halogen desorption. Photodesorption of halogens which eventually leads to desorption of alkali metals is a well-known example of radiation effects on alkali halides [32]. Such photon radiation effects which can be rather nonthermal in origin have been referred as "photon sputtering" [32,33]. Our experimental results to be presented below show that Ag etching by $Cl_2$ induced by uv-visible lasers is different from photodecomposition and desorption of AgCl. There are, in fact, strong indications that Ag-$Cl_2$ photoetching reaction may involve nonthermal excitation mechanisms. It should be pointed out, however, that with pulsed laser excitation at high intensity, photodecomposition followed by desorption of product species may play an important role and this process should be considered in some etching systems.

## III. Experimental

The experimental apparatus for the present surface etching studies consists mainly of a UHV chamber equipped with an ESCA/AES spectrometer, an ion gun, a UTI quadrupole mass spectrometer and three pulsed laser systems. The schematic diagram of the experimental arrangement is shown in Fig. 1. Basically, the x-ray photoemission spectroscopy (XPS) is used for surface chemical analyses and Auger electron spectroscopy (AES) is used for elemental analyses and chemical depth profiling in combination with ion bombardment. The mass spectrometer is used in a time-of-flight mode connected to a Tracor signal averager for determination of product and velocity distributions following a laser pulse excitation on a solid sample. An rf induction heater (not shown in the figure) is also utilized to perform sample heating for crystal annealing and for thermal desorption measurements. The sample can also be cooled to 90K with liquid $N_2$. Gaseous exposure is carried out either directly in the UHV chamber through a small stainless tubing facing the sample or in a sample preparation chamber for exposures at relatively high gas pressures. As shown in the figure, the vacuum chamber for sample preparation is connected to the UHV chamber and all surface analyses are performed in situ without ambient contamination. The laser irradiation is carried out either in the preparation chamber or in the UHV chamber. For some experiments, quartz-crystal-microbalance (QCM) are used to monitor surface adsorption and laser etching behavior. Detailed description of QCM's and their operations were published previously [4b].

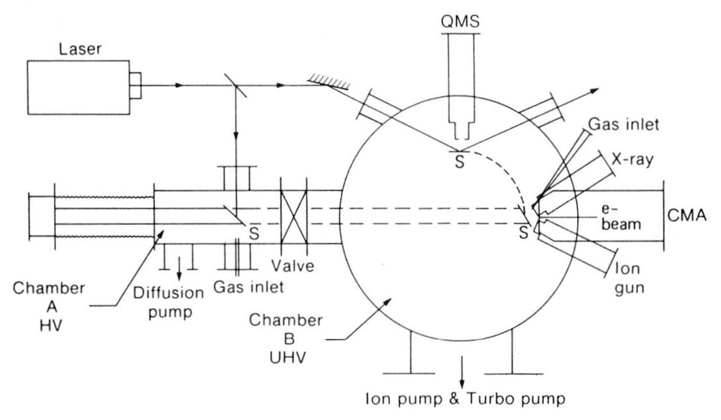


**Fig. 1.** Experimental apparatus for XPS, AES, TDS, QCM and time-resolved mass spectrometric studies on laser-induced chemical etching of solids. Laser irradiation (uv, visible or infrared) is carried out either in the UHV chamber or in the high vacuum sample preparation chamber.

The characteristics of the laser systems are briefly summarized as follows: a Nd:YAG laser (Quanta-Ray) is frequency doubled to produce 532 nm light with a 6 nsec pulse width and a maximum pulse energy of 200 mJ and 10 Hz maximum pulse rate. The laser can also be frequency tripled to generate 355 nm light with less pulse energy. The $N_2$ laser (Molectron) can product 2 mJ per pulse at 337 nm with 10 nsec pulse duration and 30 Hz pulse rate. The $CO_2$ laser (Tachisto) line-tunable between 9 and 11 $\mu m$ can generate 0.5J of pulse energy at 1 Hz pulse rate with 50-100 nsec pulse duration. Quartz lenses and windows are used in the uv-visible region. KCl or NaCl optical components are used for experiments with the $CO_2$ laser.

## IV. Results and Discussion

### 4.1 Silicon

When Si is exposed to $XeF_2$ at 25°C, surface fluorination to form a layer containing $SiF_x$ ($x \leq 3$) species readily occurs as detected by XPS [34] and photoemission excited by a synchrotron radiation source [35]. Further exposure of the solid to the gas can result in the spontaneous formation of volatile products and chemical etching of Si without external radiation [36]. The major volatile product in dark reaction has been identified to be $SiF_4$ with less F-coordinated $SiF_x$ species being the minor products [37]. In addition to XPS, we have further characterized the system by a conventional thermal desorption with an rf induction heater. Figure 2 shows the thermal desorption spectra (TDS) of $SiF_4$ adsorbed on a Si(111) crystal (0.1Ω n-type) at 90K. Apparently, $SiF_4$ can be readily desorbed from Si at about 95K. The adsorption energy for the physisorbed molecules at more than a monolayer surface coverage is calculated to be about 22 kJ/mole (5.3 kcal/mole). For chemisorbed $SiF_4$, which cannot be well resolved from the physisorbed molecules in TDS, the desorption temperature and the adsorption energy seem to be slightly higher. Clearly, $SiF_4$ molecules are only very weakly bound to Si on the surface. When the Si surface is exposed to $XeF_2$ at 90K, little reaction takes place. Instead, a relatively thick fluorine overlayer can be condensed on the solid. TDS shows that some Xe atoms are also trapped in the condensed overlayer and can readily desorb above 100K. In contrast, the $SiF_x$ surface layer obtained by exposing Si at 25°C to $XeF_2$ is fairly stable. Upon heating to 300°C, little desorption occurs and the total F(1s) XPS intensity decreases only slightly. Thus, in comparison with $SiF_4$, F and $SiF_x$ species are bound rather strongly to Si.

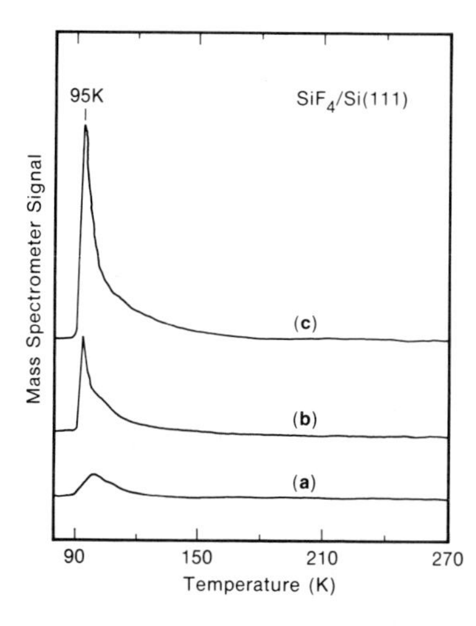


**Fig. 2.** Thermal desorption spectra of $SiF_4$ adsorbed on Si(111) at 90K: (a) $\theta$ below a monolayer coverage; (b) $\theta=1$; (c) $\theta>1$ multilayer coverage. Heating rate is about 30 K/sec.

When $SiF_4$ condensed on Si at 90K is irradiated by 532 nm light pulses, laser-induced thermal desorption readily occurs. The desorbed species is detected mainly as $SiF_3^+$ ions which are the dominant component when $SiF_4$ is cracked by the ionizer of the mass spectrometer. A clean Si(111) (0.1Ω n-type) sample is then exposed to $XeF_2$ at 25°C until the surface is covered with a few layers of $SiF_x$ species and spontaneous etching, as monitored simultaneously with a Si-QCM placed near the Si crystal, is about to begin. When the fluorine-saturated Si surface is irradiated by 532 nm laser pulses, we find that $Si^+$, $SiF^+$, $SiF_2^+$ and $SiF_3^+$ species can be detected by the mass spectrometer.

At a laser intensity of about 10 $MW/cm^2$, the observed yields for $SiF_2^+$ and $SiF^+$ are about the same. They are, however, much higher than the $SiF_3^+$ yield. It is clear that less F-coordinated species, *i.e.*, $SiF_x$ ($x \leq 3$), are the major etching products when the fluorine-exposed surface is irradiated by relatively high power laser pulses in the visible region. It is also interesting to note that at this laser intensity, the $Si^+$ mass signal can be substantially higher than the combined signals of $SiF^+$, $SiF_2^+$ and $SiF_3^+$, suggesting that some Si atoms are directly desorbed by the pulsed radiation. The probability of Si atom emission apparently increases with the laser intensity.

Figure 3 shows the typical time-of-flight (TOF) signals for $SiF_3^+$, $SiF_2^+$, $SiF^+$ and $Si^+$ species detected by the mass spectrometer as the fluorinated surface is irradiated by 532 nm light pulses at 9 $MW/cm^2$. From the maximum of TOF signal ($t_m$), the translational temperature of the desorbing species ($T_d$) can be calculated. A detailed description of the theoretical treatment assuming that the desorbed species leave the surface with a Maxwell-Boltzmann distribution has been given by Wedler and Ruhmann [38] among others. Following this approach, $T_d$ can be calculated according to:

$$T_d = \frac{m}{4k} \frac{\ell^2}{t_m^2} \tag{1}$$

where m, k, and $\ell$ are the mass, the Boltzmann constant and the distance between the sample and the middle of the ionization chamber, respectively. The average temperature rise ($\Delta T_s$) in the laser-heated surface layer can also be estimated according to the equation given by Bloembergen [39],

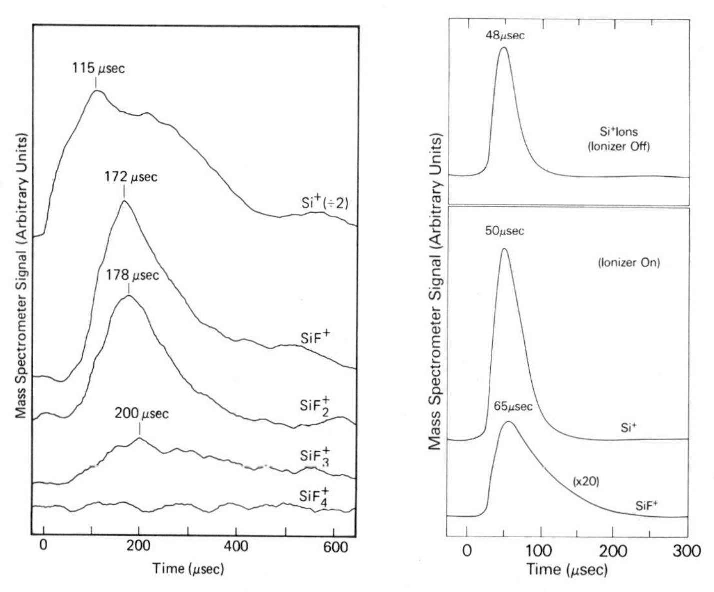


**Fig. 3. (left).** Time-of-flight (TOF) signals of $SiF_3^+$, $SiF_2^+$, $SiF^+$ and $Si^+$ detected by the mass spectrometer from $XeF_2$ exposed Si surface at 300K, irradiated by 532 nm laser pulses at I=9 $MW/cm^2$ on the surface; actual $Si^+$ signal a factor of two higher than other signals.

**Fig. 4 (right).** TOF signals of $SiF^+$ and $Si^+$ detected by the mass spectrometer from $XeF_2$ exposed Si surface irradiated by 532 nm light pulses at I=18 $MW/cm^2$; the top signal for $Si^+$ ions is detected by the mass spectrometer without using the ionizer.

$$\Delta T_s = \frac{(1 - R)It_p}{C_v \rho (2Dt_p)^{1/2}} \qquad (2)$$

where R is optical reflection coefficient, I is laser intensity, $t_p$ is pulse duration, and $C_v$, $\rho$, and D are specific heat, density, and thermal diffusivity of the material, respectively. At I=9 $MW/cm^2$, $\Delta T_s$ is estimated to be about 500K and the peak surface temperature due to the 6 nsec laser pulse could reach above 800K. The translational temperatures calculated from the observed $t_m$ for $SiF_x$ species are in the 400-560K range. These temperatures appear to be substantially lower than the estimated surface temperature during the laser excitation pulse. A lower $T_d$ than $T_s$ should not be particularly surprising in view of the fact that the surface species can desorb during the rise of surface temperature before reaching the maximum temperature. Also, a desorbing species may lose part of its energy for breaking the surface bond in the desorption process which can result in a translational temperature lower than that of the substrate. $T_d$ significantly less than $T_s$ has also been observed in pulsed laser-induced thermal desorption of CO from Cu and Fe surfaces [38,40]. It is further observed that irradiation of the fluorinated Si surface at a high laser fluence can induce the formation of plasma resulting in the ejection of both Si atoms and $Si^+$ ions (the latter are detected without using the ionizer of the mass spectrometer) in addition to $SiF_x$ species. The velocities of these ejected particles are very high as shown in TOF signals in Fig. 4. The threshold of laser fluence for plasma generation is much lower for the fluorinated Si than the clean surface. For instance, at 15 $MW/cm^2$, plasma formation giving rise to the characteristic optical emission from the surface is readily observed when Si is exposed to $XeF_2$. Yet, on a clean, well polished and annealed Si surface, plasma generation is not detectable even at the intensity of 20 $MW/cm^2$. Once the Si crystal is damaged due to either chemical etching or laser physical ablation, the laser threshold for particle emission is also substantially reduced. In short, our pulsed-laser time-resolved mass spectrometric study of the Si-$XeF_2$ has revealed interesting surface interaction characteristics quite different from the dark reaction [37] and the reaction enhanced by a cw $Ar^+$-ion laser at 515 nm [7], in which $SiF_4$ is identified as the major desorbed species with $SiF_x$ ($x \leq 3$) being the minor products.

In order to evaluate the importance of direct band-gap excitation to create electron-hole pair in influencing the radiation-enhanced etching behavior, we have also used a pulsed $CO_2$ laser at 10.6 $\mu$m to excite the $XeF_2$-exposed Si(111) surface (0.1$\Omega$ n-type). The results show that, similar to the pulsed visible laser radiation, the IR laser at 5 $MW/cm^2$ can also induce desorption of Si-$XeF_2$ reaction products, *i.e.*, $SiF_4$ and $SiF_x$ species. As shown in Fig. 5, the dominant species desorbed by the IR pulses is again not $SiF_4$. Namely, the observed yields for $SiF^+$ and $SiF_2^+$ are substantially higher than $SiF_3^+$ and $SiF_4^+$ yields. It is thus clear that less F-coordinated $SiF_x$ species are more easily produced and desorbed than $SiF_4$ under pulsed laser irradiation either in the visible or IR region. Although the product distribution induced by an IR pulse is generally quite similar to that induced by a visible light pulse, there still exist significant differences between the two types of excitation. When we compare Fig. 5 with Fig. 3, it is apparent that $CO_2$ laser pulses produce more $SiF_3^+$ and $SiF_4^+$ than the 532 light pulses. In fact, the IR pulses produce about the same amount of $SiF_4^+$ as $SiF_3^+$. This is very unusual because $SiF_3^+$ is definitely the dominant component when $SiF_4$ is cracked by electron impact ionization of the mass spectrometer. To be completely certain, we have also performed laser-induced thermal desorption of $SiF_4$ condensed on Si at 90K and irradiated the surface with $CO_2$ laser pulses. Figure 6 shows the TOF spectra of $SiF_4$ thermally desorbed from Si by the IR pulse. The figure also shows that indeed $SiF_3^+$ is the dominant fragment of $SiF_4$ under our experimental conditions. Therefore, the $CO_2$ laser excitation on a fluorinated Si surface also produces a product distribution

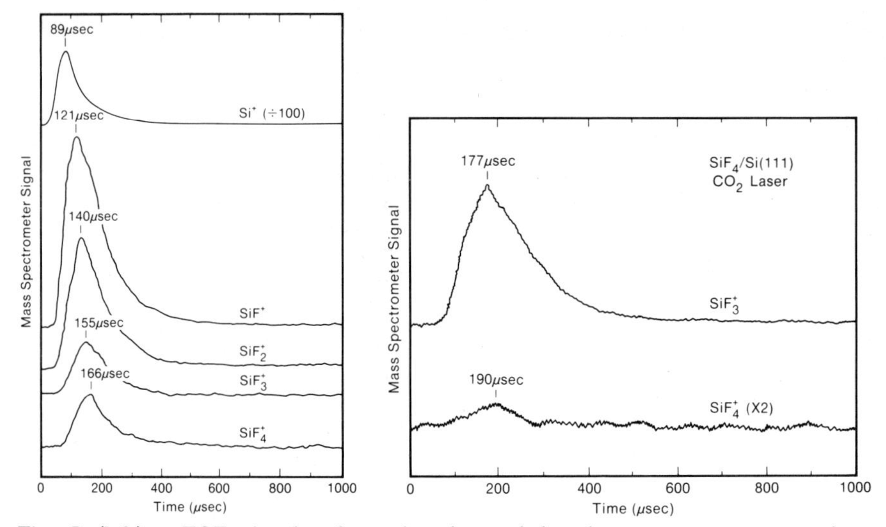


**Fig. 5 (left).** TOF signals of species detected by the mass spectrometer from $XeF_2$-exposed Si surface at 300K excited by $CO_2$ laser pulses at I=5 $MW/cm^2$.
**Fig. 6 (right).** TOF signals detected by the mass spectrometer from $SiF_4$ adsorbed on a clean Si surface at 90K irradiated by $CO_2$ laser pulses at I=5 $MW/cm^2$.

drastically different from the thermal reaction [37]. Apparently, like the visible radiation, an ir laser can also induce a nonthermal radiation effect on Si etching reaction as Chuang had suggested earlier [5]. It is interesting to note that a single $CO_2$ laser photon at 0.12 eV energy is incapable of exciting the band gap of Si. If band-gap excitation above 1 eV is necessary for electronic effect to be important, then more than eight $CO_2$ laser photons would be needed to facilitate such excitation. Whether or not such multi-photon excitation process can indeed occur on a semiconductor surface in 5-10 $MW/cm^2$ laser intensity region remains to be further elucidated. Our results also show that at 5 $MW/cm^2$, the translational temperatures of the photodesorbed particles are calculated to be in the 1000K range when the fluorinated Si is excited by the IR pulses. At this laser intensity, no genuine ionic species (as determined without the ionizer) can be detected by the mass spectrometer. It should be pointed out clearly that our studies are directly relevant to practical etching conditions with pulsed lasers. The etching condition with the present experimental procedure should be equivalent to the situation between laser pulses.

In addition to Si-$XeF_2$, we have also investigated Si-$Cl_2$ reactions excited by a pulsed $N_2$ laser at 337 nm. It is observed that for a Si(111) (0.1Ω) surface exposed to $Cl_2$ at 0.1 Torr, chemisorption readily takes place but there is no significant spontaneous etching in the absence of radiation. With the uv laser at 12 $MW/cm^2$ on the solid, chemical etching occurs and the laser-enhanced etch rate for the n-type material is higher than the p-type. Similar etching behavior has been observed by Sekine *et al.*, [20] for poly-silicon with different dopants excited by a cw Hg-Xe arc lamp. Our observed etch rate difference between the two types of semiconductors, however, appears to be substantially smaller than that obtained by Sekine *et al.* with relatively low uv intensities. It is interesting to note that with a focussed CW $Ar^+$-ion laser, Ehrlich *et al.* [6] did not detect significant differences in etch rate between the n- and p-type of Si or between samples of different conductivities, also with $Cl_2$ gas. We are carrying out further experiments on Si-$Cl_2$ system with a pulsed uv laser including studies on different Si crystal faces. The results will be reported later.

## 4.2 Nickel, Iron and Alloys

When Ni, Fe and Ni-Fe alloys are exposed to $Cl_2$ gas at 25°C, the molecule can dissociatively chemisorb on the metal surfaces. Figure 7 shows the chlorine adsorption behavior on the metals as monitored with quartz-crystal-microbalances (QCM). For exposures at 0.1 Torr, gaseous adsorption saturates to form a passivated chloride layer about 10-15Å thick. When the Fe surface is irradiated by a $N_2$ laser operated at 30 Hz pulse rate and 12 $MW/cm^2$ per pulse on the solid, chemical etching occurs in a $Cl_2$ ambient maintained at 0.1 Torr. The response of a Fe-QCM under laser irradiation is also shown in Fig. 7. As the material is chemically removed from the metal surface, the frequency of the QCM increases. The initial jump in the QCM frequency when the uv laser beam is directed onto the sample is due to the sudden temperature rise induced by the laser pulses. Under the same gaseous exposure and irradiation conditions, negligible etching is observed for a Ni surface. For a Fe(53%)+Ni(47%) alloy, the laser-induced etch rate is slightly less than half of the Fe etch rate. The relative surface etch rates for the alloys with different metal atomic ratios, as determined with a diamond stylus (Tencor Alpha-Step Profiler) on etched features, are shown in Fig. 8. The observed etch rate apparently increases with Fe concentration in the alloy, although the proportionality seems to be slightly sublinear.

The observed laser-induced etching behavior for Ni-Fe systems appears to be quite reasonable in view of the fact that the chemical reactivities of the metals with $Cl_2$ are quite similar, but the volatility of iron chloride is much higher than nickel chloride at elevated temperatures. Laser radiation on a solid can induce a severe temperature rise in the irradiated region and the thermal effect is always important even though it may not be the only contributing factor in inducing surface etching. It should be noted that Ni and Fe have rather similar metallurgical properties. For alloys composed of materials

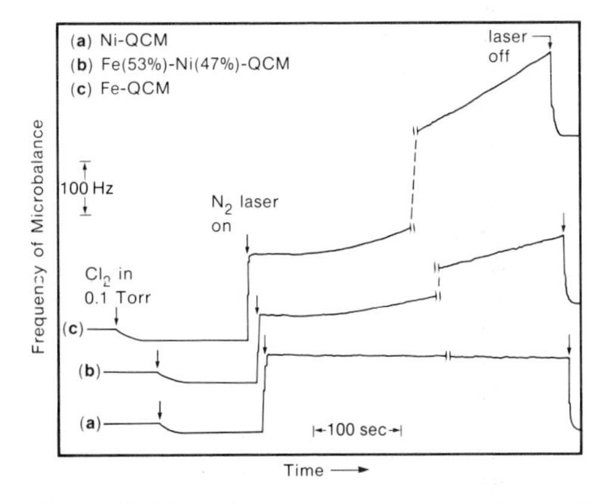


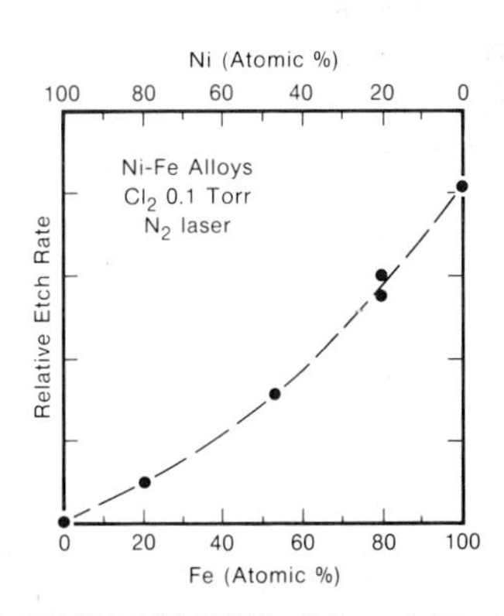


**Fig. 7 (left).** Frequency responses of Ni (a), Fe(53%)-Ni(47%) (b) and Fe (c) microbalances when the metal QCM's are exposed to $Cl_2$ at 0.1 Torr and irradiated by $N_2$ laser at 12 $MW/cm^2$ pulse intensity operated at 30 Hz pulse rate.

**Fig. 8 (right).** Relative etch rates of Ni-Fe alloys as a function of Fe atomic concentration in the solids excited by $N_2$ laser at 12 $MW/cm^2$ and 30 Hz pulse rate, in $Cl_2$ at 0.1 Torr.

with very different thermal and chemical properties, the radiation-enhanced etch rates can be strongly dependent on the atomic ratios and the surface etching behavior can be highly unpredictable. Furthermore, it would be very interesting to determine if preferential chemical etching of an element, *i.e.*, Fe in the case of Ni-Fe alloys, would occur so that the etched surface would be enriched with another element. We are using XPS to further investigate this and other alloy systems.

### 4.3 Silver

Silver represents a class of materials which strongly interact with $Cl_2$ so that chlorine not only chemisorbs on the surface but also diffuses into the bulk of the material. Figure 9a shows the chlorine adsorption and diffusion behavior on Ag surfaces exposed to $Cl_2$ at various pressures studied with QCM's. The results indicate that the initial $Cl_2$ adsorption rates at low exposures are very high. In the high-exposure region, the chlorine adsorption rate decreases apparently due to the limited Cl diffusion rate into the bulk. XPS experiments further reveal the interesting Ag-$Cl_2$ interaction behavior. When a clean Ag surface is exposed to $Cl_2$, except perhaps the top few monolayers, the surface region of the metal does not completely chlorinate to form a uniform AgCl layer. This is so even if we expose an Ag film (2 $\mu$m thick) to $Cl_2$ at 0.1 Torr for 1000 sec, *i.e.*, $10^8$ Langmuirs of exposure. Figure 10 shows the Ag($3d_{5/2}$,$3d_{3/2}$) and Cl(2p) XPS spectra as well as the Ag Auger spectra which are also obtained by x-ray excitation for an Ag film exposed to $Cl_2$. In comparison with the equivalent spectra for a solid AgCl (also shown in Fig. 10), it is evident that although the binding energies of Ag(3d) core level peaks do not shift significantly due to chlorine exposure, the Auger peaks are very sensitive to the metal bonding with chlorine. In fact, chemical shifts of about 2 eV are obtained for the Ag($M_4$VV) and ($M_5$VV) transitions when Ag is chlorinated. These chemical shifts indicate the formation of some AgCl in the surface region of the metal. Earlier studies of the system under lower $Cl_2$ exposure conditions also showed the formation of silver chloride in the surface overlayer [41-43]. We have further determined from XPS intensity analyses of Ag(3d) and Cl(2p) peaks that the average surface concentration of Cl with respect to Ag is about 0.67 (within the XPS sampling depth of about 20Å), when the metal surface is exposed to $Cl_2$ at 0.1 Torr for 10 sec. The chlorinated surface layer may be represented as $AgCl_x$ with x being 0.81 as the gaseous exposure time is increased to 100 sec and 0.95 for 1000 sec. Evidently, as long as Ag is present under the chlorinated surface layer, Ag can diffuse through the AgCl-containing layer onto the surface for reaction with chlorine under our exposure

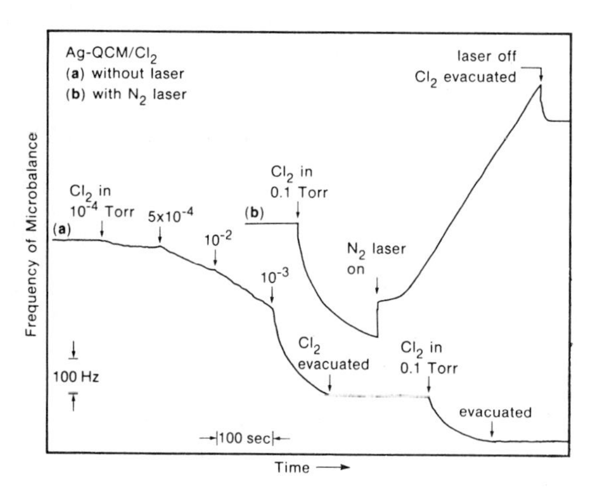


**Fig. 9.** Frequency response of an Ag-QCM exposed to $Cl_2$ at various pressures sequentially each for 100 sec as indicated (a); and exposed to $Cl_2$ at 0.1 Torr also irradiated by $N_2$ laser pulses at 12 MW/cm$^2$-30 Hz pulse rate (b).

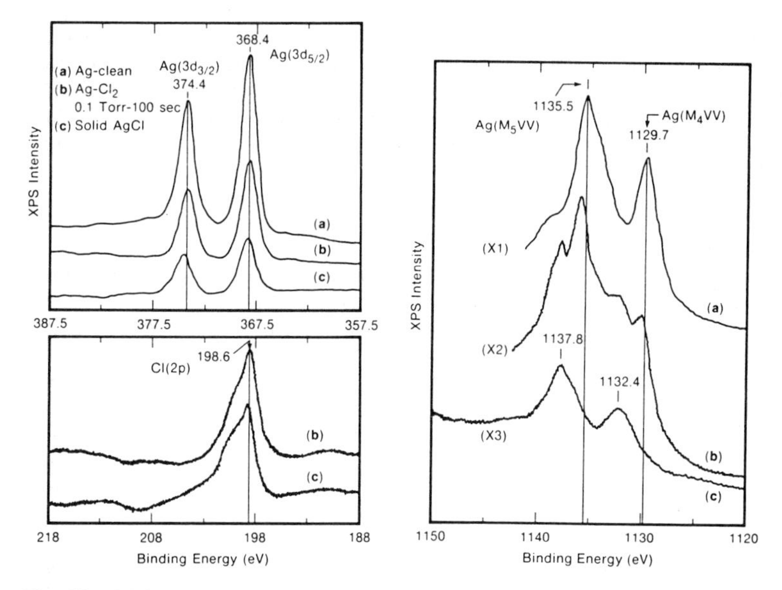


**Fig. 10.** XPS spectra of Ag(3d) and Cl(2p) of an Ag film along with Auger spectra also excited by x-ray; (a) clean Ag surface; (b) exposed to $Cl_2$ at 0.1 Torr for 100 sec; (c) a solid AgCl for comparison.

conditions. Other experiments have shown that at a lower dosage, $Cl_2$ exposure never leads to halide growth beyond the monolayer stage [42].

In spite of the incomplete surface chlorination, exposure of the surface to a uv or visible laser can result in efficient etching of the metal. Figure 9b shows the response of an Ag-QCM exposed to $Cl_2$ at 0.1 Torr and irradiated by a focussed $N_2$ laser at 12 $MW/cm^2$ pulse intensity. The laser-induced etch rate of the Ag film (2 $\mu$m thick on quartz), as determined with a diamond stylus, is shown in Fig. 11 for different $Cl_2$ pressures. Efficient etching has also been observed with 532 nm and 355 nm light pulses generated from a Nd:YAG laser [44], even under relatively low $Cl_2$ exposure conditions. These results suggest that while chlorine penetration into the surface region of Ag is necessary for the laser etching to take place, complete AgCl formation is not necessary for efficient etching to occur. Our pulsed-laser time-of-flight mass spectrometric studies of the system [44] also support this conclusion. Although solid AgCl strongly absorb photons below 400 nm, the material is practically transparent above 500 nm [45]. Yet, for Ag-$Cl_2$, we observe no major differences in the etching yield per pulse with a 532 nm and a 355 nm laser. Furthermore, the product and velocity distributions obtained by

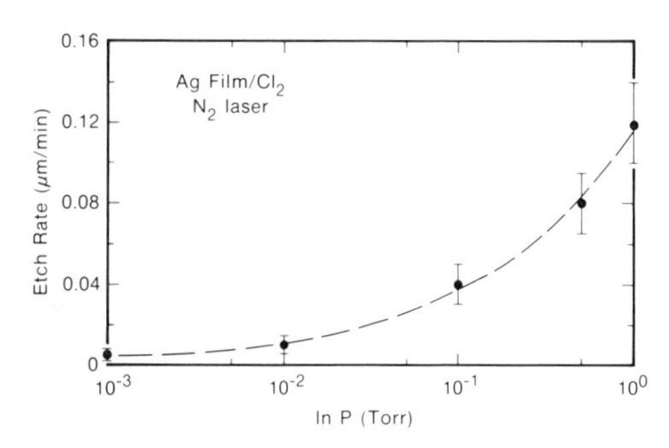


**Fig. 11.** Laser-induced etch rate of an Ag film as a function of $Cl_2$ gas pressure; $N_2$ laser at 12 $MW/cm^2$ operated at 30 Hz pulse rate.

time-resolved mass spectrometric measurements [44] show that the Ag-$Cl_2$ etching reaction induced by laser pulses is very different from thermal or laser evaporation of AgCl. There are strong indications that the laser radiation effect can be quite nonthermal in nature, *i.e.*, very likely via electronic excitation mechanisms. This particular aspect will be discussed in detail in later publications.

From the experimental results obtained with XPS, QCM and mass spectrometry, we can conclude that the following laser-gas-surface interaction steps take place in pulsed-laser-excited Ag-$Cl_2$ etching reactions: (1) dark chlorine adsorption and diffusion between laser pulses (and the extent of surface chlorination and diffusion depth depend on $Cl_2$ pressure and pulse repetition rate); (2) weakening of Ag-Ag bonds in the metal due to Cl penetration into the subsurface region; (3) laser excitation of the chlorinated surface via electronic activation as well as thermal heating effects; (4) desorption and ejection of Ag, Cl, AgCl, *etc.*, particles by a laser pulse resulting in the etching of the solid; and (5) chlorine readsorption and diffusion in the period between laser pulses and the repeat of etching cycles.

## V. Summary

In this report, we have briefly examined the basic surface processes involved in laser-assisted chemical etching of metal and semiconductor materials with particular emphasis on aspects related to photon-stimulated desorption and the important role played by photodesorption in surface etching reactions. Specifically, we have studied three solid systems which represent three different classes of surface interactions and laser etching behavior. Experimental techniques such as XPS, conventional as well as laser-induced thermal desorption, time-resolved mass spectrometry and quartz-crystal-microbalance measurements in conjection with three uv, visible and infrared laser systems are employed. New experimental results show that for Si-$XeF_2$, the product and velocity distributions of chemical species photodesorbed by 532 nm light pulses can be very different from the thermal reaction in the dark or the reaction enhanced by a cw laser. While the electron-hole pair generation by a uv-visible light beam certainly can contribute to enhancement in etch rate, $CO_2$ laser experiments demonstrate that single-photon absorption for band-gap excitation may not be essential in promoting nonthermal radiation effects. For $Cl_2$ interaction with a Si(111) crystal, it is observed that pulsed uv radiation can induce a substantially higher etch rate for a n-type material than a p-type. For Ni, Fe and the alloy system, chlorine adsorption is followed by the formation of a passivated surface layer. Laser radiation on the chlorinated surface results in the etching of these metals. The observed etch rates for Fe are much higher than Ni possibly because of the difference in volatility of the metal halides at elevated temperatures. For Ag-$Cl_2$, it is shown that chlorine can not only adsorb on Ag but also diffuse into the bulk. Chlorine adsorption results in the formation of AgCl in the surface region. Although the halide growth is never complete in the surface region, even for $Cl_2$ exposures as high as 0.1 Torr-1000 sec, Ag etching can be readily achieved by irradiation with uv and visible lasers. Time-resolved mass spectrometric measurements with lasers at different wavelengths further show that the laser etching is very different form thermal evaporation of AgCl and the radiation effects may involve electronic excitation mechanisms. Studies on these gas-solid systems have therefore provided valuable insight into the basic interaction steps and processes in laser-induced surface etching reactions.

Acknowledgments: The authors wish to thank J. Goitia for his assistance with the experiments, E. Marinero for his contribution to part of the Ag-$Cl_2$ work, and H. F. Winters, J. R. Lankard, J. H. Brannon and L. Chen for many useful discussions.

References


[1] See the reviews: (a) T. J. Chuang, J. Vac. Sci. Technol. **21**, 798 (1982); (b) T. J. Chuang, Mat. Res. Soc. Symp. Proc. **17**, 45 (1983); (c) D. J. Ehrlich and J. Y. Tsao, J. Vac. Sci. Technol. **B1**, 969 (1983).
[2] T. J. Chuang, Surf. Sci. Reports **3**, 1 (1983).
[3] L. L. Sveshnikova, V. I. Donin and S. M. Repinskii, Sov. Tech. Phys. Lett. **3**, 223 (1977).
[4] (a) T. J. Chuang, J. Chem. Phys. **72**, 6303 (1980); (b) T. J. Chuang, J. Chem. Phys. **74**, 1453 (1981).
[5] T. J. Chuang, J. Chem. Phys. **74**, 1461 (1981).
[6] D. J. Ehrlich, R. M. Osgood, Jr. and T. F. Deutsch, Appl. Phys. Lett. **38**, 1018 (1981).
[7] (a) F. A. Houle, Chem. Phys. Lett. **95**, 5 (1983); (b) F. A. Houle, J. Chem. Phys. **79**, 4237 (1983).
[8] T. Arikado, H. Okano, M. Sekine and Y. Horiike, Mat. Res. Soc. Symp. Proc. (1984, in press).
[9] (a) F. A. Houle and T. J. Chuang, (unpublished); (b) J. R. Lankard, J. H. Brannon, L. Chen and T. J. Chuang, (unpublished).
[10] I. M. Beterov, P. Chebotaev, N. I. Yushina and B. Ya. Yurshin, Sov. J. Quantum Electron. **8**, 1310 (1978).
[11] D. J. Ehrlich, R. M. Osgood, Jr. and T. F. Deutsch, Appl. Phys. Lett. **36**, 698 (1980).
[12] A. W. Tucker and M. Birnbaum, IEEE Electron Device Lett. **EDL-4**, 39 (1983).
[13] M. Takai, J. Tokuda, H. Nakai, K. Gamo and S. Namba, Mat. Res. Soc. Symp. Proc. (1984, in press).
[14] T. J. Chuang, J. Vac. Sci. Technol. **18**, 638 (1981).
[15] T. J. Chuang, IBM J. Res. Develop. **26**, 145 (1982).
[16] T. J. Chuang, Mat. Res. Soc. Symp. Proc. (1984, in press).
[17] K. Daree and W. Kaiser, Glass Technol. **18**, 19 (1977).
[18] (a) J. I. Steinfeld, T. G. Anderson, C. Reiser, D. R. Denison, L. D. Hartsough and J. R. Hallahan, J. Electrochem. Soc. **127**, 514 (1980); (b) D. Harradine, F. R. McFeely, B. Roop, J. I. Steinfeld, D. Denison, L. Hartsough and J. R. Hollahan, SPIE **270**, 52 (1981).
[19] H. F. Winters, J. W. Coburn and T. J. Chuang, J. Vac. Sci. Technol. **B1**, 469 (1983).
[20] M. Sekine, H. Okano and Y. Horiike, in Proceedings of the Fifth Symposium on Dry Processes (Tokyo, Japan, 1983), p. 97.
[21] F. P. Fehner and N. F. Mott, J. Oxidation of Metals **2**, 59 (1970).
[22] J. Gersten and A. Nitzan, J. Chem. Phys. **73**, 3023 (1980).
[23] (a) S. R. J. Brueck and D. J. Ehrlich, Phys. Rev. Lett. **48**, 1678 (1982); (b) R. M. Osgood, Jr. and D. J. Ehrlich, Opt. Lett. **7**, 385 (1982).
[24] (a) D. Lichtman and Y. Shapira, CRC Critical Rev. Solid State Mater. Sci. **8**, 93 (1978); (b) B. E. Koel, J. M. White, J. L. Erskine and P. R. Antoniewicz, American Chemical Society, Adv. Chem. Ser. **184**, 27 (1980).
[25] (a) J. Heidberg, H. Stein, E. Riehl and A. Nestmann, Z. Physik. Chem. (NF) **121**, 145 (1980); (b) J. Heidberg, H. Stein and E. Riehl, Phys. Rev. Lett. **49**, 666 (1982).
[26] (a) T. J. Chuang, J. Chem. Phys. **76**, 3828 (1982); (b) H. Seki and T. J. Chuang, Solid State Commun. **44**, 473 (1982); (c) T. J. Chuang, J. Electr. Spectr. Relat. Phenom. **29**, 125 (1983).
[27] T. J. Chuang and H. Seki, Phys. Rev. Lett. **49**, 382 (1982).

[28] R. G. Greenler, J. Chem. Phys. **44**, 310 (1966); ibid. **50**, 1963 (1969).
[29] T. J. Chuang and I. Hussla, Phys. Rev. Lett. **52**, 2045 (1984).
[30] T. J. Chuang and I. Hussla, in Proceedings of the 17th Jerusalem Symposium in Quantum Chemistry and Biochemistry: Dynamics of Molecule-Surface Interactions, ed. by B. Pullman (Reidl, Dortrecht, Holland, 1984).
[31] Z. W. Gortel, H. J. Kruzer, P. Piercy and R. Teshima, Phys. Rev. **B27**, 5066 (1983).
[32] See *e.g.*, the review by P. C. Townsend, in *Sputtering in Particle Bombardment II*, ed. by R. Behrisch (Springer, Berlin, 1983), pp. 147-178.
[33] (a) M. Hanabusa, M. Suzuki and S. Nishigaki, Appl. Phys. Lett. **38**, 385 (1981); (b) N. Itoh and T. Nakayama, Phys. Lett. **92A**, 471 (1982); (c) T. Nakayama, H. Ichikawa and N. Itoh, Surf. Sci. **129**, L693 (1982).
[34] T. J. Chuang, J. Appl. Phys. **51**, 2614 (1980).
[35] F. R. McFeely, J. Morar, G. Landgren and F. J. Himpsel, presented at MRS Symposium on Thin Films and Interfaces (November 14-18, 1983, Boston, Massachusetts), to be published.
[36] H. F. Winters and J. W. Coburn, Appl. Phys. Lett. **34**, 70 (1979).
[37] (a) Y. Y. Tu, T. J. Chuang and H. F. Winters, Phys. Rev. **B23**, 823 (1981); (b) H. F. Winters and F. A. Houle, J. Appl. Phys. **54**, 1218 (1983).
[38] G. Wedler and H. Ruhmann, Surf. Sci. **121**, 464 (1982).
[39] N. Bloembergen, in MRS Symposium on Laser-Solid Interactions and Laser Processing - 1978, AIP Conf. Proc., No. 50, pp. 1-9 (1979).
[40] D. Burgess, Jr., R. Viswanathan, I. Hussla, P. C. Stair and E. Weitz, J. Chem. Phys. **79**, 5200 (1983).
[41] Y. Y. Tu and J. M. Blakely, Surf. Sci. **85**, 276 (1978).
[42] M. Kitson and R. M. Lambert, Surf. Sci. **100**, 368 (1980).
[43] M. Bowker and K. C. Waugh, Surf. Sci. **134**, 639 (1983).
[44] W. Sesselmann, E. Marinero and T. J. Chuang, to be published.
[45] (a) M. A. Gilleo, Phys. Rev. **91**, 534 (1953); (b) H. Kanzaki and S. Sakuragi, Photogr. Sci. Eng. **17**, 69 (1973).

# Maskless Dry Etching of GaAs by Focused Laser Beam

M. Takai, H. Nakai, J. Tsuchimoto, J. Tokuda, T. Minamisono*,
K. Gamo, and S. Namba

Faculty of Engineering Science, *Faculty of Science, Osaka University
Toyonaka, Osaka 560, Japan

## 1. Introduction

There has been increasing interest in the application of laser beams to semiconductor processing such as etching and deposition because of the potential for low temperature and maskless processes [1]. Laser beams, furthermore, have a feature as a clean energy source in comparison with ion beams or plasmas, which inevitably induce lattice defects or impurity incorporation when applied to etching or deposition for semiconductor materials. Local etching of GaAs by ultraviolet laser photolysis [2], for example, is a low temperature process which does not induce lattice defects and, hence, does not need subsequent annealing processes. Dry etching by laser pyrolysis, on the other hand, induces a local temperature rise, but it realizes, by an order of 3 to 4, higher etching rates than ion-beam [3] or plasma etching.

In our recent studies[4, 5], pyrolytic local etching of GaAs with focused Ar laser beams in $Cl_2$, $CCl_4$ or $SiCl_4$ was performed and it was found that etching rates of 0.3 to 40 μm/scan and a buried carbon or silicon line in the etched groove in the special case could be obtained by a single scan of a laser beam. The etched width was found to be narrower than the laser beam diameter by a factor of 4 - 5.

In this study, the possibility of maskless etching for GaAs with a line-width less than 1 μm was investigated using fine focused laser beams by microscope optics. The chemical composition of the GaAs sample before and after laser irradiation in ambient gas atmospheres and the local temperature rise during laser irradiation were studied to clarify the mechanism of etching.

## 2. Experimental Procedures

(100)-oriented n-type GaAs wafers with a carrier density ranging from $10^{16}$ to $10^{17}/cm^3$ were mounted on the target in a vacuum chamber evacuated down to $10^{-3}$ Torr. Ambient gas was introduced into the chamber at a pressure of up to 120 Torr for $CCl_4$ and 250 Torr for $SiCl_4$. The sample surface was not stained or etched by either gas alone. The gas pressure was controlled by changing the temperature of a bath immersed with gas bottles as described elsewhere [5].

The focused 514.5 nm beam of an Ar laser with a width of 18.7 μm and a power up to 0.65 W was scanned over the sample by moving the target chamber with an electronically controlled stage [4, 5]. A microscope objective lens with a numerical aperture of 0.6 was used to obtain the minimum focal-spot size as in Fig. 1. The measured beam diameter was 1.2 μm. The working distance between the objective lens and the sample surface in this case was 3 mm. Scanning speeds were varied from 3 to 60 μm/sec, corresponding to a beam dwell time of 0.31 - 6.2 sec for 18.7 μm and 0.02 - 0.40 sec for 1.2 μm beam diameters. The laser power was controlled so that in the vacuum, i.e., without ambient gas, the GaAs surface was not etched or stained.

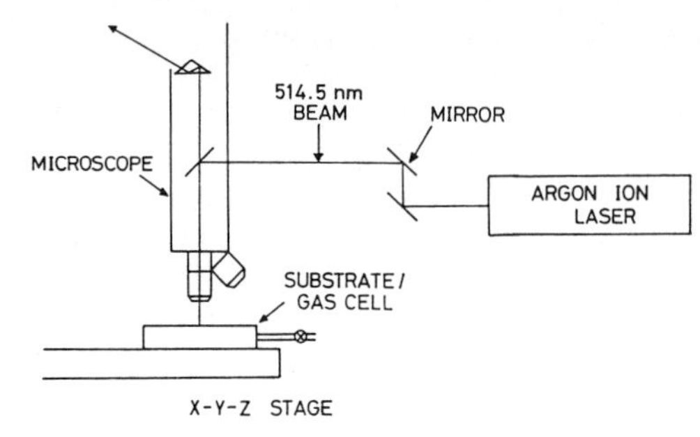


Fig. 1 Experimental Set-up for laser assisted etching with microscope objective lenses

The etching rates and etched line shapes were measured by scanning electron microscopy (SEM) observation. 2 MeV helium ion induced X-ray emission (IIXE) and Auger electron spectroscopy (AES) measurements were performed to detect the surface chemical composition of the sample before and after laser irradiation.

## 3. Results and Discussion

Figure 2 shows a typical etched line shape of the GaAs surface scanned at a speed of 9 μm/sec with a laser beam focused down to 1.2 μm at a $CCl_4$ pressure of 65 Torr, indicating a Gaussian-shaped etch pattern with a depth of 0.25 μm. The etched width was measured to be about 1.0 μm. The etched depth and width as a function of beam scanning speed or beam dwell time at a $CCl_4$ pressure of 65 Torr are shown in Fig. 3. The etched line width

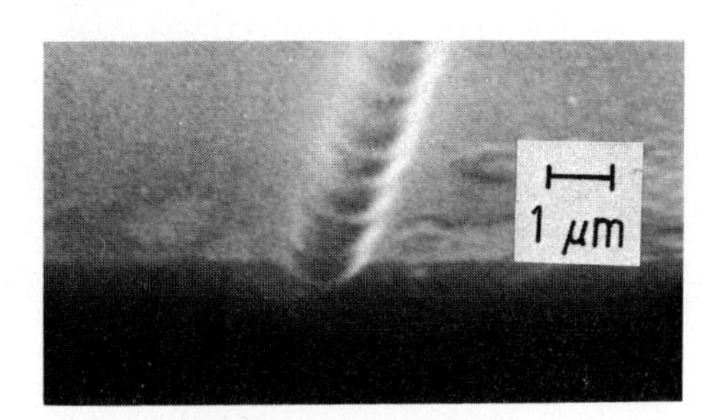


Fig. 2 A cross-sectional view of a line shape etched in $CCl_4$

Fig. 3 Etched width and depth versus beam scanning speeds

Fig. 4 Etched width versus beam scanning speeds

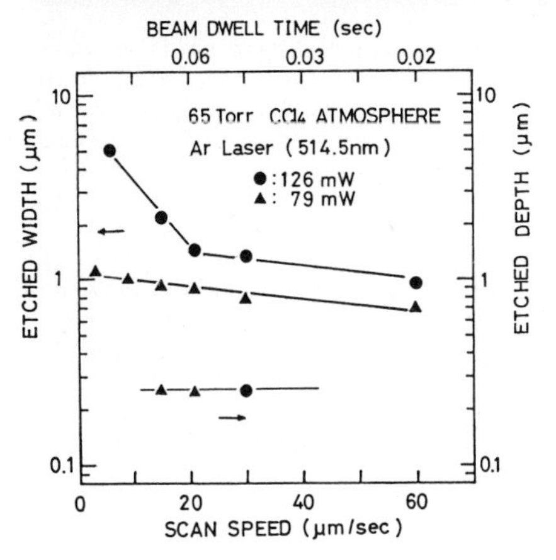


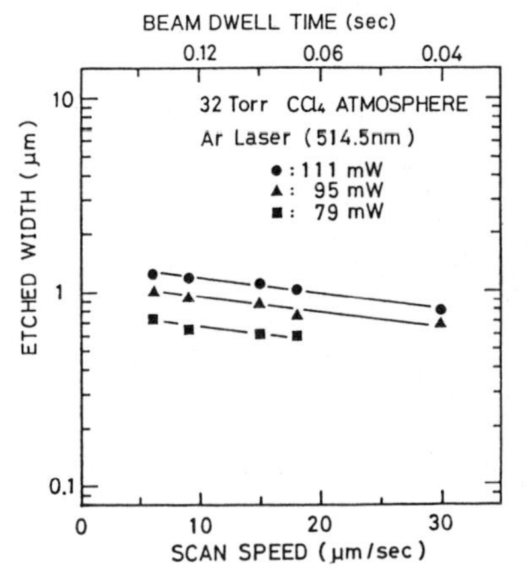

decreases exponentially from 1.2 μm down to 0.7 μm, as the beam scanning speed increases from 3 μm/sec to 60 μm/sec with a laser power of 79 mW. With a laser power of 126 mW, the etched line width increases because of the increased temperature. It should be noted that the etched width becomes broader than the laser beam diameter with a laser power of 126 mW at scanning speeds below 20 μm/sec, in which a deposited carbon layer buried in the etched groove was observed for a single scan of a laser beam as reported elsewhere [4, 5]. The etched depth obtained by a single scan of a laser beam was about 0.25 μm except in the case of buried deposition.

Further minimization of the etching line width was found to be possible by reducing the ambient gas pressure. Figure 4 shows the etched width as a function of a beam scanning speed at a $CCl_4$ pressure of 32 Torr with laser powers of 79, 95, and 111 mW, indicating the decrease in the etched line width down to 0.6 μm with the increase in beam scanning speeds or with the decrease in laser powers.

The local temperature rise induced by laser irradiation is an important parameter in laser pyrolysis, which should be minimized for processing of III-V compound semiconductors such as GaAs because of the high vapor pressure of constituent elements, and, hence, the difficulty of preserving the stoichiometry at high temperatures. The temperature profile at a moving laser spot is estimated by solving the three-dimensional heat equation using the Kirchhoff transform with the linearized temperature and the Green's function method [6, 7]. The important parameters which scatter the calculated values at high temperatures are the temperature-dependent thermal conductivity K(T) and thermal diffusivity D(T) of materials. In this study, K(T)=171/(T+100) and D(T)=163/(T+100) for GaAs was used by fitting the published values by MAYCOCK [8], and the peak temperature was calculated.

Figure 5 shows the etched depth as a function of a laser power and corresponding calculated maximum temperatures at a $SiCl_4$ pressure of 74 Torr. The beam scanning speed was 3 μm/sec with a beam diameter of 18.7 μm (at $1/e^2$ intensity) or 13.2 μm (at 1/e intensity). The etching was observed with a laser power of 0.25 W, corresponding to a peak temperature of 205°C. The etched depth increases exponentially from 2 μm up to 15 μm, as the laser power, i.e., the peak temperature, increases. It should be noted that the temperature at which the etching starts coincides with the

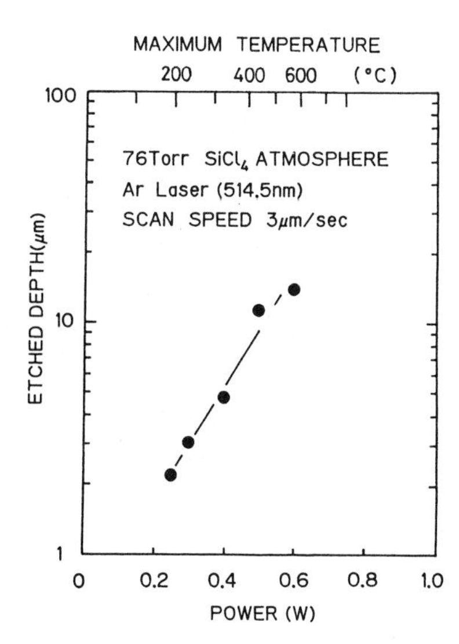


Fig. 5 Etched depth as a function of incident laser power and corresponding maximum temperature

boiling point of $GaCl_3$ (201.3 °C), where the vaporization of $GaCl_3$ is exponentially enhanced. The incident laser power of 0.6 W in this case induces a temperature rise up to 594 °C, which is a critical temperature for the decomposition of GaAs surfaces, although the etched depth of more than 10 μm by a single scan of a laser beam can be obtained.

Although the temperature rise in the case of fine focused laser beams as in Figs. 2 – 4 is estimated to be around 1000 °C, the beam dwell time is shorter by an order of magnitude than the case in Fig. 5. Therefore, the deterioration due to local heating is considered to be small. The etching rate seems to be higher for longer dwell times at low temperatures as in Fig. 5 than that for short beam dwell times at high temperatures as in Figs. 2 – 4.

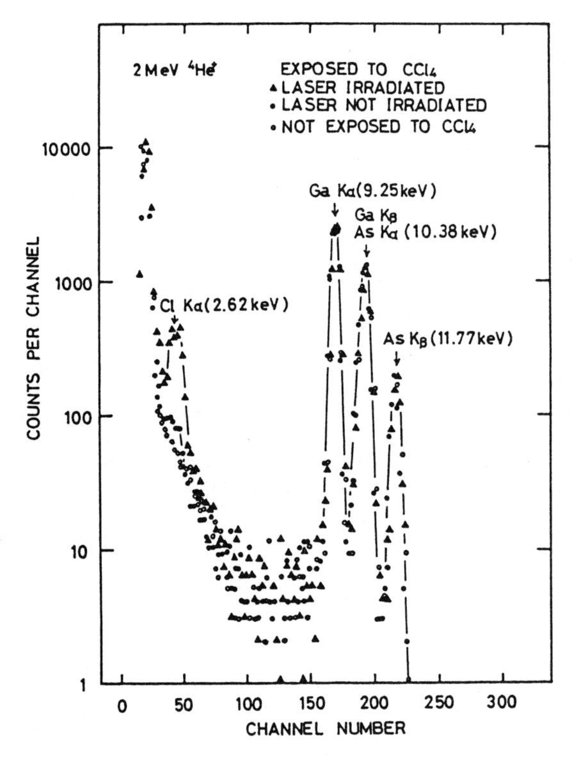


Fig. 6 Ion induced X-ray spectra for GaAs samples before and after laser assisted etching in $CCl_4$ atmosphere at a pressure of 100 Torr

Figure 6 shows IIXE spectra for GaAs samples exposed to $CCl_4$ at a pressure of 100 Torr before and after laser irradiation, indicating Cl K-shell X-rays besides characteristic Ga and As X-rays. The Cl X-ray signal is observed for the sample exposed only to $CCl_4$ gas and increases by an order of magnitude after laser irradiation. The thickness of chlorine adsorbed layers was estimated from the X-ray intensity to be one mono-layer for the sample exposed only to $CCl_4$, provided that chlorine adsorbs at sample surfaces with a form of $CCl_4$, which was confirmed by AES measurements. The content of chlorine at the surface is enhanced after laser irradiation up to 10 layers presumably because of $GaCl_3$ products, which vaporize by a local temperature rise above 200 °C due to laser irradiation.

Although the GaAs sample is locally heated by at least 200 °C, the obtained etch rate for the laser pyrolysis in this study is higher than that for the ultraviolet laser photolysis [2].

## 4. Conclusion

Maskless dry etching of GaAs by laser pyrolysis with a controlled linewidth of down to 0.6 μm was performed using Ar laser beams focused to 1.2 μm at ambient $CCl_4$ or $SiCl_4$ gas pressures ranging from 32 to 100 Torr. The obtained etch rate was higher and the minimum line width was narrower than those of laser photolysis for GaAs. The minimum local temperature for pyrolytic etching was found to be about 200°C, which corresponds to the boiling point of reaction products, i.e., $GaCl_3$.


## Acknowledgements

The authors are indebted to K. Murakami (Tsukuba University) for helpful discussions on microscope optics, to H. Aritome and Y. Yuba for continuing discussions on etching, and to K. Kawasaki and K. Mino for their help during experiments.


## References


1. D.J. Ehrlich, R.M. Osgood, and T.F.Deutsch:IEEE J. Quantum Electron. QE-16, 1233 (1980)
2. D.J. Ehrlich, R.M. Osgood, and T.F.Deutsch: Appl. Phys. Lett. 36, 698 (1980)
3. Y. Yuba, K. Gamo, X.G. He, Y.S. Zhang, and S. Namba: Japan. J. Appl. Phys. 22, 1211 (1983)
4. M. Takai, J. Tokuda, H. Nakai, K. Gamo, and S. Namba: Japan. J. Appl. Phys. 22, L757 (1983)
5. M. Takai, J. Tokuda, H. Nakai, K. Gamo, and S. Namba: in *Laser-Controlled Chemical Processing of Surfaces*, eds. A.W. Johnson and D.J. Ehrlich (North-Holland, New York, 1984) in press
6. Y.I. Nissim, A. Lietoila, R.B. Gold, and J.F. Gibbons: J. Appl. Phys. 51, 274 (1980)
7. J.E. Moody and R.H. Hendel: J. Appl. Phys. 53, 4364 (1982)
8. P.D. Maycock: Solid-State Electron. 10, 161 (1967)

# Laser Induced Reduction and Etching of Oxidic Perovskites

J. Otto[+], R. Stumpe, and D. Bäuerle
Angewandte Physik, Johannes Kepler Universität, A-4040 Linz, Austria

## 1. Introduction

In oxidic perovskites like $SrTiO_3$, $BaTiO_3$,etc. oxygen vacancies can easily be produced by first heating the material in a reducing atmosphere, e.g. in hydrogen atmosphere, up to several hundred degrees and then quenching it to room temperature. The concentration of vacancies increases with increasing reduction temperature and with decreasing oxygen partial pressure. The oxygen vacancies act as shallow donor levels and the originally insulating material (band gap typically 3eV) becomes a n-type semiconductor; the originally transparent material changes to a blue or black colour, depending on the concentration of vacancies [1,2]. Because of the fundamental role of the oxygen ion in connection with the dynamical properties of perovskites, the oxygen vacancies also strongly influence the ferroelectric and non-ferroelectric structural phase transitions observed in these materials [3,4].

In this paper we report on the local reduction and reactive etching of oxidic perovskites by means of visible $Ar^+$ and $Kr^+$ laser light. These first experiments have been performed on single crystal $SrTiO_3$ and $BaTiO_3$ and on ceramic $PbTi_{1-x}Zr_xO_3$ (PZT).

## 2. Results and Discussion

The experimental setup was similar to that described in [5]. The reducing atmosphere was 90 mbar $H_2$. When moving the oxidic perovskite with constant velocity, $v_s$, perpendicular to the laser beam, the material is locally reduced, resulting in conducting stripes with an electrical conductivity which is increased by several orders of magnitude compared to the surrounding bulk material. At higher laser powers, P, reactive etching occurs.

### 2.1 Laser Induced Reduction

In the single crystals, the width and depth of the conducting stripes corresponds roughly to the diameter of the laser focus, $2w_0$, which was varied from a few µm up to about 100 µm . With increasing laser power, at constant laser focus diameter and constant scanning velocity, the conductivity of the stripes strongly increases. For $SrTiO_3$,e.g., with $2w_0 = 42\mu m$, $v_s = 42\mu m/sec$ and a laser power in the range of $0.9\ W < P(Ar^+, \lambda = 488\ nm) < 1.3\ W$, the corresponding dc resistance per unit length of stripe was found to be $12\ k\Omega/mm \gtrsim R \gtrsim 2\ k\Omega/mm$ (this corresponds to a change in resistivity of at least a factor of $10^{12}$). Similar results were obtained for $BaTiO_3$.

+)Present address: Institut für Prozeßmeßtechnik und Prozeßleittechnik Hertzstraße 16, D-7500 Karlsruhe, FRG

The conductivity of the stripes is based on the production of oxygen vacancies and free electrons as in oven heated homogeneously reduced bulk material. The reduction process is reversible, i.e. when heating the material in $O_2$ atmosphere or in air, the conducting stripes vanish. Only a small change in surface morphology was observed. When increasing the laser power above about 1.3 W, with otherwise the same parameters, reactive etching or cutting is observed. The low power limit for which reduction is observed strongly depends on the surrounding atmosphere. It may be considered remarkable that the results for the colourless transparent $SrTiO_3$ crystals and the yellowish flux-grown $BaTiO_3$ crystals were found to be similar. This observation may be a hint that under steady state conditions, the absorbed laser light is essentially determined by the absorbance within the reduced region itself; the situation seems to be very similar to the steady growth of stripes in laser induced chemical vapour deposition [5]. The absorbance of the bulk material and the surface quality, however, determines the latent time for the beginning of the reduction process. For $SrTiO_3$ this latent time seems to be determined by local perturbations on the surface as,e.g., "dust" particles or scratches.

The conducting stripes produced on ceramic PZT show remarkable differences to those on single crystal $SrTiO_3$ and $BaTiO_3$. Two distinct regions are observable. In a relatively broad region the colour of the PZT is changed to black. In the centre of the stripe, scanning electron micrographs show an etching and destruction of the perovskite structure. A variation of the laser power in the range 200 mW $\leqslant$ P ($Ar^+$, $\lambda$= 488 nm) $\leqslant$ 600 mW yielded a dc resistance per unit length of stripe which was $10^5$ Ω/mm $\gtrsim$ R $\gtrsim$ 10 Ω/mm. In the best samples, the resistance/length decreased approximately logarithmically with laser power.

When annealing the PZT samples in an oxygen atmosphere or in air, the outer region of the stripe changes back to nearly the original colour of the bulk material, indicating that the change in colour originates from a reduction of the material. Although the resistance of the stripe is increased during annealing, it still remains much lower than the original bulk value. Because the change in the conductivity cannot be completely annealed, and furthermore,because the stripes without a centrally damaged, but with a reduced region, do not show measurable increase of the conductivity, we conclude that the increase of the conductivity is due to a metallisation, and not due to a reduction of the material. This is also supported by ac measurements, which do not show any frequency dependence of the conductivity up to the highest measuring frequency of 10 MHz. A metallisation of the central region is also confirmed by microprobe measurements. The reproducibility of the electrical measurements was much worse than for the single crystals. The reason is probably based on microcracks which often have been observed in the central part of the stripes and in particular in metallised regions.

## 2.2 Laser Induced Etching

Reactive etching and cutting of oxidic perovskites in an $H_2$ atmosphere can be performed with much lower laser powers than in air. Moreover, the depth of grooves, h, is much more uniform and the edges are much steeper than in any experiment performed in air. Scanning electron micrographs of grooves produced in air and in $H_2$ atmosphere are shown in Figs. 1a and b,c, respectively. For ceramic PZT, a focussed beam diameter $2w_0$ = 50 µm, a scanning velocity of $v_s$ = 10 µm/sec and a range of laser powers between 0.7 W $\leqslant$ P ($Kr^+$, $\lambda$= 647.1 nm) $\leqslant$ 1.8 W, the depth of the grooves was 50 µm $\leqslant$ h $\leqslant$ 400 µm. The ratio of width, d, and depth of grooves was about d/h ≈ 0.1.

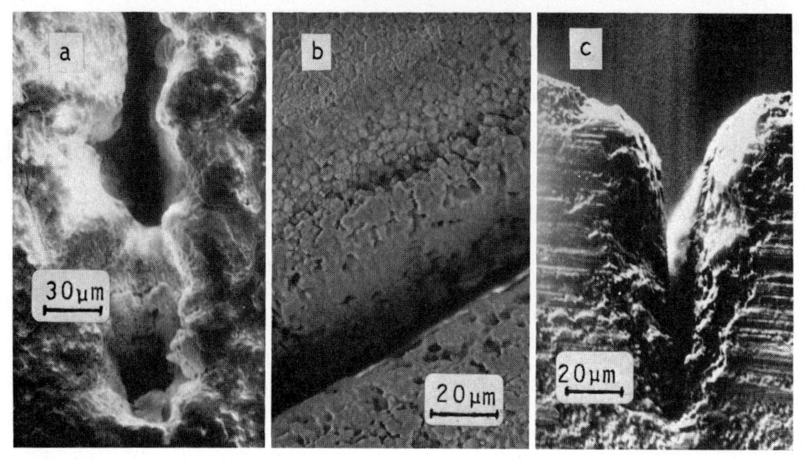


Fig.1: Scanning electron micrographs of grooves etched with 647 nm $Kr^+$ laser radiation in Nb-doped PZT (x=0.48) ceramic: a) 90 mbar air (1.7 W), b) 90 mbar $H_2$ atmosphere (800 mW), c) profile of a groove etched in $H_2$

## 3. Conclusion

Laser chemical processing of oxidic perovskites in $H_2$ atmosphere allows single-step production of conducting microstructures or micron-sized grooves within the otherwise unaffected material. The reproducibility of the reduction experiments was satisfactory for the single crystals, but not for the ceramic samples. Reactive etching of ceramic PZT could be performed with high accuracy and reproducibility.

Acknowledgements:

We wish to thank Dr E. Hammel (Austria Microsystems Int.) for performing scanning electron micrographs, and Drs. H. Thomann and W. Wersing (Siemens) for the PZT ceramics.

References:

1. see, e.g.: Landolt-Börnstein III/16a: Ferroelectrics: Oxides (Springer-Verlag, Heidelberg, 1981)
2. G. Perluzzo, J. Destry: Can. J. Phys. 56, 453 (1978)
3. R. Migoni, H. Bilz, D. Bäuerle: Phys. Rev. Lett. 37, 1155 (1976)
4. D. Bäuerle, D. Wagner, M. Wöhlecke, B. Dorner, H. Kraxenberger: Z.Physik B 38, 335 (1980), and references therein
5. D. Bäuerle: this volume

# Laser Enhanced Plating and Etching: A Review

R.J. von Gutfeld

IBM T.J. Watson Research Center, P.O. Box 218
Yorktown Heights, NY 10598, USA

Experiments on laser enhanced plating and etching are reviewed with particular emphasis on applications to microelectronic materials. Depositions of nickel, gold and copper are described, obtained by using a focused argon laser to provide maskless patterning onto premetallized glass substrates. The theory for the enhancement is discussed in terms of photothermal effects, i.e., increased charge transfer and mass transfer rates as well as a shift in the equilibrium potential with increased local temperature. The highest deposition rates have been obtained using a collinear laser-jet configuration. Results for gold and copper using this system will be described. The laser etching of stainless steel, silicon and a number of ceramics is discussed using both electroetching and chemical machining techniques.

## 2. Introduction

The ability to produce maskless patterns on conducting and nonconducting surfaces is a subject of widespread interest, particularly for applications relating to the microelectronics industry. Patterning is crucial to chip circuitization as well as the multitude of peripheral circuits comprising the circuit package. Maskless patterns can result in enormous savings in both production and labor costs by obviating the need for mask fabrication. Eliminating masks is particularly effective in the area of circuit modeling in which a design is tested and altered based on the test results until an optimum design is obtained. Generally, each design change requires a new mask. Typical turn around time for the fabrication of a mask can be from several days to several weeks. A further problem with masks is that they are often impractical or even impossible to use particularly where parts to be processed (etched or plated) have non-planar geometries or in fabrication techniques such as reel-to-reel plating where parts are moving rapidly through a plating bath.

For cases involving precious metal plating such as gold, large savings can also be realized with the aid of suitable maskless patterning techniques by preventing unnecessary deposits from occurring in those areas not requiring gold.

We have developed a maskless plating and etching technique which utilizes a focused laser beam directed onto the part requiring patterning and confines the plating (etching) to essentially that region exclusively via thermal enhancement mechanisms [1 4]. The general scheme is illustrated in Fig. 1 showing the laser and an optically transparent plating cell attached to a computerized x,y,z table. Arbitrary patterns are generated via the table movement or with the scanning mirror in combination with the table. The enhancement ratio for the laser illuminated region compared to that not illuminated can be as high $\sim 10^4$:1. This laser plating technique has been successfully applied to the plating of nickel, copper and more recently to gold. Copper lines (minimum dimensions, 2$\mu$m in width) were deposited on a variety of substrates including glass predeposited with metals such as tungsten, molybdenum, copper and gold. Nickel and electroless nickel depositions have also been successfully laser plated on similar substrates. Gold spots, on the order of ~0.5 mm - 1 mm diameter, up to ~50$\mu$m high have more recently been laser plated on bulk metal substrates [5,6].

Interest in laser enhanced gold plating over the past year and a half has centered on obtaining plating rates an order of magnitude higher than those previously reported (1$\mu$ m/s) by using a new scheme, laser enhanced jet plating [7]. The increase in plating rates must not degrade the

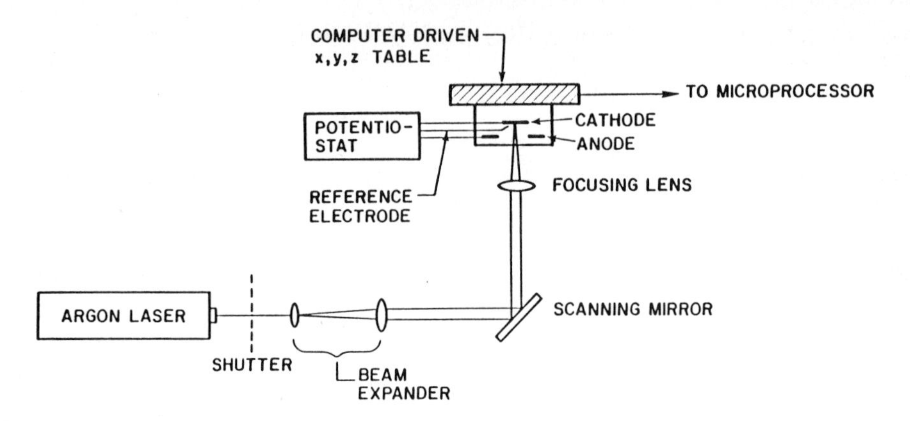


Figure 1 Schematic of laser, potentiostat and computer controlled table. Beam can also be scanned over the sample. Both laser and potentiostat can be operated CW or pulsed.

following deposition requirements, 1) pore free and dense deposits, 2) good adhesion, 3) low electrical resistivity, and 4) proper Knoop hardness. This has required a detailed study of the parameters of laser enhanced plating, in particular those pertaining to the limiting current density.

## 3. Theory

The following thermal mechanisms for laser enhanced plating have been previously identified: [1-4] 1) At low overpotentials $\eta$, the enhancement is due mainly to an increase in the charge transfer kinetics with increased temperature since charge transfer is a thermally activated process; the temperature dependence of the charge transfer term is expressed explicitly in terms of the exchange current density, $i_o$,

$$i_o = nFC_A \frac{kT}{h} \left[ \exp\left(\frac{-\Delta F^\circ}{RT}\right) \right] \exp\left(-\frac{n\alpha F}{RT}\varepsilon^\circ\right) \quad (1)$$

while the expression for the current density i in the low overpotential regime is given by the Butler-Volmer expression

$$i = i_o \left[ \exp \frac{n\alpha\eta F}{RT} - \exp\left(-\frac{n\beta\eta F}{RT}\right) \right] \quad (2)$$

Here $\alpha$ and $\beta$ are exchange coefficients, k is Boltzmann's constant, R is the gas constant, F is Faraday's constant, T is absolute temperature, $\varepsilon^\circ$ and $F^\circ$ are the equilibrium potential and free energy of the reaction respectively, and $C_A$ is the ion concentration per $cm^2$ at the cathode. 2) The equilibrium potential $\varepsilon^\circ$ is temperature dependent and shifts to a larger (more positive) value with increasing temperature for many electrolytes. This positive shift has the effect of off-setting the polarization curve to higher current densities for a fixed overpotential at the higher temperatures. This shift was measured for the $Cu/Cu^{++}$ system by Puippe et al. [3] and has been measured by us recently for the Selrex solution, Autronex 55GV [8]. A shift towards a more positive value with increasing temperature was found to occur. However, this positive shift does not occur for all electrolytes and, in fact, is negative for an interface of Ni- with a $NiSO_4$, sodium citrate electrolyte. 3) At higher overpotentials, plating rates are limited by the rate of mass transport of ions J, into the ion depleted region. The mass transport by diffusion for an unagitated solution is given by Fick's law

$$J_i = -D_i \nabla C_i \quad (3)$$

where $J_i$ is the ionic flux, $D_i$ is the diffusion constant for the ith species with $C_i$ the ionic concentration of species i. However, with agitation, increased mass transport takes place. With local laser heating, hydrodynamic stirring occurs in the local region of laser absorption. This increased mass transport can be expressed by the more complete mass transport expressions of Nernst-Planck,

$$J_i = -D_i \nabla C_i - \frac{z_i F}{RT} D_i C_i \nabla \phi + C_i v . \qquad (4)$$

Here the second term on the right expresses the field dependent mass transport in terms of the potential gradient while the last term represents forced convection in terms of the velocity component of the ith species with $z_i$ the ionic charge in electronic units. Velocity fields v for laser enhanced plating have been estimated for special boundary conditions from three-dimensional solutions to the Navier-Stokes equations by Langlois [9]. An additional plating enhancement mechanism has been observed for laser enhanced copper and shown to be due to localized boiling. This causes additional mass transport over and beyond that afforded by hydrodynamic stirring.

## 4. Laser Enhanced Electroplating

The effect of local laser heating in producing enhanced plating (etching) rates was studied in detail for the system $Cu/Cu^{++}$ using a specially designed miniature electrode [3]. This structure consisted of a premetallized glass substrate covered entirely by a layer of photoresist except for a small aperture (hole) with diameters in the range 200-600 μm. Polarization curves (current vs. overpotential) were obtained over the entire range of the kinetic and mass transport regions. These data are shown in Fig. 2a for a 550 μm diameter electrode without the laser and a 200 μm diameter electrode, Fig. 2b, with the laser applied at 50 mV intervals. A ratio of current with and without the laser of as high as 500 (enhancement factor) is observed.

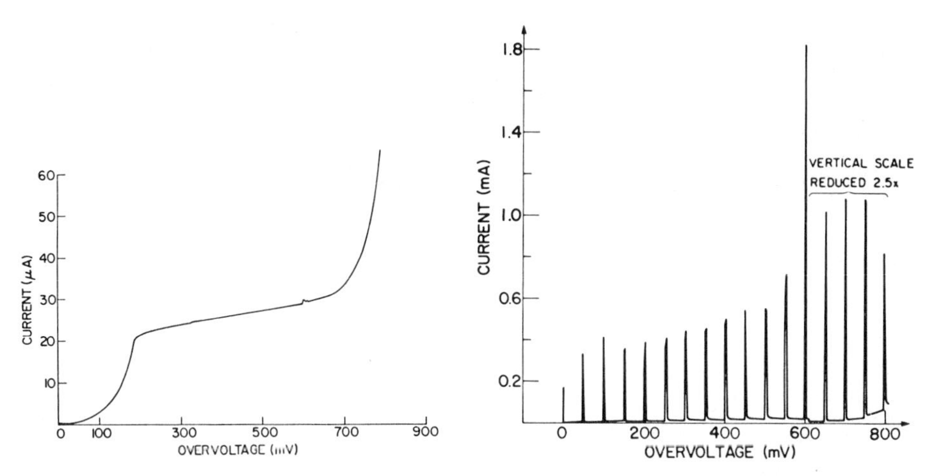


Figure 2 a) Polarization curve for a 0.05M solution of $CuSO_4$ and $H_2SO_4$ and an electrode of 550 μm in diameter. b) Polarization curve for a 200 μm diameter electrode with the laser applied at 50 mV intervals, indicated by the current spikes.

We have also utilized laser enhanced plating to produce a variety of gold spots and lines for use as contact areas on microelectronic connectors and connector material [5]. For these experiments, nickel plated Be-Cu substrates, approximately 8 mil thick, were used as the cathode material as this is the material commonly used in today's connector industry. Some experiments were also conducted using pure nickel shim stock. Since the thermal conductivity here is so much higher compared to the previously described glass substrates, considerably higher laser powers and power densities were required. We used 1.5 watts to plate small spots (~50 μm diameter) and ~20 w from an argon laser to plate 0.5 mm diameter spots (0.1-3.0 watts were used for copper plating experiments on glass substrates). By operating near the potential corresponding to the mass transport limited region, we were able to obtain ~0.5 mm diameter gold plated areas and ~200 $\mu$m wide gold lines with very little background plating. The purpose of these experiments was to determine the parameters that give rise to: (1) dense, small grained, crack free and uniform deposits, (2) good adhesion to the substrates, (3) improved plating speeds. The parameters important to these properties are: (1) high density gold concentrations of the electrolyte, (2) elevated ambient temperatures, and (3) sufficient mass transport to replenish the ionically depleted solution in the region of the cathode. Examination of the metallurgy of numerous laser plated gold deposits using SEM (scanning electron microscopy) for the surface morphology and optical microscopy of cross-sectioned samples for interior examination revealed crack-free, dense deposits. For spots, deposition rates up to 1 $\mu$m/s were obtained. Three important parameters were recognized in this study for yielding quality depositions: the use of a defocused beam to prevent overheating for spots, rapid scanning of the beam for lines, the physical displacement of the beam producing the equivalent to resupplying ions in the region of plating, and the use of a high concentration of gold (up to 4 Tr oz/gallon in these studies) [5]. An example of the surface morphology of a ~600$\mu$m diameter gold spot laser plated onto a nickel plated Be-Cu substrate is shown in Fig. 3.

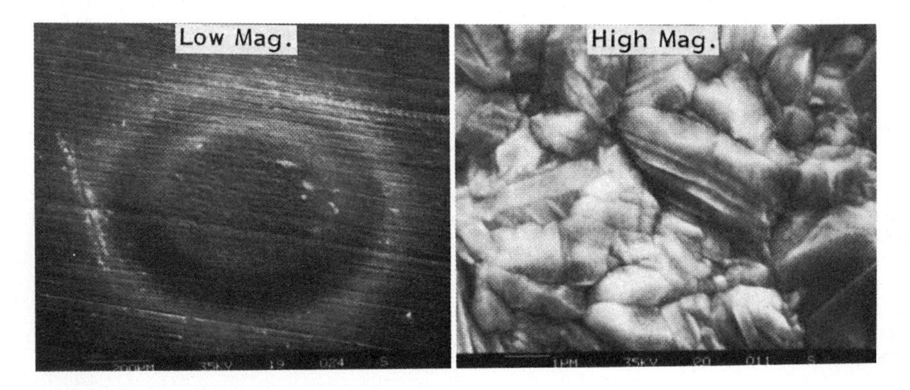


Figure 3 Gold spot deposited onto nickel plated Be-Cu substrate using high density gold solution, 4 Tr oz/gallon (Autronex 55GV).*

These experiments also showed that plating rates greater than 1 $\mu$m/s would not be possible without degrading the morphology of the deposits. Increased current density resulted in dendritic and cratered growth. This kind of morphology generally results when operating near the limiting current density, $i_\ell$ , determined by the flux of ions entering via mass transport with $i_\ell$ given by:

$$i_\ell = \frac{nFDC_o}{\delta} \tag{5}$$

where $\delta$ is the diffusion layer thickness and $C_o$ the concentration of the ion (here, gold) in the bulk of the solution with C, the concentration at the electrode interface at the boundary approaching zero.

Initial attempts to increase the mass transport of ions into the plating region included: 1) high speed mechanical stirring of the electrolyte near the laser-cathode impingement region, and 2) the use of a submerged recirculating jet with flow tangentially across the laser-cathode impingement area. The submerged jet produced some increase in the laser plating rate (20-40%) while no noticeable increase was observed from the high speed stirring.

---

*Selrex Corp., Nutley, NJ

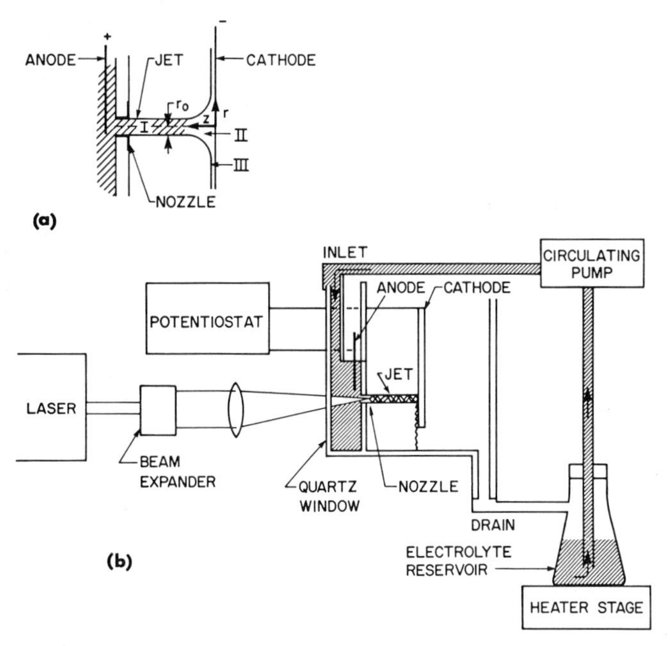


Figure 4 (a) Diagram of the free jet (no laser) showing the impingement regions as given in Ref. 10. The jet is assumed to have a radius $r_0$ in region I as well as uniform axial velocity. Electric field varies only in the *z* direction. II is the stagnation flow region. Region III constitutes the wall jet, a thin layer of fluid which during plating carries very low current densities. The fields therefore are assumed to vary only in the ***r*** direction. (b) Schematic of the laser-jet system. The laser is directed through the lens to focus approximately at the center of the jet nozzle. The cathode is attached to the ***xyz*** table via an extension arm.

A novel approach which has resulted in a substantial increase in the gold plating rate is shown schematically in Fig. 4. This arrangement has been termed by us "laser-enhanced jet plating" as it combines an earlier concept of a free standing jet with laser plating [7]. In the present configuration the jet serves three major functions: 1) To provide maskless patterning of the region of jet impingement on the substrate (cathode), 2) to deliver a rapid re-supply of gold ions to the region of plating permitting high plating current densities not possible in conventional plating, and 3) to confine the light beam within the jet, thereby using the jet as a light guide. The following experimental results have been found for laser jet gold plating onto 8 mil thick nickel plated Be-Cu substrates: 1) Plating rates up to 10 $\mu$m/s using Autronex 55GV solution for a 0.05 cm nozzle diameter, 2) excellent adhesion of the plated gold based on scotch tape pull tests, and 3) high density, crack-free deposits based on cross-sectioned SEM examination.

The jet can be divided into three fundamental regions as shown in Fig. 4a. Region I contains the jet of radius $r_0$, assumed to travel with uniform velocity over its cross-sectional area. Here electric fields have only z dependence while in region II, the stagnation region, electric fields vary in both the z and radial directions. Region III, the wall jet region, contains a relatively thin layer of fluid with velocity and electric field variation principally in the r direction. This layer produces a thin region of plating that extends somewhat beyond $r_0$ [10]. The relatively small thickness of the deposition is a result of the relatively high electrical resistance compared to that which exists in II. The high resistance in III gives rise to relatively small current densities and causes the thickest deposition to occur in region II. The laser light is focused into the center of the orifice of the jet and after diverging beyond the focal plane is maintained within the liquid column by total internal reflection until impingement on the cathode. The potentiostat for these experiments was

**TABLE I:** Gold plating solution and laser-jet cell parameters.

| Gold Solution | Sel-Rex* Autronex 55GV, Au cyanide, no additives, 4 Tr. Oz. Au/gal. |
|---|---|
| Solution temperature | 60 C |
| Jet orifice | 0.05 cm diameter, ~ 0.2 cm long |
| Linear flow velocity | $1.0 \times 10^3$ cm/s |
| Reynolds number | $5.5 \times 10^3$ |
| Nozzle-cathode spacing | ~ 0.5 cm |
| Plating current density | 1 - 16A/ $cm^2$ |
| cw Laser power into jet | ~25 W maximum |

*Sel-Rex, Div. of Oxy-Metal Industries Corp., Nutley, NJ 07110.

set to deliver constant current, i.e. to plate galvanostatically. Patterning was achieved by moving the cathode via the computer controlled xyz table. Spots were made with current densities as high as 16 A/$cm^2$. With a 0.05 cm diameter nozzle orifice and 25 W of laser power, plating rates of 10 $\mu$m/s were observed. This should be contrasted to conventional gold plating where maximum current densities are 0.25 A/$cm^2$ and plating rates are more than two orders of magnitude slower [11]. We also found that with a smaller nozzle, 0.035 cm diameter, rates as high as 20 $\mu$m/s were obtained. This increase in plating rate over that found for the 0.05 cm nozzle indicates that plating over the larger area was limited by the available power density at the cathode, in turn limited by the total available laser power. Details of the experimental parameters of the cell and plating conditions under which most of the experiments were carried out are listed in Table I. Gold spots as a function of varying plating times were produced by maintaining the jet fluid flow continuously and then simultaneously applying the plating current and laser power. The laser power was controlled by the xyz table microprocessor and was turned off between plating spots as the sample moved to new plating positions. During this time the potentiostat was left running continuously. These samples were cleaned using only detergent and acetone prior to a quick dip in concentrated HCl as opposed to the extensive precleaning and surface activation technique customarily used in the plating industry. Some examples of laser-jet plated spots are shown in cross section, Figs. 5 a-c. Examination of their morphology after metallographic etching indicates a dense deposit consisting of small grains, free of cracks and pores. Upon electroetching, the samples were found to possess a columnar structure, typical of pure soft gold deposits. In addition excellent adhesion between the gold and ~ 2 $\mu$m thick nickel was found based on the "scotch-tape" pull test. In contrast, cross-sections of depositions using the same jet and the same high current density as in Fig. 5 but without laser radiation during plating are shown in Fig. 6. Here voids are present throughout the deposit irrespective of film thickness, apparently initiated at the nickel-gold interface. This type of columnar deposit with columns physically separated from each other is typical of metal depositions near the limiting current density (Eq. 5) for a given agitated solution, particularly if deposited on substrates with incomplete oxide removal. Scotch tape pull-testing of these deposits showed poorer adhesion with the gold sometimes separating from the substrate and adhering to the tape as might be expected due to the less stringent precleaning. We also found that laser-jet plated spots sometimes contain peripheral deposition areas not subjected to laser light, i.e. in the wall jet region. These peripheral areas were also removed with scotch

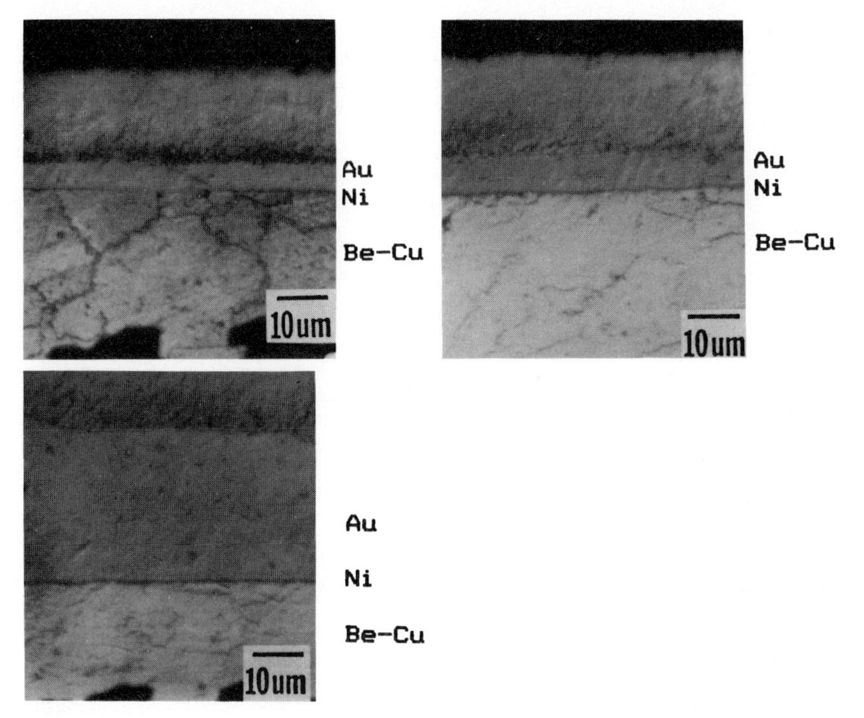


Figure 5 Cross sections of laser-jet plated gold spots on nickel-plated Be-Cu substrates, 200$\mu$m thick. The current density is 11A/ $cm^2$. In each case, the top layer is an electrodeposited nickel deposition to protect the gold during cross sectioning and polishing. Laser-jet plating times and resulting thicknesses are (a) 0.5 s, 4.5$\mu$m; (b) 1 s,8 $\mu$m; (c) 5 s,30 $\mu$m.

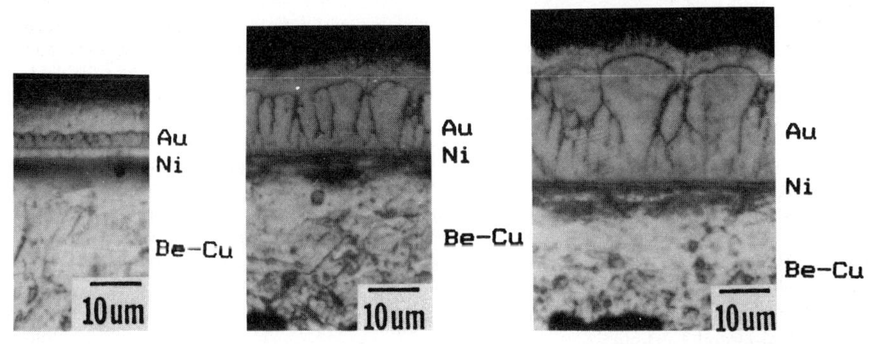


Figure 6 Cross section of jet plated areas without the use of laser power during deposition. Substrates and current densities are the same as for Fig. 4. Plating times and resulting thicknesses are (a) 1 s, 3$\mu$m; (b) 5 s, 12.5$\mu$m; (c) 10 s, 25$\mu$m. Note the cracks and voids throughout the deposits, irrespective of gold film thickness in contrast to laser-jet plating. (Fig. 5).

tape while the central laser irradiated portion remained intact. However, this peeling does not occur with properly cleaned and activated substrates. Thus, although there is some significant substrate cleaning that the laser produces, its usefulness is not clear in the present context since no peeling can be tolerated in any manufacturing plating application. Thus very clean substrates may have to be used with laser-jet plating applications to assure good adhesion over the entire plated area.

The three significant experimentally observed results from these laser-jet gold plating experiments are: 1) an increase in plating speed due to local laser heating of the cathode, 2) improved adhesion, probably caused by a cleaner cathodic surface resulting from local heating providing a gold to nickel metal bond rather than gold to nickel oxide bond, and 3) crack-free, dense deposits at much higher current density than is possible for the jet alone. This may be due to annealing of internal film stresses that occur simultaneously with the deposition process as a result of laser heating. It should be noted that it is possible to obtain gold deposits of the quality and structure of Fig. 5 from jet plating without the laser, but at current densities (hence plating rates) on the order of one magnitude smaller.

The new laser-jet technique has been demonstrated to have the highest plating rate for gold reported to date, up to 10 $\mu$m/s for a 0.05 cm nozzle and ~20$\mu$m/s for a 0.035 cm nozzle diameter. We have studied the plating rates as a function of both laser power and current density and found the speed to be linearly dependent on both sets of parameters over a wide range. Knoop hardness measurements of cross sectioned laser-jet plated samples indicate the soft gold to have values in the range 70-90 Kg/mm$^2$, [12], well within the range of values expected for conventionally plated soft gold. We have also shown that with the 0.5 mm diameter nozzle, the plating rates for gold are limited by the available laser power (power density) from the argon laser (25 W max). We have obtained thermal profiles of the Be-Cu samples during laser-jet plating as a function of position and time. The full width, half maximum of the temperature rise extends approximately two nozzle diameters. This result is very encouraging for closely spaced localized patterning of a continuous ribbon which could be utilized in a reel to reel plating machine. In addition the fast thermal rise times we have measured (less than 50 ms for 8 mil thick samples) indicate a possible throughput of 5 to 10 spots per second for plating thicknesses of 1-2 microns [8].

We have also initiated studies of other laser-jet metal systems, namely copper for the purpose of maskless circuit design and repair.

## 5. Laser Enhanced Plating without External Electrodes

Two other types of laser enhanced plating have been identified that require no external electrodes or sources of EMF. Both of these electrodeless effects have been experimentally demonstrated and described in other reports [3,4]. The first of these is electroless plating where a catalyst is contained in the plating solution to complete the reduction process and maintain charge conservation [4]. Electroless nickel has been plated at rates up to 1000Å /s using 2-3 watts of focused argon laser light incident on a glass sample containing a pre-metallization. Background plating rates were maintained at approximately 5 Å /s.

The thermobattery or laser enhanced exchange plating utilizes the positive shift in the rest potential which results in a local thermobattery [3,4]. Both copper and gold have been plated on both metal and premetallized glass samples. Enhanced plating occurs in the heated region while simultaneous etching occurs in the area peripheral to the laser heated region. However, since in many applications the peripheral area is large compared to the region undergoing deposition, localized etching effects are small and need not be deleterious to the part.

## 6. Laser Enhanced Etching:

Reversal of anode and cathode potentials from those described previously gives rise to laser enhanced etching. Several materials have been etched successfully in this manner, particularly thin stainless steel shim stock. Through holes, laser electroetched in 2 mil stainless, have been produced with extremely uniform roundness at rates on the order of 10 $\mu$m/s using a solution of $NiCl_2$ in combination with a focused argon laser [4].

A second type of laser enhanced etching utilizes intense heating to cause local melting of the substrate prior to etching [13]. This form of chemical machining also requires no external electrodes. Experimentally, the substrate is immersed in an etchant such as KOH with a focused laser beam incident on the surface. This technique has been used to etch sub-millimeter patterns in a number of ceramics and [111] silicon. We believe the high speeds obtainable with this method are related to 1) increased thermal activation at the high melt temperatures for the chemical etch process and 2) rapid microstirring of the etchant due to the intense local boiling. The latter helps to rapidly remove the reacted fluid and replenish the depleted etchant ions.

Materials that have been successfully etched by this technique include $Al_2O_3/TiC$, a very hard ceramic, WC, glass, alumina and silicon. Both grooves and holes of varying depths have been fabricated. Linear etch rates of 200 $\mu m/s$ have been observed for $Al_2O_3/TiC$ with an incident power of $10^6$ $W/cm^2$. [111] Si, a symmetry direction which under normal conditions will not etch in KOH at ambient temperatures, has been etched at rates up to 10 $\mu m/s$ using a focused beam of 15 W ($\sim 10^7 W/cm^2$). It is believed that etching occurs because the local melting destroys the crystal symmetry prior to chemical reaction with the etchant.

## 7. Acknowledgments

The work described has been in collaboration with a number of coworkers whom I wish to acknowledge for their many contributions over the years. They include Drs. L. T. Romankiw, R. E. Acosta, J-Cl. Puippe, and M. H. Gelchinski; also thanks go to E. E. Tynan and D. R. Vigliotti for their collaborative and technical assistance.

## REFERENCES

1. R. J. von Gutfeld, E. E. Tynan, R. L. Melcher, and S. E. Blum, ***Appl. Phys. Lett.*** 35, 651 (1979).

2. R. J. von Gutfeld, E. E. Tynan, and L. T. Romankiw, Extended Abstract No. 472 Electrochem. Soc. 79-2 (1979).

3. J.-Cl. Puippe, R. E. Acosta, and R. J. von Gutfeld, ***Journal of Electrochemical Society,*** 128, 2539 (1981).

4. R. J. von Gutfeld, R. E. Acosta, and L. T. Romankiw, IBM Journal of Res. & Develop. 26, 136 (1982). See also R. J. von Gutfeld in "Laser Applications", Vol. V (J. F. Ready and R. F. Erf, Eds.) Academic Press (1984) pgs. 1-67.

5. M. H. Gelchinski, L. T. Romankiw, and R. J. von Gutfeld, Extended Abstracts 82-2, pg. 206, ***Electrochem. Soc.***, Detroit, MI, October, 1982.

6. L. T. Romankiw, M. H. Gelchinski, R. E. Acosta, and R. J. von Gutfeld, Proc. of Symposium on Electroplating Engineering & Waste Recycle. New Develop. & Trends, Electrodeposition Div. Proc. Vol 83-12, ***Electrochem. Soc.***, pg. 66 (1983).

7. R. J. von Gutfeld, M. H. Gelchinski, L. T. Romankiw, and D. R. Vigliotti, ***Appl. Phys. Lett.*** 43, 876 (1983).

8. R. J. von Gutfeld and D. R. Vigliotti, (unpublished).

9. W. E. Langlois, IBM Res. Lab., San Jose, CA (unpublished).

10. R. C. Alkire, and T. J. Chen, ***J. Electrochem. Soc.*** 129, 2424 (1982).

11. D. R. Turner, Thin Solid Films 95, 143 (1982).

12. M. H. Gelchinski, R. T. Romankiw, D. R. Vigliotti and R. J. von Gutfeld, to be published.

13. R. J. von Gutfeld and R. T. Hodgson ***Appl. Phys. Lett.*** 40, 352 (1982).

# Laser Surface Modification Below a Liquid Layer

Terence Donohue

Laser Physics Branch, Naval Research Laboratory
Washington, DC 20375, USA

## 1. Introduction

Reactions at interfaces are now being examined with increasing vigor, with applications as diverse as catalyst synthesis to integrated circuit production under study. As has been found for the entire field of laser-enhanced chemistry, most such efforts have involved gas-phase reactions, for reasons of familiarity and relative simplicity. However, most conventional industrial processes use the liquid phase as the preferred medium. Thus, as advantages have been reported in employing the liquid phase as the optimum phase in elemental photochemical separation and purification work [1], similar results are now being reported in laser processing at liquid/solid interfaces. These advantages over gas/solid interactions include a much larger variety of reactants available without restrictions on volatility. Furthermore, temperatures at the interface can be kept lower and spatial resolution can be controlled through adjustment of diffusion lengths in solution.

Recent reports from a number of laboratories have discussed thermal etching processes in silicon by KOH [2], etching of InP by $H_3PO_4$ [3], and metallic aluminum by various acids [4]. Photochemical etching has also been observed in certain cases, resulting from direct excitation of a semiconductor surface [5] and by excitation of species in a solution or absorbed on the surface [6]. Features as fine as 2 μm have been reported [4], using a direct-write, "serial" processing technique. However, lasers could be even more useful and efficient if employed in large-area, wafer size "parallel" processing methods [7], where masks are used to define features. Here the advantages of the laser over mercury lamps used in current methods include a greater variety of photolytic wavelengths available, and better spatial characteristics, including a much higher depth-of-field. In the work reported here, both types of processing techniqes have been employed on several semiconductor and metal surfaces [8].

## 2. Experimental

Photochemical sources used included a Lumonics excimer laser (Model 610), as well as a Quanta-Ray neodymium YAG laser. The excimers used were KrF (249 nm), XeCl (308 nm) and XeF (351 nm), with pulse lengths of approximately 10 ns, repetition rates varied from 0.5–10 hz and pulse energies varied from 1–150 mJ. The YAG laser was doubled to operate at 530 nm, and pulse energies and rates varied as with the excimer sources.

Two optical configurations were used: In the geometry used for direct writing, the beam was focussed at the liquid/surface interface, with a spot size of about 100 μm. For parallel processing, the beam was expanded and passed through a mask before impinging on the surface. Two types of masks were used. The first was made of a thin stainless steel sheet, with features of 200 μm and larger. The second was gold deposited on a quartz substrate (allowing transmission to below 193 nm) with features as fine as 10 μm discernable. Projection distance between the mask and surface was varied from 20 μm to several mm depending on the experiment involved.

## 3. Results and Discussion

The experiments described here fall into two distinct classes. Those employing direct writing techniques by a focussed beam involved very high energy densities, typically about 100 $J/cm^2$ per pulse or $10^{10}$ $watts/cm^2$. On the other hand, the second type used mask-defined features with unfocussed or defocussed laserbeams where the energy was usually $10^4$ times smaller, 10 $mJ/cm^2$ per pulse or 1 $MW/cm^2$. These are clearly different regimes, where the first will be dominated by thermal processes, but the second will allow photochemistry to become significant if the chemistry is carefully chosen.

### A. Thermal Processing

The high peak powers used here caused thermal damage and related effects with every substrate examined. More useful were thermally activated effects resulting from transient high temperatures at liquid/surface interfaces. These included enhanced etching of $SiO_2$ on Si by sulphuric acid. Here, the liquid reduces unwanted ripple outside of the main portion of the laserbeam, while the hot $H_2SO_4$ removes $SiO_2$ at the high temperatures produced during the laser pulse, estimated to be around 100 C, close to the solvent boiling point. These effects were not observed with neat water or other acids.

A similar effect was found with a clean copper surface under a liquid. Only with hydrochloric acid was a reaction observed, where small bubbles were observed following each laser pulse, and more rapid etching of the Cu surface was observed. Here, again, the reaction is thermally enhanced, according to:

$$Cu + HCl \longrightarrow CuCl + 1/2\, H_2 . \qquad (1)$$

This reaction is endothermic at room temperature, but proceeds vigorously at elevated temperatures. Further details of some of these results can be found in Ref. 8.

### B. Photochemical Processing

At the much lower power densities used in here, thermal effects were not observed and all processes could be assigned to photochemically induced reactions. Features were produced using masks and unfocussed laser light. Several types of processes were used in attempts to etch copper. This metal was chosen for ease of study in a proof-of-principle type effort to understand what might be involved in working with other metals less amenable to conventional processing, such as iron or stainless steel. The first reaction system used cerium, which becomes a powerful oxidizing agent when it becomes electronically excited by photolysis in its f-d bands around 250 nm [9, 10],

$$Ce^{3+} \xrightarrow{h\nu} Ce^{4+} \xrightarrow{h\nu} (Ce^{4+})^* \quad . \qquad (2)$$

While $(Ce^{4+})^*$ is a powerful enough oxidizing agent to oxidize copper, we never observed significant etching rates. This is due to the fact that it was not possible to generate a large enough excited species density near the surface, since the excited state survives for less than 20 ns. A significant improvement was found when reaction (2) was used as part of a photosensitization sequence:

$$(Ce^{4+})^* + Cl^- \longrightarrow Ce^{3+} + 1/2\, Cl_2 \quad . \qquad (3)$$

In this case, the reaction sequence can produce molecular chlorine [11], which effectively oxidizes and hence removes copper surfaces. With this system, crude mask-defined features could be produced, but reaction rates were still slow.

Best results were obtained using a different photochemical system where molecular bromine dissolved in water, and sometimes in the presence of KBr, was used as the photochemical etchant. This solution shows a peak absorption at 350-400 nm, thus either a XeCl or XeF laser was found to be effective. Reactivity was also observed when using doubled YAG at 530 nm, but was slow, since this wavelength is in the tail of the $Br_2$ absorption. Figures 1-4 show scanning electron micrographs of the results of some copper etching experiments. The first two were produced using the stainless steel mask, which was placed 3 mm above the copper surface, hence the poor resolution. Interesting and unusual micron-sized grains can be seen at the edges in Fig. 2. These particulate structures are probably CuBr, which is rather insoluble in water. The reaction sequence deduced from these observations is given as

$$Br_2 \xrightarrow{h\nu} 2\,Br\cdot \,; \quad Cu + Br\cdot \longrightarrow CuBr\,;\ CuBr + Br\cdot \longrightarrow CuBr_2 \ . \qquad (4)$$

In aqueous solution, $CuBr_2$ is very soluble, and thus copper is removed from the surface as $Cu^{2+}$. The lower density of bromine radicals, Br·, at the edge reduces the rate to the extent that insoluble CuBr can build up. An obvious improvement would be finding a method for rapidly dissolving CuBr as it is

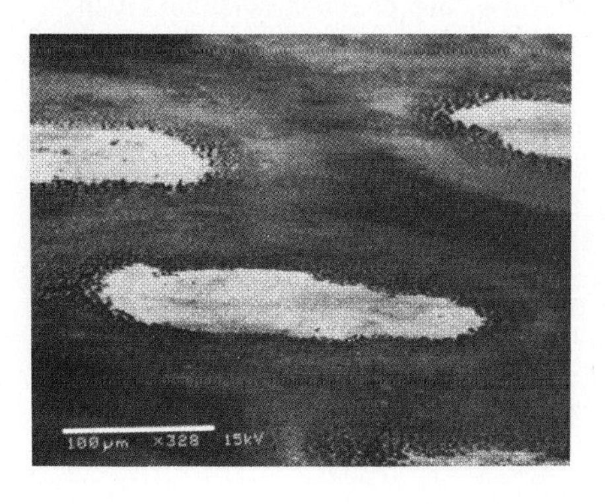

Fig. 1. Large-scale view of a copper surface following photochemical etching with a solution of bromine in water. The photolytic source used was a XeF laser.

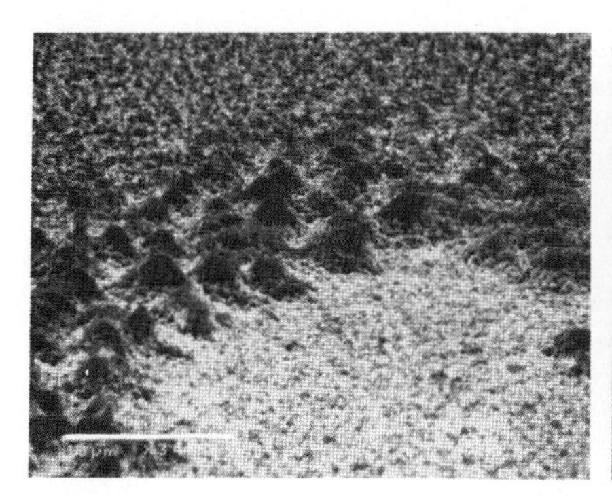

Fig. 2. A more detailed scan of a section from Fig. 1, showing structure of the grainy deposits found at the edges of photolyzed regions, probably due to CuBr.

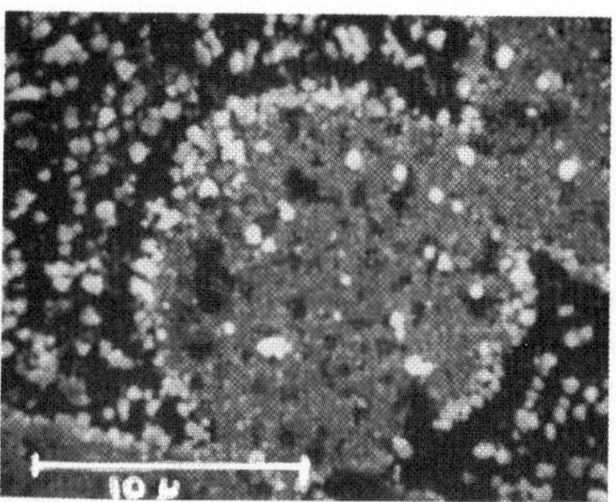

Fig. 3. Most detailed feature produced using the gold on quartz mask. Here a XeCl laser was the photolysis source.

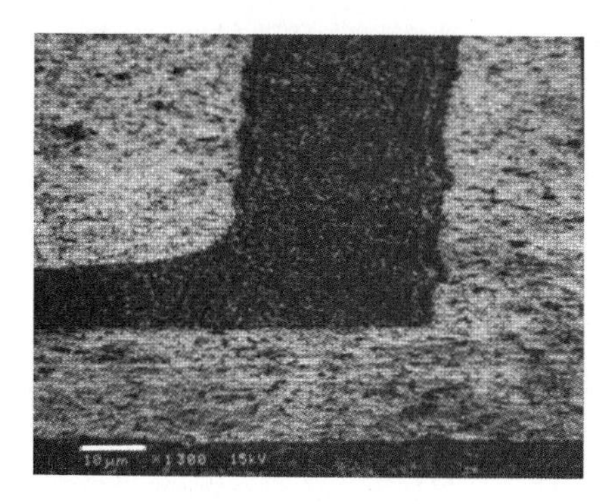

Fig. 4. Another feature produced with the same mask used in Fig. 3. The waviness is due to irregularities in the copper on fiberglas surface. These results suggest that resolution below 2 μm should easily be attainable.

formed. Thus the need for a second bromine radical would be eliminated. Bromide ions, as from KBr, should assist, but we have been unable to observe any improvement in etching rates in the presence of KBr in the solution.

The best resolutions obtained are shown in Figs. 3 and 4, and were obtained using the Au/quartz mask positioned about 15-20 μm above the surface. The resolutions observed here have been degraded by the poor mask quality, as well as the uneven copper surface (a printed circuit board cleaned in ferric chloride and nitric acid). We anticipate much higher quality when finer masks and improved surfaces are employed.

## 4. Conclusions

The liquid phase offers some clear advantages in comparison with more conventional gas-phase work in that a greater variety of reactions are possible, though more effort is necessary to find those which will be useful. The results obtained so far suggest that species which absorb on the surface can be more effectively employed than those occurring in homogeneous solution. This limitation is related to the fact that diffusion lengths in solution are very short, so that a species with a lifetime of 10 ns will diffuse only a few nm. This effect is, of course, good for high resolution but poor for efficient use of photons. Longer-lived, photolytically produced reagents will allow more efficient photon use, but with a reduction in resolution. Non-linear reactions, where two or more photons are necessary to cause a reaction, could create another class of reaction systems, and permit higher resolution features as well. We have observed features on $SiO_2$/Si under dodecane tentatively assigned to such a process. More research is needed to define the limitations of laser-controlled surface processing with a liquid phase before truly viable processes can be expected.

## References


1. T. Donohue, in Chemical and Biochemical Applications of Lasers, Vol. V, ed. C. B. Moore (Academic, New York, 1981), p. 239; Opt. Eng. 18, 181 (1979).
2. R. J. v. Gutfeld and R. T. Hodgson, Appl. Phys. Lett. 40, 352 (1982).
3. J. E. Bjorkholm and A. A. Ballman, Appl. Phys. Lett. 43, 574 (1983).
4. J. Y. Tsao and D. J. Ehrlich, Appl. Phys. Lett. 43, 146 (1983).
5. R. M. Osgood, A. Sanchez-Rubio, D. J. Ehrlich and V. Daneu, Appl. Phys. Lett. 40, 391 (1982); G. C. Tisone and A. W. Johnson, Appl. Phys. Lett. 42, 530 (1983).
6. R. W. Haynes, G. M. Metze, V. G. Kreismanis and L. F. Eastman, Appl. Phys. Lett. 37, 344 (1980).
7. D. J. Elliot, Integrated Circuit Fabrication Technology (McGRaw-Hill, New York, 1982).
8. T. Donohue, Proc. S.P.I.E. 482, 125 (1984).
9. T. Donohue, Chem. Phys. Lett. 61, 601 (1979).
10. R. W. Matthews and T. J. Sworski, J. Phys. Chem. 79, 681 (1975).
11. T. Donohue, in Photochemical Conversion and Storage of Solar Energy, ed. J. S. Connolly (Academic, New York, 1981), p. 443; J. Less Common Metals 94, 83 (1983).

# Selectivity of Etching III-V Compounds by Laser-Induced Electrochemistry

A. Wayne Johnson, L.R. Dawson, and R.V. Smilgys
Sandia National Laboratories, Albuquerque, NM 87185, USA

The laser-induced electrochemical etching of III-V compounds is a demonstrated method for the spatially defined removal of materials from surfaces [1]. A critical feature of the etching process is its selectivity: for example, the relative etch rate of p-doped compared to n-doped material or of one compound compared to another compound. A second important feature is the etching mechanism near a heterojunction or a p-n junction. We have identified the controlling mechanisms of the etching process that elucidates these features. For illustrative purpose, we will present the analysis and data on the $Ar^+$-laser-induced electrochemical etching of the compounds gallium arsenide and gallium phosphide with n and p dopants. Etching occurs in an aqueous solution of KOH. The analysis and description is also applicable to other III-V compound materials.

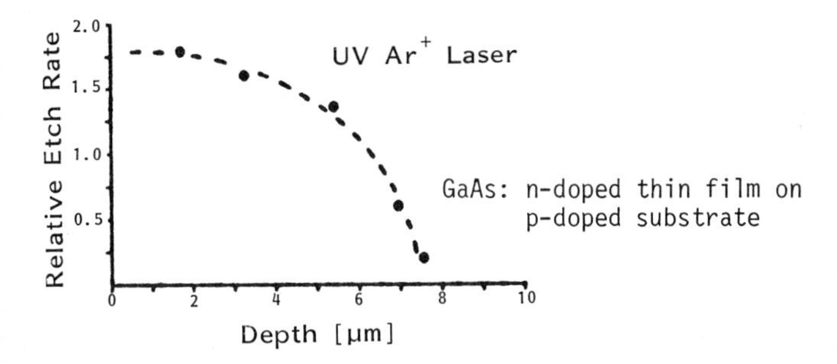


The etch rates, measured near a p-n junction in GaAs (see Fig.), illustrate how the holes, produced by the laser, control the etching. A thin film of n-doped material, 9-micrometers thick, was epitaxially grown onto a p-doped substrate. For this data, the $Ar^+$ laser was held constant (3000 $W/cm^2$), and the etch rate was measured from the top of the thin film to near the junction. At the top of the thin film, etching of the n-doped material proceeds rapid-

This work performed at Sandia National Laboratories supported by the U.S. Department of Energy under contract number DE-AC04-76DP00789.

ly ($5 \times 10^{-2}$ cm/s). As the etching nears the junction, the electric fields in the solid are such as to drive the holes away from the liquid-solid interface and the etching rate is reduced. Etching for the p-doped substrate is over 100 times slower than that near the top of the thin film. By a judicious selection of the laser wavelength, etching selectivity of over a factor of 100 has also been demonstrated for GaAs compared to GaP.

## References


1. For further details see
   A.W. Johnson, G.C. Tisone: In *Laser Controlled Chemical Processing of Surfaces*, ed.by A.W. Johnson et.al. (North Holland, New York, 1984) and references therein

# Photochemical Microetching of InP

D. Moutonnet, S. Mottet, D. Riviere, J.P. Mercier
Centre National d'Etudes des Telecommunications, B.P. 40
F-22301 Lannion Cedex, France

## 1 Introduction

For the fabrication of microwave or optoelectronic devices on InP materials, different etching techniques are used such as classical chemical etching, or preferential chemical etching following crystallographic orientation [1,2], or plasma etching and photoetching [3-7]. With our scanning optical microscope, the light spot is used to etch photochemically n-type InP samples immersed in several basic or acidic solutions.

## II Experimental

The scanning optical microetching set-up has been previously described [8]. The light source is a 632.8 nm HeNe Laser. The optical system gives a spot of 1.3 µm diameter. The sample is covered by a small quantity of aqueous solution spread into a thin film by capillary action under the cover glass. Two stepping motors, positioned by a computer, control the etching of grooves or patterns. The single crystals of InP were grown by LEC method in CNET laboratories. We used n-type substrates with a carrier concentration of $10^{16}/cm^3$. The (100) and $(\bar{1}\bar{1}\bar{1})$ or B-face samples were polished with a $Br_2$ /methanol solution. The (111) or A-face substrates were only chemically/mechanically HCl/NALCO polished. Different basic or acidic aqueous solutions have been studied. They are known to etch III-V semiconductors and contain different oxidizing agents such as HCl, $HNO_3$ , $H_2O$ , $Fe^{+++}$... [9,10,11].

## III Results

### IIIa Basic aqueous solutions

These weakly concentrated solutions are known to etch III-V semiconductors such as GaAs, for example 5 % KOH aqueous solution [8]. Only a weak attack is obtained on InP samples using a light power of $2 \times 10^7$ W/cm$^2$.
Etching occurs only on the surface illuminated for a long time (⩾5 minutes). The etching rate is too slow to record a figure by scanning the surface. If the basic concentration is increased (from 10 % to 45 %), the etching rate decreases. For the higher concentration, no etching takes place. This phenomenon can be explained by better decomposition of the active molecule in

low concentrated solution, and therefore a greater reactivity under illumination can be observed. The same phenomenon has been observed for aqueous acidic solution with HCl or $HNO_3$. These results are very different from those obtained on n-GaAs samples [8]. In this case, a light power of $4x10^4$ W/cm$^2$ give an etching rate of about 20 μm/sec.

IIIb - Acidic aqueous solutions

Various chemical etchings have been performed with aqueous acidic solutions. In order not to induce any reaction on the unilluminated sample areas, solutions with a conventionally very low etching rate (from 0.1 to 1 μm/hr) have been selected [12]. The object of the experiments is to increase the etching rate under the illuminated area. Figure 1 shows scanning electron micrographs of the n-InP surface in a $HNO_3$:HCl:$H_2O$ (3:1:6) etchant. The upper part is unilluminated. The lower part has been scanned by the laser light ($7x10^5$ W/cm$^2$) in order to etch grooves.

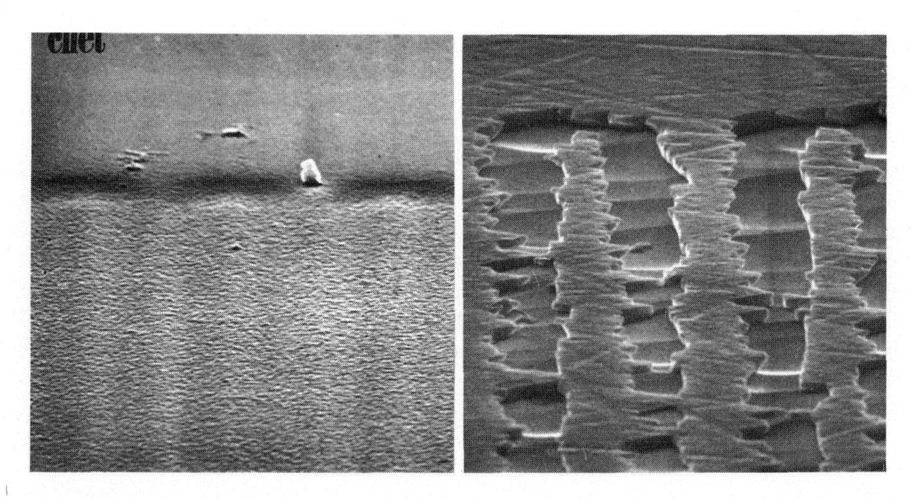

Fig.1 Scanning electron micrographs of n-InP (Scanning speed = 2 μm/sec)
(a) (100); (b) (111)

For the (100) and ($\bar{1}\bar{1}\bar{1}$) surface, the grooves present the same smooth profile (Fig. 1(a)) and the unilluminated area is unperturbed. Figure 1(b) shows, for the (111) surface, a very different surface aspect. In the unilluminated area, lines crossing the surface have been revealed, corresponding to polishing and dislocations. In the illuminated area, etching appears to proceed by sheet removing. This attack can be due to the crystal structure (zinc-blende) of the III-V intermetallic compounds [9]. The (100) and ($\bar{1}\bar{1}\bar{1}$) faces have phosphorus atoms on the surface while the (111) face has only indium atoms. So, it seems that under illumination, the solution mainly reacts with phosphorus atoms. On the (111) face, the attack seems to proceed via the surface defects which expose the phosphorus atoms. This might explain the irregularities observed along the illuminated grooves.

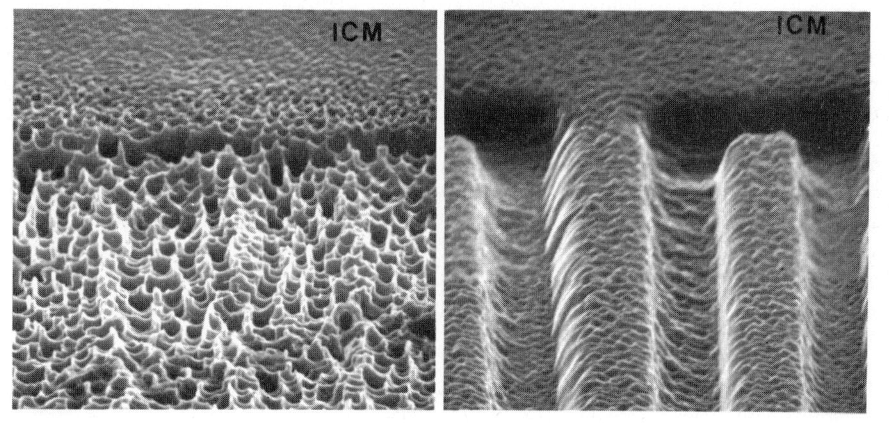


Fig. 2. Scanning Electron micrographs of n-InP (111) (scanning speed = 2 μm/sec; step = 4 μm), (a) P = $7x10^5 W/cm^2$; (b) P = $4x10^4 W/cm^2$

Figure 2 shows results obtained with 41 % $FeCl_3$ aqueous solution under the same experimental conditions. The surfaces present a rough aspect for all the orientations (Fig.2 (a)). A decrease of light power ($4x10^4 W/cm^2$) leads to a better definition of grooves (Fig. 2(b)). These results can be compared with those obtained on GaAs sample in Ref. [8].

In order to study the boundaries between illuminated and unilluminated areas, a grating of 4 μm width, 1000 μm length and 0.5 μm step has been performed. The overlapping of the etching grooves due to the spot area, changes this grating into a large groove which can be cleaved along a (110) direction. The etchant is $FeCl_3$ (41 % aqueous solution) in Fig. 3(a) (P = $4x10^4 W/cm^2$) and $HCl:HNO_3:H_2O$ (1:3:6) (P = $7x10^7 W/cm^2$) in Fig. 3(b). In Fig. 3(a), the total groove width is about 6.2 μm, corresponding to the total illuminated area. On the other hand, in Fig. 3(b), the total groove width is about 11.6 μm. The same wide profile has been observed for different incident light power. Therefore, the widening of the groove cannot only be attributed to photons. We assume that incident light creates electron-hole

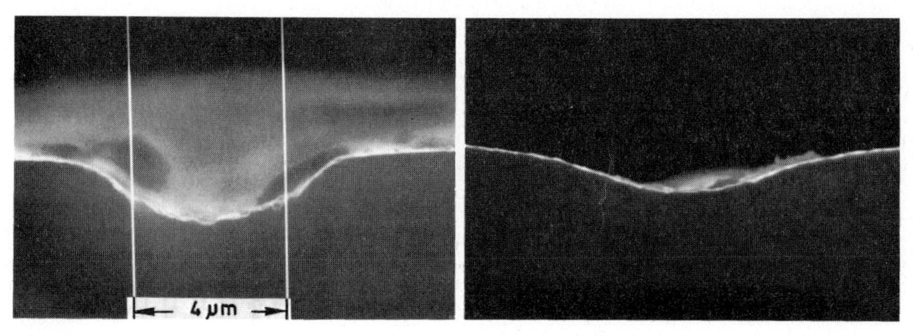


Fig. 3. Groove profile of n-InP (100) along a (110) direction (scanning rate = 9 μm/s) (a) $FeCl_3$; P = $4x10^4 W/cm^2$; (b) $HCl:HNO_3:H_2O$;P = $7x10^7 W/cm^2$

pairs which will diffuse into the bulk material. A semi-log representation of Fig. 3(b) allows to estimate the carrier diffusion length $L_D$ [13,14]. We have found a value of about $2 \times 10^{-4}$cm which is in good agreement with that of bulk material.

## IV - Conclusion

According to the results, it is more difficult to obtain a good surface aspect for InP than for GaAs. These difficulties are similar to those encountered in InP plasma etching. The etching technique, though relatively slow, might be used for via-hole technology. Different experiments are being performed with weak acids (such as $H_3PO_4$ and HI) and with other oxidizing agents.

## References


1. Z.L. Liau, J.N. Walpole and D.Z. Tsang : Appl. Phys. Lett. 44, 945(1984)
2. K. Furuya, L.A. Coldren, B.I. Miller and J.A. Rentschler : Elec. Lett. 17, 582 (1984)
3. D.J. Ehrlich, R.M. Osgood, Jr, and T.F. Deutsch : Appl. Phys. Lett. 36, 698 (1980)
4. R.M. Osgood, Jr, A. Sanchez-Rubio, D.J. Ehrlich and V. Daneu : Appl. Phys. Lett. 40, 391 (1982)
5. P.A. Kohl, F.W. Ostermayer, Jr, : "Photoelectrochemical etching of semiconductors", USA patent 4,369,099(1983)
6. F.W. Ostermayer, Jr, P.A. Kohl and R.H. Burton : Appl.Phys. Lett. 43, 642 (1984)
7. P.A. Kohl, C. Wolowodiuk and F.W. Ostermayer, Jr : J. Electrochem. Soc. Sol. St. Sci. Technol. 130, 2288 (1983)
8. S. Mottet, L. Henry : Elec. Lett. 19, 919 (1983)
9. H.C. Gatos and M.C. Lavine : J. Electrochem. Soc., 107, 427 (1960)
10. H.C. Gatos and M.C. Lavine : J. Electrochem. Soc., 107, 433 (1960)
11. G. Colomer : Private communication
12. A.R. Clawson, D.A. Collins, D.L. Elder and J.J. Monroe : "Laboratory Procedures for Etching and Polishing InP Semiconductors", NOSC TN 592(1978)
13. D. Moutonnet, M. Matabon : 2nd Conf. on "Semiconductor Injection Lasers and their Applications" Cardiff (1979)
14. S.M. Sze : In "Physics of Semiconductor Devices", 2nd edition Wiley-Interscience Publication (1981)

# Ultraviolet Laser Ablation of Organic Polymer Films

R. Srinivasan
IBM Thomas J. Watson Research Center
Yorktown Heights, NY 10598

## 1. Introduction

When a pulse (~ 14 nsec half-width) of laser radiation of 193 nm wavelength with a fluence above a threshold value falls on a polymer film, the material at the irradiation site is spontaneously etched away to a depth of 1000 Å or more.[1,2] This process has been called Ablative Photo Decomposition' [3]. The excimer laser which is the source of the 193 nm radiation is capable of providing radiation at other wavelengths such as 249 nm, 308 nm, and 351 nm. Spontaneous etching of the polymer films by the laser beam has been observed at all of these wavelengths [4-7]. But there are quantitative differences in the etching process at different wavelengths and with different polymers.

This review is meant to be:

(i) an introduction to the subject of ultraviolet laser ablation of organic polymer films,

(ii) a critical analysis of all of the published data on the subject in order to point out the directions in which further research can be undertaken, and

(iii) a discussion of the mechanisms which have been proposed to explain the phenomenon of UV laser ablation.

## 2. Interaction of Polymer Films with Ultraviolet Radiation

The ultraviolet region of the electromagnetic spectrum (Fig. 1) corresponds to electronic transitions in organic molecules. In solution phase, in non-polar solvents, organic molecules give rise to absorption spectra which are nearly free from intermolecular interactive effects. As a first approximation, polymer films can be viewed as highly viscous solutions. But as the degree of crystallinity of the films increases and some local ordering of the polymer chains is achieved, the absorption spectra can show changes in intensity and wavelength as well as anisotropy. In the near- and mid-UV region, the absorptions in organic molecules are from valence transitions from bonding to anti-bonding MOs but at 193 nm, Rydberg transitions also become important [8].

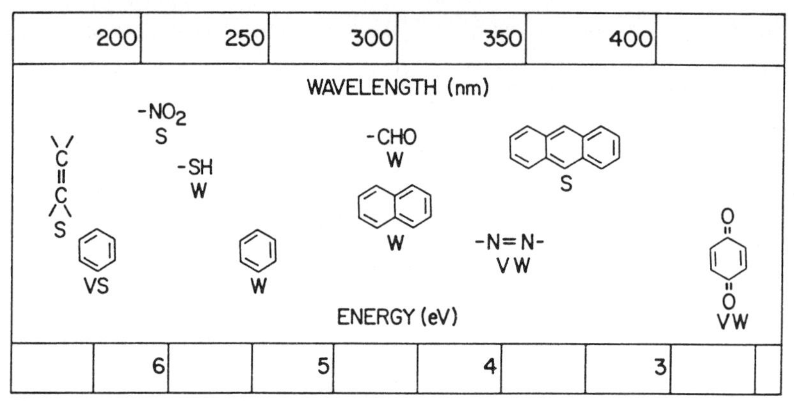


**Fig. 1 Ultraviolet Absorption Maxima of Some Typical Organic Groups**

**The maxima tend to be broad (half–width ~ 50 nm) and have very little structure. The intensities are denoted by S – strong; VS – very strong; W – weak; VW – very weak**

It is generally accepted that absorption of the excimer laser pulse will lead to an electronic transition (Fig. 2 - Step 'a') in the polymer molecule. The subsequent behavior of this excited species is well-documented in general terms in the photochemical literature [9].The excited molecule can decompose

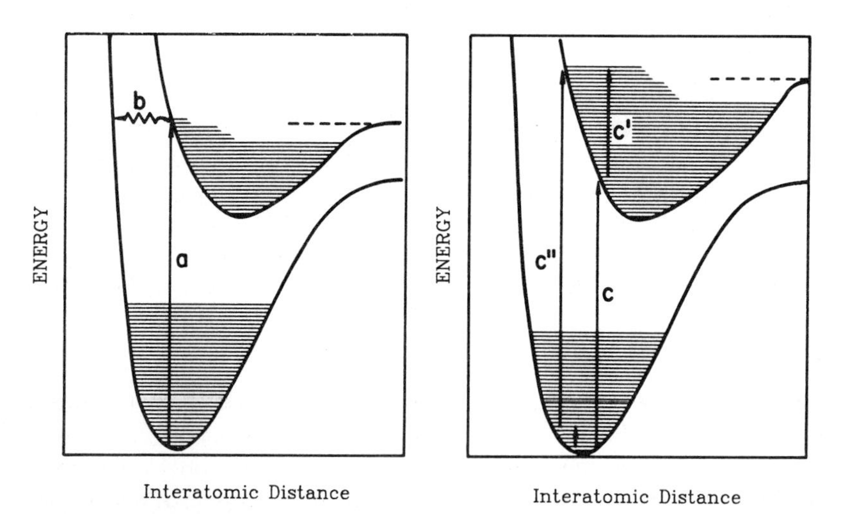


**Fig. 2 Hypothetical Potential Energy Curves of a Diatomic Species**

**The lower curve represents the ground state and the upper one an electronically excited state. The horizontal lines correspond to vibrational levels. A vertical arrow within an electronic state represents a vibrational transition which is equivalent to a thermal excitation. A vertical arrow between two electronic states represents a photoexcitation. The wiggly line b indicates an internal conversion.**

via three pathways. If the transition ('a') leads to an energy level in the excited state that is above the dissociation energy in the state, the molecule can dissociate at the very next vibration, i.e., in a matter of picoseconds. This is most likely to happen with a photon of high energy content which would be the case at the shortest wavelength. This purely photochemical process, when followed by ablation can be called 'ablative photodecomposition'. However, every excited molecule may not dissociate but instead cross over to the ground state (Fig. 2 - Step 'b') in which case the electronic energy will be internally converted to vibrational-rotational energy. In turn, this energy will be rapidly dissipated among the surrounding molecules and cause a local rise in the temperature of the film. This heating effect can cause the thermal decomposition of the weakest bond in the polymer molecule and the products can be ejected by vaporization. This would also lead to etching of the film and this mechanism has been referred to as a photo-thermal process. A third possibility involves an initial transition to an upper state (Fig. 2 - Step 'c') which lacks the energy to decompose from that state itself. If this state can be activated by a temperature rise (i.e., step 'c' is followed by c' or 'c' is replaced by c''), decomposition can occur in the excited state. The thermal energy would come from a certain number of excited molecules which would internally convert to the ground state as in the photo-thermal process described above. This mechanism obviously combines elements of the first two processes and can be termed a thermally-assisted (or activated) photoprocess. The common element to all three mechanisms is the initial excitation to an electronic transition. Therefore, an important difference between the interaction of polymer films with UV radiation on one hand and visible or infrared radiation on the other is that in the latter instances, initial excitation is unlikely to populate an upper electronic level except at fluences high enough to allow facile multiphoton transitions. It follows that long wavelength laser radiation is more likely to cause purely thermal decomposition. Since the absorption spectra of organic molecules and polymers can vary widely, it is important to emphasize that the behavior observed in one polymer (e.g., polyimide) at 308 nm may be from an initial electronic transition whereas in another case (e.g., polymethyl methacrylate) the spectrum can be entirely different and the same wavelength photons may not lead to electronic excitation.

If a sufficient number of bonds in a small volume of polymer are broken in a short time interval, there would be a considerable increase in pressure in that volume which will be caused by the volume change that can be ascribed to the reaction as well as the excess energy possessed by the fragments. Therefore it is not surprising that the fragments are ejected with high translational, vibrational, and rotational energies. What is really remarkable is that the fragments remove the excess energy so well that the substrate shows no detectable sign of heat damage even when fluences as high as 0.5 $J/cm^2$/pulse are used and extremely heat-sensitive polymers such as atactic polymethyl methacrylate ($T_g$ = 104°C)[10] or biological tissue (cornea)[11] are the substrates. The process appears to be truly an 'ablation' [12].It is this aspect of the interaction of UV laser radiation with organic polymers that has focused attention to this phenomenon and led to considerable technological interest.

In the following text the term 'ablative photodecomposition' will be used only when a purely photochemical pathway is implied. The more general term 'UV laser ablation' will be used to denote all of the processes (including ablative photodecomposition) that can occur when laser radiation of wavelength <370 nm (the conventional long wavelength limit for ultraviolet) causes the removal of material from the surface of a polymer film.

## 3. Experimental Results on UV Laser Ablation

The data that have been published are mainly concerned with

(i) The depth of the etching that can be achieved with a pulse of a given fluence at a certain wavelength in nearly a dozen polymers.

(ii) The energy which remains in the film following UV laser ablation.

(iii) The translational and vibrational energy in the ejected material as well as its angular distribution.

(iv) The spectrum of the visible radiation that can be seen above the etched surface.

(v) The chemical analysis of the low molecular weight (m/e<200) material that is ejected.

(vi) The XPS study of the surface created by ablative removal from a polymer.

Items ii - vi are more fragmentary than 'i' in that the data have been obtained in only one or two polymers. In addition, considerable attention has been paid to the morphology of the surface that is created by the laser pulse since this information is of importance to the technological application of the phenomenon. This last aspect will not be discussed here except to remark on a suggestion that has been made[13] relating the nature of the etched surface to the plasma that is created by the laser beam at fluences >1 $J/cm^2$/pulse.

We shall examine these data in order.

(i) The logarithm of the fluence when plotted against the etch depth per pulse is a measure of the effectiveness of the photons in causing ablation. In view of the utility of this information for practical applications and, more significantly, since these measurements are the easiest to make, there are as

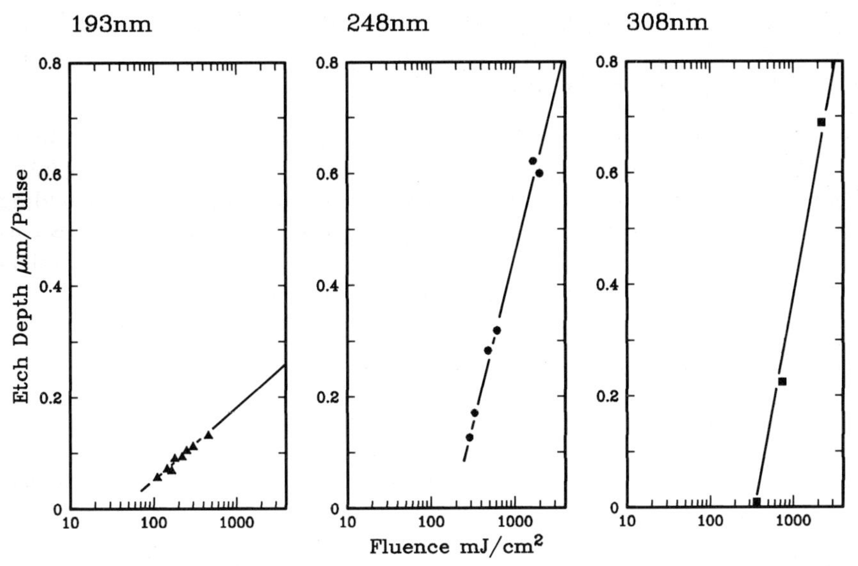


**Fig. 3** Etch Depth/ Pulse vs. Fluence at Various Wavelengths for Polycarbonate

**Data from Ref. 14**

many as three sets of such data on certain polymers and at least one set of such measurements on several polymers. In Fig. 3, the experimental data[14] for polycarbonate at three excimer laser wavelengths are plotted. Both the threshold for ablation and the slope of the etch depth vs. log fluence plot increase with increasing wavelength in this and nearly all other polymers which have been investigated [6,7,15].

It can be readily derived on a purely photothermal model[6,16] or with a photochemical model and several assumptions[17] that the etch depth per pulse ($l_f$) should be related to the logarithm of the fluence (F) by Eq. 1.

$$l_f = \frac{1}{\alpha} \log (F/F_T) \qquad (1)$$

where $\alpha$ is the absorption coefficient of the polymer at the wavelength of the laser beam and $F_T$ is the threshold fluence. The values for $F_T$ range from 0.02 to 0.05 $J/cm^2$/pulse but significant etching which can be accurately measured tends to occur at fluences in the range of 0.1 to 0.3 $J/cm^2$/pulse. At pulse energies greater than 0.5 $J/cm^2$ heating effects on the substrate become evident. Over the short range of energy fluence in which Eq. 1 has been tested, many polymers do show a linear relationship between $l_f$ and log F but polyimide at 249 nm and Mylar at 308 nm seem to be exceptional. A more serious problem is that the experimental slopes of these plots are different from the slopes that can be calculated from Eq. 1 using absorption coefficients measured in an ultraviolet spectrometer.

The $l_f$ vs. Log F plots can be criticized for more fundamental reasons. Since the absorption of photons by the polymer film extends below the level at which etching stops, there should be a portion of the energy of the laser pulse that should remain in the substrate as thermal energy. Recently, two groups have measured the value of this residual energy in polyimide film at several wavelengths. In one set of measurements[18] in which the film was attached to a pyroelectric crystal which sensed the temperature rise, there was a linear relationship between the energy of the laser pulse and the electrical output of the pyroelectric crystal at fluences below the threshold. Above $F_T$ there was a sharp fall-off from this linear correlation which showed that a large portion of the laser energy was carried away by the ablated material. However, a close examination of the data (Table 1) shows that the energy left behind in the substrate is substantially less than the value that can be calculated from Beer's Law. For example, at an incident fluence of 0.2 J/cm$^2$ per pulse, the signal would have been 165 mV if no ablation had occurred. Since ablation caused etching to a depth of 760 Å, the signal should have been 108 mV after correcting for the energy absorbed by the portion of the film that ablated. In fact, a signal of only 50 mV was detected. This discrepancy suggests that all of the energy of the laser pulse does not reach the surface of the polymer when the value of $F_T$ is exceeded.

The results of a second group[15] which used a thermocouple to measure the temperature rise in the polymer also show a direct correlation to the incident laser energy up to the value $F_T$. Above this value, the measured temperature rise is constant which would make these results even more discordant from the values that can be calculated.

TABLE I. MEASURED AND CALCULATED RESPONSE OF PYROELECTRIC CRYSTAL ATTACHED TO KAPTON FILM TO LASER PULSES (193 nm)

| Fluence Incident (mJ/cm$^2$) | Measured Etch Depth Å | $\frac{I_{Transmitted}}{I\ Incident}$ at Bottom of Etch Pit | Response of Pyroelectric Crystal (mV) | | |
|---|---|---|---|---|---|
| | | | Calculated Value if no Ablation occured | Observed Value | Calculated Value if Absorption was "Normal" |
| 100 | 350 | 0.82 | 83 | 41 | 68 |
| 200 | 760 | 0.66 | 165 | 50 | 108 |
| 300 | 1000 | 0.58 | 250 | 66 | 144 |
| 400 | 1170 | 0.52 | 330 | 82 | 173 |

Data from Ref. [18]

A reasonable explanation for these discrepancies can be found from the modelling of ablative photodecomposition at 193 nm that has been carried out [19]. According to this model, ejection of the material from the ablated volume can begin in 1 psec after the photons are deposited (it is assumed that all the photons are in place at $t = 0$) and proceeds in steps rather than in one explosive burst. The implication of this for an actual system is that the ejected material (which will travel normal to the surface and therefore exactly towards the incoming laser beam) will absorb a part of the incoming beam and partially filter out its effect on the polymer surface. The net result will be a diminution in the energy that actually reaches the polymer surface. Since excimer laser pulses have a long (~ 14 nsec) halfwidth compared to the times (~ 2 nsec) at which the first trace of a material can actually be observed to leave the surface, the prediction of the model seem acceptable. Furthermore, in Sec. v of this part it will be mentioned that some of the products of UV laser ablation which have been identified do absorb at 193 nm more strongly than the polymer from which they originate. Ideally, all of the photons from the laser should be absorbed in the polymer film in a time interval which is short with respect to the ablation time. In practice the use of laser pulses with widths of the order of 10 psecs should be acceptable. All of the data that have been obtained with pulses of 10 nsec or longer should be reexamined to see if they are free from the inner filtering effect of the products.

(ii) The measurement of the residual energy in the substrate following ablation has been discussed already in some detail. Such energy measurements can be meaningful only when the energy incident upon the film can be known accurately.

(iii) The translational energy of specific molecules in the ablated material has been measured from the intensities of the emission of a particular species (e.g. CH) at various distances from the surface [20]. In a second approach[21], an indirect measurement of the total translational energy of all of the ablated material has been made by measuring the momentum of the recoil induced in a film when material is ejected from its surface. Since the momentum of recoil = $\Sigma m_i v_i$, the momentum of fragments leaving the surface, an average translational velocity $<v_i>$ can be calculated from

$$<v_i> = \Sigma m_i v_i / \Sigma m_i \quad (2)$$

the value of $\Sigma m_i$ being measured in a separate etch measurement at the same fluence.

At 193 nm, the velocity of CH ablated from polymethyl methacrylate was reported to be $4.2 \times 10^5$ cm/sec at the surface [20]. The values for $C_2$ and CN were $2.0 \times 10^5$ cm/sec and $5.1 \times 10^5$ cm/sec respectively in the same experiment (fluence not indicated). These values may be compared to the value of $2.2 \times 10^5$ cm/sec for the average velocity ($<v_i>$) of the products from Mylar at 193 nm that was reported from recoil measurements in a vacuum in the fluence range from 0.05 to 0.3 $J/cm^2$/pulse [21]. Modelling suggests[19] a mean value of 1.3 x $10^5$ cm/sec for the velocity of methyl methacrylate monomer ejected from the surface of polymethyl methacrylate by 193 nm laser radiation. In this calculation, every monomer in the irradiated volume was assumed to be excited by one photon apiece.

It is gratifying that all of these velocity measurements and estimates suggest a perpendicular ejection velocity in the range of 1 - 5 x $10^5$ cm/sec. It should be pointed out that the calculation of the velocity from recoil measurements does not give any information about the distribution of velocities among the ejected particles. This information is needed in order to understand the process of ablation in a detailed way. The direct measurements of velocities of specific molecules from their emission lines are in all probability influenced by the absorption of a second photon followed by secondary decomposition of the primary ablation product. It is unlikely that diatomic species such as CH, CN or $C_2$ are formed through photolysis which uses only one photon per monomer.

The most desirable approach to the study of the ablated material would be a combination of fluorescence probing of the material and time-of-flight mass spectrometry since this would provide information on both the masses and structures of the ablated fragments.

(iv) The spectrum of the visible radiation that can be seen above the surface that is undergoing UV laser ablation has been the subject of several investigations. At fluences <0.15 $J/cm^2$ per pulse, at 193 nm, in a vacuum the emission is weak, but in air, under otherwise identical conditions, there is a structureless visible spectrum. The principal source of this radiation is probably the chemiluminescence from the oxidation of the ablated fragments [20]. At higher fluences, CH, CN, $C_2$, and C have been detected [20]. The vibrational, rotational spectrum of CH has been used to calculate its internal temperature to be 3200 ± 200 K in contrast to its translational temperature which was estimated to be 11,000 K [20]. At fluences greater than 1 $J/cm^2$/pulse, a plasma emission has been observed over polyimide film [13]. For these extreme values of the fluence, a mechanism for the etching of the surface of the polymer by the plasma has been proposed. It is, at present, not possible to relate these data or the mechanism to any of the other published data which were obtained at fluences <1 $J/cm^2$/pulse.

(v) At first sight, the analysis of the material that is ablated from a polymer surface by a laser pulse may seem to be a simple problem in mass spectrometry. In reality, it is greatly complicated by the nature of the absorption of light by the polymer. The logarithmic decrease in the (laser) photon intensity with the depth below the surface of the film - a consequence of Beer's Law - will lead to vastly different compositions of the products as a function of depth. A preliminary separation of the products by an analytical method such as gas chromatography is essential before mass spectrometry can be employed. A theoretical analysis of the distribution of products with depth in the case of polymethyl methacrylate has been carried out [17].If the decomposition process is photothermal, a temperature gradient should prevail as a function of depth. A purely thermal decomposition process may give a less complex mixture of products than a photochemical process.

Volatile products from UV laser ablation fall under two categories. The small molecules such as CO, $CO_2$, or CH are as likely to be formed by a secondary photolysis of the primary products as by primary photolysis. Their identification is relatively simple by spectroscopic methods but their relationship to the decomposition pathways of the polymer may not be direct. An exception is a highly energetic polymer such as nitrocellulose which can decompose exothermically (following photoexcitation) to give mainly gaseous products[2,16].Products in the range of m/e of 30 to 200 can generate information on the primary decomposition pathways. But it was found that no less than 30 compounds in this mass range were formed in the ablation of polyethylene terephthalate with a 193 nm laser pulse [3].A look at the structure of the repeating unit in the polymer and the structures of the three ablation fragments which have been identified shows the complex nature of the rearrangement reactions that have occurred during the ablation process. Products in the range of m/e of 200 to 3000 are formed from nearly all polymers although they are a larger fraction from highly condensed polymers such as polyimide than a linear addition polymer such as polymethyl methacrylate. These fragments are difficult to capture in sufficient quantity for analysis by the standard techniques used in polymer science.

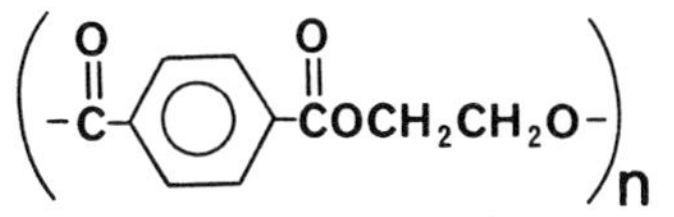

$(-CO-C_6H_4-COCH_2CH_2O-)_n$

MYLAR

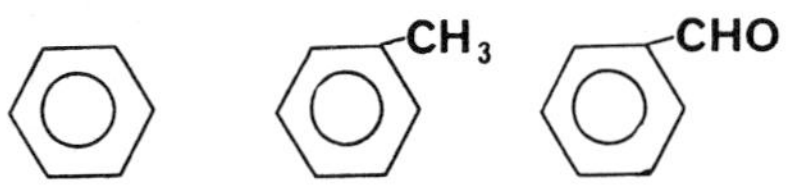

Three Products of UV Laser Ablation (Ref. 3)

(vi) Under any set of experimental conditions, the irradiation or a polymer surface by a UV laser pulse does not etch way the entire depth (for 95% absorption) of the film to which photons penetrate. There must therefore be a significant thickness of the substrate which had been exposed to photons and which may have been chemically modified. There has been little investigation of the chemical composition of the substrate after laser ablation.

Two studies[22,23] in which X-Ray Photoelectron Spectroscopy (XPS) and wet chemical techniques have been used show that in the first 100 Å of the material (which is the depth of penetration of XPS) the oxygen-to-carbon ratio had changed significantly. This may be attributed to the loss of CO and/or $CO_2$ from this layer. This is an indication that chemical processes have occurred even below the bottom of the etched pit. Since the UV absorption spectrum of the polymer can be expected to change when any chemical modification of the structure occurs, one has to contend with a change in the response of the polymer to the second pulse after a first pulse has caused ablation!

## 4. Theoretical Analysis of UV Laser Ablation

There are three theoretical investigations[17,19,24] into the details of ablative photodecomposition. In each instance many assumptions have been necessary regarding the details of the ablation process in order to reduce the problem to tractable proportions. We will examine each approach to the problem individually.

(i) The first approach[17] was based on the kinetics of the photochemical degradation of polymers. If the quantum yield for the photochemical bond-breaking in the polymer chain is unity then the rate of breaking of main chain links equals the number of photons absorbed per unit volume per unit time. The number of photons in a small volume element in the irradiated area can be calculated from Beer's Law. The volume ejected is proportional to the number of main chain links that are broken. The equations which express these relationships are combined and integrated between $l = 0$ (the top of the etch pit, i.e., the surface of the polymer) and $l = l_f$ (the bottom of the etch pit). Noting that $F_T$ (the threshold fluence) equals the fluence at the bottom of the pit, Eq. 1 in Sec. 3 (i) is obtained. As has already been noted, this expression fits the results in a qualitative way but the slopes obtained experimentally do not match the calculated slopes.

This kinetic approach, in spite of the limitations imposed by the assumptions, is useful for the insight it yields on the significance of the depth at which etching stops. The reader is referred to the original article for this analysis.

(ii) A second approach[19] to ablative photodecomposition was based on the following boundary conditions.

The polymer is approximated by an array of structureless monomer units. Initially all monomer units interact with a potential that makes the sample stable at its normal density. The photochemical reaction then corresponds to a switch in the potential surfaces such that the monomer occupies a larger volume. The motion of the ensemble of monomer units is followed in time by integrating the classical equations of motion. In an actual experiment, as many as 500 layers of material may ablate per pulse. In a calculation, it is not feasible to include so many monomers. Only a small sample was used.

The predictions of this model have already been alluded to in earlier sections. The principal conclusions were that the reacted material will ablate without melting the remainder of the sample, the average perpendicular velocity of the ejected material will be ~ $1.3 \times 10^5$ cm/sec, and the angular spread will be small and peaked in the direction normal to the surface.

(iii) A third approach[24] which was based on the energy balance in the polymer film did not automatically assume a mechanism but dealt with the interaction of UV laser radiation with polymer surfaces in a general way. Full details of this work can be found in an article by the author of this theory in this volume.

## 5. Conclusions

UV laser ablation of polymers promises to be an exceedingly interesting phenomenon for further study. Numerous variations in the composition of the polymer used, in the characteristics of the laser pulse, and in the irradiation conditions are possible. These variations should produce scientific results which would bear on fast kinetics, transient chemical species, synthesis of novel compounds, and analysis of bulk organic material. The potential applications to technology seem equally vast and varied.

## References


1. R. Srinivasan and V. Mayne-Banton: Appl. Phys. Lett. 41, 576 (1982)

2. M. W. Geis, J. N. Randall, T. F. Deutsch, P. D. DeGraff, K. E. Krohn, and L. A. Stern: ibid. 43, 74 (1983)

3. R. Srinivasan and W. J. Leigh: J. Am. Chem. Soc. 104, 6784 (1982)

4. J. Brannon, J. Lankard, F. Burns, and J. Kaufman: Private communication

5. M. Murahara, Y. Kawamura, K. Toyoda, and S. Namba: Ohyo Butsuri (Appl. Phys.) 52, 83 (1983)

6. J. E. Andrew, P. E. Dyer, D. Forster, and P. H. Key: Appl. Phys. Lett. 43, 717 (1983)

7. R. Srinivasan and B. Braren: J. Polymer Sci. (in press)

8. For a concise review of electronic spectra of organic molecules, see F. P. Schäfer: Dye Lasers (Topics in Applied Physics, Vol. I, Springer-Verlag, New York 1973)

9. For a review of photochemical primary processes in organic molecules, see J. P. Simons: Photochemistry and Spectroscopy (Wiley-Interscience, New York 1971)

10. R. Srinivasan: J. Vac. Sci. Tech. B 1: 1, 923 (1983)

11. S. L. Trokel, R. Srinivasan, and B. Braren: Amer. J. Ophthalmology, 96, 710 (1983)

12. "To ablate" (verb transitive) is defined by Webster's Collegiate Dictionary (G. C. Merriam: Springfield, 1981) as "to remove by cutting, erosion, melting, evaporation, or vaporization."

13. G. Koren and J.T.C. Yeh: Appl. Phys. Lett. 44, 1112 (1984)

14. B. Braren and R. Srinivasan: Unpublished research

15. P. E. Dyer and J. Sidhu: CLEO '84, Abstract THK 4

16. T. F. Deutsch and M. W. Geis: J. Appl. Phys. 54, 7201 (1983)

17. H.H.G. Jellinek and R. Srinivasan: J. Phys. Chem. 88, 3048 (1984)

18. G. Gorodetsky, T. G. Kazyaka, R. L. Melcher, and R. Srinivasan: CLEO '84, Abstract THK 5

19. B. J. Garrison and R. Srinivasan: Appl. Phys. Lett. 44, 849 (1984)

20. G. M. Davis, M. C. Gower, C. Fotakis, T. Efthimiopoulos and P. Argyrakis: J. Appl. Phys. (in press)

21. R. Srinivasan and S-H. Liu: ibid. (in press)

22. S. Lazare, P. D. Hoh, J. M. Baker, and R. Srinivasan: J. Amer. Chem Soc. 106, (1984)

23. R. Srinivasan and S. Lazare: Polymer (in press)

24. R. L. Melcher, this volume

# 3.4 Compound Formation

## Laser-Induced Synthesis of Compound Semiconductors

L.D. Laude

Université de l'Etat, 23 Av. Maistriau, B-7000 Mons, Belgium

### 1. INTRODUCTION

Interest in dependable semiconducting compounds has been revived recently with respect to a number of applications in optoelectronics and photovoltaics, in particular to 3D thin film devices onto insulating substrates. Although known for thirty years, stoichiometry difficulties have always hampered the development of these III-V or II-VI compounds. It is only since the advent of molecular beam epitaxy (MBE) that new hopes have emerged both in terms of scaling down the devices and achieving high quality materials (cf. carrier mobility). Nevertheless, MBE might be considered to be a rather sophisticated and expensive technique leaving room for cheaper and simpler alternatives. Within this challenging background, it will be shown in this paper that laser-processing of semi-conducting compound films on insulator is probably a most attractive way a) to circumvent the composition problems of the compound, and b) to prepare it in a most useful and competitive form.

In this respect, a technique has been set up by which binary and ternary semiconducting compounds are synthesized via laser irradiation of multi-layered metallic films containing proportions of atomic species corresponding to given over-all compositions. After delineating the main characteristics of the irradiation products, an approach to the physics involved in these laser-induced ordering processes is developed with respect to the energy balance of the atomic system under non-equilibrium conditions. The presentation then proceeds to a development of the process in multi-phase systems, namely Ge-Se and In-Cu-Se.

### 2. LASER SYNTHESIS OF A COMPOUND: EXPERIMENTAL

Fabrication of a compound film on an insulator may be performed in many ways which can be classified into two types: either by evaporating the compound and depositing already formed compound aggregates, or by condensing vapors of the constituents in the appropriate ratios. Of the two, the second type (synthesis) is by far the most effective if proper controls of deposition rates and temperatures (sources, substrate) are at hand throughout the film deposition. Processing of the film is in general performed thermally during deposition by maintaining the substrate at a moderate temperature, a compromise between increasing the mean free path of ad-atoms and keeping a low rate of desorption. Synthesis is then achieved during the film growth, layer by layer, allowing both lateral and in-depth tailoring of the film (cf. superlattices).

When evaluating the eventual shortcomings of this technique, one of the most critical parameters would be time: the growth proceeds at near equilibrium conditions so that any accidental excess of one of the constituents would be difficult to eliminate by diffusion or compensation within the film.Only a drastic control of all parameters makes epitaxial growth possible. Producing relatively large and thick films (1μm or more) also presents difficulties: stability of the sources, contamination of the film (ultra-high vacuum is required since condensation rate is very small). Nevertheless, films of exceptional quality are prepared in this way, and a technique such as MBE is in the process of being integrated into production lines for very high-value-added materials. However, quality requirements vary with the needs, and alternatives to these delicate and expensive processes would probably be much welcomed. One of these is laser-induced synthesis (1).

Basic materials to be laser-processed consist of multi-layered structures. Each layer contains atoms of one element only, and proportions between atoms of different elements are adjusted to conform to overall stoichiometric amounts. Let us note that in this work such proportions are obtained to not better than ± 1% by quartz monitoring electron beam evaporation sources in vacuum. Other film preparation (electro-deposition, for instance, (2)) can be used as well with an even larger departure from stoichiometry. In any case, such inaccuracy would be detrimental in any slow (or near-equilibrium) processing. We will see in the following that this is not the case in laser processing.

Once the film is formed, laser processing may be carried out in either CW or pulsed regimes, over a very wide range of energy densities. In CW mode, the beam is scanned over the target at velocities typically between $1 cm sec^{-1}$ to $20 m sec^{-1}$. Since the beam has a Gaussian profile in general, the processed volume is also precisely known. Adding the possibility of reducing injection time to $10^{-9}$sec or less makes lasers unique tools for depositing energy at all rates into films and, therefore, to perform and study ordering mechanisms, nucleation, growth, phase mixing or segregation, at near or far from equilibrium conditions. In the following, some examples of CW $Ar^+$ laser processing will be given aiming at demonstrating a) the extreme versatility of the laser tools in promoting phase transformations, b) the wealth of physical mechanisms associated with such transformations which can be studied in detail, and c) the simplicity of laser-induced synthesis compared to others in the field.

## 3. THERMODYNAMICS OR DYNAMICS ?

What we are concerned with is the phase transformation which is observed when laser irradiating a film as described above, at and above a given power threshold. There is not much mystery about the phase itself: it may be obtained in general (but not always) in different ways, for instance, in an oven. The trouble is rather in the circumstances of the move and in the "quality" of the end product. The onset of the new phase is in practice extremely sharp in terms of energy density necessary and concerns the whole of the irradiated material at once: nothing like an "activated" process which progressively gains strength along an Arrhenius-like law. The transformed film consists of relatively large crystallites (1μm) when supported on a glass substrate, or extremely large ones in non-supported films (3). In the latter case, films are first deposited on NaCl and then floated off and mounted on microscope Cu grids. Irradiation occurs once the films are on the grid. Portions of the film are not "supported" (no substrate) and crystallize into 20 to 50 μm crystals over 0.1 μm thickness. The interest of such free-standing films lies in the fact that all of the energy optically absorbed by the material more or less remains in the film, minimizing thermal losses to the grid bars. Energy threshold is also extremely sharp in this case. Either supported or non-supported, films exhibit optical properties comparable to those of single crystals. Transport properties of supported films reveal a semiconductor band-gap devoid of deep centers and an intrinsic conductivity down to room temperature (4). This is typically the case for III-V and II-VI compounds processed in CW or pulsed mode. The same materials, thermally annealed in vacuum, become extrinsic at about 500°C. Similar processing has been performed on more complex systems (IV-VI, ternaries) presenting several phases in their phase diagrams. It will be shown in the last section of this paper that individual phases can be produced depending on the laser parameters, whilst heat treated films of the same elements consist in general of a mixture of such phases.

Therefore, there is a number of reasons to believe that the physics involved in such laser processing, which includes phase transformation and synthesis, is unusual in many respects and may not be just another way to heat, melt and crystallize films. Being themselves the direct consequence of an atomic instability (the "inversion of population") laser beams may be thought to have required energy and power to destabilize in turn other atomic systems. This may well be the case for isolated, non-interacting systems like the free standing films mentioned. There, the energy transfer to the atoms is quasi adiabatic. For supported films (or single crystal surface regions), this overall non-equilibrium energy transfer is obscured by diffusion processes, i.e. a general slowing down of energy and mass transport is observed which is controlled by the heat capacity of the substrate (i.e. the optically inert material). A thermodynamic material equilibrium results which can be traced and characterized as such, in particular regarding crystal growth and impurity diffusion.

In fact, what is thermodynamic equilibrium in such multi-layered structures? Let us consider a classical diffusion problem: a thin layer of atoms A is deposited on a single-crystal of atoms B and the set is heated up to a temperature T. Fick's equations can predict concentration profiles of atoms A into crystal B at any time following the onset of annealing. Conditions for such predictions to hold are that under all circumstances, the concentration of atoms A into crystal B would be negligible compared to the atomic density in crystal B, i.e. cohesion of the latter should not be affected by the diffusion process. This clearly restricts evaluation of the diffusion of atoms A to regions deep in the crystal and after very long diffusion times. This also sets a limit of validity to the diffusion constant D for atoms A into crystal B. The displacement of atoms A very close to the A/B boundary is non-linear and may not be predicted at all. Thermodynamic equilibrium is reached when the concentration of atoms A is homogeneous in crystal B. This means that atomic transportation within the crystal is exactly reversible, and that the atoms can compensate each other a long time (hours!) after the beginning of the diffusion process at temperature T. Such an equilibrium is best characterized by T, representing more or less the average vibrational energy of each atom B. The atoms A would be allowed to move around with an "activation energy" representing the potential barrier each atom A would have to pass in the vicinity of atoms A already in the lattice.

Other parameters are used to label this equilibrium: energy , pressure, entropy, composition. They all appear in thermodynamic equations which help describing (small) reversible changes of the system. In the case of irreversible changes, such macroscopic thermodynamic parameters vary in space and time. Their local values are restricted to small domains containing however large numbers of atoms. Here, the equilibrium equations become inequalities: as an example, the increase in entropy during an adiabatic irreversible process provides information only about the direction of the change and not on its intensity. To know the actual entropy created upon an irreversible transformation would require knowledge of local pressure, temperature, chemical composition within restricted domains of the system, and the faster the transformation the smaller the domains. It is clear that within the phenomenology of the thermodynamics of irreversible processes, local equilibrium should be attained very rapidly and it should not be too different from the overall thermal equilibrium: the free path for energy transfer must be much smaller than distances over which the temperature varies (5).

In pulsed laser processing, temperatute variations of 1500 K (melting) may be achieved in some $10^{-9}$ sec and the resulting melt front velocity may attain or exceed 10 $msec^{-1}$, i.e. a temperature shift of 1-2 K between adjacent atoms every $10^{-12}$sec! Obviously, temperature and entropy are difficult to quantify here. The only reliable parameter is energy which, in any case, is conserved globally in the system. The problem is further complicated by the fact that these synthesis reactions are exothermal. Such quantities like the heat liberated during the formation of a compound are evaluated macroscopically in kcal per mole; it would be hazardous to extrapolate them to very small quantities such as 200 Å thick layers,or at film interfaces.

Altogether, a plain thermodynamic approach to laser synthesis of a compound seems inappropriate. As we shall see in the following, there are clear indications that materials do melt prior to forming the compound. On the other hand, it has been shown that Cd-Te and Cd-Se films can be synthesized in two configurations (6): cubic (blende) or hexagonal (wurtzite) in the CW or pulsed (1μsec) regimes, respectively. Here we postulate that the system should transfrom via an intermediate state. Such a state, as in a number of non-equilibrium systems (laser cavity, superconductors below $T_c$, high energy plasma) would sustain long lifetimes exceeding the lifetime of excited individual particles. In the present situation, this intermediate state would be a liquid-like medium of possibly ionized atoms, maintained in activity along the irradiation time. Upon interrupting the excitation (or external energy) source, the system would relax first into the highest energy state. Further relaxation to the lower state would depend on the actual time and temperature the system remains at the higher level $E_1$ (Fig.1). In a pulsed irradiation scheme, the energy gradient may be large enough to prevent the system from increasing the thermal energy above $E_1$ and crossing the activation energy barrier ΔE. The system would then be trapped into Phase 1 at level $E_1$ upon cooling. In CW regime, the system would decay in a cascade from E* into $E_1$ and subsequently into $E_2$, the most stable phase available.

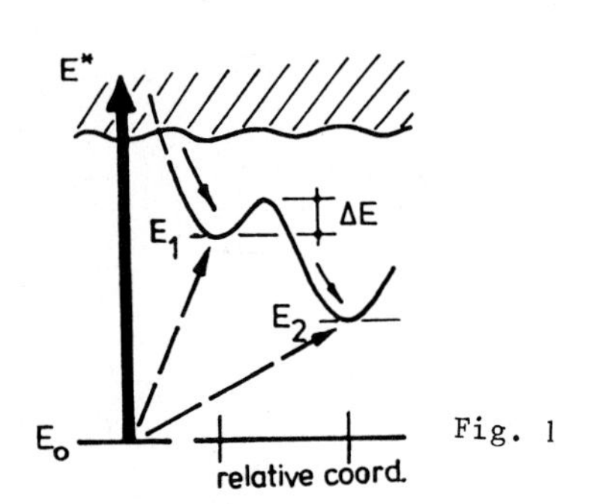

Fig. 1

As a matter of fact, the non-equilibrium state need not be real but virtual the energy absorbed by the system corresponding to either $(E_1-E_o)$ or $(E_2-E_o)$. The model can be tested for more complicated systems like Zr-O, and also Cu-O etc.

The issue on the melting of the individual layers prior to synthesis of the compound is further raised from structural arguments (7). The interface between adjacent crystallites A and B would develop grain boundaries consisting of AB compound aggregates. These are formed by thermal diffusion at low temperatures but require time. Such aggregates tend to inhibit complete melting of the constituents if (slow) thermal annealing is to be used for synthesis. Laser processing is much too fast (scanning is performed at some $1msec^{-1}$) to allow the growth of compound grain boundaries. In addition, these individual films are very thin (2 to 300 Å each) and formed from a collection of defect-rich crystallites. These arguments strongly suggest that the actual melting temperature of the films might well be below that of the individual bulk materials quoted in literature.

Should this be the case, synthesis would in effect follow the melt of both constituents, in support of the model of Fig.1. Note that this procedure is in contrast with all other non-equilibrium techniques (MBE,CVD). Here, injection time and decay time (the quenching) are both extremely sharp in pulsed laser processing, contrary to the others where the decay is extremely long (no quenching) where there is no possibility to "pick up" a metastable phase.

When devising the non-equilibrium intermediate state at level $E^*$, it was not intended to place it at or very close to the liquid-solid interface. It could stand clearly above the highest melting point of the constituents. The system is then assumed to be in the hydrodynamic regime. This latter regime plays an important role in industrial crystal growth. It is in fact responsible for the impurity segregation in the Czochralski technique. Instabilities are produced within the bulk melt for a number of reasons which develop into convection roles or Rayleigh-Bénard cells. Evaluation of such possibilities occurring in laser irradiated multi-layered films of the sort used in laser-induced synthesis has been made by H.Müller-Krumbhaar (8). Among many other hydrodynamic instabilities, two are of particular interest since they are common to a variety of laser processings. One is due to the density difference between the liquid and the rigid boundary solid (substrate).The second relates to a gradient in surface tension produced by an inhomogeneous heating (Marangoni effect). Estimates of the flow velocity in the case of silicon are of the order of the melt front velocity. One would expect such role patterns to be quenched upon interrupting the cause of the instability.

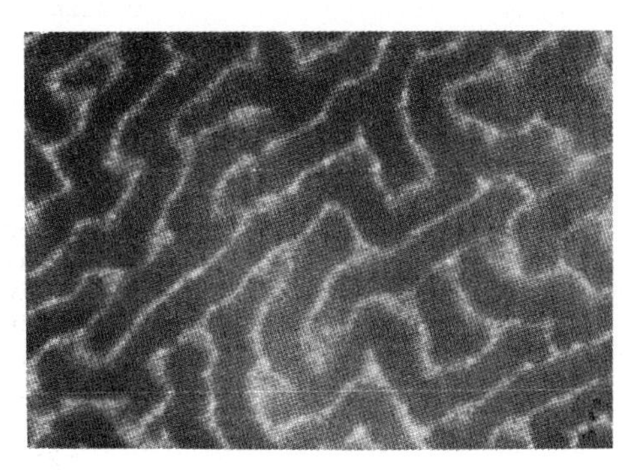

Fig.2

In Fig.2 is shown a transmission photograph of a Cd-Se sandwich film which has been irradiated in the CW regime for several seconds. Cells over 5μm wide are formed well outside the irradiated spot but their orientation is independent of any temperature gradient developing radially from the center of the spot. Atomic species have been segregated microns apart although they were initially distributed in layers parallel to the plane of the figure, over 0.1μm thickness.

Other examples of hydrodynamic instabilities produced in laser processed films are presented in the next section.

One should note that although the film is obviously molten during the process, Fig.2 (the calculated temperature agrees with a direct measurement at around 350°C), the compound is not formed.

Conclusions to these overviews on the laser-synthesis process are both simple and complex: laser synthesis is not thermally controlled and proceeds through melting of the constituents. An instability regime is then induced which is difficult to parametrize but certainly is responsible for a) the large crystallites which are produced and which exceed by far the size of those obtained by slow annealing, b) the quality of such large crystallites which is similar to that of zone-refined single crystals in terms of impurity content, c) the ability to produce metastable phases which are out-of-reach by conventional non-equilibrium processing techniques.

More studies are obviously required to understand and model the various puzzling aspects of the physics involved here. To convince the reader of the generality of these conclusions, more complex atomic systems are envisaged in the last section of this paper with no added difficulties with respect to points a) to c).

## 4. MULTIPHASE SYSTEMS

The variety of compounds which have been synthesized until now is extremely wide. They include: AlSb,AlAs, CdTe, CdSe, ZnSe, ZnTe,CdO, ZnO, $Cu_2O$, and there seem to be no factors limiting the formation of others (9). Most of these have simple phase diagrams with one stable single phase. Many more, however, may present practical interest and require more advanced processing in order to justify a deeper evaluation. Two of these atomic systems are Ge-Se and Cu-In-Se. Preliminary results have been obtained which open new horizons in compound synthesis (10).

### 4.1 Ge-Se

Ge-Se is known to present two crystalline phases: GeSe with an orthorhombic structure, and $GeSe_2$ with a monoclinic one, i.e. much less symmetric structures compared to the previous materials. In addition, amorphous phases (glasses) are known to exist in Se-rich mixtures, like $GeSe_3$. The microscopic structure of the latter is thought to consist of $GeSe_2$ tetrahedra weakly coupled via Se atoms. Since this $GeSe_3$ is seriously considered for inorganic resin applications in sub-micron geometry microelectronics, a proper control of its stability is necessary.

The challenge of synthesizing any of these phases is to avoid the simultaneous and competing formation of one or more of the other phases. GeSe and $GeSe_2$ are semiconductors with direct forbidden band gap width of 1.5 and 2.3 eV, respectively. Phase mixing of these two compounds would then be immediately evident from optical absorption measurements.

The study of the Ge-Se system requires, in view of the complexity of the phase diagram, both a reliable film composition and a reliable lasing procedure. $Ge_{1-x}Se_x$ films are prepared classically as a stack of elemental layers with x varying in the range 0 to 1 by 0.1 increments, within 1% accuracy. To avoid oxidation or other contamination during laser processing in air, films are encapsulated between two SiO layers. The substrate may be either plain glass or NaCl crystal for studying adiabatic synthesis in free-standing films. Irradiation is performed in this work with a CW $Ar^+$ laser: maximum power is 25 W; the beam profile is Gaussian with mid-width of 40μm, and scanning is performed at a constant velocity of $1msec^{-1}$ but could be varied from $1cmsec^{-1}$ to $20msec^{-1}$ at will.

The scanning procedure which is used is based on the technique of G.Auvert, and further developed by P.Pierrard. The sequence adopted has been adjusted to provide for a maximum amount of information in the shortest time. Films on glass, for instance 2x8 $cm^2$ and 0.1 m thick, are scanned at normal incidence, constant speed and constant profile, along parallel paths 120 μm apart. A delay time between consecutive paths, typically 1sec, is arranged to avoid cumulative heating. From one path to the next, the beam power is varied by 14.3 mW increments by a closed-loop control between exit power in the beam and the laser power supply. Under normal conditions, stability of the source and the recurring adjustment guarantee reproducibility of absolute exit power to better than 1%.

For each film composition, the above sequence is programmed from 0 to 1 W, over some 70 scans. Along the program, films are observed to transform abruptly from one path to the next into one phase or another which can be controlled in

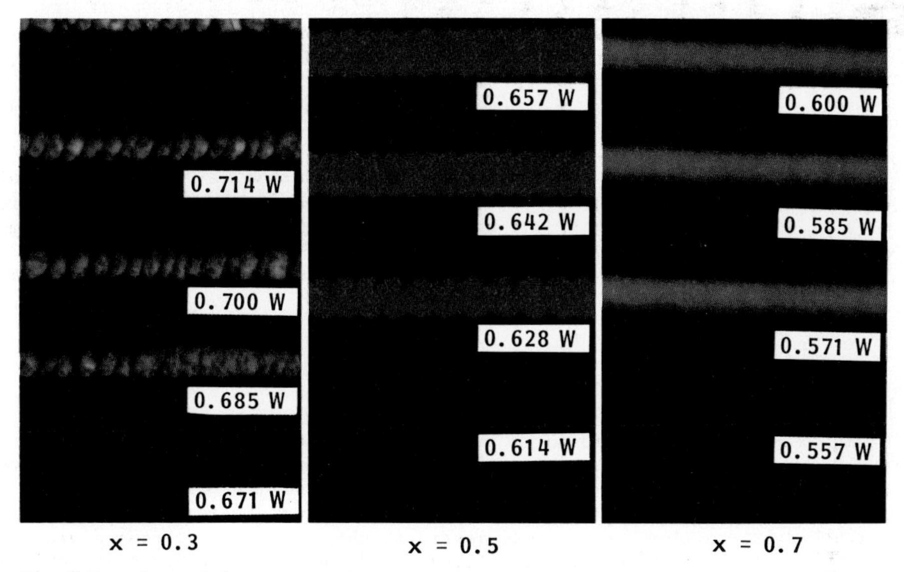


Fig.3 Results of laser scanning three $Ge_{1-x}Se_x$ films at compositions x = 0.3 (left), 0.5 (center) and 0.7 (right), for various powers.

first approximation by optical transmission means in a microscope. In a matter of some 70 sec, a given composition is completely scanned and this eventually provides for analysis work taking several weeks. An example of the resulting evidence is shown in Fig.3 for three compositions at x = 0.3, 0.5 and 0.7, respectively from left to right.

A general observation is that transformation power is extremely well delineated between two consecutive scans, whatever the product obtained. This power onset is quickly transformed into an energy onset knowing the beam profile and dwell time: 1 W is here equivalent to 3.2 $Jcm^{-2}$. At x = 0.5, crystallization progresses "explosively", to follow the accepted terminology. The crystallites being formed are GeSe ones of some 12µm dimension. Increasing the scan speed to some $15msec^{-1}$ would extend this crystal growth indefinitely. Although not shown here, the ends of the trace reveal more precisely the energy onset due to a slight spread of the energy density in the beam. More specifically, energy liberated upon synthesis of the compound can be directly measured in the free standing version of the scanning procedure at energy densities some 10 times lower. One should note also that the volume being processed does follow the energy increment. Below the onset of synthesis, wiggles are observed which do not show up in the photograph. Such wiggles are much better evidenced at x = 0.7, Fig.3. Here, crystallites are not formed at all but an amorphous phase is formed at 0.571 W or 1.827 $Jcm^{-2}$ (i.e. onset at 1.81 ± 0.02 $Jcm^{-2}$). Apparent in this photograph are the wiggles within the transformed material. An onset for the formation of these cells is detectable at much lower power, 0.285 W (or 0.89 ± 0.02 $Jcm^{-2}$). The same composition crystallizes into $GeSe_2$ + Se at a larger power, 0.657 W (or 2.08 ± 0.02 $Jcm^{-2}$). At x = 0.7, amorphous formation never occurs (Fig.3 left). First hand indication shows a probable phase demixing between Ge and Se at 0.685 W.

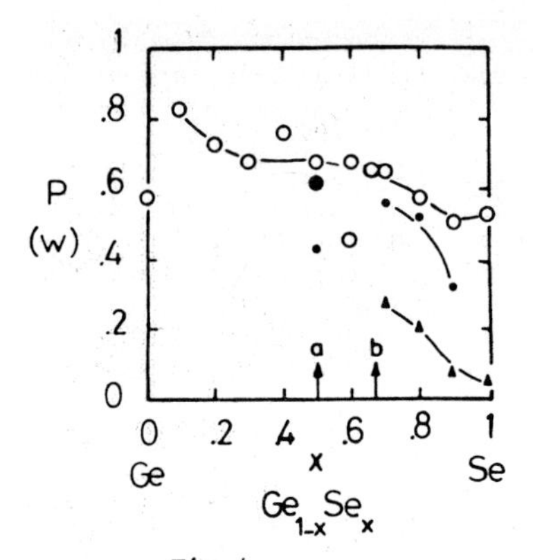


Fig.4
Triangles refer to the onset of "wiggle" formation, small dots to the onset of amorphous phase and large circles (open and dark) to a proposed crystalline phase formation

A more complete evaluation of the behaviour of the films with composition is shown in Fig.4. a and b denote phases GeSe and $GeSe_2$, respectively. On the right the cell formation and amorphous synthesis are traced. They are totally absent in the Ge-rich films. Note also that Ge films crystallize at a much lower power than at $x = 0.1$, possibly indicating inhibition of the Ge nucleation by the Se atoms as the concentration of these decreases in the films.

One particular point requires more detailed discussion. At $x = 0.5$, three levels of transformation are quoted: the small dark point and the open circle refer respectively to the onset of the amorphous phase formation and nucleation of GeSe in films deposited with the sequence Ge + Se + Ge +...+ Ge. The large dark circle refers to the onset of GeSe formation in films deposited with the sequence Se + Ge + Se +...+ Ge, i.e. Se first on the substrate. In this latter case, no amorphous phase is formed in contrast with the other sequence but with the same overall composition. Clearly, this indicates that surface tension asymmetry (perhaps in relation with the better wetting of the substrate surface by Se atoms due to a lower melting point than

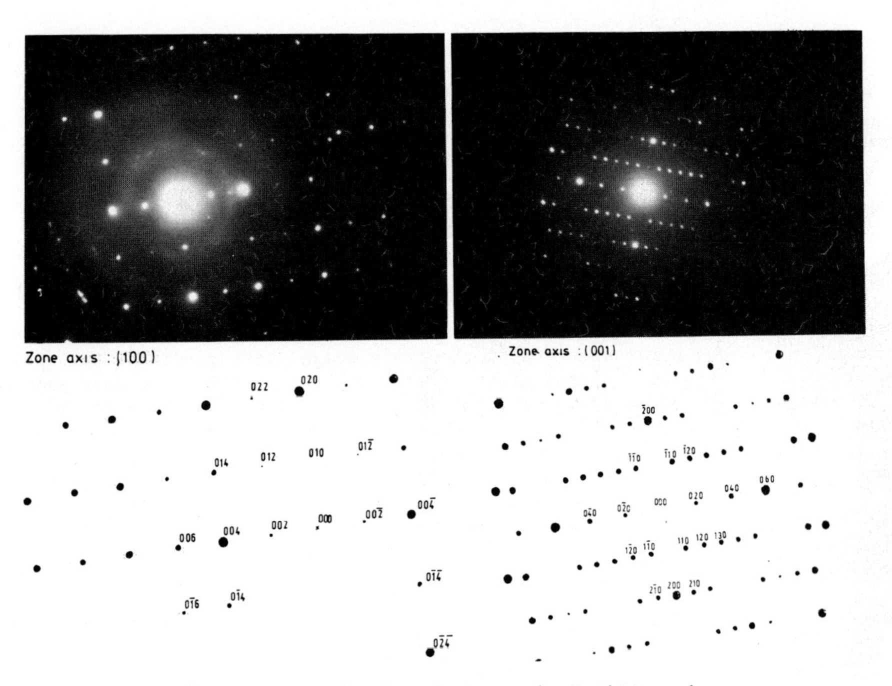


Fig.5 Diffraction patterns (top) and theoretical diffraction diagrams (bottom) for GeSe (left) and $GeSe_2$ (right) films.

Ge) plays an important role not only in the onset of the instability but also in the nature of the stable phases which form upon relaxing this instability.

An electron diffraction characterization of the two crystalline phases of the system has been carried out on films deposited and laser processed on a glass sustrate. After detaching the processed films from their substrate, high resolution analysis reveals the single-crystal growth obtained on the nominal compositions of GeSe and $GeSe_2$ (Fig.5). Original diffraction prints are shown together with theoretical diffraction diagrams (11). The area covered by the electron beam on the film is of the order of 5-7μm.

### 4.2 Cu-In-Se

If the Ge-Se system may be considered complicated compared to III-V and II-VI compounds, any ternary system is even more so. The ternary phase $CuInSe_2$ is a tetragonal structure of particular interest in photovoltaics since its optical absorption coefficient equals $2x10^5cm^{-1}$ above 1eV photon energy. This means that the complete solar spectrum would be absorbed over a 2000 Å thickness, to compare with the 10μm required for silicon with the same band gap. Evidently, one would like to produce large grained, 2000 Å thick $CuInSe_2$ layers and evaluate them against photovoltaics applications. The challenge here is

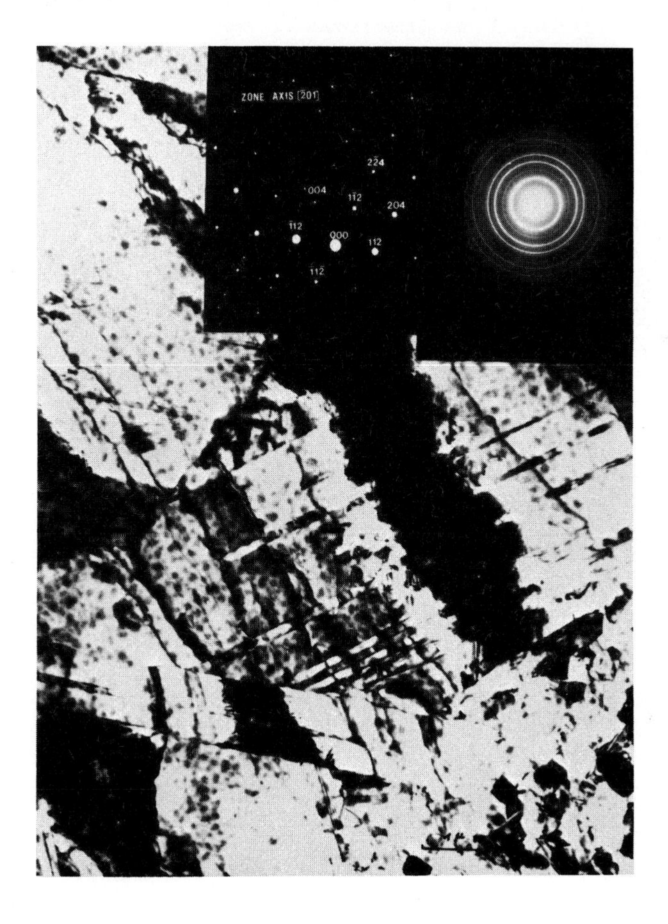


Fig.6

enormous. Other phases are present in the phase diagram of the system: CuSe and $Cu_2Se$ on one hand, $In_2Se$, InSe and $In_2Se_3$ on the other hand. All of them crystallize and have very similar chemical compositions. With 1% uncertainty for each layer, an overall non-stoichiometry of 4-5% is to be expected at best. Also, it is most likely that binary formation is the most probable, with the apparent result of a strong mixture of all five binaries to be expected from laser processing sandwich films of nominal composition corresponding to the hypothetical $CuInSe_2$ phase.

Fig.6 is a Transmission Electron Microscope photograph of a film of nominal composition corresponding to the ternary. The film was deposited on glass, irradiated and detached before analysis. The actual power of the $Ar^+$laser beam was 5.6W and irradiation time was about 0.7sec; beam cross-section was diaphragmed to 1mm. Large crystallites are evident. On top of the figure, diffraction patterns from 80µm Ø spots on the film (right) and 5µm Ø spots (left) are shown which demonstrate the formation of the compound (interpretation of the diffraction pattern is given) to near perfect form. A more detailed analysis, not shown here, reveals that a) no binary is formed simultaneously, b) no oxide is formed, and c) no phase segregation of elemental species is evidenced.

It is fair to say that a)such a result is not understood, and b) it was not envisaged that one could "pick up" the most improbable phase to be synthesized to such a level of perfectness! Yet, the result is there and has become a routine test in fact to check stoichiometry of the initial films.

When talking of non-equilibrium phase transformations, this is what one may expect for other ternaries as well: a completely new way to envisage synthesis. This work is currently performed in air.

## 5. CONCLUSIONS

It is the hope of the author and of his colleagues in Mons that the arguments presented here will encourage more people to engage in similar work. It is evident that the fundamentals of the laser-induced synthesis is far more appealing to theoreticians today, because non-linear thermodynamics of irreversible processes is emerging as a success story of the years to come. On the other hand, research and development activities may not require in the beginning a full understanding of the physics controlling a process. Since theoretical arguments rest on experimental facts, let us provide facts, and a proper modelling of laser synthesis will show up progressively along the lines mentioned in this presentation.

## ACKNOWLEDGEMENTS

It is a pleasure to the author to thank his colleagues in the Mons group for fruitful and enthusiastic discussions on this subject. Part of the work outlined here on Ge-Se and $CuInSe_2$ will be presented elsewhere in full details. Thanks are also due to G.Auvert for the use of his splendid machinery at an early stage of the Ge-Se work, and to P.Pierrard for his collaboration in this same work at a latter stage.

This work is currently carried out within Project IRIS and the National Energy Program, both run by the Ministry for Science Policy in Brussels.

## REFERENCES

1. R.Andrew, M.Ledezma, M.Lovato, L.D.Laude and M.Wautelet, Appl.Phys.Lett., 35, 418 (1979); R.Andrew et al., J.Appl.Phys.53, 4862 (1982);
2. F.Hanus et at., to be published;

3. L.Baufay, A.Pigeolet and L.D.Laude, J.Appl.Phys.54, 660 (1983);

4. L.Baufay et al., 4th Int. Photovoltaic Conf., eds. W.H. Bloss and G. Grassi (D.Reidel, Dordrecht 1982), p.839;
5. J.W.Christian, "The theory of transformations in metals and alloys", (Pergamon, Oxford 1968), p.95;
6. L.Baufay et al., J. of Cryst. Growth 59, 143 (1982);

7. M.Wautelet, private communication ; M.Wautelet and L.D.Laude, to be published;
8. H.Müller-Krumbhaar, in "Cohesive Properties of Semiconductors under Laser Irradiation", NATO ASI Series E: Applied Sciences No.69 (L.D.Laude, ed., M.Nijhoff, The Hague 1983), p.197-236;

9. R.Andrew et al., in Proc.MRS Symposium, Boston 1982;

10. C.Antoniadis, M.C.Joliet, L.D.Laude and P.Pierrard, to be published; C.Antoniadis, M.C.Joliet, L.D.Laude and R.Andrew, to be published;
11. C.Antoniadis and M.C.Joliet, Thin Solid Films 115, 75 (1984).

# Laser Synthesis of Thin Film $CuInSe_2$

M.C. Joliet, C. Antoniadis, R. Andrew, and L.D. Laude
Université de l'Etat, B-7000 Mons, Belgium

## 1 INTRODUCTION

The technique of laser irradiation of multilayer elemental films for the production of binary semiconductor thin films has previously been applied to the systems AlSb, AlAs, CdTe, CdSe (1-3) GeSe & $GeSe_2$ (4). In this work the technique is extended to the ternary compound $CuInSe_2$. The films of $CuInSe_2$ are formed by laser irradiation of multilayer films of the components in the appropriate atomic ratio. The individual layers are deposited by E-beam evaporation onto glass or salt substrates; films detached from the latter are then mounted on TEM grids. Irradiation is performed in air using all green lines of an $Ar^+$ laser.

For both grid mounted and glass supported films the compound $CuInSe_2$ is formed on irradiation, with no evidence of other phases. Characterization of the films is made by TEM, electron diffraction and optical spectrometry.

## 2 FILM PREPARATION

1000Å thick films made up of Cu-In-Se layers in 1:1:2 atomic proportion are prepared by sequential vacuum evaporation onto glass or cleaved salt substrates using a multi-crucible E-gun source in a vacuum of $\sim 10^{-6}$ torr. Film thicknesses are controlled by a quartz monitor to a precision of ~1-2%. The films are encapsulated between two SiO layers ~150Å thick. Films evaporated onto salt are detached and mounted onto TEM grids with a 80μm x 80μm hole size.

Variations in the layer sequence do not detectably influence the film resulting from irradiation, although the threshold irradiation power may vary with film reflectivity.

## 3 IRRADIATION

All films are irradiated in air using an $Ar^+$ laser operating on all green lines. Grid mounted films are irradiated for 0.7s with varying power density via a 1mm dia. aperture. Films on glass substrates are irradiated using a raster scan with $v_x$=2mm/s and $v_y$=40μm/s, at various power densities, through a cylindrical lens, thereby producing irradiated areas several square cm in extent. Portions of such films are detached by a collodion pull, and mounted on TEM grids for subsequent analysis.

## 4 RESULTS

### Grid Mounted Films

Irradiation of a grid mounted film above a threshold of ~3W results in the formation of a polycrystalline film as depicted in the left part of

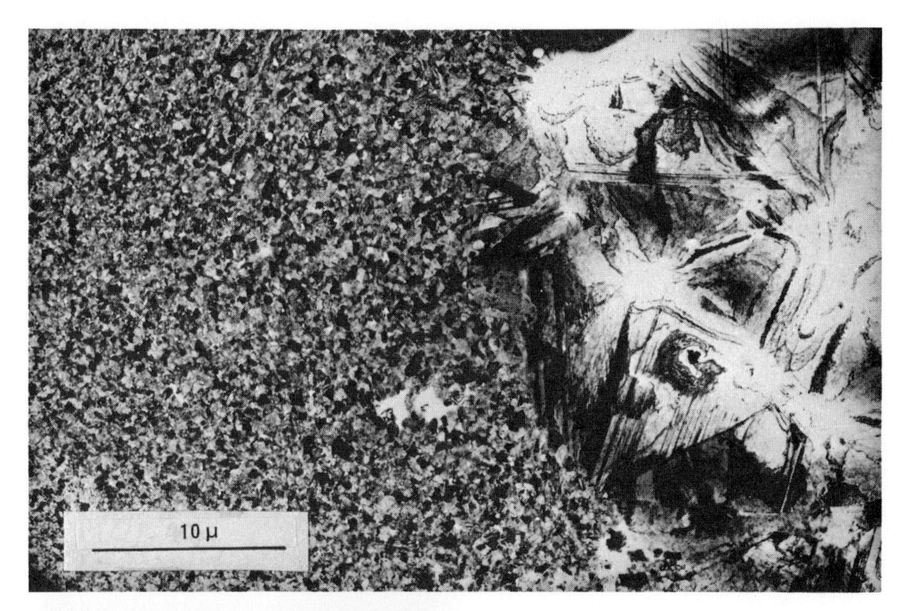


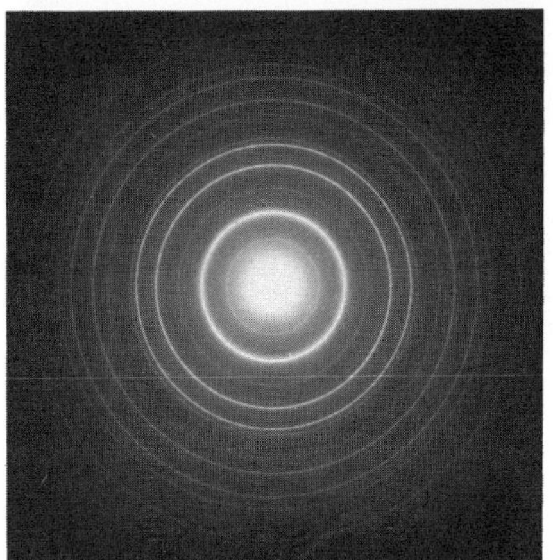

Fig.1. Multilayer Cu/In/Se film after laser irradiation.

Fig.2. Diffraction from 80µm x 80µm irradiated zone.

Fig.1. Crystal size is between 0.1-1µm depending on laser power from 3-5W. The high resolution electron diffraction pattern from an 80µm x 80µm grid hole is shown in Fig.2., with the associated microdensitometer trace in Fig.3. Analysis here shows that the film is composed of the chalcopyrite (tetragonal) structure of $CuInSe_2$ (5). We see no evidence of any remaining elemental constituents, nor any of the various possible binary compounds in this system.

At a beam power exceeding ~5W the central part of each grid hole is composed of much larger, heavily twinned, crystals, as appearing at the right side of Fig.1. Crystal dimensions here can reach 20µm and electron diffraction from this zone also clearly identifies $CuInSe_2$.

Fig.4., for example, has $\bar{2}01$ zone axis parallel to the electron beam and obvious twin reflections.

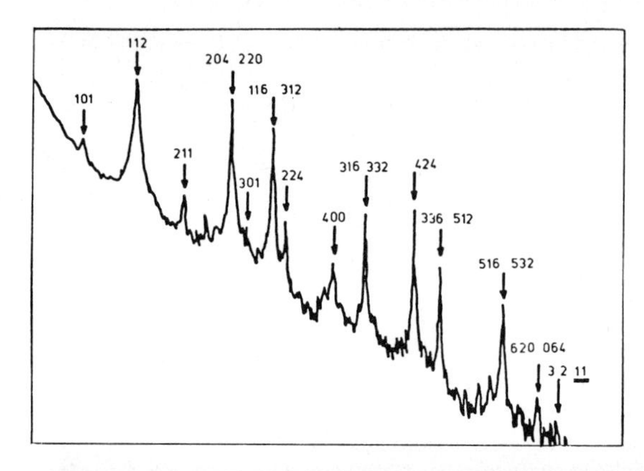


Fig.3. Microdensitometer trace of Fig.2.

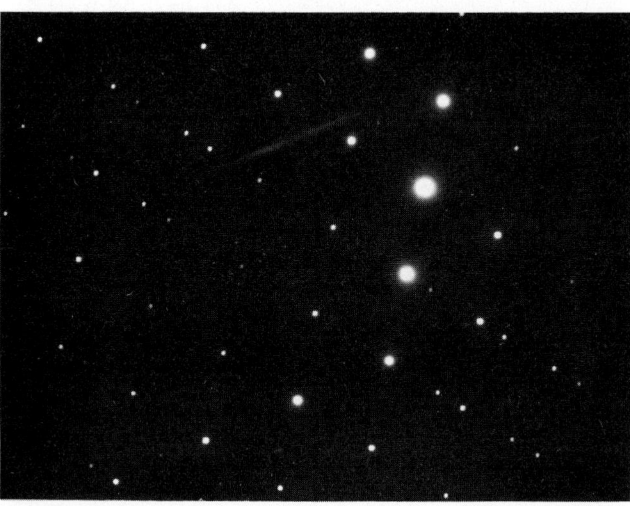

Fig.4. Diffraction from right portion of Fig.1.

Glass Mounted Films

Detached fragments of scan-irradiated films are polycrystalline with grain sizes ~1000Å, this size being essentially independent of beam power. Diffraction data, however, are as Fig.2., and show reflections due only to tetragonal $CuInSe_2$.

Areas of scan irradiated films were examined by optical spectrometry. Fig.5. shows the plot of $(\alpha h\omega)^2$ vs $h\omega$, indicating a direct gap at around 0.95eV.

## 5 DISCUSSION

Quite clearly the irradiated films are composed of the ternary compound $CuInSe_2$. Since these were the ingredients of the deposited film this might not appear unusual, though the phase diagram of this system is not particularly simple and it is surprising that the compound seems to form so easily without traces of the alternative binary compounds even when the layer order is such that, for example, In and Se are in contact. Either InSe, $InSe_2$ or $In_2Se_3$ might be formed here, but apparently they are not.

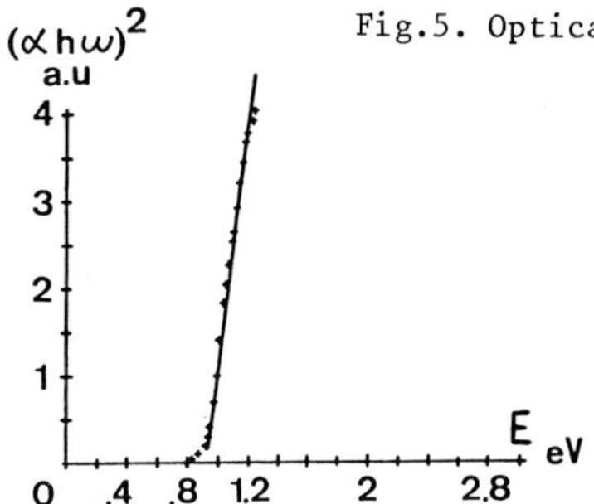


Fig.5. Optical absorbance of scan-irradiated $CuInSe_2$ film.

As with the binary systems previously studied, the final result is controlled by the overall stoichiometry of the film and any slight excesses due to the inherent inaccuracy of the deposition method are presumably swept to the grain boundaries where they are so widely dispersed that they show no trace in electron diffraction.

The temperature achieved during the irradiation is not easily calculated since both the reflectivity, transmission and thermal conductivity during irradiation are time dependent in an unknown way.

Irradiation of grid mounted films above ~5W produces particularly large $CuInSe_2$ crystals, with a rather sharp boundary between these and the surrounding polycrystalline zone. The situation is not dissimilar to the creation of explosively crystallized regions in a poly matrix when amorphous Ge films are irradiated above a certain threshold, and the heat of formation of $CuInSe_2$ can be expected to play a similar role to the heat of crystallization in the case of Ge.

Though substrate supported films exhibit, in these preliminary experiments, a disappointingly small crystal size, the fundamental absorption edge at 0.95eV is in good agreement with the gap reported for $CuInSe_2$(6-8), which is known to be direct.

In conclusion, these promising results, allied to the current interest in $CuInSe_2$ as a photovoltaic material, suggest that further work along these lines is appropriate.

## 6 ACKNOWLEDGEMENTS

This work was performed as a part of project 'Energy' of the Belgian Ministry for Science Policy.

## 7 REFERENCES

1. R.Andrew, M.Ledezma, M.Lovato, M.Wautelet & L.D.Laude Appl. Phys. Letters 35, 418 (1979).
2. R.Andrew, L.Baufay, A.Pigeolet & L.D.Laude, J.Appl. Phys. 53, 4862 (1982).
3. L.Baufay, A.Pigeolet, R.Andrew & L.D.Laude, Proceedings MRS Boston 1982.
4. C.Antoniadis & M.C. Joliet, Thin Solid Films 115, 75 (1984).
5. Power Diffraction File, ASTM, Philadelphia, PA, 1962, card 23-209.
6. K.Löschke, H.Neuman, R.D.Tomlinson, W.Hörig, E.Elliott, N.Avgerinos & L.Howarth, Phys. Stat. Sol(a) 61 K39 (1980).
7. C.W.Bates, K.F.Nelson & S.A.Raza, Thin Solid Films 88, 279 (1982).
8. C.Rinson, J.Gonzalez & G.Sanchez Perez, Phys. Stat. Sol.(b) 108, K19(1981).

# Metal/Silicon Reactions Using Pulsed Excimer and Ruby Lasers

E. D'Anna, G. Leggieri, A. Luches, and M.R. Perrone
Università di Lecce, Dipartimento di Fisica, I-73100 Lecce, Italy
G. Majni
Università di Modena, Dipartimento di Fisica, I-41100 Modena, Italy
I. Catalano
Università di Bari, Dipartimento di Fisica, I-70100 Bari, Italy

The formation of metal silicides was studied by irradiating thin metal films deposited on Si single crystals with laser and electron beams. It was observed that in the Si/Pt system reactions occur at relatively low energy fluences, corresponding to temperatures well below melting point. On the basis of a numerically solved heat diffusion equation, it is shown that reaction starts when the Si/Pt interface reaches the lowest eutectic temperature of the binary Si/Pt system. The growth rate of the reacted layers is of a few m/s.

## 1. Introduction

Metal silicides are of great importance in integrated circuit technology. They can provide ohmic or rectifying contacts, interconnections, barriers to interdiffusion, etc. The formation of metal silicides by solid phase reactions was extensively studied by heating thin metal films, deposited onto single crystal silicon wafers, in conventional vacuum furnaces [1]. Very often the result is metal-silicon interpenetration to depths in excess of those allowable in integrated circuit technology.

In the last few years much interest has arisen in metal-silicon reactions induced by pulsed laser, electron and ion beams. Because of the very short pulse width, a depth of only a few microns is heated and very shallow silicide layers can be formed. The high cooling rates ($\sim 10^{10}$ K/s) allow also the formation of thermally metastable phases, unobtainable with conventional furnace heating. Moreover, pulsed heating can be used for a time-resolved study of the physical mechanisms responsible for alloy formation.

In preceding papers [2,3] we studied the reaction of silicon with near-noble and refractory metals under pulsed ruby laser and electron beam annealing. It was noted that partial and even complete reaction of the thin (100-300 nm) metal film occurred at so low energy fluences that liquid phase formation should not be expected from temperature calculations.

To explain silicide formation we supposed that a quasi-liquid layer is formed when the temperature T of the metal/silicon interface reaches the lowest eutectic temperature $T_e$ of the binary metal/silicon system. The thickness of the quasi-liquid layer increases as long as $T \geq T_e$.

To verify the validity of this assumption we irradiated Si/Pt samples with different energy sources. We used ultraviolet (UV) light (KrCl excimer laser), visible light (ruby laser) and charged particles (electrons). The use of charged particles allows confidence in the temperature calculations, since the energy loss and penetration ranges into the samples are readily predictable and they do not depend on the surface characteristics.

## 2. Experimental Apparatus

Our KrCl excimer laser, which emits at 222 nm, was described previously [4]. It is of the capacitive discharge type. It can deliver up to 230 mJ in 16 ns pulses.

The ruby laser is a commercial device. It can produce up to 1.5 J in 20 ns pulses.

The electron source consists of a field emission diode, fed by a Marx circuit and a pulse-forming coaxial line [5]. The electron energy is variable, but usual operating energy is 25 keV. The pulse length is 50 ns. The current intensity can be varied from 100 A up to a few kA.

The analysis of the irradiated samples was made using the Rutherford backscattering (RBS) technique with 2 MeV $^4He^+$ particles.

The samples considered in the present work consist of a thin (100 nm) Pt film deposited on a Si single crystal wafer.

## 3. Results

Figure 1 shows the RBS spectrum of a sample irradiated at 0.3 J/cm$^2$ with the KrCl laser. The Si/Pt reaction is evident. A second shot at the same energy increases the thickness of the reacted layer and changes the silicide composition.

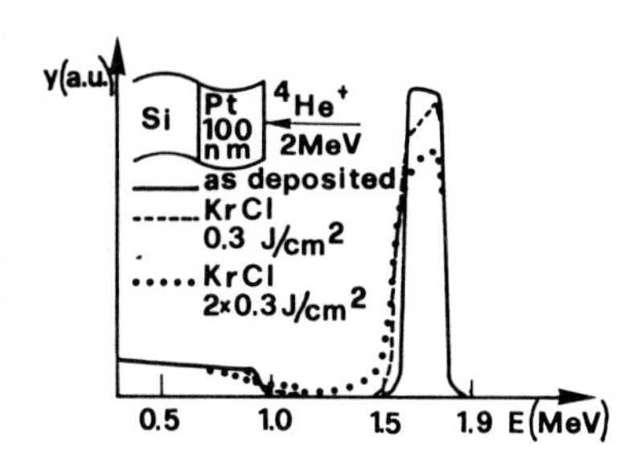


Fig.1: RBS spectrum of a Si/Pt (100 nm) sample irradiated with an excimer laser (KrCl, 222 nm).

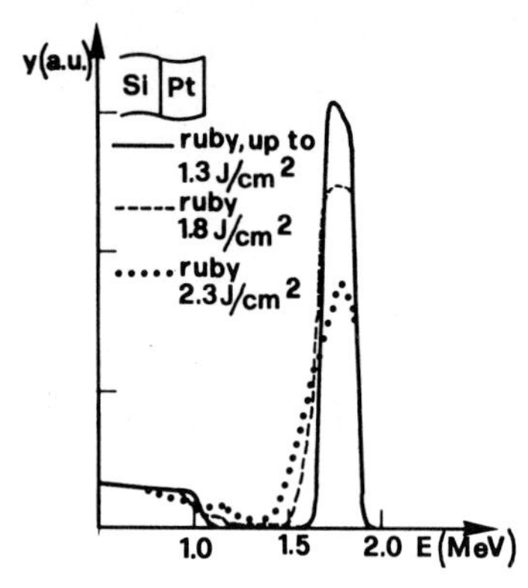


Fig.2: RBS spectrum of a Si/Pt (100 nm) sample irradiated with a ruby laser.

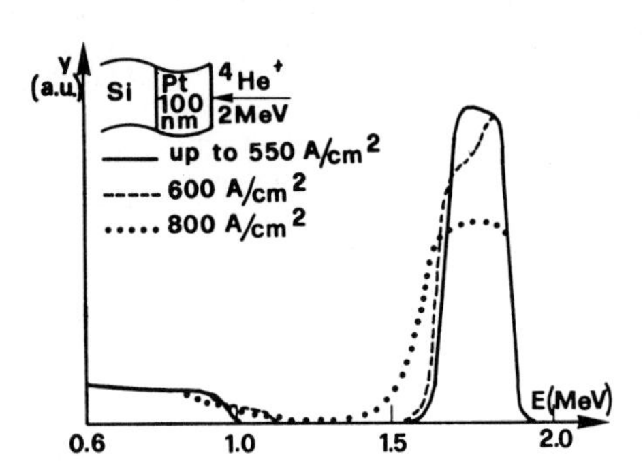


Fig.3: RBS spectrum of a Si/Pt (100 nm) sample irradiated with a pulsed electron beam (25 keV - 50 ns).

Figure 2 shows the RBS spectrum of a sample irradiated with the ruby laser. No reaction is detected up to 1.3 $J/cm^2$. At 1.8 $J/cm^2$ the Pt film has completely reacted. At 2.3 $J/cm^2$ surface damage and non uniform penetration of Pt is evident.

Figure 3 shows the RBS spectrum of a sample irradiated with electron beam pulses. No reaction is detected up to a current fluence of 550 $A/cm^2$ (0.69 $J/cm^2$). Si/Pt reaction with formation of a Pt/Si layer occurs at 600 $A/cm^2$ (0.75 $J/cm^2$). At 800 $A/cm^2$ (1.0 $J/cm^2$) surface damage and non uniform penetration of Pt is evident from the RBS spectrum.

## 4. Discussion

The energy fluence of each irradiation was correlated to the temperature of the Si/Pt interface by numerically solving the unidimensional heat diffusion equation [6]:

$$\rho(z,T)C(z,T)\ \frac{\partial T(z,t)}{\partial t} = \frac{\partial}{\partial z}\left\{k(z,T)\ \frac{\partial T(z,t)}{\partial z}\right\} + W(z,t)$$

where z is the direction of propagation of the beam (z=0 at the sample surface); $\rho(z,T)$, $C(z,T)$ and $k(z,T)$ are the density, specific heat capacity and thermal conductivity, respectively, at position z and temperature T; $W(z,t)$ is the energy loss rate per unit volume.

Figures 4, 5 and 6 show the temperature evolution at the interface of the Si/Pt (100 nm) sample under the different kinds of irradiation. It is evident that energy fluences of 0.3 $J/cm^2$ (KrCl laser), 1.3 $J/cm^2$ (ruby laser) and 0.75 $J/cm^2$ (e-beam) are too low to produce melting of the irradiated samples. But under all these fluencies, the interface temperature gets over

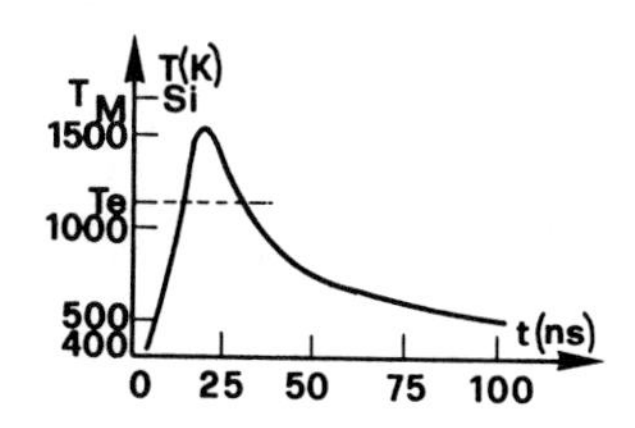


Fig.4: Temperature evolution at the interface of the Si/Pt (100 nm) sample irradiated with the KrCl laser at 0.3 $J/cm^2$.

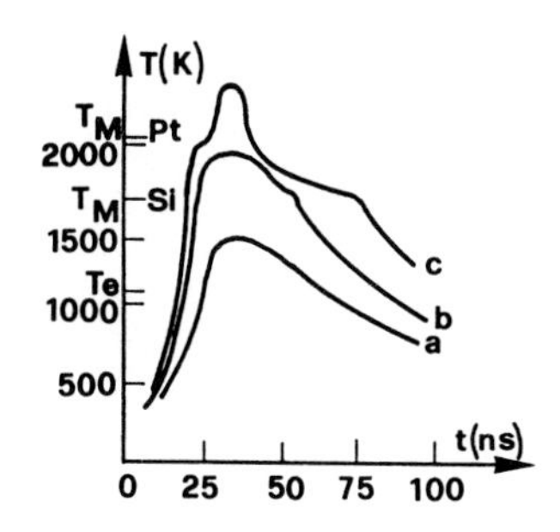


Fig.5: Temperature evolution at the interface of the Si/Pt (100 nm) sample irradiated with the ruby laser: a) 1.3 $J/cm^2$; b) 1.8 $J/cm^2$; c) 2.3 $J/cm^2$.

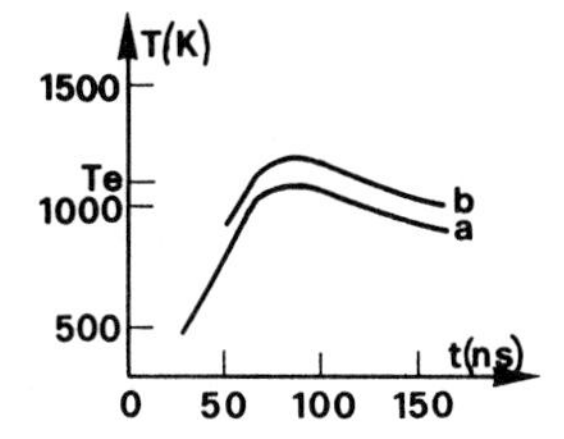


Fig.6: Temperature evolution at the interface of the Si/Pt (100 nm) sample irradiated with the 25 keV-50 ns electron beam: a) 550 $A/cm^2$ (0.69 $J/cm^2$); b) 600 $A/cm^2$ (0.75 $J/cm^2$).

the lowest eutectic temperature $T_e$. So we can affirm that Si/Pt reactions occur whenever the Si/Pt interface exceeds $T_e$. This is clearly confirmed by the comparison of Figs.3 and 6. From Fig.3 we see that Si/Pt reaction occurs at 600 $A/cm^2$ but not at 550 $A/cm^2$. From Fig.6 we see that the temperature T of the Si/Pt interface at 550 $A/cm^2$ does not exceed $T_e$, while at 600 $A/cm^2$ $T>T_e$ for about 40 ns.

## 5. Conclusions

The assumption that a quasi-liquid layer is formed at the Si/Pt interface when $T \geq T_e$ is supported by the results obtained with both laser and electron beam pulses. It results also from the comparison of the RBS spectra with the corresponding temperature profiles that the growth rate of the reacted layers is of a few m/s.

We also observed that the KrCl laser is a very efficient tool for semiconductor annealing, due to the strong coupling of the UV (222 nm) radiation with matter. In fact, at energy fluences as low as 0.6 $J/cm^2$ we reacted thin (100 nm) films of Mo deposited on Si single crystal. With the ruby laser the Si/Mo reaction was attained only at an energy fluence of 1.7 $J/cm^2$ and after covering the Mo film with an antireflecting Si layer (30 nm). Moreover, SEM pictures showed that while the samples irradiated with the ruby laser presented ripple patterns [7], the sample irradiated with the KrCl laser looked very smooth. This is probably due to the poor monochromaticity ($\Delta\lambda \simeq 1.5$ nm) of the KrCl excimer laser.

Work supported in part by C.N.R. (Consiglio Nazionale delle Ricerche). We thank G.Ottaviani for many helpful suggestions and F.De Donno and V.Nicolardi for technical assistance.

## References

1. G.Ottaviani: J.Vac.Sci.Technol.16, 1112 (1979).
2. F.Nava, G.Majni, A.Luches, V.Nassisi and E.Janniti: J.Physique 41C4, 97 (1980).
3. G.Majni, F.Nava, G.Ottaviani, A.Luches, V.Nassisi and G.Celotti: Vacuum TAIP 32, 11 (1982).
4. A.Luches, V.Nassisi and M.R.Perrone: Appl.Phys.Lett.42, 860 (1983).
5. A.Luches, V.Nassisi, A.Perrone and M.R.Perrone: Physica 104C, 228 (1981).
6. E.D'Anna, G.Leggieri, A.Luches and F.Nava: Thin Solid Films 110, 83 (1983).
7. J.F.Joung, J.S.Preston, H.M.van Driel and J.E.Sipe: Phys.Rev. B27, 1155 (1983).

# Structural Investigation of Laser Processed PZT Ceramics

M. Popescu, I.N. Mihailescu*, M. Dinescu*, and P. Nicolau

Institute of Physics and Technology of Materials ,
Bucharest - Magurele, Romania

## 1. Introduction

Materials with the composition $Pb(Zr,Ti)O_3$, or PZT ceramics, are very important for industrial applications because they exhibit piezoelectric properties. $PbTiO_3$ is a ferroelectric with a perovskite structure of tetragonal symmetry. $PbZrO_3$ is antiferroelectric with orthorhombic structure. Solid solution ceramics based on $PbTiO_3$ and $PbZrO_3$ can be synthesized for all composition ratios [1]. A morphotropic phase boundary (MPB) exists near the composition of 52 mol% $PbZrO_3$ [5]. Solid solutions containing less than ~48 mol% $PbTiO_3$ are rhombohedral while those containing more than ~48 mol% $PbTiO_3$ are tetragonal. The piezoelectric activity reaches a maximum when ceramic compositions are situated near the MPB. These ceramics are therefore the most useful for practical applications. In such PZT ceramics the coexistence of the two ferroelectric phases has been thoroughly demonstrated [2].

This paper deals with the investigation of the structure of some ceramic compositions when laser processed,i.e. heated up to melting and quenched.
The very high heating rated minimized the possible stoichiometry changes.

## 2. Experimental

The formation of PZT by laser irradiation was investigated on two powder samples consisting of mixtures of $PbTiO_3$ and $PbZrO_3$.
The first sample corresponds to a composition near MPB and is labelled PZT-45: 45 mol% $PbTiO_3$ + 55 mol% $PbZrO_3$.

The second sample is a composition far away from the MPB and is labelled PZT-73: 73 mol% $PbTiO_3$ + 27 mol% $PbZrO_3$.
A PZT sample (labelled PZT-La) was prepared by classical ceramic technology. It is a doped PZT ceramic having the chemical formula: $Pb_{0.98}La_{0.02}Zr_{0.51}Ti_{0.443}Fe_{0.02}Nb_{0.02}Li_{0.007}O_3$.
The samples were processed by a TEA-$CO_2$ laser with a beam power of 0.5 kW ($\lambda$ = 10.6 μm). The laser spot of ~0.5 cm diameter heated the powdered samples for some seconds and the droplets thus formed were quenched against a steel block. The sin-

*Institute of Physics and Technology of Radiation Apparata
Bucharest - Măgurele, ROMANIA

tered powder of PZT - La (labelled PZT - La (S)) was laser processed and a chip (labelled PZT - La(P)) was obtained. A sample of identical composition, prepared by hot pressing (950°C/2 h, 1000 kgf/cm$^2$) and labelled PZT-La(H) was also investigated.

The structure of the samples was determined by X-ray diffraction. A Siemens Kristalloflex IV diffractometer was used for measurements. The copper $K_\alpha$ radiation was monochromatized by a curved graphite crystal monochromator mounted in the diffracted beam. The X-ray diffraction data were recorded using a step by step method and the calculation of the lattice parameters was undertaken using the carefully determined angular positions of the X-ray lines, corrected for the distortion factors by means of a reference corundum sample.

## 3. Results

The X-ray patterns of the initial PZT-45 powder sample and of the same sample after laser processing are shown in Figure 1. After laser beam action a diphasic structure consisting of a rhombohedral and a tetragonal phase is obtained, the tetragonal phase being predominant. The lattice parameters of these crystallographic phases are given in Table 1. The structure looks similar to that of a sintered PZT compound of the same composition. Therefore laser treatment allows a PZT compound to be formed.

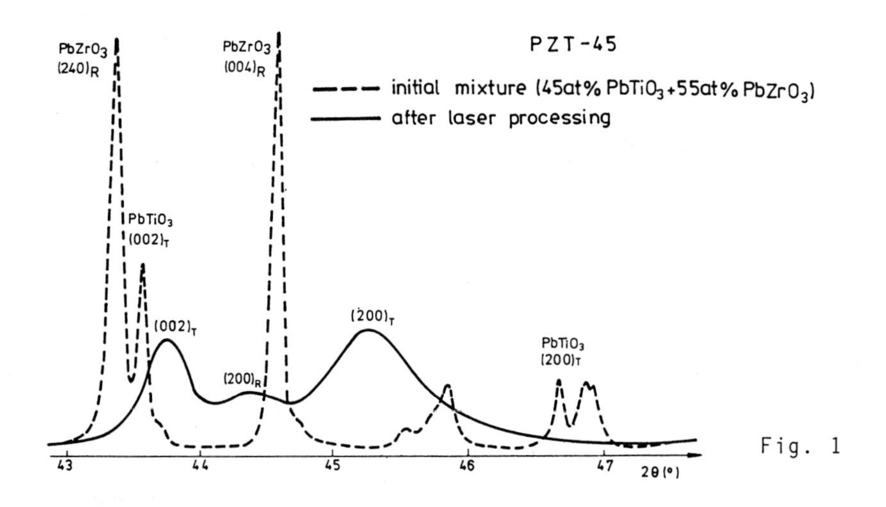


Fig. 1

The X-ray diagram of the PZT-45 processed sample shows a much stronger broadening of the (200) peak compared to that of the (002) peak in the tetragonal phase. Because it is unlikely this effect can be ascribed to the differences in the crystallite sizes along the two crystallographic directions, the only plausible explanation is the formation of microphases with large fluctuations of "a" and the distribution of c/a ratios near a central mean value.

Table 1 - Structural data on PZT ceramics

| Sample | Tetragonal phase | | | Rhombohedral phase | | Obs. |
|---|---|---|---|---|---|---|
| | c(Å) | a(Å) | c/a | a(Å) | α( °) | |
| PZT-45 | 4.140 | 4.005 | 1.0336 | 4.088 | 89.19 | T+R* |
| PZT-73 | 4.154 | 3.943 | 1.0536 | - | - | T |
| PZT-La(S) | 4.123 | 4.040 | 1.0205 | - | - | T+R** |
| PZT-La(P) | 4.132 | 3.970 | 1.0407 | 4.038 | 87.76 | T+R* |
| PZT-La(H) | 4.130 | 4.012 | 1.0294 | 4.089 | 89.98 | R+T* |
| $PbTiO_3$[3] | 4.532 | 3.899 | 1.0642 | - | - | |
| $PbZr_{0.53}$[4] $Ti_{0.47}O_3$ | 4.120 | 4.053 | 1.017 | 4.078 | 89.83 | T+R |

T=tetragonal phase; R=rhombohedral phase;
* minor phase ; ** very small amount.

After laser processing the sample PZT-73 shows an X-ray pattern characteristic for the tetragonal phase (Figure 2). The formation of the PZT compound leads to a lower tetragonality (c/a) than that of $PbTiO_3$, as revealed by the change of positions of the peaks (002) and (200) (see also Table 1). A strong contrast in the widths of the peaks (002) and (200) is in favour of fluctuations in the ratio c/a due to the local compositional variations. The fluctuations are not large enough to give rise to a rhombohedral phase although a very faint peak at ∿45°, which may be ascribed to this phase, can be seen on the X-ray diagram (Figure 2).

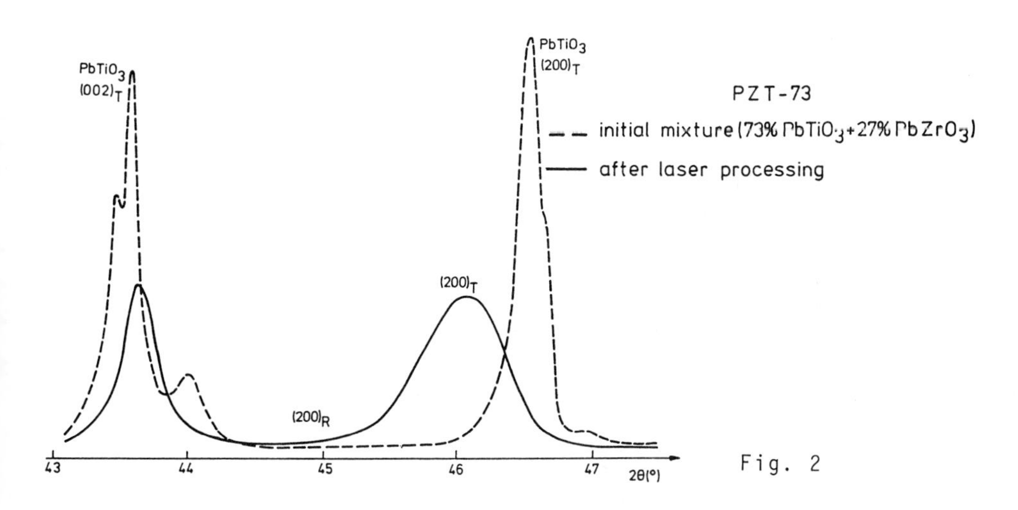

Fig. 2

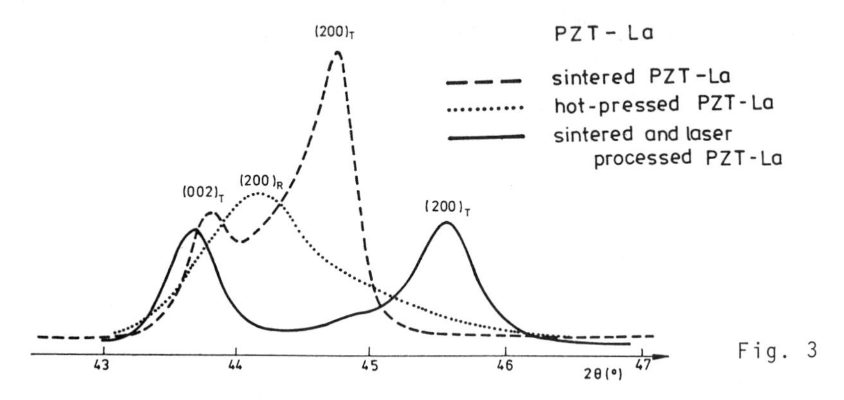

Fig. 3

The sample PZT-La(S) shows a tetragonal structure with low c/a ratio (see Table 1 and Figure 3). After laser processing the c/a ratio increases and a small amount of the rhombohedral phase is revealed. Contrary to the other samples, in this case no difference in the width of (002) and (200) peaks can be observed. Therefore the homogeneous tetragonal composition seems to be preserved after laser processing.

The hot pressed sample gives a diffraction pattern which reveals the formation of mainly rhombohedral phase.

## 4. Conclusions

The laser melting followed by quenching allows to get PZT materials with structural characteristics similar to those of classical PZT starting from powder mixtures of lead titanate and lead zirconate. A peculiar feature of laser processing is the high content of rhombohedral phase and local fluctuations of compositions reflected in the fluctuation of the lattice parameter "a" and of the tetragonality c/a.

The doped PZT ceramic situated at MPB and processed by laser exhibits lower "a" and higher tetragonality "c/a" than in the case of both classical ceramic and hot pressed ceramic. As opposite to the hot pressed ceramic which is mainly rhombohedral, the laser processed ceramic is mainly tetragonal.

Preliminary results have shown that thermal annealing of the laser processed samples significantly improves the densities and mechanical properties, challenging problems for the PZT ceramists.

1. B. Jaffe, R,S. Roth, S. Marzullo: J. Appl. Phys. 25, 809 (1954)
2. K. Okazaki: Ceramic Engineering for Dielectrics (Gakkenska Co., Ltd., Tokyo 1969)
3. ASTM, Powder diffraction file, Fiche No. 6-0452
4. F. Vasiliu, P.G. Lucuţa, F. Constantinescu, Phys. Stat. Sol. (a), 80, 637 (1983)
5. D. Bäuerle: Ferroelectrics 21, 555 (1978)

# Light-Induced Sublimation of Cadmium Sulphide

C. Arnone, C. Calì, and S. Riva-Sanseverino

Dipartimento di Ingegneria Elettrica, Università di Palermo
and
IAIF-CNR, Viale delle Scienze, I-90128 Palermo, Italy

It has recently been shown that single crystal CdS, illuminated by light whose photon energy exceeds the bandgap, can eject particles from its surface while the temperature is well below the value required for vacuum sublimation. This phenomenon has obvious applications to the fabrication of surface structures as well as to the production of thin films that can show good CdS stoichiometry. This work will present several data on the morphology of the etched surface and its dependance on crystal orientation; results of an analysis of the recondensed thin film phase from the ejected material will also be shown. Emphasis will be devoted to examples of high resolution surface structures fabricated with this technique.

## 1. Introduction

Recently much attention has been paid to the possibility of extracting material from a CdS crystal surface, at temperatures lower than those required for vacuum thermal sublimation, by illuminating the samples with monochromatic light. This effect has been observed in other research laboratories at different wavelengths above the CdS bandgap [1], [2], [3]. Our work concerns CdS surface processing by radiation at $\lambda$ = 4880 A from an Ar laser. In what follows several experiments will be reported, suggesting a photo-induced sublimation mechanism, associated with a thermal "bias" of the sample.

A threshold temperature around 400 °C has been found to be necessary for observing the light induced sublimation. A power density of 3.5 $W/cm^2$, associated with that minimum temperature and exhibiting a digging speed of about $10^5$ $\mu m^3/sec$, has been used in many of our experiments. Previous results showed a dependence on temperature of the minimum power density, to ensure a visible etching, roughly as $e^{-T/T_0}$ where T is the crystal temperature and $T_0$ is around 180 °C. It shows that photosublimation can also occur at temperatures much below 400 °C. Moreover other researchers [3] have measured average temperatures below 200 °C during the sublimation, by operating with focussed laser beams. We suppose, however, that in such conditions both the localized heating of the sample up to the threshold temperature and the photo-induced evaporation should be attributed to the laser "writing" beam.

(*) Work supported by Italian MPI and CNR (contr. 83/01437.02).

## 2. Laser Etching of CdS

We have performed three kinds of experiments on CdS crystals, differing from one another in laser power densities and in the techniques adopted for delimiting boundaries:

a - processing with high power density, by focussing the 4880 Å light on small areas, to engrave deep grooves or holes;

b - processing without focussing the radiation, but illuminating the crystal surface through masks;

c - maskless grooves engraving, using as a tool the interference pattern created by two interfering beams.

In the first set of experiments, run at atmospheric pressure or under moderate vacuum conditions ($10^{-2}$ torr), it has been possible to cut arbitrary shapes on CdS thin plates, opening holes or slots through the sample thickness. Sharp edges and no noticeable damage (i.e. no modification in the fluorescence properties or in the external aspect of the crystal), in the areas surrounding them, have been observed. Figures 1 and 2 show three different depth holes and also a cross section of one of them. This experiment had to be performed under vacuum, to allow the generated CdS particles to leave the crystal, without stopping a further penetration of the radiation. However some fallen back CdS powder can be observed all around the holes, due to the poor vacuum level. A non-perfect Gaussian laser beam, with two maxima in the intensity profile, was intentionally used in this "drilling" experiment; figure 2 shows a hole whose shape follows the transverse intensity distribution of the beam. Figure 3 is related to an array of 1 micron deep and 0.7 micron large grooves fabricated with light power densities just above the threshold; the corrugations that can be observed along the groove sides are due to discrete movements produced by the stepping motors of the translators used to steer the laser beam.

The second set of experiments has been carried out maintaining at very low level the heating due to photon absorption and generating the threshold temperature by putting the CdS sam-

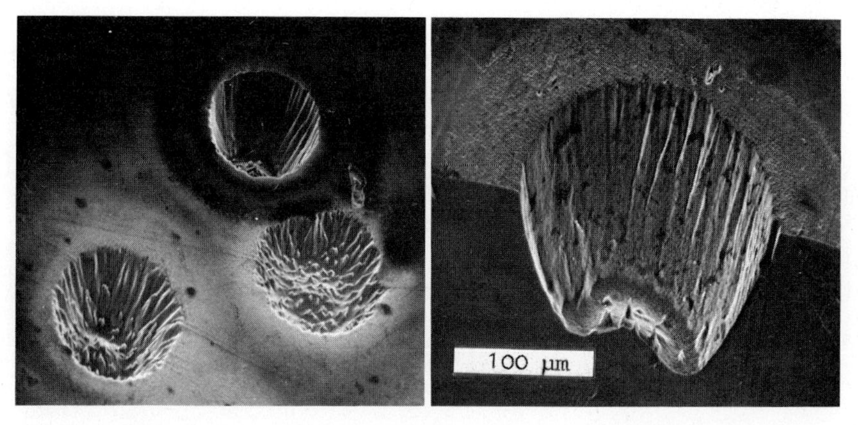


Fig.1 SEM picture of laser-drilled holes in a CdS crystal plate by Ar laser

Fig.2 Cross section of a laser-drilled hole

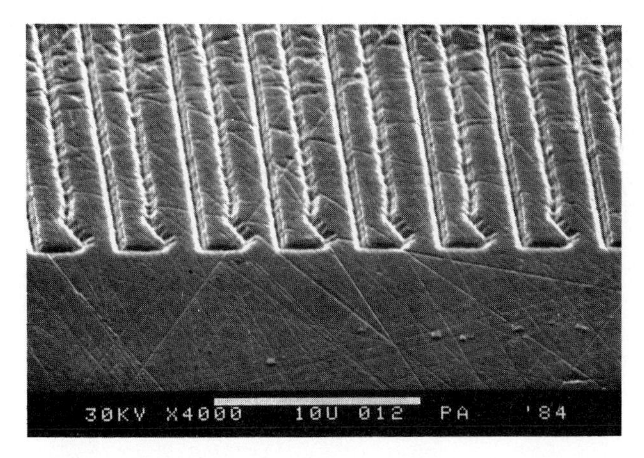

Fig.3 SEM picture of 0.7 micron grooves

ple on an electrically heated holder. The simplest experiment consisted of light etching using a laser beam power density as low as 10 $mW/mm^2$. This result suggested the possibility of fabricating a fine structure by selectively etching the crystal surface using a mask. For this purpose a stainless steel fine grid was placed directly onto the sample illuminated surface. A uniform heating of the crystal and an accurate temperature measurement was obtained with the device of Fig. 4. Moreover the experiment was run in high vacuum conditions ($10^{-6}$ torr). The masking action of the grid has produced an erosion only in the exposed areas, as it is shown in the SEM picture of Fig. 5, where the sides of the etched squares are 50 microns in length.

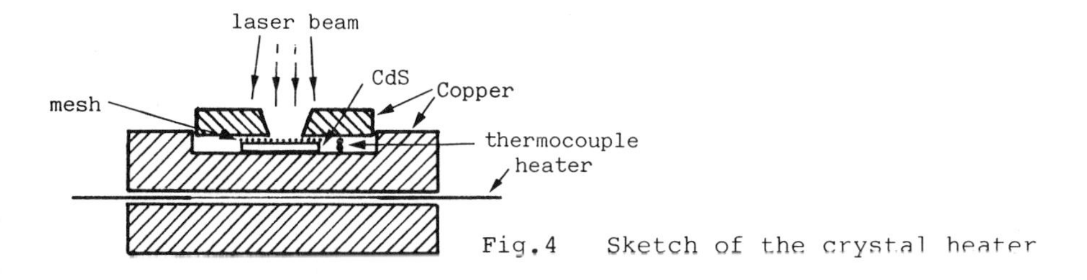

Fig.4 Sketch of the crystal heater

With the adopted light power density of 35 $mW/mm^2$ and an "exposure time" of 500 sec a 10 micron deep structure has been obtained. Referring to the wurtzite structure of CdS, such etching speed has been measured for the "sulfur" face of the (0001) crystallographic orientation of the sample. Digging speed was less than half in experiments performed under identical conditions on the "cadmium" $(000\bar{1})$ face.

From a morphological point of view, the effect of laser light on (0001) and $(000\bar{1})$ surfaces is very much like that of usual chemical etchants for CdS [4]. In Fig. 5, hexagonal pits can be seen in the bottom of the squared areas, created on a sulfur

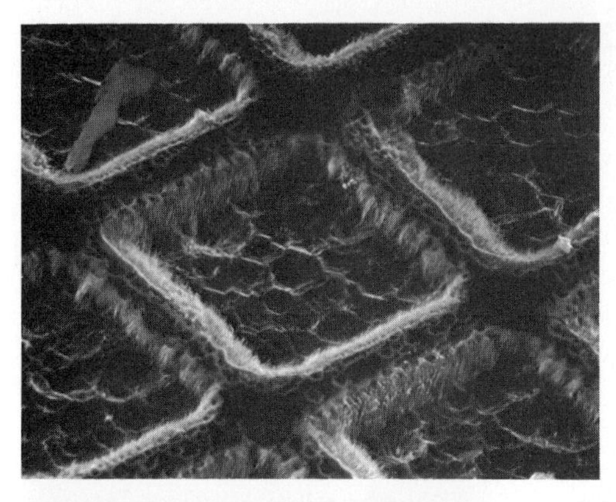

Fig.5 SEM view of squared areas etched by laser light, with hexagonal pits shown.

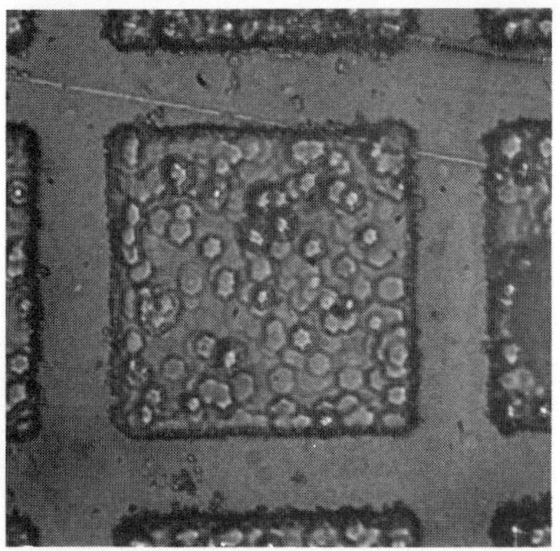

Fig.6 Optical microscope view of photoetched "S" face

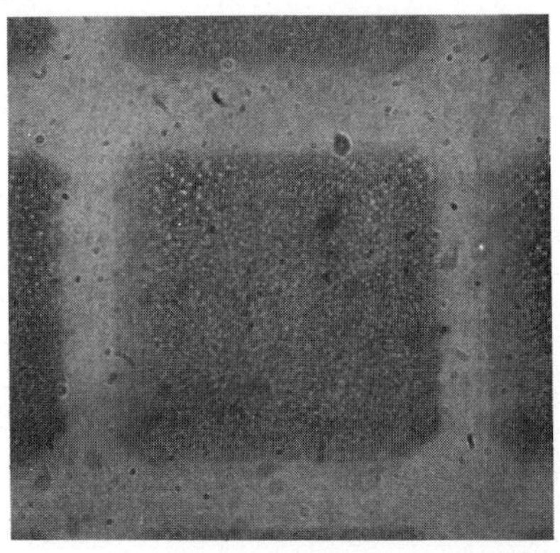

Fig.7 Optical microscope view of photoetched "Cd" face

surface. The pictures reported in Figs. 6 and 7, obtained using an optical microscope, allow a direct comparison between the photoetching of sulfur and cadmium faces. As expected from the action of a chemical etching, no particular regular structure can be detected on the cadmium side of the crystal.

The purpose of the third set of experiments was to write gratings directly on CdS surfaces bypassing the usual photolithographic step. The optical apparatus used is shown in Fig. 8. Particular care had to be devoted to the elimination of vibrations during the experiments, where two beams from the Argon laser were overlapped at an angle of about 3 degrees on a polished CdS crystal surface, preheated at about 250 °C, under vacuum. A simple observation of diffracted beams, arising as soon as the creation of the surface grating starts, allowed the dynamics of the experiment to be monitored. Figure 9 shows a microprofilometer plot of a surface modulation obtained.
The low ratio between grating depth and pitch is attributed to the thermal expansion of the sample, appreciable only at micrometric scale, because of the high power density of the laser light used in the experiment, where laser heating was added to

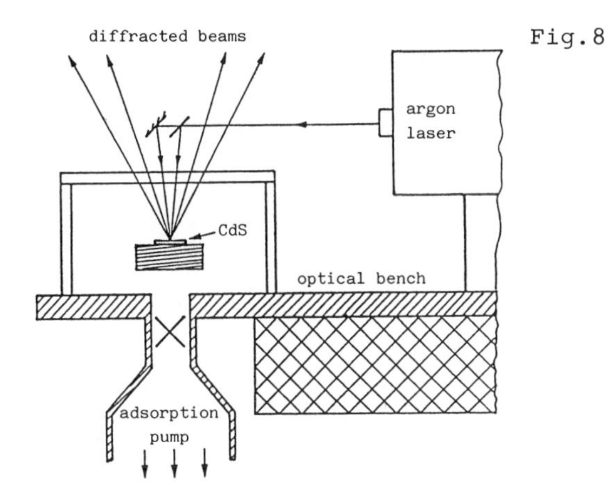


Fig.8 Sketch of the optical apparatus used for direct gratings engraving

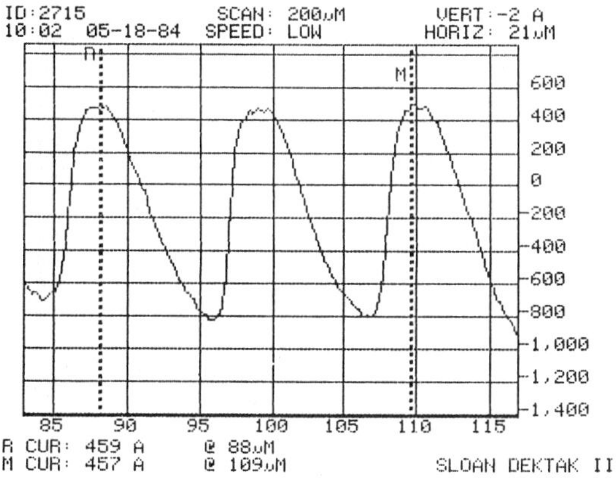


Fig.9 "Dektak" stylus scan of a photo-etched grating

the previous 250 °C "bias". In this case good monitoring of crystal temperature could be accomplished by observing in white light the color of the sample, **knowing the variation** of CdS bandgap with temperature (roughly 1 Å/°K). This experiment of laser photo-engraving was performed on CdS surfaces variously oriented with respect to the direction of the interference pattern, and different surface finishings were achieved. Very uniform etching was produced with the pattern at 90 degrees with the c axis of the crystal, i.e. in the (0001) plane, independently from its direction. On the contrary, such direction strongly influenced the etch uniformity on the $(10\bar{1}0)$ plane, because of the rising of new preferential crystalline orientations, according to [5].

## 3. Thin Film Production

A completely different application of the photostimulated ejection of molecules from CdS concerns the possibility of CdS thin film deposition under vacuum. By focussing an Ar laser beam, at $\lambda$ = 4880 Å, on bulk CdS single crystal inside an evaporation chamber, high stoichiometry films could be fabricated.

This evaporation technique is very "clean" and efficient, with respect to conventional methods, because of the possibility of localizing the evaporated areas, and the strong radiation coupling with the crystal in its first layers, the absorption length being around 120 nm at the wavelength used.

We have performed several tests on the films obtained. Auger electron spectroscopic analysis showed variations in stoichiometry less than 4%, throughout the film. Grazing X-ray analysis indicated that polycrystalline films were obtained, independent of the substrates used (glass, sapphire, silicon). By SEM inspection of the films deposited on glass, a grain size increasing with the substrate temperature used during film deposition has been observed, in the 20-200 °C range, with sizes up to 0.15 μm. Finally, by optical measurement during and after film depositions, a refractive index of 2.45 at $\lambda = 633$ nm has been found, for substrate temperatures ranging from 20 to 300 °C. The absorption length, at the same wavelength, was strongly dependent on the substrate temperature during the deposition. Values of 2.5 and 8 μm for 20 and 100 °C respectively, have been measured with no appreciable absorption, for thicknesses up to 0.25 μm, at temperatures above 150 °C.

## 4. Conclusions.

The results reported above on various experiments of light induced sublimation suggest a possible explanation of the observed phenomena. First of all it is recognized that both thermal and light sources are necessary to obtain a localized etching. In order to get high resolution engraved patterns it seems convenient to use high thermal bias (i.e. 400 °C) and moderate laser power density. The possibility of achieving fine-geometry structures, characterized by high spatial resolution and sharp edges, together with the observation of hexagonal pits etched on the sulfur face, indicates a slight non-thermal nature of the CdS sublimation induced by Ar laser light at 4880 Å.

Photons seem to be very useful for surface machining in order to modify selectively the surface morphology with a low energy interaction. Applications are envisaged whenever chemical or mechanical processing of CdS cannot be used.

The authors wish to thank V. Daneu and A. Sanchez of MIT Lincoln Laboratories for the stimulating discussions about the subject of this work and C. Sunseri of Palermo University for his cooperation in using the SEM facility.

## References

1 - A.Namiki, K.Watabe, H.Fukano, S.Nishigaki and T.Noda: "Ejection of atoms and molecules from highly excited CdS" - Surface Science, 128 (1983) L243-248.

2 - G.A.Somorjai and J.E.Lester: "Charge-transfer-controlled vaporization of cadmium sulfide single crystals. I. Effect of light on the evaporation rate of the (0001) face" - The Journal of Chemical Physics, 43,5 (1965) 1450.

3 - V.Daneu, J.Peers, A.Sanchez: "Laser fabrication of micron-size structures on CdS" - 1983 MRS Symposium on Laser-Controlled Chemical Processing of Surfaces, Boston (USA) 14-16 November 1983.

4 - E.P.Warekois, M.C.Lavine, A.N.Mariano and H.C.Gatos: "Crystallographic polarity in the II-VI compounds" - Journ. of Appl. Phys., 33, 2 (1962) 690.

5 - G.A.Somorjai and N.R.Stemple: "Orientation dependence of the evaporation rate of CdS single crystals" - Journ. of Appl. Phys., 35, 11 (1964) 3398.

# 3.5 Applications

## Laser Direct Writing Applications [1]

D.J. Ehrlich and J.Y. Tsao

Lincoln Laboratory, Massachusetts Institute of Technology
Lexington, MA 02173-0073, USA

### 1. Introduction

In this article, we survey research carried out at Lincoln Laboratory on the application of laser-microchemical direct-write processes. Practical refinement of these processes is still at an early stage, although a variety of techniques has already been demonstrated for specific applications and recent experiments have shown that a spatial resolution of ~ 0.2 μm is feasible for a range of direct-write processes. It is clear that a significant effort, comparable to that required for practical acceptance of any new microfabrication technology, will be required to bring instrumentation, material characterization and control, and process tolerances to a stage necessary for regular use. At this early stage, we can only guess at first areas of major technological importance. We can, however, give a reasonable picture of the range of processing possibilities and illustrate possible generic areas of application. For the purpose of this review it is convenient to divide laser direct-writing applications into two categories. First, those in which the laser process is a maskless substitute for a conventional planar fabrication step. Second, those in which the laser process has no planar fabrication equivalent, and therefore addresses a unique set of nonplanar fabrication difficulties. Many of the specific examples cited are from previously described, but recent, studies [1,2].

### 2. Planar Fabrication

In these applications, direct-write techniques have been adopted to address planar fabrication problems. Since they simplify or avoid entirely the multistep processing sequences necessary for even small-volume integrated circuit production used in the early stages of design, direct-write techniques can offer a means to speed the iterative process of circuit design and testing. Rapid implementation and testing may be particularly important as designs become more complex and more subject to errors. In addition, laser direct writing can restructure circuits and correct local fabrication-related defects. The potential in these areas has been explored in rapid prototype fabrication and testing at both the device [3,4] and the circuit levels of complexity [5-7]. In some situations it is possible to produce device or circuit prototypes, to carry out testing, and to alter the structures *in situ* within the fabrication chamber [3,7].

[1]This work was supported by the Defense Advanced Research Projects Agency, the Department of the Air Force (in part under a specific program sponsored by the Air Force Office of Scientific Research), and the Army Research Office.

## 2.1. Device Restructuring and Customization

As a first demonstration of real-time prototype fabrication at the device level, Si MOSFETs were metallized through the use of laser photodeposition [3]. In one study, dimethylcadmium (DMCd), because of its large photodissociation cross section, was used to write Cd gate electrodes. An example of two laser-deposited gates are shown in Fig. 1. These gates, as well as prepatterned sources and drains, are connected to bonding leads that are attached via vacuum feedthroughs to an external I-V curve tracer for *in situ* testing.

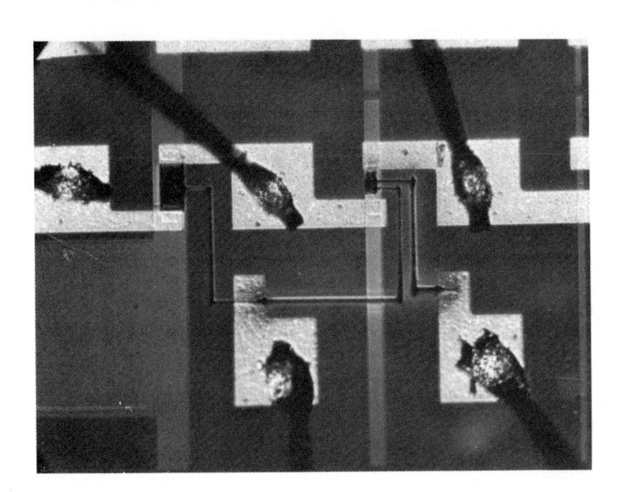

Fig. 1. Optical micrograph of laser-metallized Si MOSFETs. The two central blackened in regions and the conductors that lead to the pads on the right were photodeposited. The two vertical stripes are Si active channel regions, and are 20 micrometers wide.

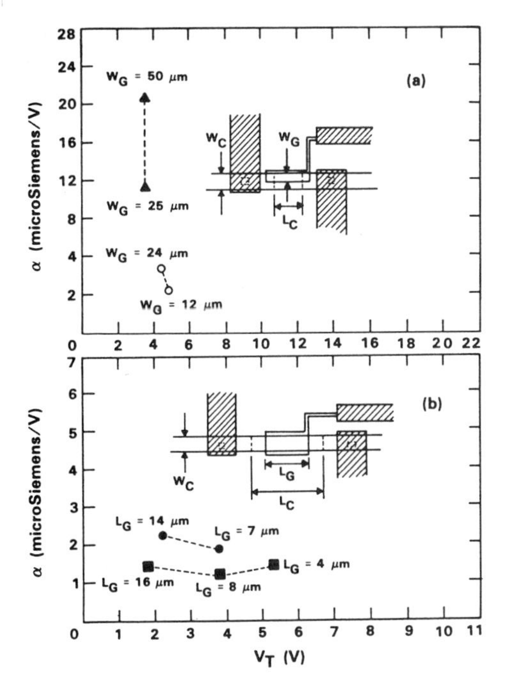


Fig. 2. Electrical characteristics of laser-metallized Si MOSFETs. Parameter adjustment by direct *in situ* deposition is demonstrated. (a) Dependence of transistor characteristics on gate width for gates that cover the entire channel length but variable portions of the channel width. For the device indicated by ▲, the channel dimensions were $W_C$ = 44 μm and $L_C$ = 4 μm. For the device indicated by o, the channel dimensions were $W_C$ = 21 μm and $L_C$ = 11 μm. (b) Dependence of transistor characteristics on gate length for gates that cover the entire channel width but variable portions of the channel length. For the device indicated by ●, the channel dimensions were $W_C$ = 10 μm and $L_C$ = 12 μm. For the device indicated by ■, the channel dimensions were $W_C$ = 3.5 μm and $L_C$ = 11 μm.

The geometries of the laser-deposited gates were varied systematically in two distinct experiments. In the first experiment, the results of which are shown in Fig. 2a, gates were laser deposited so as to cover the entire channel length but variable portions of the channel width. Since the differential transconductance, $\alpha$, is proportional to the gate width, it can be modified by adjusting the gate coverage of the channel width. In the second experiment, the results of which are shown in Fig. 2b, gates were laser deposited so as to cover the entire channel width but variable portions of the channel length. For complete overlap of the length of the gate over the length of the channel, the threshold voltage depends on material parameters such as surface states, doping and gate-channel work-function differences, and geometrical parameters such as oxide thickness. For incomplete coverage of the channel by the gate, however, the threshold voltage increases, because fringing fields are then required to invert the device at the uncovered ends of the channel. More details can be found in Ref. 3.

In another study, laser photodeposition has also been used to form local thin films of poly(methyl methacrylate) (PMMA), by polymerizing methyl methacrylate (MMA). These PMMA films are chemically resistant, and can be used as etch masks for subsequent pattern transfer. Figure 3 shows a result in which an Al gate on the same MOSFET structure described above has been defined by PMMA photodeposition followed by Al etching. In all of these studies, the variations in device characteristics were consistent with the expectations of established MOSFET behavior. MOSFETs have also been defined by thermal deposition.

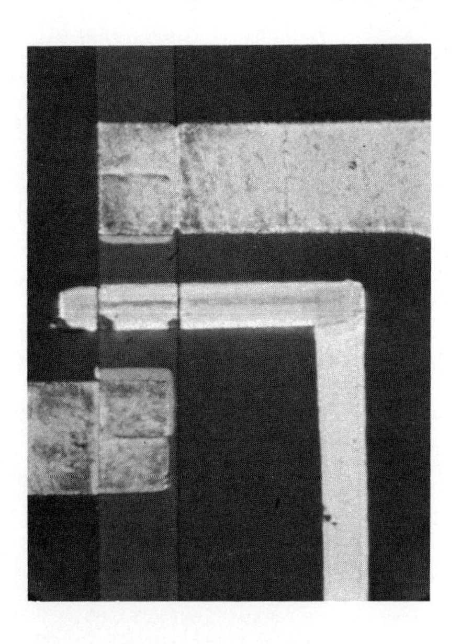

Fig. 3. Optical micrograph of Si MOSFET similar to that shown in Fig. 1, but with an Al gate defined by using laser direct-write polymerized PMMA as a mask for Al etching.

## 2.2 Circuit Restructuring

Laser direct writing can also be useful on the circuit level, for example, by modifying interconnect metallization. Applications here include real-time circuit designing and prototyping as well as fault correction by restructuring circuits. Along these lines, nonchemical laser techniques

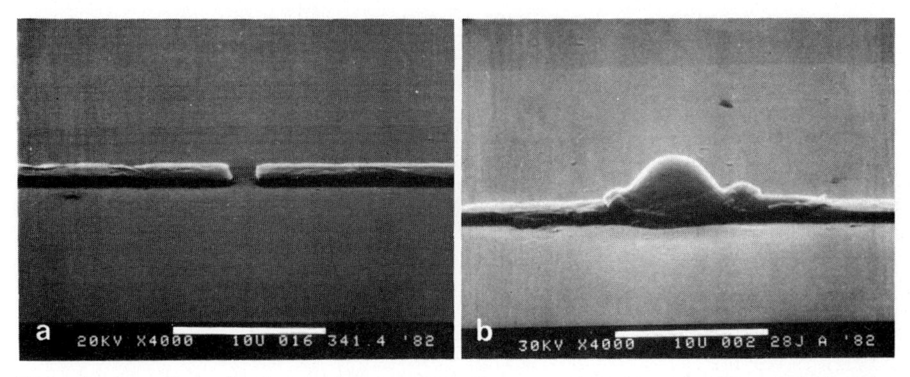


Fig. 4. Scanning electron micrographs of a gap structure in Al metallization (a) before and (b) after laser deposition of a conducting link. The link is formed with a 20-ms pulse in a $B(CH_3)_3/SiH_4$ vapor ambient (see the text). Shown are 10-μm scale markers.

that use photoresist, ablation, or local alloying of prefabricated structures have been described by KIANG et al. [8]. Recently, we have begun exploring applications using laser-chemical techniques [5-7].

In one example, laser-pyrolytic deposition makes use of pulsed $Ar^+$-laser radiation for direct deposition [from $B(CH_3)_3/SiH_4$] of poly-Si links [9,10]. Ohmic contact can be made, without postprocessing, between Si and Al gap structures. A typical link, deposited with a single 20-ms laser pulse, is shown in Fig. 4. These same links or other, prefabricated poly-Si, links can also be laser etched by using $Cl_2$ vapor. This allows the restructuring process to be reversed, if necessary. A strong chemical selectivity in etching permits rapid elimination of the conductor with a minimal disturbance of the underlying dielectric layer.

In another example [5-7], gate-array test circuits have been reconfigured by severing discretionary Al interconnects using laser-controlled chemical etching and by adding doped-poly-Si interconnects using laser-controlled chemical vapor deposition. The starting circuit for this work was a 500-gate commercial CMOS gate array manufactured using 5-μm design rules. This chip makes use of 1-μm-thick aluminum-alloy (2-percent Si) metallization combined with poly-Si gates. The $SiO_2$ dielectrics are 500 and 80 nm thick in the field and gate regions, respectively. A metal interconnect pattern, fabricated by conventional photolithography and dry etching, personalized the array into simple test structures such as ring oscillators, comparators, and logic gates.

The laser etching [1,2,11] and deposition processes have been described previously. Briefly, the etching process for Al involves localized modest (< 200-C) laser heating of a surface bathed in a capillary liquid etchant (0.15-percent $K_2Cr_2O_7$ in 10-percent phosphoric-acid/90-percent nitric-acid solution) layer trapped between the Si wafer and a thin cover glass. The liquid is normally cooled to retard background etching. Contrast ratios have been designed to be > $10^6$ between laser-enhanced (~ 0.5 μm/s and background etch rates. The spatial resolution is ~ 1.5 μm for typical metallizations [11]. Due to its low temperature and high chemical selectivity, the process leaves underlying insulating oxide layers damage free. The deposition process [9] is by localized laser heating of a surface in a 200-Torr ambient of diborane-doped silane

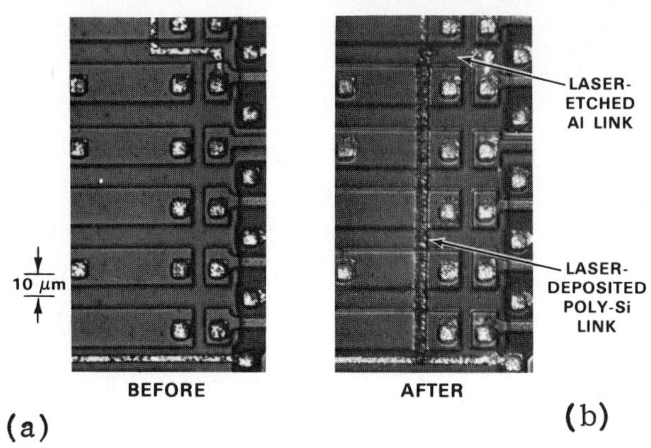


Fig. 5. Optical micrographs of a portion of a ring oscillator. (a) Before laser-microchemical restructuring. (b) After laser-microchemical restructuring. One short vertical Al link has been removed and one long horizontal poly-Si link has been added.

vapor. This induces the chemical vapor deposition of heavily B-doped poly-Si, suitable for forming ohmic contacts to Al. Laser scan rates for deposition of 1.5-μm-thick conductors are ~ 75 μm/s.

Figure 5 shows optical micrographs of a section of a ring-oscillator circuit before and after restructuring. The Al metallization at the top of Fig. 5(a) connects the eighth to the ninth gate in the ring-oscillator. In Fig. 5(b), this conductor is shown severed by laser etching. Also shown in Fig. 5(b) is a laser-deposited poly-Si conductor which connects the eighth to the thirteenth gate in the oscillator, thereby decreasing the number of stages from 23 to 19. The step coverage is very good, and is characteristic of laser deposition processes over even higher steps [1,2]. Al/poly-Si contact resistances were measured to be $< 10\ \Omega$ for a typical 3-μm x 3-μm contact area. Sheet resistances for 1.5-μm-thick films are 20-30 Ω/cm. This implies a resistivity $\approx 3 \times 10^3\ \Omega \cdot cm$, comparable to that of conventionally formed B-doped poly-Si. No furnace annealing or other treatment was used after any of the laser operations.

Electrical characteristics of a representative ring oscillator before and after a 23-19-stage restructuring are shown in Fig. 6. Similar oscillation waveforms are observed both before and after [Fig. 6(b)] the laser modification. Typical delays are ~ 4 ns per stage. The before and after oscillation period versus supply voltage plots [Fig. 6(a)] are identical except for a proportionate reduction by the ratio 23/19. Similar proportionate reductions were found for 23-15-stage restructurings.

These studies indicate that the laser-chemical restructuring operations do not adversely affect circuit performance. The measurements of ring-oscillator periods are a sensitive measure of damage at the device level, and of increased interconnect impedance. The laser modifications are rapid and can be applied directly to single-step modification of standard circuit structures with no need for prefabricated test nodes or switches. By using additional microchemical steps, it is possible to return the circuit to its original function with no degradation in performance. This ability to perform multiple restructuring may be particularly useful for

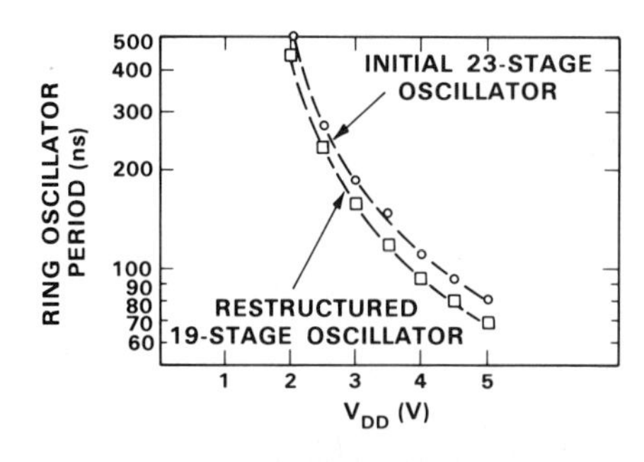


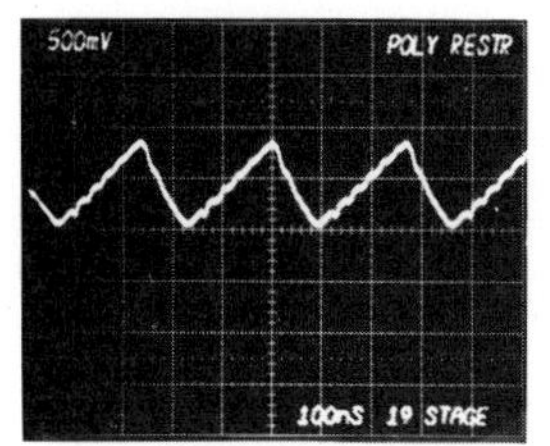


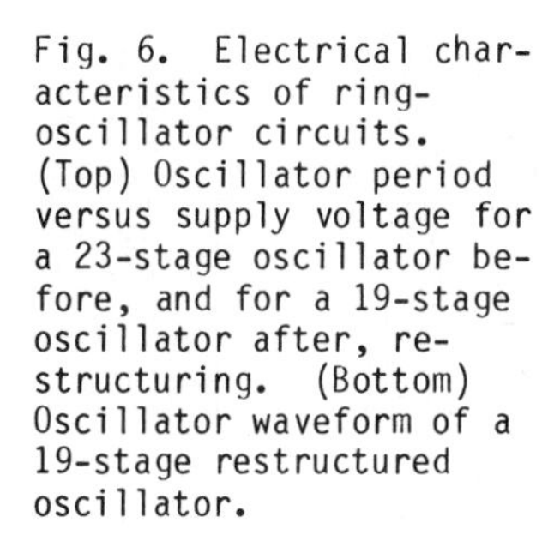
Fig. 6. Electrical characteristics of ring-oscillator circuits. (Top) Oscillator period versus supply voltage for a 23-stage oscillator before, and for a 19-stage oscillator after, restructuring. (Bottom) Oscillator waveform of a 19-stage restructured oscillator.

comparison and optimization of circuit architectures and layouts for semi-custom or gate-array chips. The techniques have application as a development tool for circuit prototypes, as a testing tool to isolate, provide access, and reconfigure circuit subfunctions on IC chips, and as a yield-enhancement tool in situations where photoresist or metal patterning on even the original circuit layout are problematical.

## 2.3 Fault Correction

As mentioned in the introduction, increases in the densities of integrated circuits are reflected as reduced and unacceptably low yields resulting from the random occurrence of nonrepeating defects. The importance of fault correction has been made clear, for example, in the recent development of large-capacity random-access memories that depend on redundant columns and rows. Electrical fusing and laser ablative techniques have been essential to the commercial production of these devices. Analogous randomly occurring faults are introduced in fabrication and by wear, after repeated use, of masks for optical and x-ray lithography. The correction of such faults is a problem not easily addressed with conventional multi-step lithographic techniques.

For example, the Al-etching process described above is well suited to repairing a particularly prevalent class of faults in VLSI circuits in which metallization shorts are introduced by surface contaminants, resist failure, or poorly controlled etching of circuit conductors. When shorts occur in certain areas of a chip, they may sometimes be repaired by using laser ablation of the excess metal although only with relatively low spatial resolution and with a high risk of damage to dielectric layers and nearby structures. More precise removal of the excess metal is possible by using laser-chemical etching (see Fig. 7). It should be emphasized that Al is a particularly problematic metal to etch chemically, due to its tough native oxide. For some applications, more convenient dry etching of Al can be accomplished through the use of thin-film oxidation barriers. In addition, other metals that do not form such tough oxides can be etched easily in a $Cl_2$ ambient.

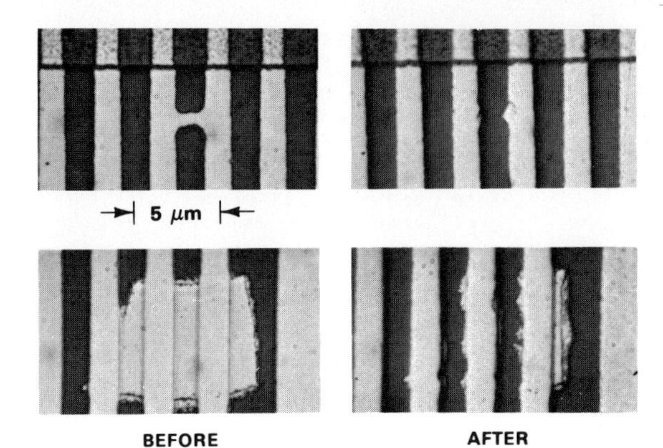


Fig. 7. Optical micrographs of Al bridging effects on an integrated-circuit-metallization pattern before (left) and after (right) correction by laser-microchemical etching.

An example of a problem that perhaps requires a laser-photochemical process is that of transparent defects on masks for optical or x-ray lithography. In a previous demonstration [12], photodeposition was applied with sufficient accuracy to repair ~ 15-μm pinholes of breaks in photomask patterns; an accuracy of < 1 μm has since been demonstrated. More recently, photodeposition has been applied to the repair of membrane masks for x-ray lithography [13]. An example is shown in Fig. 8. By photodeposition, metal (typically Cd or Ti) is deposited to a thickness of ~ 1000 Å in pattern breaks; no subsequent processing is necessary. Among laser direct-write techniques, photodeposition is chosen because it is particularly nonperturbing to the existing metallization pattern and because the deposition rate is insensitive to the differences in surface properties between clear and opaque regions of the photomask. The repairs made are adherent and able to withstand normal mask-handling and mask-cleaning procedures [13].

## 3. Nonplanar Fabrication

Further varied applications arise in the use of laser direct writing for microfabrication tasks not well addressed by planar fabrication technology, for example, patterned deposition or etching of highly three-dimensional structures or production of laterally graded structures. The latter are possible by variations of scanned-laser dwell times or beam in-

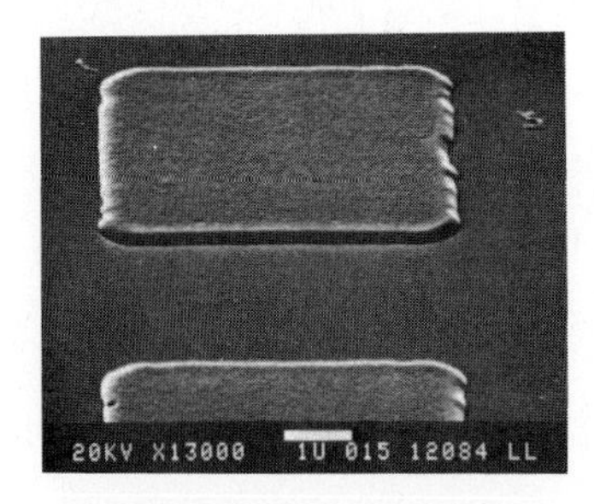


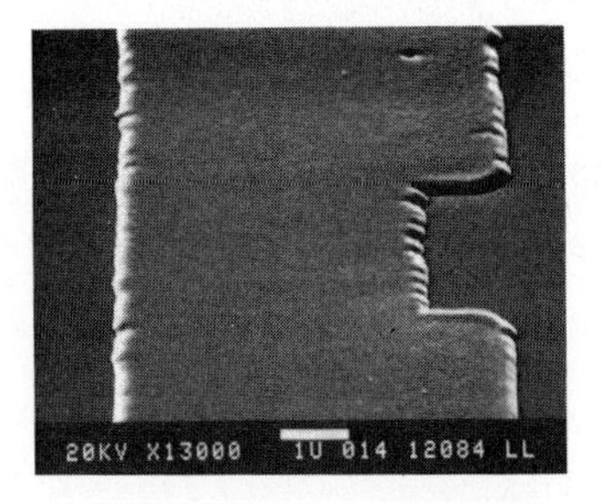


(a) X-RAY EXPOSURE OF POLYIMIDE MASK WITH Au ABSORBER (b) X-RAY EXPOSURE OF MASK REPAIRED BY LEAD DEPOSITION

Fig. 8. Scanning electron micrograph of the replication of an X-ray mask on which lead was not photodeposited.

tensities. Such structures are often prohibitively difficult to produce by lithographic patterning and full-area processing. The simplest examples are the patterned deposition of mid-thickness (greater than several micrometers) films or the processing of surfaces of extended area or of variable topography. Many such problems exist; two are described in the following two subsections.

## 3.1 Through-Wafer Via Conductors

Through-wafer via conductors have many applications in the bonding and interconnecting of novel integrated-circuit device structures. For example, in fast GaAs circuits, via connections can significantly reduce lead inductances. Silicon via holes are also used in the fabrication of mechanical components, for example, as nozzles for ink-jet printing. Previous methods of fabrication have relied on the anisotropic wet etching of single-crystal substrates; a large opening angle, associated with the intersection of slow-etching crystallographic planes of the substrate, limits these methods to making low-aspect-ratio via holes. To illustrate this limitation, a typical closest spacing for a via wet etched in a 10-mil wafer is ~ 15 mils. Fabrication based on laser-chemical etching can reduce via dimensions and spacings substantially.

Recently, laser etching and deposition methods have been applied to via formation for both Si [14] and GaAs [15,16] wafers. For Si, etching in $Cl_2$ was used to define conical (40-50-μm-diameter) via holes in 250-μm-thick wafers, as shown in Fig. 9. Laser photodeposition was then used (and found to compare favorably with alternative methods) to apply a conductive plating base in order to metallize the vias. Grazing-incidence UV radiation is sufficient to give good film coverage even on the nearly vertical walls of the via hole. More details of the process for Si vias are given in Ref. 14.

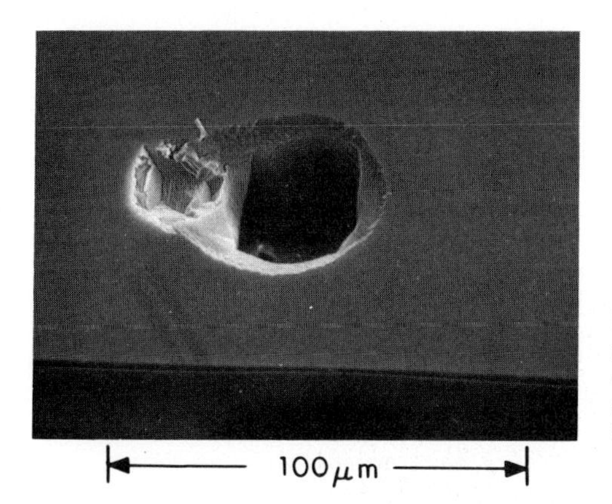


Fig. 9. Top surface scanning electron micrograph of a 40 x 50 micrometer-diameter conical via through a Si wafer.

## 3.2 Ti-Diffused Optical Waveguides

As an additional example, one that demonstrates an application for graded, laser-written films, Ti-indiffused $LiNbO_3$ optical waveguides have been fabricated recently [17] by photodeposition of Ti from $TiCl_4$. Metal films several hundred angstroms thick were deposited on $LiNbO_3$ in curved or straight lines 3 to 4 μm wide and 1 to 1.5 cm long. Photochemical deposition was used, because deposition by laser pyrolysis is not workable due to the fragility of $LiNbO_3$ to thermal shock. The deposited Ti was then indiffused under argon and oxygen, according to usual procedures, to form optical waveguides. Low optical scattering losses and high-mode confinement were obtained [17].

As a potentially important extension, preliminary experiments have used smooth, functional variations of the laser exposure along the guides. A preliminary result is shown in Fig. 10. The process suggests new possibilities for $LiNbO_3$-waveguide structures and integrated optics by providing a simple method to vary smoothly the refractive index of indiffused guides. Such structures have several applications. For example, waveguide-bend losses associated with guided-wave modulators and switches could be decreased considerably by increasing the mode confinement in the bend regions. In another example, the photodeposition technique allows one to optimize separately the guide parameters for both fiber-to-guide coupling and active-device geometry by first optimizing the geometry of the active electrooptic devices and then gradually increasing both the Ti thickness and the channel width such that at the $LiNbO_3$ sample edge the waveguide mode closely approximates that of the optical fiber. More details of this study can be found in Ref. 17.

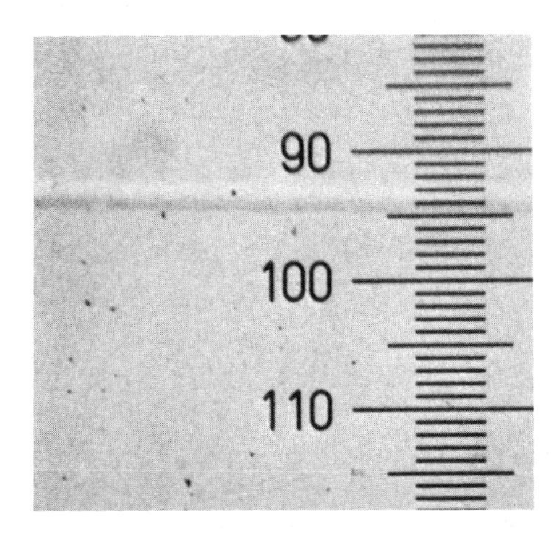


Fig. 10. Nomarski optical micrograph of a laser-photodeposited Ti line on $LiNbO_3$ after indiffusion to form a channel optical waveguide with functionally curved bends. The scale indicates 2 micrometers per division.

## 4. Summary and Future Directions

In this article we have surveyed recent applications of laser-chemical direct writing in which microscopic chemical reactions are used to modify surfaces. Specific methods have been described for addition and deletion of structures by local deposition, etching, and doping of various thin-film and substrate materials.

We can expect, as applications become more complex, the instrumentation and process engineering also to become more complex. Compared with presently available laser-based commercial equipment such as wafer scribers and laser trimmers, however, the much broader range of surface modifications possible with microchemistry should justify the additional investment.

We have stressed the unique potential of laser direct writing as a means for one-step local modifications of devices and circuits and for intrinsically nonplanar fabrication problems in such areas as packaging and bonding. Both types of problem are likely to become increasingly important in VLSI manufacturing, though neither is well addressed by lithographic patterning. It is important, however, to realize the fundamental differences in thought processes necessary to take advantage of laser writing within the framework of an advanced, lithography-based fabrication technology. The assimilation of laser direct writing into practical production will depend not only on the refinement of these new techniques but also on the inventiveness with which direct-writing and lithographic processes can be combined on the production line.

Acknowledgments

We should like to acknowledge stimulating conversations with D. J. Silversmith and to thank D. J. Sullivan, B. E. Duquette, J. Sedlacek, S. Fiorillo, R. W. Mountain, D. M. Klays and P. M. Nitishin for technical contributions.

1. D. J. Ehrlich and J. Y. Tsao, "Laser Direct Writing for VLSI" in VLSI Electronics: Microstructure Science, Vol. 7, N. G. Einspruch, ed., (Academic Press, N.Y., 1983).
2. D. J. Ehrlich and J. Y. Tsao, J. Vac. Sci. Technol. B1, 969 (1983).
3. J. Y. Tsao, D. J. Ehrlich, D. J. Silversmith and R. W. Mountain, IEEE Electron Device Lett. EDL-3, 164 (1982).
4. B. M. McWilliams, I. P. Herman, F. Mitlitsky, R. A. Hyde and L. L. Wood, Appl. Phys. Lett. 43, 946 (1983).
5. D. J. Ehrlich, J. Y. Tsao, D. J. Silversmith, J. H. C. Sedlacek, R. W. Mountain and W. S. Graber, Electron Dev. Lett. EDL-5, 32 (1984).
6. W. S. Graber, D. J. Ehrlich, J. Y. Tsao, D. J. Silversmith, J. H. C. Sedlacek and R. W. Mountain (to be published in IEEE Proceedings of the 1984 Custom Integrated Circuits Conference, Rochester, New York, 21-23 May 1984).
7. D. J. Silversmith, D. J. Ehrlich, J. Y. Tsao, R. W. Mountain and J. H. C. Sedlacek, "Laser Direct Write Technologies as Tools for Gate-Array Circuit Development" in Laser-Chemical Processing of Surfaces, A. W. Johnson, D. J. Ehrlich and H. R. Schlossberg, eds., (Elsevier, N.Y., 1984).
8. Y. C. Kiang, J. R. Moulic, W. K. Chu and A. C. Yen, IBM J. Res. Dev. 26, 171 (1982).
9. D. J. Ehrlich, R. M. Osgood, Jr. and T. F. Deutsch, Appl. Phys. Lett. 39, 957 (1981).
10. J. Y. Tsao, D. J. Ehrlich, B. P. Mathur and G. H. Chapman (to be published).
11. J. Y. Tsao and D. J. Ehrlich, Appl. Phys. Lett. 43, 147 (1983).
12. D. J. Ehrlich, R. M. Osgood, Jr., D. J. Silversmith and T. F. Deutsch, IEEE Electron Device Lett. EDL-1, 101 (1980).
13. J. N. Randall, D. J. Ehrlich and J. Y. Tsao, J. Vac. Sci. Technol. B (to be published, September, 1984).
14. D. J. Ehrlich, D. J. Silversmith, R. W. Mountain and J. Y. Tsao, IEEE Trans. Parts, Hybrids, Packag. CHMT-4, 520 (1982).
15. A. W. Tucker and M. Birnbaum, IEEE Electron Device Lett. EDL-4, 39 (1983).
16. R. M. Osgood, Jr., A. Sanchez-Rubio, D. J. Ehrlich and V. Daneu, Appl. Phys. Lett. 40, 391 (1982).
17. J. Y. Tsao, R. A. Becker, D. J. Ehrlich and R. J. Leonberger, Appl. Phys. Lett. 42, 559 (1983).

# Laser Fabrication of Integrated Circuits

Irving P. Herman

University of California, Lawrence Livermore National Laboratory,
Department of Physics, P.O. Box 808, L-278, Livermore, CA 94550, USA

The techniques used to fabricate integrated circuits have evolved rapidly during the past two decades, resulting in faster circuit speeds, smaller feature sizes, greater device density, a larger number of devices per chip, higher die yields, shorter fabrication times and lower costs. Current process research will continue promoting this trend of improved integrated circuit manufacturing performance in coming years. Recent research in laser processing of semiconductors has also been impressive, impacting each established fabrication method. Surely, selected elements of laser processing will be included in the rapidly expanding technology base of successful production techniques. This wide-ranging spectrum of laser-based candidate steps for the fabrication of silicon-based planar integrated circuits will be critically surveyed here. Emphasis will be placed on direct-laser writing fabrication steps in which a laser focused to $\sim 1\ \mu m$ induces local gas-surface pyrolytic reactions.

## 1. Introduction

To best appreciate the potential impact of lasers in planar device fabrication it is instrucive to briefly review the rudiments of conventional processing.[1,2] In classical photolithography the integrated circuit layout is encoded in a series of chrome-on-quartz (or glass) masks. A typical process step may begin with deposition of either an insulating or conducting film on the substrate by chemical vapor deposition (CVD), evaporation, sputtering, plasma deposition, or a surface reaction. A resist is then spun on the substrate and appropriately baked. The mask design is transferred to the resist by contact or projection printing, utilizing spatially selective transmission of incoherent ultraviolet light through the mask. The irradiated (non-irradiated) regions of the positive (negative) resist are then removed by either wet (i.e., solvent) or dry (i.e., plasma) etching. With the remaining resist as a barrier, the exposed underlayer can be appropriately doped or etched, as desired. After the remaining resist is removed, the next process step begins. Several such steps may be necessary for each phase of integrated circuit fabrication: device layout, interconnection and packaging. Many variations in this overly simplified process sequence are currently in use or under active study, such as the use of the lift-off technique[1] (film deposition following resist patterning), multi-layered resists,[2] and self-aligning procedures.[1] In photolithography, attaining acceptable product yields demands utmost care in applying, baking, developing and etching the resist in a particulate-free environment, as well as equally stringent care in the other parts of the process.

In silicon-based unipolar and bipolar transistors, boron (p-type) and phosphorous/arsenic (n-type) dopants are used in the active source/gate/drain and emitter/base/collector regions, and also in inter-transistor isolation regions. Spatially delineated insulator films of silicon dioxide, silicon nitride, phosphosilicate glass (PSG), polyimide, etc.,are used for insulation between interconnect layers, as passivation/encapsulation layers, and (for some of these materials such as $SiO_2$ and $Si_3N_4$) as gate insulators (for MOSFET's).[1] Interconnect materials include near-degenerately doped polysilicon, aluminum, tungsten, tungsten silicide, and gold; some of these conductors are also suitable for gates.[1-4] Other metals such as platinum and titanium are used in some process steps to improve the conductivity of ohmic contacts or for adhesion.[1] Direct-laser writing has been used to demonstrate the deposition of (or doping by) virtually each of these materials (with the exception of polyimide and PSG deposition). Furthermore, laser etching of some of these materials has also been sucessfully investigated. It would be fair to say that a complete set of laser-based (silicon) integrated circuit fabrication techniques has already been demonstrated, in the sense that each conventional step has a suitable direct-laser processing analog for both local ($\sim 1\ \mu$m dimension) and non-local (substrate-scale) writing. However, immediate inclusion of practically any of these laser methods into production lines would be premature indeed. More research and development of each promising laser technique is needed to demonstrate possible economic superiority compared to present day methods. The process physics and applications of these laser-writing methods will be addressed here. No extensive review of research in laser-writing will be attempted, though many relevant studies will be emphasized. For a more thorough review of laser-initiated surface processing, the reader is referred to Refs. 5-10.

The broad range of laser processing candidates for possible replacement of their respective photolithography counterparts is illustrated in Table 1. One or more of these laser-based steps may join the optimized sequence for manufacturing a given circuit. In the order listed, these process steps show several trends. The trend down the chart is toward a greater deviation from conventional processing philosophy. The highest listings (Nos. 1-3) represent the least radical changes. In these steps a laser is used either without a mask to prepare the surface of an entire wafer before the mask-patterning step, or else with a mask to locally prepare the surface by either contact or projection printing. In either case, the design layout is transferred to all regions on the wafer simultaneously, i.e., there is parallel processing of the wafer. One significant change from current technology occurs in laser photochemical projection printing, in which resist is not used at all (No. 3), though masks are still

**Table 1**

Candidate Laser Processing Steps

1. Laser Annealing, Recrystallization (excimer, $Ar^+$, $CO_2$ lasers)
2. Patterned Development/Ablation of Resist (ArF, $F_2$)
3. Mask Patterning of Doping, Thin Film Deposition/Etching (excimer, $CO_2$)
4. Direct-Laser Writing/Repair/Rerouting of Masks, Interconnects ($Ar^+$, cw UV)
5. Laser Linking in Restructurable Logic ($Ar^+$, pulsed)
6. Direct-Laser Interconnection of Gate Arrays, etc. ($Ar^+$, cw UV)
7. Localized Direct-Laser Thin Film Preparation ($Ar^+$, cw UV)
8. Localized Direct-Laser Microelectronic Device Fabrication/Alteration ($Ar^+$, cw UV)
9. Fabrication of Integrated Circuits Exclusively by Direct-Laser Writing ($Ar^+$)

employed. Since these steps (Nos. 1-3) represent relatively minor changes in current practice, they may be more quickly accepted in the semiconductor community than the other laser techniques listed in Table 1. The lasers used for Nos. 1-3 are geared for rapid wafer-scale processing, i.e., either high powered pulsed lasers, such as (though not exclusively) excimer lasers, or rapidly scanned, focused cw lasers, such as $Ar^+$ or $CO_2$ lasers. In contrast, the processes summarized in the lower listings in Table 1 (Nos. 4-9) are very different from conventional photolithography methods. They entail a serial or sequential transfer of design information to the substrate using a focused, and in many cases a temporally modulated, cw laser by localized direct-laser writing, also known as laser pantography. Listings 5-9 are processing steps that entirely avoid the use of resists and masks. With these methods the circuit design resides in software that directly controls the progress of the local direct-laser writing step. These lower listings represent successively more radical deviations from current practice.

Each process listed in Table 1 entails at least one of three basic laser-substrate interactions. In purely laser-surface processing the laser heats predeposited films inducing diffusion, melting, ablation or thin film reactions. The substrate is either in vacuum or an effectively inert atmosphere. In pyrolytic and photolytic processing the irradiated substrate is bathed in a particular gas or liquid of interest. A surface reaction is driven between the cold (transparent) gas/liquid and the laser-heated substrate in pyrolytic processes. In photolytic processes gas-phase or surface-adsorbed molecules absorb radiation, decompose, perhaps react further, and then the products (if formed above the substrate) diffuse to and adsorb on the cold, transparent surface. For a given set of experimental conditions two or three of these elementary mechanisms may simultaneously drive the reaction. Ultraviolet lasers with $\lambda \lesssim 2500$ Å (excimer, frequency doubled $Ar^+$) are usually required to stimulate photolytic processes. Wavelength requirements for pyrolytic and purely surface reactions are usually less restrictive than for photolytic reactions because commonly used substrates and overlaying films absorb in the visible and ultraviolet and sometimes also in the infrared. For silicon surfaces, visible and ultraviolet lasers can be used (argon-ion, krypton-ion, ruby lasers, etc.), since the absorption depth is $\lesssim 2\ \mu m$ for $\lesssim 6000$Å.[11]

Several market needs have spurred research in laser semiconductor processing. Some device material requirements appear to be best attained with laser processing, such as recrystallization of polysilicon films on SOI (silicon-on-insulator) wafers (Table 1, No. 1). In other cases, process times can be shortened and yields improved by reducing the number of process steps, while still following currently successful parallel processing philosophy (Nos. 2-3). Direct-laser mask processing can improve yields and can permit rapid discretionary changes in design layout (No. 4). Finally, the requirement of rapid turnaround times for small-volume customized and prototype circuits has spurred studies involving localized-direct laser writing (Nos. 4-9). These studies are also driven by the prospect of wafer-scale integration (WSI) of circuits.

Naturally, production cost will be the only final judge of the commericial success of any laser-based semiconductor processing step. Since it is difficult to reliably estimate the ultimate manufacturing costs based on reported pioneering research, the criteria used here for assessing the prospects of partial or complete laser fabrication of integrated circuits will be more qualitative in nature. These criteria are addressed by answering the following questions for each candidate laser process. What are the definitive advantages of the laser method vis à vis conventional methods and other developing technologies (e.g., electron beam, X-ray, ion beam lithography)? Can cheaper non-laser sources be used as well? Is it easy to include proposed sequence of laser steps into current processing lines? What are the speed and yield of the laser step? What are the physical and electrical properties and spatial dimensions (ultimate design rules) of the laser-processed material and device? And most important, is the laser-based step compatible with previous substrate processing?

## 2. Non-Local Laser Processing

Laser annealing, recrystallization of thin polysilicon films on insulators, and thin film excimer laser processing are three most important elements of non-local laser fabrication of integrated circuits. Recent highlights of these latter two areas will be presented here. The reader is referred to Refs. 12-13 for a discussion of laser annealing.

Device fabrication using laser-recrystallized thin films of polysilicon is under active investigation (Table 1, No. 1).[14,15] In one approach to recrystallization, a focused $Ar^+$ laser (5145Å) is scanned over a small-grained CVD polysilicon film insulated from a silicon substrate by an $SiO_2$ film (silicon-on-insulator, SOI). As needed, this recrystallization can be seeded by the crystalline substrate through windows in the $SiO_2$.[16] (Other common thin film/substrate combinations include polycrystalline Si on sapphire (SOS), fused quartz, or glass substrates; scanned $CO_2$ lasers can also be used for recrystallization in these cases.) Device quality of MOS transistors fabricated with these films approaches that of crystalline Si-grown devices, moreover, with superior device isolation.[17-19] Fabrication of dynamic RAM cells with increased storage capacitance compared to cells in bulk silicon has been demonstrated on laser-recrystallized SOI.[20,21] Perhaps even more exciting is the current effort in the fabrication of non-planar CMOS structures using recrystallized SOI. In efforts to date, a laser-beam-recrystallized n-channel MOS transistor is constructed on top of a p-channel MOS device which is fabricated in the silicon substrate.[21-25] Extension to many layers of devices is promising. This prospect of manufacturing chips with extremely high memory packing densities (per unit area) and other 3-D structures may well be the most important impact of SOI techniques. More details concerning laser-recrystallized SOI devices may be found in Refs. 14-15. Though laser recrystallization has been quite successful, alternate means of polysilicon heating (by electron beams, blackbody radiation from graphite strips, light from incoherent sources) must also be considered. However, the laser technique may be the only one to offer sufficient three-dimensional temperature control to reliably prevent substrate melting (in SOI)[26] and the associated non-annealable material damage.[27]

Research in semiconductor processing with excimer lasers is currently very active. The high peak intensity, high average power and multimode output (and hence "speckle-free" characteristics) of these ultraviolet lasers combine to make them quite versatile for thin film processing both with and without masks. Some highlights of recent studies will be cited here. For more detailed reviews see Refs. 28 and 29.

The current resolution limit in optical lithography is $\sim 1.5\ \mu m$,[30] and the ultimate limit using conventional light sources is thought to be $\sim 0.75\ \mu m$[30,31] with step-and-repeat projection printing. Use of excimer lasers along with the mask and resist technologies in photolithography may further improve resolution and reduce the number of processing steps (Table 1, No. 2). Features as small as $0.15\ \mu m$ have been observed in MMA/MAA copolymer and PMMA/Ge/polyimide resists employing an $F_2$ excimer laser (157 nm) and an e-beam written mask in contact lithography.[32] Resist features as small as 0.3 $\mu$m have been made in nitrocellulose using an ArF laser and contact printing.[33] Using ArF lasers (193 nm)[34-36] and other longer wavelength excimer lasers,[29,36-38] submicron resist features have been made via contact and projection lithography in several materials. In one study of laser development of several conventional organic polymers and resists, [29,38] only small deviations from exposure reciprocity were observed (KrF laser, 249 nm; XeCl, 308nm), i.e., resist modification was found to depend essentially only on exposure dose (energy/area) and only mildly on radiation intensity for $\lesssim$ 5 MW/cm$^2$. However, striking reciprocity failure has been observed in the self-developing resists nitrocellulose[33] and in PMMA,[34,35] and in the (normally insensitive) inorganic resist $Ag_2Se/GeSe_2$ (KrF laser).[39] For this inorganic resist, increasing the dose rate from very low values to 520 KW/cm$^2$ decreased the required dose from 130 to 5.2 mJ/cm$^2$. The short wavelength and high peak intensity of the excimer laser combine to make it vastly superior to incoherent ultraviolet sources for processing such inorganic and self-developing organic resists.

This self-development of resists using excimer lasers has been termed "ablative" photodecomposition.[34] In this process bonds in the exposed material are broken by the short wavelength radiation and the products are vaporized leaving no evidence of thermal effects. Under certain experimental conditions (for $\lambda$ = 0.19 - 10 $\mu$) analogous behavior is observed which can be attributed to thermal effects. Details may be found in Ref. 40. Ablative photodecomposition is particularly well suited for semiconductor processing since it combines resist exposure and subsequent resist etching into a single step. Features as small as 0.3 $\mu$m have been observed by ArF laser photoetching of resists and polymers (0.3 $\mu$m for AZ 2400 and nitrocellulose; 0.5 $\mu$ for PMMA) using contact lithography.[33,35]

Numerous examples of thin film etching, doping and deposition of insulators, semiconductors and metals have been demonstrated using photolytic and/or pyrolytic reactions stimulated by excimer lasers, as reviewed in Ref. 28 (Table 1, No. 3). In one notable study, submicron resist-free etching of Si was noted using a KrF laser incident on a Si wafer in $Cl_2$ gas (with patterned CVD-deposited $SiO_2$ serving as the etch mask).[41] This method is free from the radiation damage sometimes observed using plasma etching.[41] Careful spatial control of n- and p-type doping of silicon wafers has been accomplished using excimer laser-induced dissociation of boron and phosphorus-containing molecules and subsequent laser-induced diffusion into the substrate;[42-44] simple bipolar devices have been made using this procedure.[42-44] Also, $SiO_2$ and $Si_3N_4$ thin films of encapsulation, and perhaps field oxide, quality have been deposited on various substrates using excimer laser photolytic reactions and densification;[45-47] in these demonstrations the substrate temperatures were below those used in conventional processing.

Many elements of these non-local laser fabrication techniques are commercially attractive. Accordingly, the already active research effort in these areas is rapidly expanding.

## 3. Local Direct Laser Writing

### 3.1 Overview

Integrated circuit fabrication steps employing localized-laser writing involve mask-free, sequential processing of the circuit layout. Consequently, these steps are fundamentally different from those used in optical lithography. This laser pantography approach may be used for one, some, or all process steps in device fabrication, device interconnection and die packaging; only the first two areas will be considered here. Use of direct laser writing in some or even all processing steps in no way implies abandonment of current thin-film processing (deposition or etching) techniques. In many local direct-writing steps both technologies may be needed. For example, spatially discretionary deposition of a material may prove to be inferior to thin-film (bulk) deposition followed by localized laser etching[48] as judged by the criteria of processing speed and electrical quality. The rapid, discretionary interconnection of prefabricated arrays of transistor blocks (gate arrays) or higher-order transistor configurations (such as programmable logic arrays and restructurable logic) using laser pantography is well suited for either developing prototype circuits or filling low-volume custom orders of large-area circuits. It appears to be the most practical near-term application of this technology (Table 1, Nos. 5 and 6). Discretionary fabrication of high performance devices (Table 1, No. 8) and the subsequent goal of die-scale or wafer-scale discretionary device fabrication and interconnection are technically much more demanding applications of laser pantography. If the versatility afforded by discretionary device fabrication is demanded in making certain custom circuits, significantly more research and development will be necessary before practical implementation. Other possible applications, such as in packaging (via formation, input/output connections, etc.) will not be discussed here. Furthermore, applications of only gas/surface microreactions will be addressed. (Liquid/surface reactions are described in Refs. 5-8.) Progress and future prospects in these applications of laser pantography will be considered after reviewing the basic methods and interactions in direct-laser writing.

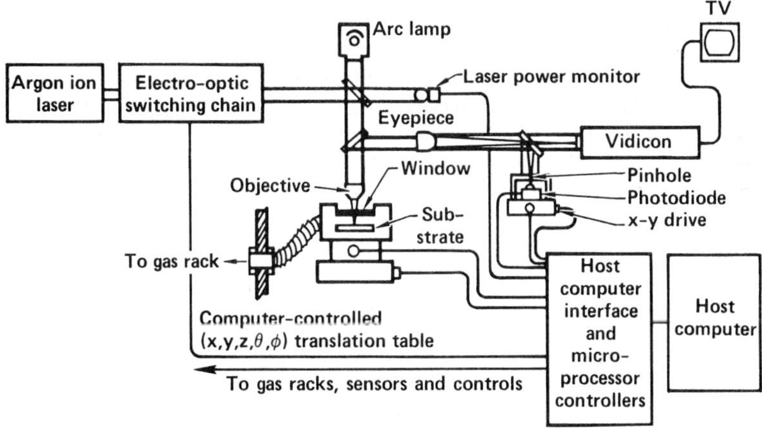


**Fig. 1** The experimental arrangement for direct-laser writing; see text for details.[48]

The essential elements of the apparatus used in laser pantography are shown in Fig. 1.[48] A cw laser, in this case an argon-ion laser, can be temporally modulated before entering the laser microscope. In the laser microscope, the laser is focused by a microscope objective through the entrance window of the reaction chamber and onto the wafer. As in an ordinary microscope, a source of incoherent light also impinges on the substrate to allow real-time viewing of the process, in this case using a vidicon. The reaction chamber is mounted on an x-y translation stage and is attached to a gas manifold and vacuum system. Both the time-dependent position of this stage and the timing of laser amplitude modulation are under computer control. This experimental apparatus is flexible, and may be adapted to the specific demands of the application. More details may be found in Ref. 48.

Both pyrolytic and photolytic microreactions have been used to deposit VLSI-type microstructures using the type of experimental arrangement in Fig. 1. For a given application, one of the two approaches is usually clearly superior. Photolytic techniques have the advantage that they can be used without constraint in choice of substrate or fear of thermal modification, and therefore are more suited for some applications, such as the repair or rerouting of quartz masks[49] (Table 1, No. 4). However, they lack the versatility demanded in many applications. High quality interconnect materials of choice, such as polysilicon, aluminum, tungsten, gold, and metal silicides, either cannot be deposited by the gas-phase photolytic techniques demonstrated to date or else are deposited too slowly for applications such as gate array wiring. This lack of versatility is in part due to the wavelength (2573Å) and low average power (~1 mW) of the frequency doubled argon-ion laser, which has been the most common photon source used to induce photolytic microreactions. (Future studies using higher power and shorter wavelength cw lasers may help overcome some of these shortcomings.) Other problems with ultraviolet-laser photolytic circuit fabrication include the relatively underdeveloped state of optics for $\lambda \lesssim$ 2500Å and ultraviolet radiation-induced damage to exposed silicon dioxide layers[50] (which in many cases can be healed by thermal annealing). Moreover, each material deposited by photolysis (such as various metals from their respective alkyls or carbonyls) can be deposited by pyrolysis on an appropriate substrate, though the converse of this statement is not true at present. In some applications rapid writing speed is a crucial process criterion (Table 1, Nos. 6-9).[51] Micron-dimension structures can be deposited faster on silicon substrates or thin films by pyrolytic reactions than by the analogous photolytic reactions using state-of-the-art lasers.[52] In general, this would be true even if much higher power cw ultraviolet lasers were available for inducing photolytic microreactions. At higher ultraviolet powers pyrolytic effects begin to dominate photolytic contributions in silicon processing.[52] For these reasons, the following discussion will focus on pyrolytic reactions, mentioning only the isolated, yet important demonstrations of laser-photolysis steps in integrated circuit fabrication.

### 3.2 Pyrolytic Processing of Integrated Circuits

Pyrolytic laser writing of micron-scale structures utilizes the same set of thermochemical reactions as used in conventional non-local chemical vapor deposition. In most cases the reaction mechanisms are very similar. However, the operating philosophies of the two techniques differ in many ways. Whereas low pressures are preferred in classical CVD (~ 1 Torr in low pressure CVD, LPCVD) to optimize film properties, in laser CVD much higher operating pressures (~ 1 atm) are often necessary to attain sufficiently rapid writing speeds. During a given LPCVD cycle either the substrate alone or the substrate and chamber both are maintained at a specified temperature for several minutes, for example at 800°C for depositing ~ 1 $\mu$m of polysilicon in ~ 10 min (~ 1 Torr $SiH_4$). In laser CVD a substrate area of only ~ 1 $\mu m^2$ is heated, usually to a higher temperature (up to the melting point of silicon 1420°C), for a very much shorter time, ~ 10-100 $\mu$sec.

**Table 2**

Representative Demonstrated Pyrolytic Gas/Surface Microreactions

| *Deposition on Si* | *From (vapor pressure at 20°C)* | *Refs.* |
|---|---|---|
| Si | Silanes (> 1 atm, doped using $PH_3$, $AsH_3$, $B_2H_6$) | 48, 53, 54 |
| W | $WF_6+H_2$, $WF_6$+Si(s)(> 1 atm) | 48, 55 |
| Ni | $Ni(CO)_4$ (~ 350 Torr) | 51, 56 |
| Al | $Al_2(CH_3)_6$ (~ 10 Torr) | 51, 57 |
| Au | Gold Acetylacetonate (~ 0.1-1 Torr) | 58 |
| $SiO_2$ | $SiH_4+N_2O$ (> 1 atm) | 59 |
| *Etching of* | *By* | |
| Si | $Cl_2$, HCl (> 1 atm) | 60 |
| $SiO_2$ | vacuum, $HCl/H_2$, $Cl_2$(> 1 atm) | 48, 61 |
| *Doping of Si with* | *Using* | |
| P | $PH_3$, $PCl_3$ (> 1 atm) | 48, 62 |
| B | $BCl_3$, $B_2H_6$ (> 1 atm) | 62 |

Table 2 lists a series of investigated local pyrolytic reactions induced by focused visible lasers which are potentially important in integrated circuit fabrication (Table 1, No. 7). Some involve the surface-mediated unimolecular decomposition of one reactant such as, $SiH_4$, $PH_3$, $Al_2(CH_3)_6$ or $Ni(CO)_4$, while others are based on "bimolecular" reactions, such as $WF_6 + H_2$. In each case the surface is probably an active reaction participant; it is not merely a non-reactive high temperature binding template.

Some other thermal microdeposition processes fall into the laser-surface processing category defined in the Introduction (and therefore are not listed with the local "pyrolytic" reactions of Table 2). One technique involves local heating of adjacent metal/silicon layers by a focused argon-ion laser to form metal silicide[63] microstructures. After this spatially selective maskless laser processing step, the unreacted regions can be selectively removed by dry or wet etching. Another thermal process is local curing of spun-on organosilicate films with 5145Å radiation to form silicon dioxide microstructures with controllable thickness.[64] Analogous laser processing of spun-on metalorganics may prove to be effective in depositing Au, Ag, and other metal microstructures.[65]

It is profitable to review the basic mechanistic features of laser CVD to best understand the care required in applying direct-laser writing to circuit fabrication. One proposed model[51,66] of laser microchemical reactions approaches this complex process by first treating the laser-induced temperature profile of the substrate and the local CVD dynamics separately, trying to combine these two features into a more self-consistent, time-evolutionary picture.

The local CVD part of the model incorporates the time-dependent reaction sequence of (1) three-dimensional transport of reactants to the substrate, (2) adsorption, (3) surface reaction, (4) volatile product desorption, and (5) three-dimensional transport of product gases away from the substrate. Depending on the overall reaction molecular balance, ambient pressure and local topography, transport may be dominated by molecular flow, diffusion, convection or turbulent flow. At low laser powers (and temperatures) the limiting factor in the reaction speed is the Arrhenius behavior of the reaction rate:

$$R \, \alpha \, \exp(-T/T_{act}) \tag{3.1}$$

where T and $T_{act}$ are the substrate and reaction activation temperatures, respectively. At high pressures and high laser powers, slow diffusion rates will choke the reaction. For 1 $\mu$m-scale traces, gas-limited deposition rates may saturate in the neighborhood of 1 cm/sec.[66]

Though the details of surface reaction dynamics are not completely understood for most examples of conventional CVD (especially during early reaction times), present understanding is sufficient for practice. Reaction rates in CVD are usually exponential in temperature as in Eq. 3.1 in regimes in which gas transport does not dominate. The quality of material produced by conventional and laser CVD is usually quite good. Si (from $SiH_4$), W ($WF_6$), Ni ($Ni(CO)_4$) and other materials have been deposited by laser CVD with only small levels of impurities (H, F, C, O) remaining from the starting materials.[52] Several outstanding questions regarding the early stages of laser writing (and classical CVD) remain. The roles of (laser) surface cleaning, surface diffusion, seeding and nucleation, as well as a possible required build-up of gas phase or surface reaction intermediates,[67] in laser CVD require further study.

The laser-induced rise in the surface temperature must be characterized. The temperature profile of the laser-irradiated substrate is determined by the time- and position-dependent reflectivity and absorption of the substrate, thermal diffusion in the substrate and the temporal and spatial profile of the incident focused laser. Substrate topography is a very critical factor in determining the temperature profile.

Three common substrate conditions are illustrated in Figs. 2a-c. The scanning laser may initially irradiate (a) a bulk silicon substrate, (b) an insulator-overlayed substrate or (c) a multi-film combination such as polysilicon film/insulator film/Si substrate (SOI). Each of these representative topographies is encountered in wiring gate arrays, as illustrated in Fig. 3 which depicts the respective analogs for (a) vias to source and drain regions (Fig. 3a), (b) overlaying field oxide regions (Fig. 3b),

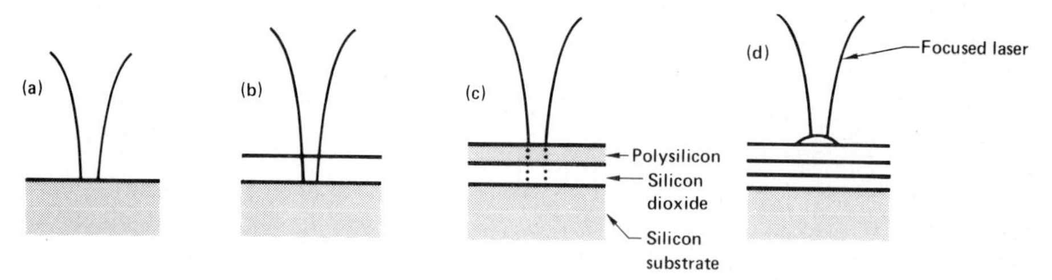


**Fig. 2** Substrate topographies encountered in direct laser writing. Examples include (a) a bare silicon wafer, (b) silicon dioxide film on silicon, (c) polysilicon/silicon dioxide/silicon (SOI), and (d) a more general arrangement on a multi-layered film after initial laser deposition of a feature.

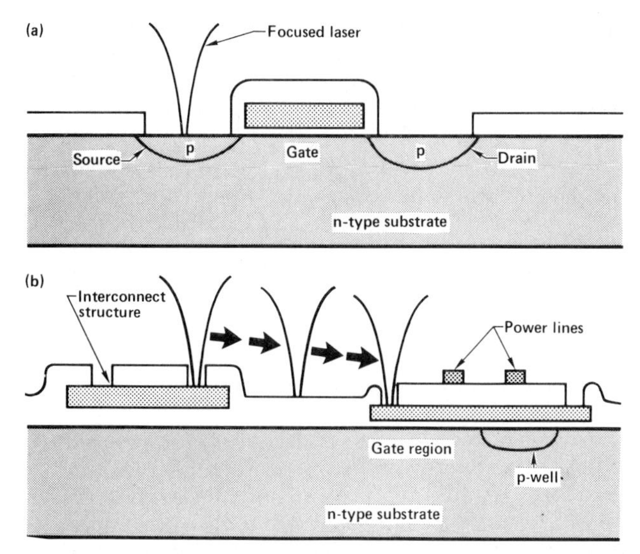


**Fig. 3** Substrate topography in a CMOS gate array illustrated by perpendicular cross-sectional profiles. In (a) the focused laser irradiates the substrate in the p-channel MOSFET structure as in Fig. 2a (corresponding to a vertical cut in Fig. 4). In (b) examples of Fig. 2b and 2c-type topographies are depicted in wiring the interconnect structure to the gate (horizontal cut in Fig. 4).

and (c) vias to gate and interconnect regions (Fig. 3b). The temperature profile due to laser heating can be obtained for each case by lengthy, though conceptionally straightforward calculations using either a Green's function or finite-element numerical approach. (When using the Green's function method implicit time variations in the thermal conductivity must not be ignored.[66]) These calculations are strictly valid only during the initial phases of laser writing, since after laser pyrolysis begins the optical and thermal diffusion properties of the substrate and gas transport change (Fig. 2d). Still much insight can be gleaned from the model cases in Figs. 2a-c. In general, for a given incident laser on these three substrates the outer surface in Fig. 2c will be the hottest, because of the (transparent) insulator layer under the absorbing film, while the surface in Fig. 2b will be the coldest (ignoring the complication due to multiple, thin film reflections). Furthermore, the thermal profile on the outer surface will be narrowest for case a and broadest for case c.

The following discussion assumes that a circular (or elliptical) gaussian beam irradiates the substrate. In most cases the microstructure morphology resulting from the surface chemistry is satisfactory. If a more flat-topped profile is required (and the surface reaction is not self-limiting as it is for some pyrolytic reactions), transverse phase modulation of the laser[68] can produce a flat-topped intensity profile at the focus which will tend to flatten the thermal profile on the surface.

The temperature profile induced by a scanning circular laser irradiating a uniform substrate, such as silicon, has been investigated by numerous authors.[69-71] Several silicon properties help determine this temperature distribution. One is the reflectivity of bulk silicon, $R_s$, which is 37% for 5145Å at room temperature and increases monotonically with temperature;[11] for molten silicon the reflectivity increases to ~ 70%.[72] At room temperature the "1/e" absorption depth at 5145Å is

0.80 $\mu$m; it decreases with increasing temperature, and at 900°C for example, the absorption depth is very small, 0.11 $\mu$m.[11] Thermal diffusion in silicon is quite fast; the thermal diffusion constant D is 0.9 $cm^2$/sec at room temperature, falling rapidly with increasing temperature as D=128 $cm^2$K/sec/(T-159 K).[70] Consequently, the characteristic equilibration time for 1 $\mu$m spatial features in the thermal profile is ~ 10 nsec near room temperature and ~ 100 nsec near melting. Therefore, for scanning speeds much slower than 1 $\mu$m/100 nsec = $10^3$ cm/sec, the temperature profile is roughly that for a fixed beam.[70] Examples of the results of these calculations may be found in Refs. 69-71. Some key insights are provided by the following observations. For sufficiently slow scanning speeds, the peak silicon surface temperature may be found using this approximate expression:[51,70]

$$T_c(K) = 99 + 201\exp\{\frac{P(1-R_s)/r_0}{106}\} \tag{3.2}$$

for a gaussian beam of radius $r_0(\mu m)$ (1/e intensity) and incident power P (mwatts). Using the calculated fall-off of laser-induced temperature with radial distance in the exponential dependence of the surface reaction rate (Eq. 3.1), the initial effective reaction radius is found to be smaller than the laser spot size $r_0$, being typically ~ 0.4 $r_0$.[51] Consequently, pyrolytic structures much smaller than the wavelength of the laser employed can be fabricated,[51] due to this non-linearity in the writing process. In fact ~ 0.25 $\mu$m wide doping features (p-type from $BCl_3$),[73] polysilicon lines (from $SiCl_4$ + $H_2$),[73] and etched lines ($Cl_2$)[6] on silicon substrates have been fabricated using local pyrolytic reactions (5145Å). (It is important to remember that in most VLSI applications even ~ 1 $\mu$m feature sizes are satisfactory; however, the tolerance in positioning is usually much more strict (~ 0.1 $\mu$m).)

The two-layer structure consisting of a transparent film on an absorbing substrate (as $SiO_2$ on Si in Fig. 2b) or an absorbing film on a transparent substrate (as Si on sapphire (SOS)) has been treated, though less extensively than for the case of bulk substrate heating.[74-76] For an $SiO_2$ film on Si (of Fig. 2b), absorption occurs at the interface, and thermal energy diffuses to the outer $SiO_2$ surface. Thermal diffusion in (amorphous) $SiO_2$ is 10-100 times slower than in silicon (D ~ 0.01 $cm^2$/sec).[77] Consequently, the width of the temperature profile on this outer surface for $SiO_2$ on Si can be significantly larger than the beam spot size,[59] especially for thicker oxide layers. To properly treat laser absorption, multi-reflection interference effects must also be included in the analysis. For this two-layer structure the substrate optical and thermal properties change rapidly once a feature is deposited.

The three-layer substrate depicted in Fig. 2c, the silicon-on-insulator SOI structure described above, is quite important in laser pantography. In SOI recrystallization, very little laser radiation is transmitted through the typically 0.5 $\mu$m thick polysilicon layer because the absorption depths are small at the 500°C substrate temperature used in recrystallization (0.19 $\mu$ depth for 4880Å radiation, 0.27 $\mu$ for 5145Å).[27] As with two-layer thermal calculations, in three-layer calculations interlayer thermal transport must be properly treated. In one calculation[76] (in which interlayer transport is in fact purposely treated in an approximate manner) the laser-induced temperature increase was determined as a function of depth for various oxide thicknesses assuming a static 40 $\mu$m radius laser incident on the 0.5 $\mu$m polysilicon/$SiO_2$/silicon structure at ambient temperature. For 1.0 $\mu$m thick $SiO_2$ the temperature rise at the lower $SiO_2$/Si interface was found to be only ~0.7 times that at the upper interface. With much thinner (or even no) $SiO_2$ layers, an equally large temperature drop is predicted only 10 $\mu$m deep into the Si substrate, due to faster thermal diffusivity in silicon. For spot sizes smaller than the 40 $\mu$m used in this calculation, approaching the insulator thickness, even greater temperature drops across the insulator are expected.

Model calculations of laser deposition rates using this combined CVD/laser heating approach may be found in Ref. 51. Since substrate optical and thermal diffusion properties and gas transport drastically change after laser pyrolysis begins (Fig. 2d), a more sophisticated self-consistent treatment of laser CVD is required. This important post-initial behavior has not been well examined, though some early work in this area is promising.[78]

### 3.3 Compatibility of Laser Pantography with Device Fabrication

A comprehensive understanding of the compatibility of laser pyrolytic writing with previously performed device processing is essential for commercially viable laser fabrication of integrated circuits. Though a specific CVD step may be successfully employed in a processing scheme, it is not immediately clear whether its laser analog will also be compatible with device fabrication. The trade-off between higher temperatures and shorter processing times ($\sim 10^{-3}$ sec) in laser CVD vis à vis lower operating temperatures and longer reaction times ($\sim 10^{3}$ sec) in LPCVD must be examined. Perhaps the two most important process issues to be addressed are dopant redistribution and possible damage to $SiO_2$/Si and other interfaces.

The solid-state diffusion coefficients[79] for boron and phosphor silicon are $\sim 5 \times 10^{-11}$ cm$^2$/sec and $\sim 10^{-11}$ cm$^2$/sec for arsenic at 1400°C (near melting). For each, the diffusion coefficient decreases with decreasing temperature as $D \sim \exp(-46,000/T(K))$. For $\sim 1$ $\mu$m circuit design rules, unintended dopant diffusion of more than $\sim 0.1$ $\mu$m by laser irradiation may be intolerable. Such a large dopant redistribution will occur only with solid-state diffusion times as long as $\sim 1$ sec (at 1400°C). Since typical laser processing times (at each 1 $\mu$m "pixel") are much shorter ($10^{-6}$ - $10^{-3}$ sec), solid-state dopant diffusion is not significant.

Liquid phase diffusion is very much faster than solid-state diffusion. Upper limit values for B, P, As diffusion in molten silicon are 2.4, 5.1, 3.3 $\times 10^{-4}$ cm$^2$/sec.[80] If the shape of the dopant profile again has a tolerance of $\sim 0.1$ $\mu$m, the effects of liquid phase diffusion may well be important if the silicon is molten for $>10^{-7}$ sec. Consequently, care must be exercised not to inadvertently melt critically profiled regions during laser processing.

Damage to Si/$SiO_2$ interfaces has been visually observed in experiments with very high laser intensities incident on $SiO_2$-on-Si (Fig. 2b) structures, even in vacuum.[81] The Si + $SiO_2 \rightarrow$ 2SiO (volatile) etching reaction may be responsible for these changes. Equivalent damage is expected in local pyrolytic deposition at roughly the same laser intensities. Even use of laser intensities below the observable damage limit in pyrolytic processing may still induce unwanted changes in material properties, manifest as poor electrical characteristics of fabricated devices. In this context, the compatibility of laser techniques in device production can be addressed by fabricating capacitors by localized laser deposition of the desired conductor on thin films of $SiO_2$ overlaying Si substrates and subsequently, performing capacitance-voltage (C-V) measurements on these devices. Oxide fixed charges, surface states and mobile ionic charges arising from laser writing can be measured by standard high frequency, quasi-static, and bias-temperature stress C-V tests, respectively.[50] Oxide leakage can be measured using the quasi-static technique or by direct measurement. Fixed and mobile charges can change the threshold voltage of transistors.[82] High fixed oxide charge density can also contribute to subthreshold leakage currents in MOSFET's.[83] Fast states can degrade transistor transconductance (and thus gain and speed) and subthreshold behavior.[82]

In early experiments on direct-laser writing of highly n-type doped polysilicon capacitor structures on 1000Å $SiO_2/Si$,[84] little leakage and no apparent change in fixed-oxide charge density (compared to conventionally fabricated $Al/SiO_2/Si$ capacitors) are seen. Work is continuing in this area.

C-V studies of laser-recrystallized SOI structures (Fig. 2c) can provide insight into potential substrate modification in direct-laser writing because the thin film arrangements and laser-induced processing temperatures are virtually identical in both techniques. Laser-recrystallized $Si/SiO_2/Si$ SOI capacitors exhibit only a slight increase in oxide fixed charge density and no appreciable change in fast surface charge density compared to conventionally prepared capacitors if the substrate does not melt during processing.[82,85,86] (Recrystallized polysilicon/$Si_3N_4$/Si capacitors have much poorer characteristics.[82]) In another investigation, the recovery time needed to form the inversion layer after pulsing these $Si/SiO_2/Si$ capacitors from accumulation to deep depletion was tested.[27] A longer recovery time (generation lifetime) signifies relatively fewer surface states. Recovery times were found to decrease after laser recrystallization. However, after subsequent furnace annealing (equivalent to continuing normal device processing), the recovery times were found to increase to their pre-laser processing values, unless the laser intensity was high enough to melt the substrate during recrystallization.[27] These results suggest the laser-pyrolytic writing techniques should be compatible with processing even delicate gate oxide structures, as long as the underlying substrate does not melt.

### 3.4 Applications of Laser Pantography in the Fabrication of Integrated Circuits

Perhaps the most important current application of direct-laser writing is discretionary interconnection of transistor blocks in gate arrays (Table 1, No. 6). Using state-of-the-art gate arrays, containing as many as ~ 13,000 CMOS gates or ~ 3,500 ECL gates per ~ 0.5 $cm^2$ die,[87] complex circuits can be wired using laser-deposited low-resistivity doped polysilicon, metal or metal silicide. The rapid writing speeds required in this application favor pyrolytic processes over their respective photolytic counterparts. The design of these gate arrays demands only ~ 2-6 μm interconnect linewidths; this specification is easily attained via laser pantography. This gate array-based approach can be extended to the fabrication of discretionary large-area integrated circuits (wafer-scale integration).

Laser-wiring of gate arrays demonstrates many of the important characteristics of laser pantography in microelectronic fabrication, such as overall process compatibility, control of the material and electrical properties of the deposited material, and variable substrate topography (Fig. 3). These characteristics have been examined in Refs. 66 and 84. Degenerately doped n-type polysilicon interconnects deposited on CMOS gate arrays by local pyrolytic surface reactions have a smooth, symmetrical morphology (~ 2 μm high × ~ 4 μm wide), with a grain structure indicative of reflowed silicon (Fig. 4). The polysilicon microstructures have good adhesion and step coverage, and follow the various gate array topographies quite well. The electrical properties of the interconnects is quite good. Electrical resistivity of the polysilicon is ~ $1 \times 10^{-3}$ Ω-cm, which is as low as the best CVD polysilicon;[66,84] for typical interconnect dimensions this corresponds to ~ 5 Ω/square.

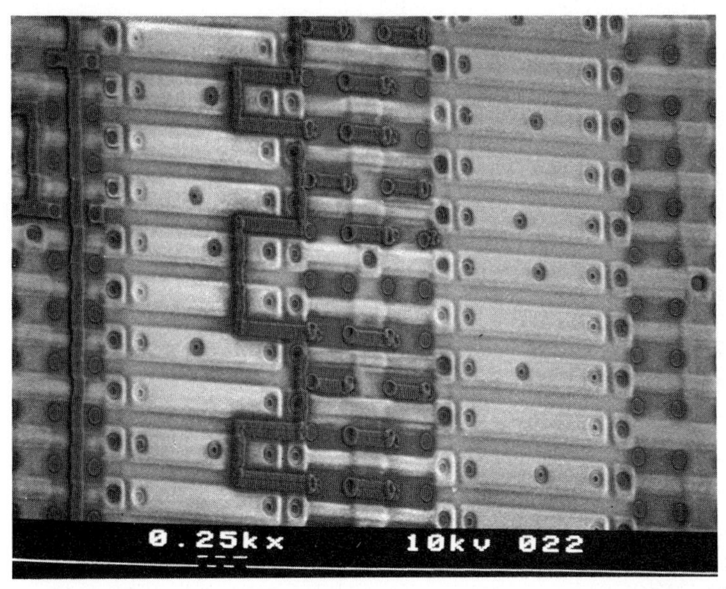


**Fig. 4** Gate array structures interconnected with laser-deposited doped polysilicon.[66]

Contact resistance of these laser-deposited lines to polysilicon tunnels ($< 10$ $\Omega$) and aluminum are suitably low. The demonstrated electrical isolation of non-connected polysilicon features suggests that there is no significant (if any) damage to the underlying $\sim 1$ $\mu$m thick silicon dioxide layer. Furthermore, the measured dc characteristics of laser-interconnected transistor blocks (such as inverters) are those expected.[66,84]

Complex CMOS gate array structures have been fabricated using this polysilicon interconnect procedure as outlined in Refs. 52, 66 and 84. Polysilicon writing speeds as fast as 3 mm/sec have been demonstrated.[66,84] Gate arrays have also been wired using p-type polysilicon.[88] Furthermore, conventionally wired gate arrays have been restructured by local laser etching of the interconnects at specified points in the circuit, followed by discretionary laser writing.[88]

As alluded to above, discretionary laser interconnection of gate arrays is one approach to very large area integration. An alternate approach, involving laser "restructuring" of circuits (Table 1, No. 5) is briefly described here. In this technique lasers are used to link or disconnect pre-fabricated conductor interconnects at a select few of the many possible provided linking points in the circuit. In this application local laser heating of thin film combinations induces a "purely laser-surface" process, as described in the Introduction; no reactive gas or liquid atmosphere is employed. Several laser linking approaches have been studied.[8,89,90] In restructable VLSI designing,[91] a square grid of prewired (MSI/LSI) cells are mounted on a substrate, which are each separated by horizontal and vertical arrays of two layers of metal bus lines. Discretionary laser linking at some of the many possible contact points between the upper and lower metal busses and between the metal busses and the cell inputs and outputs specifies the circuit configuration. Using this approach, a working 130,000 transistor wafer-scale CMOS digital integrator has been fabricated.[92]

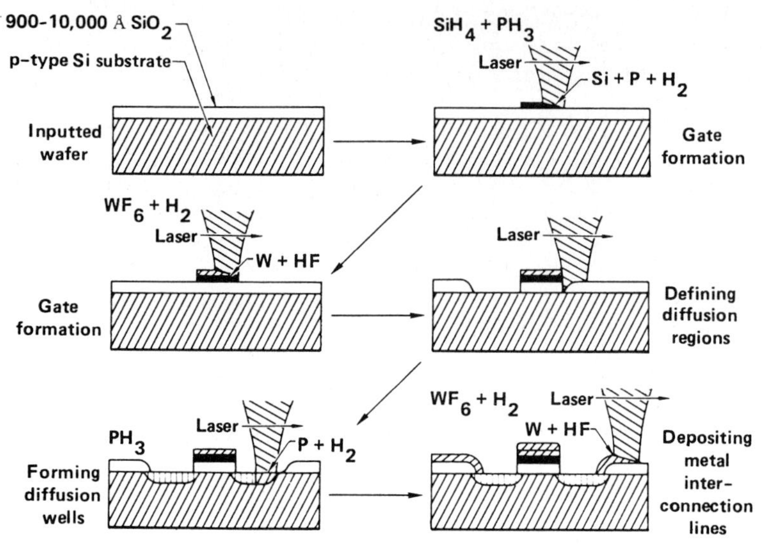


**Fig. 5** Steps in fabricating an n-channel MOSFET using direct-laser writing. Details may be found in the text and in Ref. 48.

The first fabrication of an entire transistor using only direct-laser writing techniques to define each active device area (Table 1, No. 8) is described in Ref. 48, in which n-channel MOSFET's were produced using the laser pantography apparatus of Fig. 1. The schematic in Fig. 5 illustrates the fabrication steps. The input substrate was a silicon wafer overlayed with a $SiO_2$ film (0.1-1.0 $\mu$m thick) grown by conventional means. A polysilicon gate region was defined using local pyrolytic deposition of silanes laced with phosphine. At times tungsten, from the laser-induced micro-reaction of $WF_6 + H_2$, was deposited on the polysilicon gate. The silicon dioxide film overlaying the source and drain regions was removed by local-laser heating either in vacuum or accelerated in an $HCl/H_2$ atmosphere. Afterwards, the n-type source and drain regions were doped by initially depositing either a thin phosphorus surface layer (by laser surface pyrolysis of $PH_3/He$) or a thin layer of doped polysilicon ($PH_3/SiH_4$); then the dopants were driven into the surface by heating the surface with the laser. This last step, which was performed in a vacuum, also improved the crystal structure of the source and drain regions.

The dc I-V characteristics of a 1 $\mu$m thick gate oxide transistor fabricated in this manner exhibited an ~30 V gate threshold, as expected from theory.[48] Since, to first order, the gate threshold voltage is linear with gate thickness, the observed threshold corresponds to a 1-3 V threshold for the 400-1000Å gate oxide thickness range common in state-of-the-art devices. Following these procedures, fabrication of small-scale integrated circuit structures is conceptually straightforward, as shown in Ref. 48. Preliminary work on thinner gate oxide devices suggested lower gate thresholds but larger leakage currents.

Though the device fabrication strategy outlined in Fig. 5 is by no means a unique route to MOSFET fabrication using laser pantography, it well illustrates the complete set of available laser-direct writing technologies. When combined with conventional thin film processing (e.g., formation of the gate oxide layer), there are numerous potentially successful approaches to the direct-laser writing of devices. Virtually each conventional transistor design can be fabricated by direct-laser writing. One example of this versatility is the use of laser pantography to define JFET and lateral pnp transistor structures on silicon-on-sapphire.[52]

Another application of direct-laser writing in silicon MOSFET production is described in Ref. 93, in which a frequency doubled argon-ion laser (2573Å) was used to photolytically deposit cadmium (from $Cd(CH_3)_2$) to define the gate on an otherwise prefabricated n-MOS transistor structure. By varying the gate length and width respectively, the threshold voltage and the derivative of the saturated transconductance with respect to gate voltage of the transistor could be varied independently. Use of this technique in real-time monitoring of tuned transistor characteristics is prevented by the production of UV-induced surface states at the $Si\text{-}SiO_2$ surface; nonetheless, this damage can be annealed away. Use of cadmium as a gate material in VLSI processing is inadvisable because of its low melting (321°C) and boiling (765°C) points. Still, such analog tuning of MOSFET's can be accomplished using other photolytic and pyrolytic methods.

One proposed goal[52] of laser pantography research is the discretionary fabrication of wafer-scale integrated (WSI) circuits (Table 1, No. 9), in particular leading to the fabrication of an entire supercomputer on a single wafer. Depending on the requirements of the specific application, WSI may be pursued by discretionary interconnection of gate arrays or, in some cases, by the much more demanding task of discretionary fabrication of both devices and interconnects. Using either approach laser pantography is best suited for small volume custom orders or the prototyping of very large area circuits.

Short wafer-scale fabrication times are necessary for prototyping applications, say roughly one day. The process parameters required for a one day turnaround can be estimated as follows. Assume that the actual direct-laser written area including devices and several layers of metalization can be approximated by the wafer area. Then a 5 inch wafer could be fabricated in one day with a laser processing rate of $\sim 10^{-5}$ sec per $(1\ \mu m)^2$ feature. If each device (and associated interconnects) occupies a 100 $\mu m^2$ area, this 5 inch wafer would have $10^8$ devices. These estimates are quite crude because they critically depend on the details of the process and application. Fabricating fewer devices on wafers places less of a constraint on the writing speed, as does using the laser only to interconnect prefabricated gate arrays. Furthermore, several day turnaround may be satisfactory for some prototyping applications. Simultaneous, multiple-laser microprocessing on different regions on the wafer can further decrease fabrication times and relax the writing speed requirement.

Direct laser fabrication of integrated circuits requires the same stringent tolerance on process chemistry and spatial positioning as is necessary in photolithography. This important point must be duly emphasized. In wiring gate arrays positional tolerances are $\sim 0.5\ \mu m$, while they are more exacting $\lesssim 0.1\ \mu m$ for more critical applications such as fabricating VLSI devices. Careful relative laser-substrate positioning must be maintained over the entire die or wafer, requiring very accurate and reproducible measurement procedures. To attain expected circuit performance fine control of process optical and chemical operating parameters is also essential. Equally careful positional optical and chemical control is required in conventional photolithography; however, because of the early stage of development and the sequential nature of the process, at present fine control in direct-laser fabrication of integrated circuits is quite challenging.

Circuit yield is one true measure of process control. With decreasing device size and increasing number of devices on a die, yield decreases exponentially. Yield is a serious potential problem for both conventional and laser-assisted fabrication of large-area integrated circuits. Tight process control, fault detection and correction are necessary in both. One relative advantage of the laser process is reduced handling, and correspondingly reduced dust contamination, because many (or all) of the laser processing steps can take place in a single reaction chamber. Improved handling methods currently being introduced to conventional processing lines may bridge this gap. Laser circuit fabrication is particularly well suited to state-of-the-art in situ testing procedures and on-line laser fault correction methods. These diagnostic and laser-repair procedures can also be applied to photolithographic processing with some additional effort. Still, circuit yield in fabricating large-area integrated circuits with laser processing (in all or in only some crucial steps) is potentially higher than with photolithography.

## 4. Concluding Observations

The future for implementing laser-based steps in the fabrication of integrated circuits is quite promising. Prospects for including selected non-local laser processing steps into manufacturing lines are good because in these steps the parallel design transfer philosophy of photolithography is retained. The sequential nature of local direct-laser writing offers a complementary set of technologies for applications in circuit and mask repair, device fabrication, interconnection, packaging, and large-area integration. Some of these laser pantography applications are attractive even using the current state of development. Each potential application must be considered in light of its specific requirements, addressing the suitability of laser pantography vis à vis conventional optical lithography and other emerging technologies including direct electron-beam resist writing, use of electron-beam written masks, X-ray and ion-beam lithography, etc.

This survey has concentrated on laser-assisted gas-surface pyrolytic processing of silicon-based circuits. Liquid-surface and photolysis-based methods in silicon technology and applications in non-silicon substrates, such as GaAs, must be recognized in assessing the versatility of fabricating integrated circuits with lasers. This entire field is currently very active, and promises many new exciting developments.

## 5. Acknowledgments

The author wishes to thank Prof. R. M. Osgood and Dr. Frank Magnotta for comments on this manuscript and Ms. C. Ghinazzi for assistance in manuscript preparation. Discussions with collaborators and colleagues, Drs. L. L. Wood, B. M. McWilliams, F. Mitlitsky, J. C. Whitehead, and R. A. Hyde, have been very helpful.

This work was performed under the auspices of the U.S. Department of Energy by the Lawrence Livermore National Laboratory under contract No. W-7405-ENG-48.

## 6. References

1. S. K. Ghandi: *VLSI Fabrication Principles* (Wiley, New York 1983)
2. D. J. Elliot: *Integrated Circuit Applications* (McGraw-Hill, New York 1982)
3. T. P. Chow and A. J. Steckl: *IEEE Electr. Dev.* **30**, 1480 (1983)

4. K. C. Saraswat, D. L. Brors, J. A. Fair, K. A. Monnig and R. Beyers: *IEEE Electr. Dev.* **30**, 1497 (1983)
5. R. M. Osgood, Jr: *Ann. Rev. Phys. Chem.* **34**, 77 (1983)
6. D. J. Ehrlich and J. Y. Tsao: *J. Vac. Sci. Technol.* **B1**, 969 (1983)
7. D. J. Ehrlich and J. Y. Tsao: In *VLSI Electronics: Microstructure Science* **7**, pp. 129-164, N. Einspruch, ed., (Academic, New York 1984)
8. R. J. von Gutfeld: In *Laser Applications* **5**, pp. 1-67 (Academic Press, New York 1984)
9. T. J. Chuang: *Surf. Sci. Rep.* **3**, 1 (1983)
10. W. W. Duley: *Laser Processing and Analysis of Materials* (Plenum, New York 1983)
11. G. E. Jellison, Jr. and F. A. Modine: *Appl. Phys. Lett.* **41**, 180 (1982)
12. M. Balkanski: "Fundamentals of Laser Annealing", (this volume)
13. J. Götzlich and H. Ryssel: "Application of Laser Annealing", (this volume)
14. V. T. Nguyen: "Laser Processing in SOI Technologies", (this volume)
15. Symposium on the Comparison of Thin Film Transistor and SOI Technologies, *Proc. of the Materials Research Society, 1984 Spring Meeting*, Feb. 1984 ed. by H. W. Lam and M. J. Thompson (Elsevier, New York, in press)
16. T. I. Kamins, T. R. Cass, C. J. Dell'Oca, K. F. Lee, R. F. W. Pease and J. F. Gibbons: *J. Electrochem. Soc.* **128**, 1151 (1981)
17. K. F. Lee, J. F. Gibbons, K. C. Saraswat and T. I. Kamins: *Appl. Phys. Lett.* **35**, 173 (1979)
18. K. Kugimiya, G. Fuse, S. Akiyama and A. Nishikawa: *IEEE Electr. Dev. Lett.* **3**, 270 (1982)
19. J. P. Colinge, E. Demoulin, D. Bensahel, G. Auvert and H. Morel: *IEEE Electr. Dev. Lett.*, **4**, 75 (1983)
20. R. D. Jolly, T. I. Kamins and R. H. McCharles: *IEEE Electr. Dev. Lett.* **4**, 8 (1983)
21. J. C. Sturm, M. D. Giles and J. F. Gibbons: *IEEE Electr. Dev. Lett.* **5**, 151 (1984)
22. J. P. Colinge and E. Demoulin: *IEEE Electr. Dev. Let.* **2**, 250 (1981)
23. J. F. Gibbons, K. F. Lee, F. C. Wu and G. E. J. Eggermont: *IEEE Electr. Dev. Lett.* **3**, 191 (1982)
24. T. I. Kamins: *IEEE Electr. Dev. Lett.* **3**, 341 (1982)
25. S. Kawamura, N. Sasaki, T. Iwai, M. Nakano and M. Takagi: *IEEE Electr. Dev. Lett.* **4**, 366 (1983)
26. T. I. Kamins: In *Proc. of Int. Electr. Dev. Meeting* Dec. 1982 (IEEE, 1982) p. 420
27. T. I. Kamins and C. I. Drowley: *IEEE Electr. Dev. Lett.* **3**, 363 (1982)
28. T. F. Deutsch: "Excimer Laser Processing", (this volume)
29. K. Jain: *Lasers and Applications* p. 49 (Sept. 1983)
30. P. L. Shah and R. H. Havemann: In *VLSI Electronics: Microstructure Science* **7**, pp. 40-127 (Academic Press, Orlando, Florida 1984)
31. P. R. Thornton: In *VLSI Electronics Microstructures Science* **7**, pp. 1-38 (Academic Press, Orlando, Florida 1984)
32. J. C. White, H. G. Craighead, R. E. Howard, L. D. Jackel, R. E. Behringer, R. W. Epworth, D. Henderson and J. E. Sweeney: *Appl. Phys. Lett.* **44**, 22 (1984)
33. T. F. Deutsch and M. W. Geis: *J. Appl. Phys.* **54**, 7201 (1983)

34. A. R. Srinivasan: J. Vac. Sci. Technol. **B1**, 923 (1983) and "Dynamics of Ablative Photodecomposition of Polymer Films", this volume
35. S. Rice and K. Jain: *Appl. Phys. A* **33**, 195 (1984)
36. Y. Kawamura, K. Toyoda and S. Namba: *J. Appl. Phys.* **53**, 6489 (1982)
37. K. Jain, C. G. Willson and B. J. Lin: *IEEE Electr. Dev. Lett.* **3**, 53 (1982)
38. S. Rice and K. Jain: *IEEE Electr. Dev.* **31**, 1 (1984)
39. K. J. Polasko, D. J. Ehrlich, J. Y. Tsao, R. F. W. Pease and E. E. Marinero: *IEEE Electr. Dev. Lett.* **5**, 24 (1984)
40. P. E. Dyer and J. Sidhu: In *Technical Digest of the Conference on Lasers and Electro-optics*, June 1984; presentation ThK4
41. T. Arikado, M. Sekine, H. Okano and Y. Horiike: In *Proc. of the Materials Research Society* Nov. 1983, Boston, Symposium on Laser-Controlled Chemical Processing of Surfaces (Elsevier, New York, in press)
42. T. F. Deutsch, D. J. Ehrlich, D. D. Rathman, D. J. Silversmith and R. M. Osgood, Jr.: *Appl. Phys. Lett.* **39**, 825 (1981)
43. M. L. Lloyd and K. G. Ibbs: In *Proc. of the Materials Research Society* Nov. 1983, Boston, Symposium on Laser-Controlled Chemical Processing of Surfaces (Elsevier, New York, in press)
44. K. G. Ibbs and M. L. Lloyd: *Opt. and Las. Technol.* p. 37 (Feb. 1984)
45. P. K. Boyer, G. A. Roche, W. H. Ritchie and G. J. Collins: *Appl. Phys. Lett.* **40**, 716 (1982)
46. P. K. Boyer, C. A. Moore, R. Solanki, W. K. Ritchie, G. A. Roche and G. J. Collins: In *Proc. of the Materials Research Society* **17**, Nov. 1982, Boston (Elsevier, New York), p. 119
47. T. F. Deutsch, D. J. Silversmith and R. W. Mountain: In *Proc. of the Materials Research Society* **17**, Nov. 1982, Boston (Elsevier, New York), p. 129
48. B. M. McWilliams, I. P. Herman, F. Mitlitsky, R. A. Hyde and L. L. Wood: *Appl. Phys. Lett.* **43**, 946 (1983)
49. D. J. Ehrlich, R. M. Osgood, Jr., D. J. Silversmith and T. F. Deutsch: *IEEE Electr. Dev. Lett.* **1**, 101 (1980)
50. E. H. Nicollian and J. R. Brews: *MOS Physics and Technology* (Wiley, New York 1982)
51. I. P. Herman, R. A. Hyde, B. M. McWilliams, A. H. Weisberg and L. L. Wood: In *Proc. of the Materials Research Society* **17** Nov. 1982, Boston (Elsevier, New York), p. 9; see also D. Bäuerle ibid p. 19 and Ref. 59
52. I. P. Herman, B. M. McWilliams, F. Mitlitsky, H. W. Chin, R. A. Hyde and L. L. Wood: In *Proc. of the Materials Research Society* Nov. 1983, Boston, Symposium on Laser-Controlled Chemical Processing of Surfaces (Elsevier, New York, in press)
53. D. J. Ehrlich, R. M. Osgood, Jr. and T. F. Deutsch: *Appl. Phys. Lett.* **39**, 957 (1981)
54. D. Bäuerle, P. Irsigler, G. Leyendecker, H. Noll and D. Wagner: *Appl. Phys. Lett.* **40**, 819 (1982); and *Appl. Phys. Lett.* 39, 921 (1981)
55. S. D. Allen and A. B. Tringubo: *J. Appl. Phys.* **54**, 1641 (1983)
56. W. Kräuter, D. Bäuerle and F. Fimberger: *Appl. Phys.* **A31**, 13 (1983)
57. Y. Rytz-Froideraux, R. P. Salathe, H. H. Gilgen and H. P. Weber: *Appl. Phys.* **A27**, 133 (1982)

58. F. A. Houle, C. R. Jones, T. H. Baum and C. A. Kovac: In *Technical Digest of the Conference on Lasers and Electro-optics*, June 1984; presentation ThH2
59. D. Bäuerle: In *Proc. of the Materials Research Society* Nov. 1983, Boston, Symposium on Laser-Controlled Chemical Processing of Surfaces (Elsevier, New York, in press)
60. D. J. Ehrlich, R. M. Osgood, Jr. and T. F. Deutsch: *Appl. Phys. Lett.* **38**, 1018 (1981)
61. F. A. Houle and T.J. Chuang: *J. Vac. Sci. Technol.* **20**, 790 (1982)
62. D. J. Ehrlich and J. Y. Tsao: *Appl. Phys. Lett.* **41**, 297 (1982)
63. T. Shibata, T. W. Sigmon, J. L. Regolini and J. F. Gibbons: *J. Electrochem. Soc.* **128**, 637 (1981)
64. R. R. Krchnavek, H. H. Gilgen and R. M. Osgood, Jr.: *J. Vac. Soc.* **B**, in press (1984)
65. S. Dutta, P. G. McMullin, P. Rai-Choudhury and B. D. Gallagher: In *Technical Digest of the Conference on Lasers and Electro-optics*, June 1984; presentation ThH5
66. B. M. McWilliams, H. W. Chin, I. P. Herman, R. A. Hyde, F. Mitlitsky, J. C. Whitehead and L. L. Wood: *Proc. of the SPIE/'84 Conference*, Los Angeles, Jan. 1984 (in press)
67. R. Robertson, D. Hils and A. Gallagher: *Chem. Phys. Lett.* **103**, 397 (1984)
68. W. B. Veldkamp: *Rev. Sci. Instrum.* **53**, 294 (1982)
69. Y. I. Nissim, A. Lietoila, R. B. Gold and J. F. Gibbons: *J. Appl. Phys.* **51**, 274 (1980)
70. J. E. Moody and R. H. Hendel: *J. Appl. Phys.* **53**, 4364 (1982)
71. A. A. Iranmanesh and R. F. W. Pease: *J. Vac. Sci. Technol.* **B1**, 91 (1983)
72. K. M. Shvarev, B. A. Baum and P. V. Gel'd: *Sov. Phys. Solid State* **16**, 2111 (1975)
73. D. J. Ehrlich and J. Y. Tsao: *Appl. Phys. Lett.* **44**, 267 (1984)
74. M. L. Burgener and R. E. Reedy: *J. Appl. Phys.* **53**, 4357 (1982)
75. J. P. Colinge and F. Van de Wiele: *J. Appl. Phys.* **52**, 4769 (1981)
76. I. D. Calder and R. Sue: *J. Appl. Phys.* **53**, 7545 (1982)
77. *Thermophysical Properties of High Temperature Solid Materials* **4**, Ed. Y. S. Touloukian (MacMillan, New York 1967)
78. S. D. Allen, J. Goldstone, R. Y. Jan, S. Vernon and J. Ung: In *Technical Digest of the Conference on Lasers and Electro-optics*, June 1984; presentation ThI3 and private communication
79. S. M. Sze: *Physics of Semiconductor Devices*, 2nd Ed. (J. Wiley, New York 1981) p. 68
80. R. F. Wood, J. R. Kirkpatrick and G. E. Giles: *Phys. Rev.* **B23**, 5555 (1981)
81. I. P. Herman, B. M. McWilliams, F. Mitlitsky and J. C. Whitehead: unpublished
82. T. I. Kamins, K. F. Lee and J. F. Gibbons: *Sol. St. Electr.* **23**, 1037 (1980)
83. H. W. Lam, Z. P. Sobczak, R. F. Pinizzotto and A. F. Tasch, Jr.: *IEEE Electr. Dev.* **29**, 389 (1982)
84. I. P. Herman, B. M. McWilliams, F. Mitlitsky, J. C. Whitehead and D. S. Peters: In *Technical Digest of the Conference on Lasers and Electro-optics*, June 1984; presentation ThO3

85. T. I. Kamins, K. F. Lee and J. F. Gibbons: *IEEE Electr. Dev. Lett.* **1**, 5 (1980)
86. H. P. Le and H. W. Lam: *IEEE Electr. Dev. Lett.* **3**, 161 (1982)
87. *Proc. of the 1984 Custom Integrated Circuit Conference* May 1984, Rochester (IEEE, 1984)
88. D. J. Ehrlich, J. Y. Tsao, D. J. Silversmith, J. H. C. Sedlacek, R. W. Mountain and W. S. Graber: *IEEE Electr. Dev. Lett.* **5**, 32 (1984)
89. J. A. Yasaitis, G. H. Chapman and J. I. Raffel: *IEEE Electr. Dev. Lett.* **3**, 184 (1982)
90. J. I. Raffel, J. F. Freidin and G. H. Chapman: *Appl. Phys. Lett.* **42**, 705 (1983)
91. J. I. Raffel, A. H. Anderson, G. H. Chapman, S. L. Garverick, K. H. Konkle, B. Mathur and A. M. Soares: In *Proc. of the IEEE 1983 Int'l. Symp. on Circuits and Systems*, May 1983, p. 781
92. G. H. Chapman, A. H. Anderson, K. H. Konkle, B. Mathur, J. I. Raffel and A. M. Soares: In *Technical Digest of the Conference on Lasers and Electro-optics*, June 1984; presentation FD3
93. J. Y. Tsao, D. J. Ehrlich, D. J. Silversmith and R. W. Mountain: *IEEE Electr. Dev. Lett.* **3**, 164 (1982)

Part 4

# Diagnostics of Laser Processing, Materials, and Devices

# Thermal and Acoustic Techniques for Monitoring Pulsed Laser Processing

R. L. Melcher

IBM T. J. Watson Research Center, Yorktown Heights, NY 10598

A variety of thermal and/or acoustic techniques have been developed over the past few years to monitor and study laser initiated processes used in the microelectronics industry. A review of some of these will be given with examples from the work of the author and his collaborators, as well as from other laboratories. In many processes, lasers are valuable tools because they are capable of delivering controlled amounts of energy at specific times to localized regions of space. Processes such as hole drilling and laser enhanced etching or photochemical ablation involve a variety of complex physical and chemical processes. The understanding of these requires knowledge of the energy balance between chemical excitation (bond breaking, chemiluminescence, combustion, etc.), kinetic energy of expelled particles, heat in the substrate, and heat transmitted to the surroundings through radiation or conduction. Information concerning this energy balance can be obtained using steady state and time resolved calorimetry, infrared detection of thermal radiation, and steady state and time resolved photoacoustic techniques, and through the study of high frequency ultrasonic waves generated in the substrate. The advantages and disadvantages of each technique will be discussed within the context of specific examples. A better fundamental understanding of the processes involved is achieved as well as the development of practical process monitors.

## INTRODUCTION

With the increasing interest in the use of pulsed lasers for the deposition of energy during the processing of electronic circuits and packages, techniques for the monitoring and understanding of these processes has assumed increased importance. In this short review, the use of thermal sensors and acoustic monitors is described. Optical diagnostic techniques are described elsewhere in this conference proceedings.

In the following discussion, acoustic and thermal monitors used in two types of pulsed laser processing ($CO_2$ laser drilling and excimer laser ablation) are described in detail. The third section of this review discusses several new types of transient thermal techniques which are currently under development. They include high speed pyroelectric, infrared and photothermal techniques.

### A. Pulsed $CO_2$ Laser Drilling

Pulsed and continuous wave $CO_2$ lasers have been used for a variety of "machining" processes. These generally make use of the laser's ability to efficiently and with precision, deliver energy locally to the part being machined causing thermal vaporization of unwanted material. In one specific application, holes are drilled through an approximately 200$\mu$m thick epoxy-glass composite to a copper sheet laminated to one side of the composite. The holes need to be approximately 100$\mu$m in diameter. Typically, the process uses two 25 watt, one millisecond pulses to drill the hole. An acoustic monitor has been developed[1] to sense and make use of the acoustic signal emitted in the air by the interaction of the laser pulse with the epoxy-glass/copper part. The monitor consists of a hollow cylinder of PZT piezoelectric ceramic which is mounted concentric to the optical axis and one to two centimeters from the hole to be drilled. The bandwidth of the detector and subsequent electronics is set to extend from essentially dc to 10 kHz. The signal received by the sensor lasts approximately 10-20 milliseconds, rising sharply during the laser pulse and decreasing monotonically thereafter as $t^{-2}$ where t is time measured from the laser pulse.

A model developed to understand the source of this acoustic signal[1] provides not only a clearer picture of the laser drilling process, but also provides the knowledge necessary to use the acoustic signal as a measure of the amount of material drilled by each laser pulse. The $CO_2$ laser pulse ($\lambda \sim 10.6\mu$m) is absorbed by the epoxy-glass composite and converted to heat causing a large temperature rise which results in volatization of the material. This volatile material combusts on interacting with air, causing the release of the heat of combustion, Q, in the form of heat into the air. The heat of combustion is approximately an order of magnitude greater than the heat supplied by the laser and required for volatization. Thus, this process results in net gain of thermal energy. The temperature distribution in the air is given by the solution to the thermal diffusion equation:[2]

$$\delta T(r,t) = \frac{Q}{8(\frac{\pi}{2})^{3/2}\mu^3(t)} \exp\left[-\left(\frac{r}{\mu(t)}\right)^2\right] \tag{1}$$

where $\mu(t)$ is the thermal diffusion length in air. The resulting adiabatic expansion and pressure increase of the air is related to $\delta T(r,t)$by

$$\delta P(r,t) = \left(\frac{\gamma}{\gamma - 1}\right) \frac{P}{T} \delta T(r,t) \tag{2}$$

where P and T are, respectively, the ambient pressure and temperature and $\gamma$ is the heat capacity ratio. The pressure experienced by the sensor at the position $r_s$ can be deduced from the wave equation in the near field limit to be:

$$\delta P(r_s,t) = \frac{Q}{8(\frac{\pi}{2})^{3/2}} \left(\frac{3I\gamma}{\gamma - 1}\right) \frac{P}{T} \frac{1}{r_s} \frac{1}{2\kappa t} \tag{3}$$

where $\kappa$ is the diffusivity and I is a numerical constant of order one. The piezoelectric equation of state leads to the following expression for the voltage produced across the sensor by the pressure $\delta P(r_s,t)$ in the limit that the circuit time constant, $\tau_{CKT} = R_L C$, where $R_L$ is the local resistance and C the capacitance, is much less than the characteristic time of the pressure change.

$$V(t) = dAR_L \frac{\partial}{\partial t}[\delta P(r_s,t)] \sim \frac{Q}{t^2}. \tag{4}$$

Here, d and A are, respectively, the piezoelectric constant and effective area of the sensor.

The proportionality to $t^{-2}$ is in excellent agreement with the measured signals. The proportionality to the heat of combustion demonstrates that the acoustic signal is a good measure of the amount of material volatilized by the laser pulse. A number of tests have been carried out to confirm this fact. Thus, the progress of the drilling process can be followed quantitatively by monitoring the amplitude of (and/or the area under) the acoustic signal. This information can be used with the aid of a computer to adjust the number, the amplitude and the width of the pulses to optimize the drilling process for a given hole in real time.

B. Excimer Laser Ablation

In contrast to infrared $CO_2$ lasers, excimer lasers provide energy in the far ultraviolet region of the spectrum. This form of energy thus has the potential of photochemically affecting the bonding of a solid without the need for first undergoing conversion to heat. However, both photochemical and photothermal processes are expected to occur. Sorting out which process dominates in a given application is an interesting and, at present, open question. Here, we discuss the ablation of polymeric material by excimer lasers.[3]

In order to have a better framework within which the excimer laser ablation process can be discussed, a very much simplified model of the process for ablating polymeric materials has been developed. It is based on a photochemical rate equation, conservation of energy and conservation of momentum. This model is found to be consistent with the dependence of the ablation depth as a function of laser fluence,[4] with the thermal energy contained in a polymer, or single crystal silicon on excimer laser irradiation[5] and with the ultrasonic signals generated in the polymer by the process.[5] The polymer is assumed to consist of long chains of monomer units connected by bonds which can be broken by the absorption of far UV laser photons (e.g. $\lambda \sim 193$nm). As the photons are absorbed by breaking the bonds, there is a probability, $\tau_R^{-1}$, that the bonds are remade. If, however, a critical number density of bonds, $n_c$, are broken, the resulting fragments are volatilized and hence ablated from the material. The linear rate equation for the number of broken bonds, n (z,t) in this process is

$$\frac{dn(z,t)}{dt} = \left\{ k_B N_B n_L(z) - \frac{n(z,t)}{\tau_R} \right\} \left[ 1 - \theta(n - n_c) \right], \qquad (5)$$

where $N_B$ is the density of bonds, $n_L(z)$ is the photon density (proportional to the laser fluence) $k_B$ is a rate constant for bond breaking and $\theta(n - n_c)$ is the unit step function, $\theta(x) = 1, x > 0$ and $\theta(x) = 0, x < 0$. The step function is included to account for the ablation threshold found experimentally. [ One should note that n(z,t) in the rate equation (5) and in the ensuing discussion can be interpreted as the number of optically excited molecular units rather than as the number of broken bonds. This different interpretation of the model in no way affects the validity of the results. However, this ambiguity of interpretation demonstrates clearly that the precise ablation mechanism is hidden in the origin of the critical number density, $n_c$ ]. Beer's law for the photon absorption takes the form

$$n_L(z) = n_L(0)e^{-\alpha Z} \qquad (6)$$

where $n_L(0)$ is the incident photon density and $\alpha$ is the optical absorption coefficient. These two equations (5 and 6) lead to the following expresison for the depth, $Z_c$, of ablation as a function of the incident fluence, $F_0$, and the fluence at the ablation threshold, $F_0^c$:

$$Z_c = \frac{1}{\alpha} \ln \frac{F_0}{F_0^c} . \qquad (7)$$

This result is consistent with the logarithmic dependence of $Z_c$ on $F_0$ found experimentally.[4,6]

The conservation of energy for the process can be written as

$$\begin{aligned} -\frac{\partial F(z)}{\partial z} &= n(z,t)\, E_B \\ &+ \rho C_p \delta T(z,t)\left[1 - \theta(n - n_c)\right] \\ &+ 1/2 m_p v^2 n(z,t) \theta(n - n_c) \end{aligned} \qquad (8)$$

Here, $F(z)$ is the fluence at the depth z in the material $E_B(\sim 4eV)$ is the bond energy of the polymer chain, $\rho$ and $C_p$ are the density and specific heat of the polymer, $\delta T(z,t)$ is the temperature distribution within the polymer, and $m_p$ and v are, respectively, the mass and velocity of the ablated particles. The left hand side of this expression represents the loss of energy per unit volume from the laser pulse. The three terms on the right hand side represent the energy which has gone into bond breaking, the thermal energy deposited during the process, and the kinetic energy of the ablated particles. Integrating this expression over the sample volume and taking the limit $t >> \tau_R$, an expression for the heat energy (per unit area) remaining in the polymer, $F_H$, is obtained:

$$F_H = F_0 \qquad ; \; n < n_c \qquad (9a)$$

$$F_H = F_0 - (E_B + 1/2 m_p v^2) \frac{n_c}{\alpha} \ln \frac{F_0}{F_0^c} \; ; \; n > n_c . \qquad (9b)$$

Below threshold the entire fluence, $F_0$, is converted to heat whereas above threshold the remaining heat is reduced by the bond energy and the kinetic energy of the ablated material. A calorimeter based on the pyroelectric effect has been used[5] to measure $F_H$ as a function of $F_0$. The data are in quantitative agreement with Eq. (9a) and clearly show the onset of ablation as indicated by the second term in Eq. (9b). Similar experimental results have been obtained using a calorimeter based on a thermocouple.[7]

During ablation, fragments of the polymer leave the polymer with the momentum $m_p v$ giving rise to an impulse (stress) on the polymer of the form:

$$P_M = \frac{d}{dt} \int_0^\infty m_p v n(z,t)\, \theta(n - n_c) dz . \qquad (10)$$

Evaluating this expression gives:

$$P_M = 0 \; ; \; n < n_c \qquad (11a)$$

$$P_M = \frac{m_p v}{\Delta} \frac{n_c}{\alpha} \ln \frac{F_0}{F_0^c} \; ; \; n > n_c \qquad (11b)$$

where $\Delta$ is the laser pulse width. This impulse has a band width extending to $\sim \Delta^{-1} \approx 70$ MHz.

Measurements of the ultrasonic waves thus emitted in the polymer at ultrasonic frequencies during excimer laser irradiation have been carried out.[5] These show that below threshold a thermoelastically[8] generated ultrasonic wave is excited by the laser. However, above threshold ($F_0 > F_0^c$) an additional contribution to the ultrasonic wave is found which can be as large as 30 times greater than the thermoelastic contribution. Order of magnitude estimates of the momentum transfer and the thermoelastic contributions are consistent with this result. In addition, Eqs. (9) and (11) can be used to give a good fit to the fluence dependence of the momentum transfer ultrasonic wave above threshold.[5]

The energy balance equation (8) can be used to evaluate the maximum temperature rise below threshold at the surface of the polymer (averaged over the optical absorption length) at the end of the laser pulse.

$$\delta T = \frac{\alpha F_0}{\rho C_p}\left[1 - \frac{E_B}{h\nu}\frac{\tau_R}{\Delta}(1 - e^{-\Delta/\tau_R})\right] . \qquad (12)$$

Here, $h\nu$ is the photon energy. Note that the thermal diffusion length in a polymer irradiated by a 10 ns pulse is typically shorter than the optical absorption length. Depending upon $\Delta/\tau_R$, this expression ranges from:

$$\delta T = \frac{\alpha F_0}{\rho C_p}\left[1 - \frac{E_B}{h\nu}\right] \quad : \Delta/\tau_R \rightarrow 0 \qquad (13a)$$

to

$$\delta T = \frac{\alpha F_0}{\rho C_p} \quad : \Delta/\tau_R \rightarrow \infty . \qquad (13b)$$

The calculation of temperature can be useful in helping to distinguish between different physical mechanisms for the ablation process. At least three independent mechanisms can be distinguished. (i) Thermoelastic expansion and fracture of the polymer due to large strain gradients of order $\alpha\beta\delta T$ where $\beta$ is the thermal expansion coefficient. (ii) Thermal degradation of the polymer giving rise to volatile particles due to the high temperature at and near the surface. (iii) Photoelastic expansion of the polymer due to the increased volume and volatilization of the fragments after bond breaking over that of the polymer itself. This latter mechanism is independent of the temperature. At present, the available information is insufficient to conclusively determine which model is dominant. It is quite possible that two or more mechanisms take part in any given process.

### C. New Transient Thermal Techniques

One of the reasons that it is difficult in many cases to arrive at an unambiguous understanding of the mechanisms contributing to pulsed laser processes is the absence of universal and reliable techniques for measuring temperature on the time scale of interest. Several new methods for high speed temperature measurement are being developed and may prove to be valuable in monitoring and studying pulsed laser processes.

1. Pyroelectric Calorimetry - The pyroelectric calorimeter described above in Section B is essentially a dc technique. However, pyroelectric detectors are capable of extremely high speed operation limited only by the electrical time constant of the detector and the associated

electronics. The calorimeter consists of thermally bonding the sample to a pyroelectric crystal. The outer surface of the sample absorbs the laser energy which diffuses through the sample to the detector. If the electrical time constant (usually dominated by the detector capacitance and the input impedence of the high speed amplifier) is shorter than the diffusion time, the received voltage signal will rise to a maximum at $t_{peak} \approx l^2/6\kappa$ and then slowly decrease.[9] Here, l is the sample thickness and $\kappa$ is the sample diffusivity. This technique has been used to measure thermal diffusivity in samples of known thickness.[9] However, if this technique is to be used to monitor rapid phase changes induced by a laser pulse, then $t_{peak}$ must be less than or comparable to the time scale of the phase change. For a typical metal film ($\kappa \sim 1\mathrm{cm}^2/\mathrm{s}$ $l = 1\mu\mathrm{m}$) a time resolution of $t_{peak} \approx 2\mathrm{ns}$ can be achieved. Higher speeds will require thinner samples. COUFAL and coworkers[10] have observed rapid phase transitions in thin Te films deposited directly on a high speed $PVF_2$ pyroelectric detector.

2. Fast IR Radiography - The speed and sensitivity of low temperature, photoconductive and photovoltaic infrared detectors has increased such that high speed transient measurements of surface temperature can be made. TAM and coworkers[11] have demonstrated submicrosecond time resolution using a liquid nitrogen cooled HgCdTe detector sensitive to near room temperature radiation. This method can be used either to measure the transient temperature rise on the laser irradiated surface or, in the case of thin samples, the temperature rise on the back surface of the sample. Theoretical calculations based upon thermal diffusion and the laws of thermal radiation enable one to do time resolved measurements of the thermal properties of materials in a variety of applications. High speed detectors together with good collection optics should make possible time resolved measurements of this type in the nanosecond regime. This technique has the distinct advantage that in contrast to the pyroelectric calorimeter, it does not require contact to the sample. It also places no requirements on the sample thickness. The sensitivity and speed of time resolved IR radiography as compared to the pyroelectric calorimeter are not yet clear.

3. Photothermal Deflection - A new technique which has shown promise for sensitive optical spectroscopy and microscopy can, in principle, be modified to be a sensitive and high speed monitor of surface temperature. Photothermal deflection is based upon the time and position dependent heating of a sample with a modulated or pulsed laser. This heating causes a localized time dependent thermal expansion and hence deformation of the sample surface. A second probe laser which reflects from the heated region is deflected by the surface deformation. The deflection is detected by a position sensitive detector. The deflection angle, $\theta$ is proportional to:

$$\theta \sim \frac{\beta Q \Delta}{K}, \tag{14}$$

where $\beta$ is the thermal expansion, Q the heat absorbed from the pump laser, $\Delta$ the pulse width (or inverse of the modulation frequency) and K is the sample thermal conductivity.

This technique has been successfully applied to the measurement of the polarization dependence of the optical absorption by surface states on the 2 × 1 reconstruction of single crystal silicon and germanium surfaces.[12] Consideration of the material constants in Eq. (14) leads to the conclusion that time resolution significantly less than $10^{-6}$ s should be possible during pulsed laser processing of polymers.

### D. Conclusions

Thermal and acoustic monitoring during pulsed laser processing can lead to valuable information and increased understanding of the mechanisms involved. In most cases, the value of the monitors will be closely related to the development of models which help to quantitatively interpret the measurements and to provide a framework for interpretation.

New transient thermal techniques are being developed which hold the promise of providing reliable high speed temperature measurements.

## ACKNOWLEDGEMENTS

I am indebted to my collaborators G. Gorodetsky, S. S. Jha, T. Kazyaka, R. Srinivasan and C. E. Yeack without whose insights and experiments this review could not have been written.

## REFERENCES

1. C. E. Yeack and R. L. Melcher, Appl. Phys. Lett. **41**, 1043 (1982).
2. H. S. Carslaw and J. C. Jaeger, *Conduction of Heat in Solids*, Oxford Univ. Press, Oxford (1959).
3. R. Srinivasan and V. Mayne-Banton, Appl. Phys. Lett. **41**, 576 (1982); R. Srinivasan and W. J. Leigh, J. Am. Chem. Soc. **104**, 6784 (1982); R. Srinivasan J. Vac. Sci. Tech. **B1**, 923 (1983).
4. R. Srinivasan and Bodil Braren, J. Polymer Sci. (Chem.), (in press).
5. G. Gorodetsky, T. G. Kazyaka, R. L. Melcher and R. Srinivasan, CLEO 1984, Anaheim, CA.
6. H. H. G. Jelinek and R. Srinivasan, J. Phys. Chem. **88**, 3048 (1984).
7. J. E. Andrew, P. E. Dyer, D. Forster and P. H. Key, Appl. Phys. Lett. **43**, 717 (1983); P. E. Dyer and J. Sidhu, CLEO 1984, Anaheim, CA.
8. R. M. White, J. Appl. Phys. **34**, 3559 (1963).
9. C. E. Yeack, R. L. Melcher and S. S. Jha, J. Appl. Phys. **53**, 3947 (1982).
10. H. Coufal, Appl. Phys. Lett. **44**, 59 (1984).
11. A. C. Tam and B. Sullivan, Appl. Phys. Lett. **43**, 333 (1983); Wing P. Leung and Andrew C. Tam, Optics Letters **9**, 93 (1984).
12. Marjorie A. Olmstead and Nabil M. Amer, Phys. Rev. Letters, **52**, 1148 (1984).

# Temperature Diagnostics for Laser Writing

R.P. Salathé

Generaldirektion PTT, Technical Center, CH-3000 Bern 29, Switzerland

H.H. Gilgen

Department of Electrical Engineering, Columbia University,
New York, N.Y. 10027, USA

Infrared (IR ), Raman , and luminescence measurements are discussed with respect to their application as temperature probe during laser writing. IR measurements on the high energy side of the Planck distribution can be applied to a large variety of materials and large temperature ranges. This technique is characterized by a good temperature (~ 1 deg C) and reasonable spatial (~ 3 μm) resolution. Raman measurements require long integration times. The evaluation of temperature from such measurements is difficult: for intensity measurements the spatial and temporal averaging and the (unkwown) scattering cross-sections have to be considered whereas pressure effects induced by nonuniform heating are a major problem for interpreting Raman frequency measurements. The application of luminescence measurements to temperature evaluation is limited to a few materials, e.g. III-V semiconductors. A high spatial resolution (⩽ 1 μm) allowing evaluation of temperature profiles is demonstrated in (Al,Ga)As.

## 1. Introduction

A profound understanding of laser deposition processes can only be acquired with a detailed knowledge of the laser processing parameters (i.e intensity profiles, scan speed, temperature distribution on the surface), on the reactive species (concentration, cross-section), on the reaction paths, and on the dynamics of the reactions. Most of these parameters can be evaluated by standard techniques used with vacuum and thin film technology [1], CVD processes [2], dry etching [3] or molecular beam epitaxy [4]. A problem specific to laser processing is the evaluation of the laser induced temperature distribution on the substrate surface. This parameter is important for the description of pyrolytic and photolytic reactions. The local heating is the main "driving force" for the reaction under pyrolytic processing conditions and it can lead to modified reaction rates or unwanted side reactions in the case of photolytic reactions. The reaction rates can be estimated in most cases if the maximum temperature rise is known. An understanding of the spatial features in deposition or etching requires also knowledge of the temperature profile.

The laser induced temperature rise and the profile can be evaluated from model calculations. For cw illumination of a semi-infinite solid the temperature rise is in a first order approximation proportional to the absorbed laser power and inversely proportional to the focal beam diameter and the thermal conductivity. With simple calculations the temperature profile in different depth can be calculated according to LAX [5] and the same author also indicates a straightforward extension of the calculations to the case of a temperature dependent thermal conductivity [6]. The transient heating under pulsed illumination can also be evaluated under similar conditions with simple calculations [7,8]. However, the situation is more complicated for most laser processing conditions: the surface reflectivity changes drastically during deposition, large changes in the thermal resistance occur because of changes in material and geometry, phase transitions may occur, or the substrate could consist of a layered structure. Attempts to include the description of only one additional effect into the model, e.g. the diffusion of carriers in semiconductors, results in rather tedious calculations [9]. Calculations of temperature distributions in cw-laser induced pyrolytic deposition have been performed recently [30].

In this paper we discuss some experimental techniques which can be used for in situ temperature measurements during laser processing. Of special interest are passive and non-destructive techniques which do not require a special preparation of the sample. The simplest possibility consists here in measuring the onset of melting, by, e.g., optical reflectivity [10] or photoacoustic detection [11]. The known melting point of a given material and the laser power necessary for melting constitutes the reference points on one side, room temperature and zero laser power on the other side. The scaling of laser power is then translated into a temperature scale by linear or logarithmic interpolation depending whether the temperature dependence of the thermal conductivity is neglected or included in a first order approximation [5,6]. Considerable errors in the temperatures evaluated from this method can occur if the basic assumptions used for derivation of the temperature scales are not valid. More reliable results can be obtained if the interpolation is based on the experimental measurement of a parameter with a known temperature dependence. No special probing is necessary if parameters are selected which describe an interaction mechanism between processing laser and sample or deposit. Reflection and transmission measurements have been used in laser annealing experiments [10]. For laser deposition processes their application is rather limited. Here, we focus on parameters obtained from measuring the infrared (IR ) radiation emitted from the laser heated zone (Sect. 2), Raman measurements (Sect. 3), and luminescence measurements (Sect. 4). Different methods of temperature evaluations from these optical methods have been investigated experimentally. In some cases the results from different approaches could be directly compared. The conclusions from these experiments and possible improvements are discussed in the last section (Sect.5).

## 2. Infrared Measurements

The temperature can be evaluated from measurements of the infrared radiation emitted by the laser heated zone. In principle, four different methods could be used: (1) measurements of the power integrated over the whole spectrum, P, and evaluation of the temperature based on Stefan-Boltzmann's law ($P \propto T^4$); (2) Evaluating the wavelength of the emission peak, $\lambda_m$, and calculating the temperature according to Wien's law ($T \propto 1/\lambda_m$); (3) Measuring the spectral emissivity, $P\lambda$, on the low energy side of the Planck distribution and evaluating the temperature with the Rayleigh-Jeans formula ($T \propto P\lambda$); (4) Measuring $P\lambda$ on the high energy side and evaluating T from Wien's approximation ($T^{-1} \propto \ln P_\lambda$).

Standard pyrometer measurements are based on method 1. The temperature is evaluated from an assumed Planck distribution. However, laser heated semiconductors are generally not in thermal equilibrium with the IR emission at energies below the bandgap. Deviations from the assumed Planck distribution would be expected in the bandgap region and the assumed $T^4$ scaling becomes questionable. Moreover, since this technique includes also the measurements at long wavelengths, a poor spatial resolution has to be expected. This latter disadvantage does also apply to method 3. Here, another drawback exists in the lack of sensitive detectors. Method 2 involves spectrometer measurements. Because of the broad maxima at low temperatures a poor resolution is expected here. The precision of this method is also strongly affected by deviations from the Planck distribution. Method 4 has the disadvantage that the IR-power levels are very low at low temperatures. For measurements in the near infrared, however, the most sensitive detectors are available and the best spatial resolution can be expected. Since the IR power depends exponentially on temperature, method 4 is more sensitive to temperature variations than to volume variations in the heated zone. This property is particularly useful in nonuniformly heated materials characterized by temperature dependent thermal conductivities. For these reasons method 4 has been applied for temperature measurements in our laser processing applications [12,13].

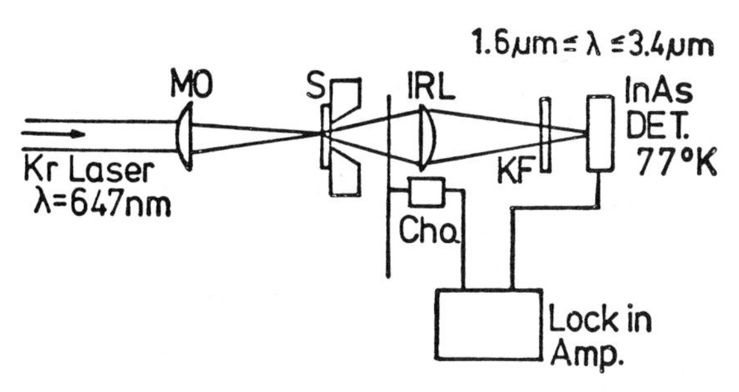


Fig. 1: Experimental arrangement for IR measurements. MO: microscope objective, S: sample, IRL: IR lens, KF: IR filter, Cho: chopper.

The experimental arrangement is schematically shown in Fig. 1. For the laser heating experiments a cw Kr-ion laser (Spectra Physics Mod. 171-17) has been used. The laser was operated at 647 nm in the $TEM_{00}$ mode together with an electrooptical feedback system for noise reduction. The laser beam is focused by means of a microscope objective MO (20x, F.L.=12.6 mm) onto the surface of the sample S. The laser spot radius on the surface was about $w_0$=1.5 μm. The samples consisted either of single crystal semiconductor wafers or of Au or Ge films evaporated onto glass. An IR lens IRL (NA=1, F.L.=12.5 mm) was used to focus the IR power on an InAs diode, operated in the photovoltaic mode at 77 K. A Ge filter (KF) of 5 mm thickness screened the detector from radiation at wavelengths shorter than 1.6 μm. An upper wavelength limit of 3.4 μm was given by the cutoff wavelength of the detector. A mechanical chopper and a lock-in amplifier (PAR Mod. 124 A) were used for signal processing. The NEP of the detection system was about $10^{-12}$ W, the time resolution ~ 0.3 s. No spatial filtering was applied to achieve best resolution: the detectors field of view on the sample surface was limited by the diameter of the detector to about 100 μm. It should also be noted that instead of measuring the transmitted IR light, the backward scattered light could be measured in a slightly modified configuration.

Fig. 2 shows the measured IR power as a function of laser power P for 200 nm thick Au and Ge films on glass (solid lines). The melting points MP could be easily detected in both materials from changes in laser light reflection and transmission. These well defined temperatures have been used to correlate the laser power with the temperature scale. The higher IR powers emitted from the Au film are explained by the larger area of the heated zone due to a higher thermal conductivity. The dashed line shows results from numerical calculations for the two films. For the detection

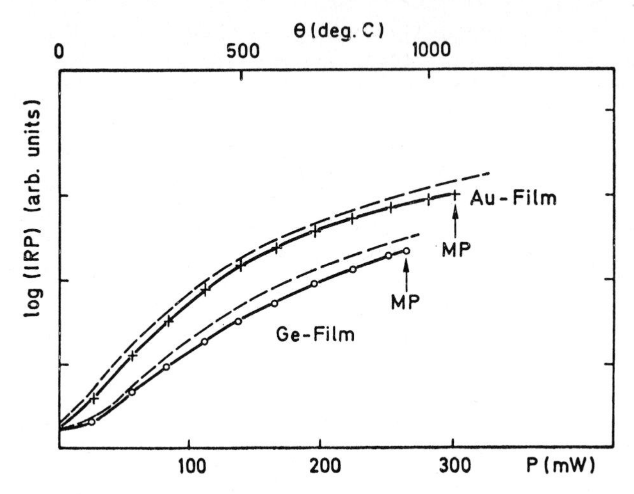


Fig 2: IR power IRP vs. laser power P for Au and Ge films on glass. Dashed line and temperature scale applies to model calculations.

system described above the Wien approximation is expected to give useful results for temperatures up to ~ 600°C. The results of the calculations shown in Fig. 2 are based on the Planck formula to give correct results also at higher temperatures. The detector response has also been included in the calculations. The adjustable parameter is the halfwidth of the temperature profile. The corresponding diameters are 15 μm for the Au and 6 μm for the Ge film. A linear temperature scale has been used for the theoretical curves. The agreement with the measurements indicates that the temperatures can be linearly interpolated between melting points and room temperature in these cases. For the Au film an increase in IR power by a factor of 400 between room temperature and melting point is shown in Fig. 2. This indicates that a measurement precision of 1 deg. C or lower could be achieved without difficulties.

Fig. 3 shows the same measurement for a Si single crystal wafer of ~ 300 μm thickness. At low temperatures the measured IR power increases more rapidly as compared to the film measurements. This is due to an increase in depth of the laser heated volume. The dashed line indicate again results from numerical calculations for two temperature profiles with different halfwidths. A logarithmic temperature scale has been used to this case. The disagreement between measurement and calculations indicates that one or several of the following assumptions for the model are questionable: the temperature depends exponentially on laser power, the temperature profile does not change with laser power, or, the emissivity of IR radiation within the detected energy range is constant.

Similar measurements have also been performed on a Ge crystal and on (Al,Ga)As multilayer structures [13]. Reasonably good agreement between measurement and theory was found for Ge indicating that the model assumptions discussed above are correct in this case. The (Al,Ga)As measurements did not agree with the results from model calculations for temperatures above 350°C. The deviations could be explained in this case by additional changes in the temperature profile due to creation of defect centers in the temperature range of 350 - 500°C and by surface reactions occurring at temperature above 500°C [13].

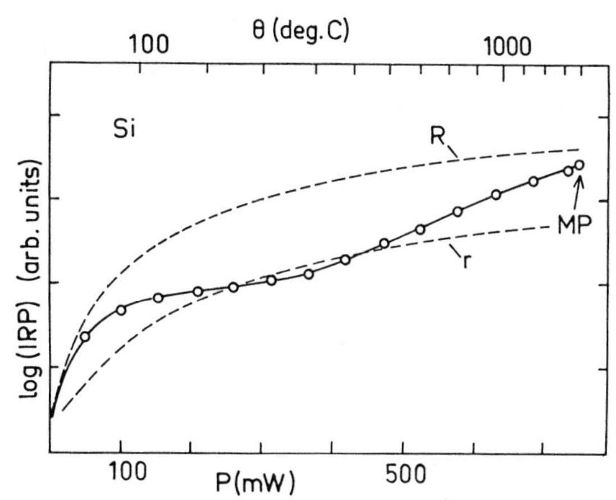


Fig. 3: IR power IRP vs. laser power P for a (100) Si crystal. Dashed lines indicate results from calculations based on temperature profiles with different radii. ($r_1 \approx 3\mu m$, $r_2 = 0{,}85\ \mu m$)

## 3. Raman Measurement

Laser Raman spectroscopy is a well-known technique to study a variety of excitations in solids including optical phonons, plasmons, color centers,etc. [14]. From Raman measurements the temperature can be evaluated from the intensity ratio of the anti-Stokes (AS) to Stokes (S) Raman peaks or from the temperature induced frequency shift or line broadening of one of the Raman lines. The very low efficiency of Raman scattering constitutes a disadvantage of these methods. Generally long time constants ($>$ 1s) are involved in measuring Raman spectra and the scattered light has to be collected from the whole irradiation zone. The signals are thus averaged over the radial and longitudinal temperature profiles. Correction factors, deduced,e.g.,from model calculations, have to be introduced in order to evaluate the maximum temperature rise [15].

The intensity ratio of the AS to S peaks depends exponentially on temperature, $I_{AS}/I_S \propto \exp(-\hbar\omega_0/kT)$, with $\hbar\omega_0$ the optical phonon energy. Precise temperature measurements seem possible with this technique. However, the proportionality factor depends on the S and AS Raman scattering cross-sections and on the absorption coefficients at the laser and Raman lines [16]. The temperature dependence of all of these parameters is not known for most materials. Using room temperature values or rough estimates of the temperature dependence for these parameters could result in considerable errors in the evaluated temperatures. Finally, the evaluation with this technique is based on the assumption of equilibrium phonon distribution. This assumption can be incorrect in special cases, e.g., if the laser irradiation is performed with psec pulses [17].

Most of these disadvantages do not apply to temperature evaluations based on the frequency shift or the line broadening of Raman spectra. Here, temperature variations of the Raman cross-sections and the absorption coefficients do not affect the evaluation and a calibration of the method is easily obtained by measuring the temperature dependence of the Raman spectra on a uniformly heated reference material. Even the averaging over the temperature profiles could be eliminated to some extent with frequency measurements by measuring the high frequency tail of the Stokes Raman line. However, the temperature induced frequency shifts and line broadening effects are generally small in semiconductor materials. For the first Stokes line in Si, e.g., the shift is about - 2 $cm^{-1}/100^oC$ and the linewidth broadening is ~ 1 $cm^{-1}/100^oC$ [18]. The resolution obtained with standard Raman equipment, e.g.,a 0.5 m double monochromator, is on the order of 0.2-0.4 $cm^{-1}$. This illustrates that the precision in temperature evaluation achieved with these techniques is not very high. Moreover, the linewidths and the frequency depend also on pressure. In nonuniformly heated solids the heated zone can expand freely only in the direction perpendicular to the surface. The expansion parallel to the surface provokes a pressure building up from the nonheated surrounding. These pressure effects can be of the same order of magnitude as temperature effect and are superimposed on the latter. They severely limit the application of these techniques for laser processing of semiconductor wafers.

For thin film processing the build up of pressure is reduced since thin films are more easily deformed. We have investigated the possibility of using Raman frequency measurements for temperature evaluation in thin films consisting of 200 nm thick polycrystalline Ge (grain size ~ 10 μm) on BK-7 glass substrates [19]. The Raman spectra were generated with the 488 nm line of an Argon ion laser (Spectra Physics Mod. 164). The samples were irradiated under Brewster's angle with the laser light polarized parallel to the plane of incidence and focused to a spot diameter of 10 μm. The light scattered perpendicular to the surface was collected by a lens (F.L.=16 mm, N.A.=0.25) and focused with a cylindrical lens (F.L.=22 mm) onto the slit of 0.5 m double grating monochromator (Jobin Yvon HRD 11). For wavelength calibration the light of a Ne spectral lamp was superimposed onto the Raman light by means of a thin foil beam splitter between the two lenses. An optical multichannel analyzer (B & M spektronik) consisting of an image intensifier with an S-20ER photocathode and a cooled Si-vidicon target was used at the output of the spectrometer. The accuracy of frequency measurements with this arrangement was given by the dispersion of the spectrograph and the spacing of the Si elements of the detector and amounted to ± 0.5 $cm^{-1}$.

The frequency shift of the Stokes line has been measured as a function of incident laser power. Fig. 4 shows the results of the measurements on two

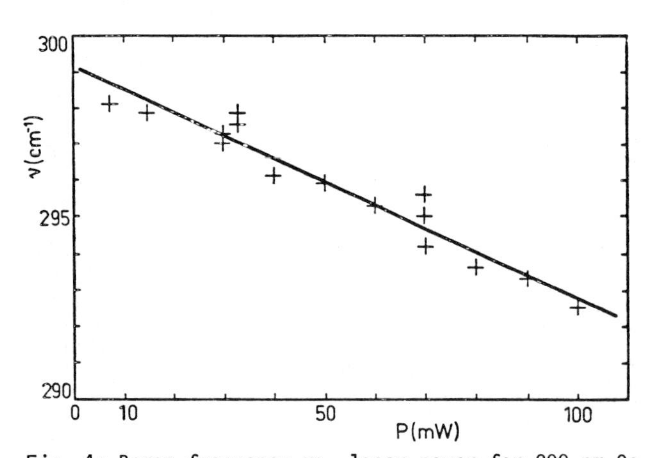

Fig. 4: Raman frequency vs. laser power for 200 nm Ge film on glass.

different spots of the same film. A shift of 64.2 $cm^{-1}$ per Watt of applied laser power is evaluated from this measurement. From the IR measurements a thermal resistance of 2100°C/W has been evaluated for the same film structure. Based on this value a shift of 3 $cm^{-1}$/100°C is calculated. This value should be compared with the 2.15 $cm^{-1}$/100°C shift measured in homogeneously heated Ge crystals by RAY et al. [20]. Neglecting stresses in non-uniformly heated thin films could thus also lead to considerable errors in temperature evaluation with this technique.

## Luminescence Measurements

The application of luminescence measurements for temperature evaluations during laser processing of semiconductors is restricted to direct gap materials. These materials exhibit efficient radiative transitions between states located near the conduction and valence band edges. The bandgap energy and the energy distribution of carriers within the bands depend on temperature. Both parameters can be evaluated from luminescence measurements and if their dependence on temperature is known the latter is determined too. In contrast to the Raman measurements discussed before, in situ luminescence measurements do not require photon counting techniques, because of the much higher transition probabilities involved. As compared to the pyrometric techniques discussed, an advantage of luminescence measurement consists in the higher spatial resolution which can be achieved in most cases. Here, we describe the application of luminescence measurement to evaluate temperature distributions which are generated during laser processing of (Al,Ga)As [13].

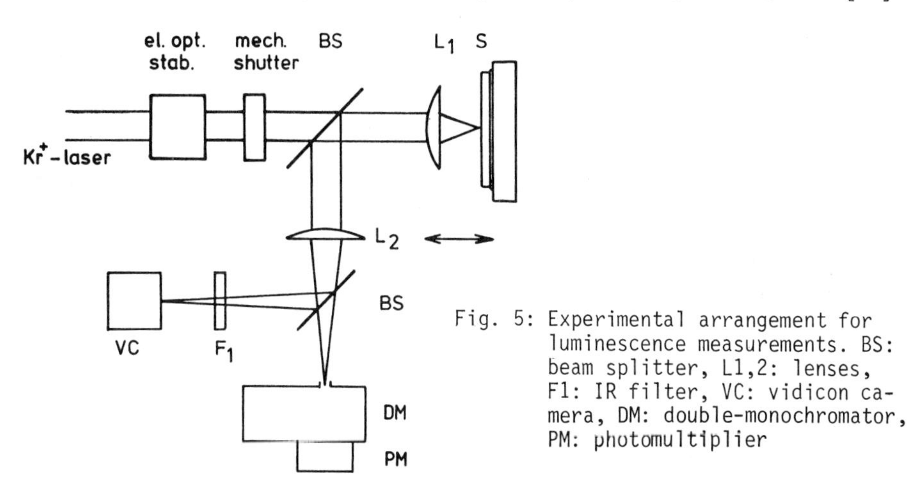


Fig. 5: Experimental arrangement for luminescence measurements. BS: beam splitter, L1,2: lenses, F1: IR filter, VC: vidicon camera, DM: double-monochromator, PM: photomultiplier

The experimental arrangement is shown schematically in Fig. 5. A Kr-ion laser (Spectra Physics Model 171-1) operating at 647 nm in the $TEM_{00}$ mode was used in the experiments. The laser beam is focused by means of a microscope objective L1 (100x, f = 2.09 mm) onto the sample S. A beamsplitter (BS) and a lens L2 are used to direct the photoluminescence collected by the microscope objective onto an infrared sensitive vidicon camera (VC) (Philips XQ 1176) and on a 1/2 m double monochromator (DM). The luminescence mapping system is protected from reflected laser light by an IR transmission filter F1 (Schott RG 715). The mapping system is used to control the focal length by minimizing the radius of the luminescence pattern. A pinhole of 100 $\mu$m diameter at the entrance of the spectrometer discriminates spatially against the luminescence from less heated regions. A diffraction limited resolution of ~ 1 μm within the second layer was obtained with the spectral system. The lens L2 was mounted on a translation stage. Profiles of luminescence light were recorded by moving L2 perpendicularly to the optical axis and the slit of the spectrometer. The light was detected at the exit of the spectrograph by a photomultiplier (PM) (Hamamatsu R 955). The PM signal was processed with a lock-in amplifier (PAR Mod.124A) and measured with an x-y recorder. A calibrated tungsten lamp was used to measure the spectral response of the system and all measurements were corrected with this calibration curve.

Three-layer $Al_xGa_{1-x}As$ heterostructures grown by liquid-phase epitaxy on p-type GaAs substrates [21] have been used in the experiments. The laser light is focused into the $Al_{0.22}Ga_{0.78}As$ layer. The top layer of $Al_{0.6}Ga_{0.4}As$ is transparent at the red Kr-laser wavelength. It protects the underlying $Al_{0.22}Ga_{0.78}As$ layer from As losses and eliminates unwanted photochemical surface reactions in our case. Of course, this layer is not necessary in most cases. The same methods can also be used to investigate surface processing. In such cases, however, the luminescence efficiency would be reduced by about one order of magnitude because of surface recombination.

Fig. 6 shows a typical luminescence spectra on a logarithmic intensity scale. The laser power is about 0.5 mW, the corresponding density ~ 50 kW/cm$^2$. The temperature can be evaluated from the position of the peak and from the low or the high energy side of the spectrum. At constant laser excitation the peak energy of the spectrum shifts with temperature according to the shift in band gap energy. The latter can be described by the Varshini formula [22]. Thus, the temperature can be evaluated directly from the measured shift of the luminescence peak. In laser heating experiments, however, the excitation increases with increasing temperature. Under such conditions the measurements of peak shifts are no longer useful: the shift to lower energies with increasing temperature is counteracted by a shift to higher energy due to band filling. The magnitude of this latter shift depends on density of states near the band edges. In the case of $Al_{0.22}Ga_{0.78}As$, e.g., the absolute value has the same size as the temperature induced shift and the position of the luminescence peak does not change [13].

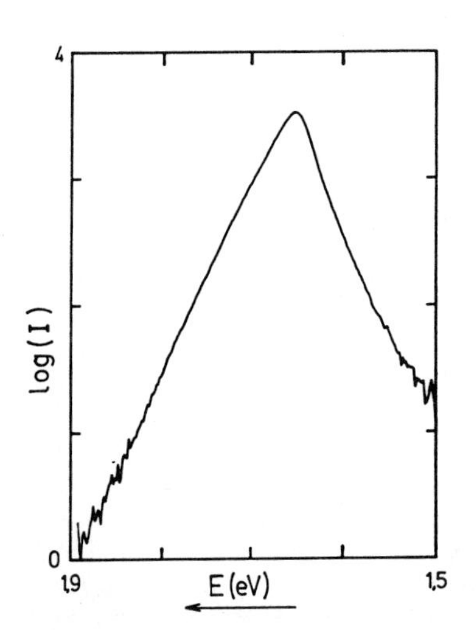


Fig. 6: Luminescence spectrum of Al 0.22 Ga 0.78 As

The shape on the low energy side of the spectrum is determined by the density of states at and below the bandgap due to impurities. The pronounced band tailing shown in Fig. 6 results from a Ge acceptor band which broadened into the valence band. The same shift as for the peak should also occur for the band edge. Since temperature variations of the separation between acceptor level and valence band edge can be neglected as a second order effect, the shift should also occur on the low energy side. In a separate measurement we measured the shift on the low energy side as a function of substrate temperature under constant irradiation condition. A shift of 0.23 nm/$^{o}$C, close to the reported values of the bandgap shift [23], was evaluated by comparing equal intensities at different temperatures. This method is also useful at variable excitation density since the measurement is not obscured by the band filling effect. At very high excitation intensities leading to carrier densities in excess of $10^{18}cm^{-3}$, an additional band gap shrinkage introduced by the high carrier density is observed [24,25]. This effect leads to an overestimate in the temperatures evaluated by this method.

At the high energy side of the spectrum shown in Fig. 6 the intensity is $I(E) \alpha E^2 \exp(E-Eg/kT_e)$ with $E_g$ the bandgap energy and $T_e$ the temperature of the electrons [26]. At liquid He temperatures the electron and lattice temperatures can differ considerably at high excitation levels [27]. However, at room temperature and higher temperatures the average energy relaxation time for carriers is extremely small. From Hall mobility measurements performed at 300-400 K in similar samples a time of $\sim 4 \cdot 10^{-14}$ s has been estimated [28]. This is about two orders of magnitude lower than relaxation times measured at 80 K in GaAs [29]. We therefore assume that the electron temperature does not deviate from the lattice temperature. The temperature can thus be evaluated from the slope of the luminescence spectrum at the high energy side.

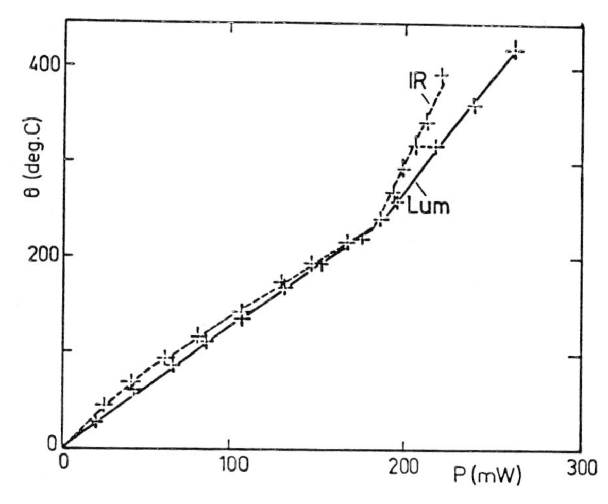


Fig. 7: Maximum temperature rise θ vs. laser power P.

Fig. 7 shows the maximum temperature rise for a (Al,Ga)As three-layer structure as a function of laser power. The temperatures have been evaluated from measuring the shift in luminescence spectra at the low energy side (solid line). The temperature increases linearly with laser power. At ~ 90 mW a slight change in the slope is observed. We attribute this change to an increased absorption in the focal zone. At the corresponding temperature (~ 230$^{o}$C) the $Al_{0.3}$ $Ga_{0.7}$ As layer becomes opaque for the 6.47 nm laser radiation. Also shown in Fig. 6 are temperature measurements performed on the same sample with the IR detection system described in Sect. 2 (dashed line). Good agreement with the luminescence technique is found at low laser powers. The increase in slope is also observed at 90 mW. However, a larger gradient is observed for the temperature curve based on the IR measurements. This is probably due to the increase in volume of the laser heated zone. The IR power measurements are sensitive to changes in volume and such corrections have not been considered in the temperature evaluation.

The spatial resolution of the luminescence techniques for measuring temperature profiles has been investigated using a 100x microscope objective (F.L.=2.09 mm, N.A.=0.95) for focusing. The resulting diameter of the laser spot was ~ 1.6 μm. Stimulated emission and thus efficient carrier recombination is significantly reduced within such small dimensions. This allowed to achieve carrier concentrations $> 2 \cdot 10^{18} cm^{-3}$. Fig. 8 shows temperature profiles evaluated for an excitation of 15 mW. The profiles have been obtained by calculating the temperatures from the bandgap shift at the low energy side and from the slope of the luminescence curve at the high energy side of the spectra. The measurements demonstrate a spatial resolution of about 1 μm which can be achieved with this technique. The halfwidths of both profiles are about 4 μm and agree with values calculated from the theory of LAX [5,6]. The temperatures evaluated with the two methods differ by nearly a factor of two. The difference in the maximum temperature rise is ~ 100°C or $\Delta E_g \simeq 48$ meV. This difference is due to neglecting the influence of bandgap shrinkage due to the carriers in case of the evaluation at the low energy side of the spectrum. For our experimental conditions we expect a carrier density of $n \approx 8 \cdot 10^{18} cm^{-3}$. Since this additional bandgap shrinkage scales with $n^{1/3}$, we would expect an overestimate of $\Delta E_g \approx 56$ meV corresponding to $\Delta\theta \approx 130°C$ for the temperature evaluated from the low energy side of the spectrum.

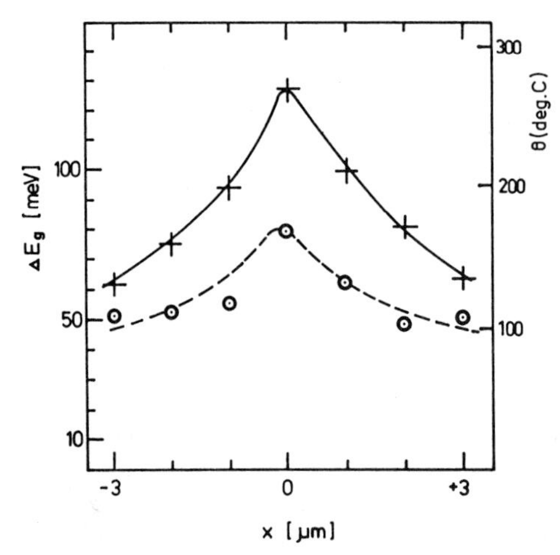


Fig. 8: Local variation of temperature θ and band gap $\Delta E_g$ of $Al_{0.22}Ga_{0.78}As$ under focused laser irradiation. Crosses and circles indicate results from measurements on the low and high energy side of spectrum, respectively.

## 5. Conclusions

The IR measurements at the high energy side of the Planck distribution are a useful and quite universal technique for temperature monitoring on thin films and solids. The influence of changes in volume of the laser heated zone on the measured IR-power are less pronounced compared with other pyrometric techniques. This can be explained by the high spatial resolution achievable and by the exponential dependence of IR power on temperature. However, measurements on Si and (Al,Ga) As at the limit of resolution (laser spot diameters $\leqslant$ 3 μm) indicate that the evaluation of temperature can be disturbed by volume changes in these cases. A reduction of this effect is expected, if the spatial resolution of the IR measurement is further improved. This could be achieved in many cases by a further decrease in the cutoff wavelength of the detection system. In the wavelength range below 2 μm the decrease in IR power could be compensated to some extent by the increased sensitivity of detectors and problems in alignment of the detection system could be eliminated by using IR imaging systems.

Raman frequency measurements are not affected by changes of the laser induced temperature profile. Here, pressure effects in the laser heated zone disturb the interpretation of the results and it has been shown that this disadvantage does also exist for thin film measurements.

Luminescence measurements are limited to semiconductor materials with a direct energy gap. The temperature can be evaluated from the shift of the luminescence spectra at the low energy side or by evaluating the carrier temperature at the high energy side of the spectrum. The latter method is not disturbed by bandgap shifts at high carrier densities or changes in the temperature profiles and a spatial resolution of ~ 1 μm for temperature profiles has been demonstrated.

Acknowledgement:
Most of the experimental work was done while the authors were with the university of Berne. The authors are grateful to Prof. Weber for the opportunity to perform this work and to B. Wicki for technical assistance. Thanks are also due to Mlle Müller, GD PTT, for preparing the manuscript.

1 Methods of Experimental Physics Vol. 14, "Vacuum Physics and Technology" (ed. G.L. Weissler and R.W. Carlson, Academic Press N.Y. 1979), p. 541

2 O.J. Elliott, "Integrated Circuit Fabrication Technology", (Mc Graw Hill, New York 1982), p. 9

3 Y. Horiike, "Dry etching: An Overview", in Semiconductor Technologies Vol. 8, (ed. J. Nishizawa, North Holland, Amsterdam 1983), p. 55

4 A.Y. Cho and J.R. Arthur, "Progress in Solid State Chemistry Vol.10, (J.O. Mc Caldin and G. Somorjai, eds., Academic Press, New York 1975) p. 157

5 M. Lax, J. Appl. Phys. 48, 3919 (1977)

6 M. Lax, Appl. Phys. Lett. 33, 786 (1978)

7 C.M. Surko, A.L. Simons, D.H. Auston, J.A. Golovchenko, R.E. Slusher, T.N.C. Venkatesan, Appl. Phys. Lett. 34, 635 (1979)

8 D.M. Kim, R.R. Shah, and D.L. Crostwait, J. Appl. Phys. 51 (6), 3121 (1980)

9 D.M. Kim, D.L. Kwong, R.R. Shah, D.L. Crosthwait J. Appl. Phys. 52 (8), 4995 (1981)

10 D.H. Auston, J.A. Golovchenko, P.R. Smith, GM. Surko, and T.N.C. Venkatesan, Appl. Phys. Lett. 33, 539 (1978)

11 J.F. McClelland and R.N. Kniseley, Bull. Am. Phys. Sec. 24, 315 (1979)

12 H. Gilgen, R. Salathé, and Y. Rytz-Froidevaux Helv. Phys. Acta 53, 638 (1980)

13 R.P. Salathé, H.H. Gilgen, and Y. Rytz-Froidevaux IEEE J. Quantum Electron., QE-17 (10), 1989 (1981)

14 S.P.S. Porto in "Light Scattering Spectra of Solids", (ed. G.B. Wright, Springer Verlag N.Y. 1969), p. 1

15 H.W. Lo and A. Compaan, J. Appl. Phys. 51 (3), 1565 (1980)

16 H.W. Lo and A. Compaan, Phys. Rev. Lett. 44 (24), 1604 (1980)

17 D. von der Linde, J. Kuhl, and H. Klingenberg, Phys. Rev. Lett. 44 (23), 1505 (1980)

18 T.R. Hart, R.L. Aggarwal, and B. Lax, Phys. Rev. 1B (1), 638 (1970)

19 R.P. Salathé, H.P. Weber, and G. Badertscher, Phys. Lett. 80A (1), 65 (1980)

20 R.K. Ray, R.L. Aggarwal, and B. Lax, Bull. Am. Phys. Soc. 16, 334 (1971)

21 R.A. Logan and F.K. Reinhart, J. Appl. Phys. 44, 4172 (1973)

22 Y.P. Varshini, Physica (Utrecht) 34, 149 (1967)

23 H.J. Lee, L.Y. Juravel, J.C. Woolley, and A.J. Spring Thorpe, Phys. Rev 21B , 659 (1980)

24 O. Hildebrand, E.O. Goebel, K.M. Romanek, H. Weber, and G. Mahler, Phys. Rev. B17, 4775 (1978)

25 J. Shah, R.F. Leheny, and W. Wiegman, Phys. Rev. B16, 1577 (1977)

26 A. Mooradian and H.Y. Fan, Phys. Rev. 148, 873 (1966)

27 J. Shah, Solid-State Electron. 21, 43 (1978)

28 S. Zukotynski, S. Sumski, M.B. Panish, and C. Casey, Jr., J. Appl. Phys. 50, 5795 (1979)

29 C.V. Shank, R.L. Fork, R.F. Leheny, and J. Shah, Phys. Rev. Lett. 42, 112 (1979)

30 K. Piglmayer, J. Doppelbauer, D. Bäuerle: In Laser Controlled Chemical Processing of Surfaces, ed. by A.W. Johnson et al. (North Holland, New York, 1984); see also D. Bäuerle, this volume

# Laser Selective Photoionization Technique: Photoion Beam Epitaxy and Semiconductor Trace Impurity Diagnostics

Georgii I. Bekov, Vladilen S. Letokhov, and Vyacheslav I. Mishin
Institute of Spectroscopy, USSR Academy of Sciences
SU-142092 Troitsk, Moscow Region, USSR

In this paper we report a method of laser resonance ionization of atoms to obtain intense Al, Ga, and In photoion beams and to measure the content of impurities [B] in Ge crystals.

## LASER PHOTOION BEAM TECHNOLOGY

### 1. Background

Recently, the ion beam deposition (IBD) method [1] to fabricate thin (a few nanometers thick) films of various substances differing in chemical composition has been intensively developed. The method is capable of meeting such requirements for the beam deposition process as (1) high beam purity, (2) precise controllability of the deposition dose rate, and (3) continuous variability of the kinetic energy of incident particles.

With this method, beam purity is as vitally important as it is in molecular beam epitaxy, for it is exactly this deposition parameter that largely determines the electrical and physical properties of the deposited films. To obtain ions, the existing ion sources make use of an electrical discharge sustained in the vapor of the substance to be deposited. The ion beams generated by the sources are purified by means of electromagnetic mass separators, but in a number of instances such separators cannot provide adequately pure beams. For example, $CO^+$ and $N_2^+$ are often present in $Si^+$ beams, since they have roughly the same mass as $Si^+$. Additionally, under electrical discharge conditions, such substances as Al, Ga, and Si become reactive towards structural materials.

Considering the above circumstances, the method of laser selective multistep photoionization looks promising for generating ultrahigh-purity ion beams of various elements. Since 1975, the idea of using this method for deep purification of materials in microelectronics has been a long-standing subject of discussion [2-4]. In principle, purification of substances by the method of laser resonance ionization of atoms does not differ from isotope separation.

The general scheme for the production of pure substances with the use of laser radiation is as follows. The atoms of the element to be treated, which may be in the form of an atomic vapor or beam, are first excited to some intermediate atomic state and then photoionized by laser radiation.
The photoions of the plasma thus produced are then extracted from the atom-radiation interaction region by means of an electromagnetic field, collected to form an ion beam, and deposited onto a substrate.

The method is advantageous in that the photoionization process is highly element-selective. This is explained by the fact that the atomic absorption linewidths of various elements are a factor of $10^3$ to $10^5$ smaller than the distances between their respective absorption lines. With this method, the selectivity of photoion production is governed by nonlinear multiphoton processes or by secondary physical and/or chemical processes such as recharge, associative ionization, and electron attachment.

Another advantage of the method is that photoionization can be performed in an atomic vapor or beam obtained by heating the desired substances in a simple, small-sized device which does not contaminate the vapor or beam in the course of atomization.

## 2. Capabilities of the Method and Photoionizing Laser Operating Mode

If all the ionizing laser photons are absorbed by atoms, and the probability of photoionization of the excited atoms is equal to unity, the maximum ion current will be

$$I_{max} = eP/\hbar\omega$$

where e is the electronic charge and $\hbar\omega$ and P the photon energy and average power of the laser radiation, respectively.

In the field of quantum electronics, the most important elements that can be used, for example, to fabricate superlattices and structures of the metal-barrier-metal type are silicon, gallium, aluminum, indium, and arsenic. The resonant absorption lines of these elements are in the near ultraviolet. The average laser power output in this spectral region, which can at present be attained by doubling the frequency of dye lasers, amounts to 50 mW. The maximum ion current in this case will be $I_{max} \approx 10$ mA and will provide for an atomic deposition rate of 150 atomic layers per second and square centimeter.

A high quantum yield of photoions can be attained by making use of pulsed laser radiation with a repetition frequency as high as a few times $10^4$ pps. In this case, a single laser pulse produces a plasma of not too high a density, so that there are no problems associated with the extraction of the ions. Although the concentration of parent atoms may not be very high, the efficiency of using the material increases with laser pulse repetition rate.

The high repetition rate lasers required with this method may take the form of dye lasers pumped by the emission of metal (copper in particular) vapor lasers. Copper-vapor lasers are capable of producing an output power of up to 100 W [5] at a typical pulse repetition rate from $5 \times 10^3$ to $20 \times 10^3$ pps [6].

## 3. Spectral Properties of Al, Ga, and In Atoms

All these elements have similar atomic energy level structures. For example, Fig. 1 shows the energy level diagram of the Ga atom.

The $^2P_{3/2,1/2}$--$^2D_{5/2,3/2}$ transitions in Al, Ga, and In can be excited by the second harmonic output of a dye laser pumped by the emission of a copper-vapor laser ($\lambda_1$ = 510.6 nm, $\lambda_2$ = 578.2 nm).

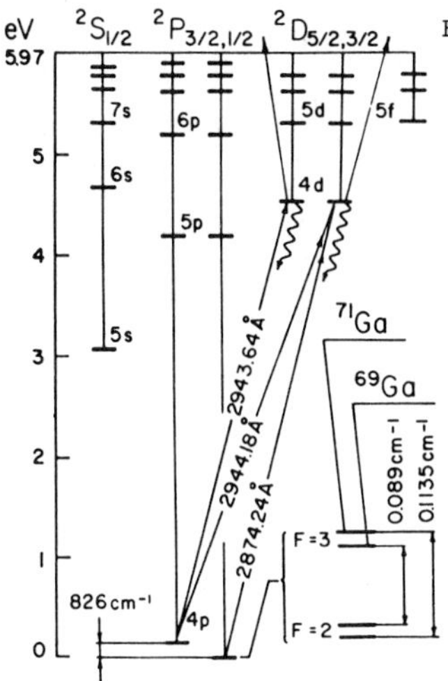


Fig. 1. Energy level diagram of the gallium atom

The ground state of these atoms is split into two components with $\Delta\nu_{f.s.}$ equal to 112.04 cm$^{-1}$ for Al, 826.19 cm$^{-1}$ for Ga, and 2212.56 cm$^{-1}$ for In. At a vapor temperature of T = 1600 K, the population density of the $^2P_{3/2}$ state comes to 60% in Al, 32% in Ga, and 10% in In. Because of hyperfine interaction, the $^2P_{1/2}$ state is split into two components with $\Delta\nu_{hf.s.}$ equal to 0.048 cm$^{-1}$ for Al, 0.113 cm$^{-1}$ for $^{71}$Ga, and o.38 cm$^{-1}$ for $^{115}$In.

With the laser linewidth being in excess of the hyperfine splitting, the effect of the latter on the excitation kinetics can be disregarded.

The radiation wavelength corresponding to the first transitions is approximately equal to 309 nm for Al, 294 nm for Ga, and 325 nm for In.

The transition from the excited $^2$D state into the continuum can be induced by a radiation with a wavelength shorter than 630 nm for Al, 736 nm for Ga, and 725.8 nm for In. The ionization of these atoms can also be effected through the Rydberg states, but in this case, a powerful, narrow-band radiation of a longer wavelength is necessary. In our experiments, we have ionized these excited atoms through the continuum by using the copper-vapor laser emission.

## 4. Experimental Setup

A schematic of the experimental setup is shown in Fig. 2. To pump the dye oscillator-amplifier system, use was made of a commercial copper-vapor laser [7] operated in an oscillator-amplifier mode. The average pump power reached 26.5 W at a pulse repetition frequency of 8 pps (pulse duration = 16 ns). The beam divergence was less than $10^{-4}$ radians.

The copper-vapor laser emission at 510.6 nm was used to pump the dye laser and that at 578.2 nm, to photoionize the selectively excited atoms. The laser cavity was formed by a glass wedge and a Littrow grating. A transverse pumping scheme was used to excite the dye. Arranged in the cavity were a six-prism beam expander, a Fabry-Perot interferometer, and a spherical lens to correct the beam divergence. With the interferometer base equal to 2 mm, the oscillation linewidth was $\Delta\nu_{osc}$ = 0.1 cm$^{-1}$.

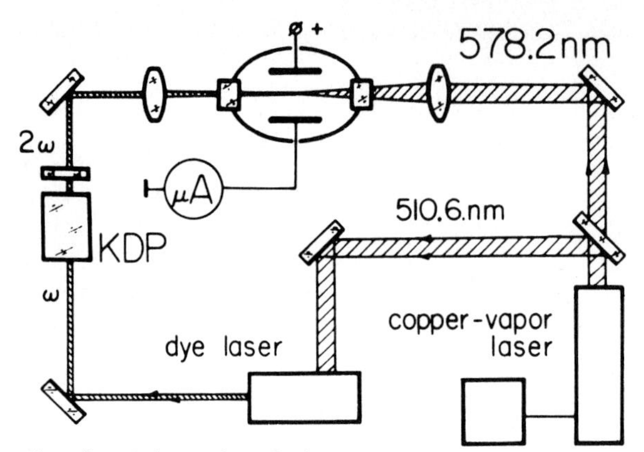


Fig. 2. Schematic of the experimental setup

The dye laser emission was amplified, so that the average output power could reach 1 W. The conversion efficiency typically was 10%. This emission was frequency-doubled by means of a KDP crystal. The UV radiation power was 20 mW at a conversion efficiency of 5%.

The yellow-line emission of the copper-vapor laser and the UV radiation emerging from the KDP crystal were focused into a vacuum chamber, so that both beams were 1 mm in diameter in the region of their interaction with the atomic source shown in Fig. 3. A BN crucible 8 mm in diameter and 23 mm high was placed in a tantalum heater supplied with an alternating current via water-cooled conductors. The crucible was covered by a graphite diaphragm with a rectangular slit 0.5 x 5 $mm^2$ in size. Boron nitride is not wettable with molten Ga or In, but is wettable with molten Al. Therefore, in the case of Ga and In, there was no metal escaping up the crucible walls. A metal shield with a 2 x 20 $mm^2$ slit was arranged 5 mm distant from the graphite diaphragm.

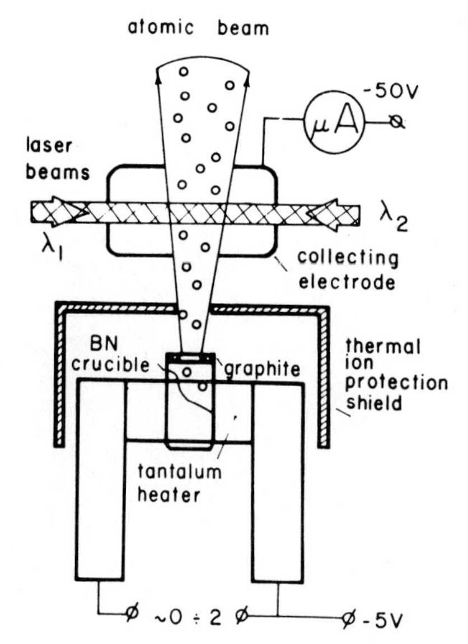


Fig. 3. Evaporator for producing atomic vapor and the photoion detection system

A 4 V dc voltage was applied to the shield to trap thermal ions. The laser beams were made to pass 5 mm above the shield. Photoions were collected on an electrode and the photocurrent was measured with a microammeter. The vacuum chamber was evacuated to $10^{-7}$ Torr by means of a magnetodischarge pump.

## 5. Results

Figure 4 shows the dependence of the In ion current on the evaporator temperature. The current was governed by the degree of radiation absorption at the first stage. With complete absorption of the first-stage photons, the average ion current amounted to 100 μA. Note that the ion current attained is acceptable for thin-film applications, since it provides a film deposition rate of around one monoatomic layer per second per square centimeter.

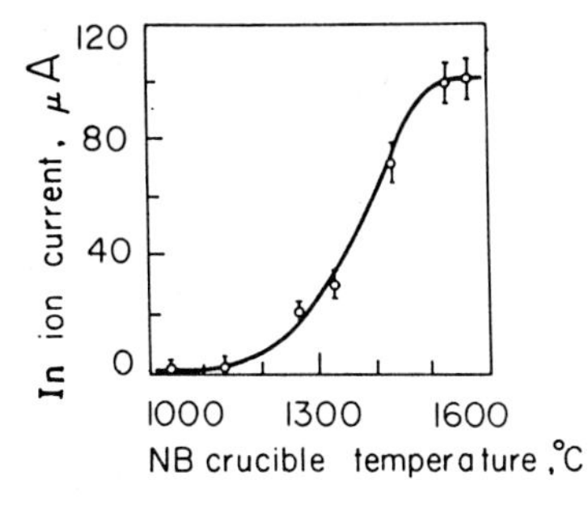


Fig. 4. Dependence of In photoion current on the crucible temperature*

The photoion current for Ga and Al was about 1.5 μA. In the case of Ga, only a small photoion current resulted from the insufficient average power of the exciting and ionizing laser radiations used at the first stage of the work [9]. The Al photoion current was low because of the Al atomic vapor density being limited as a result of the molten metal escaping up the crucible walls.

The selectivity of photoionization was investigated using Ga, with the dye laser wavelength being detuned from resonance by an amount much in excess of the laser linewidth. In this case, the photocurrent signal was detected by means of a secondary electron multiplier. With the laser wavelength out of resonance, the photocurrent was reduced by a factor of around $10^{10}$.

To determine the degree of purification, the crucible was charged with a series of samples containing 50% In and 50% Me, where Me stands for a metallic impurity. The photoion-beam-deposited In films were investigated by Auger electron spectroscopy and low-energy ion backscattering analysis. The concentrations of Ba, Ga, and Al in indium films were below the sensitivity level of the investigation methods used, i.e. they were below 0.1%. The separation factor thus exceeded $10^3$.

The crystalline structure of the photoion-beam-deposited In films [10] was also studied. An $In^+$ photoion beam with an ion energy of 200 eV was focused onto the surface of a single-crystal NaCl substrate. The photoion

---

*These data were obtained by Mikhail A. Muchnik [8].

current density was in the range 2-5 μA/cm$^2$, and the deposition time was such that films around 5000 Å in thickness were formed, which was adequate for electron microscopy investigations. The residual gas pressure in the vacuum chamber was maintained at $10^{-4}$ Torr. Indium films deposited from ion beams always had a polycrystalline structure, even with the substrate at room temperature. In contrast, similar films deposited from atomic beams onto a cold substrate were amorphous, and it was only when the temperature of the substrate was as high as 400 K that the films showed a crystalline structure.

## LASER RESONANCE PHOTOIONIZATION DETECTION OF IMPURITIES

The method of laser atomic photoionization analysis in a vacuum [11], which has been intensively developed in the last few years, has considerable promise for checking the content of impurities in high-purity substances. With direct analysis by this method, the threshold of detectability attained was as low as $10^{-10}$% for the Na content in CdS [12] and $10^{-9}$% for the Al content in Ge [13]. The factors limiting the sensitivity of the method were the nonselective ion background resulting from the laser multiphoton ionization of the atomic or molecular beams of substances being analyzed and, in part, the source-generated thermal ions that had managed to pass by the ion protection shield. Also where the absorption lines of the impurity and the host substance are relatively close, multistep photoionization of the host atoms or molecules due to line-wing absorption is inevitable, resulting in an additional ion background.

Proposed in this work is a method for substantially increasing the selectivity of laser photoionization detection of a small number of some atoms against the background of a large number of other atoms or molecules. In essence, the method consists in the following. Referring to Fig. 5, the atoms of the desired species that are present in a beam or vapor of atoms of another species are excited in several steps to the Rýdberg state by laser pulses. Following the laser action, the medium between the electrodes will contain the Rydberg atoms of the desired element along with extraneous ions, such as thermal ions and ions produced as a result of the laser multiphoton or multistep ionization of undesirable atoms. A negative pulse is then applied to the electrodes to produce an electric field with a strength lower than the critical field strength required to ionize the Rýdberg atoms. Under the effect of this pulse, all the extraneous ions accelerate towards the

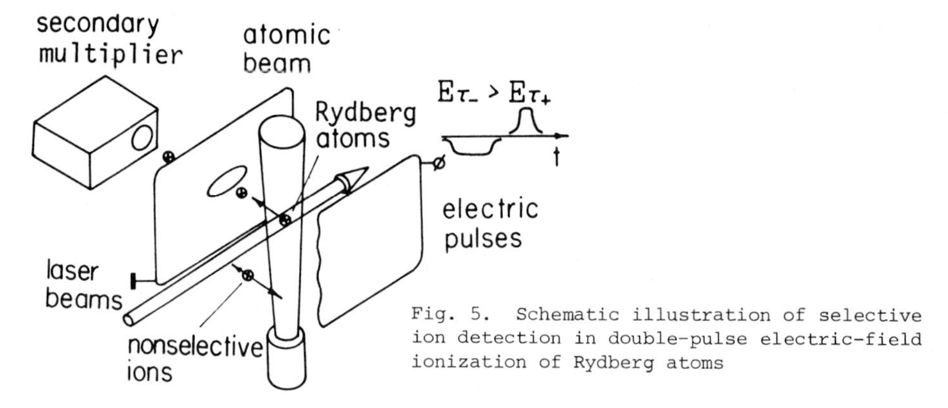


Fig. 5. Schematic illustration of selective ion detection in double-pulse electric-field ionization of Rydberg atoms

solid electrode. The influence of such a pulse on the Rydberg atoms is negligible. A short time after the negative pulse has ceased, a positive pulse is applied to the electrodes, the spacing between the negative and positive pulses and their durations being much shorter than the Rydberg state lifetime. The amplitudes $\mathcal{E}$ and durations $\tau$ of the pulses are selected so as to satisfy the condition

$$\mathcal{E}_- \tau_- > \mathcal{E}_+ \tau_+ \,.$$

In this case, under the effect of the second pulse, the nonselective ions will merely slow down their movement, and it is only the ions produced from the Rydberg atoms that will accelerate in the field of the second pulse, pass through the slit in the other electrode, and reach the ion detector. Thus, extracting from the excitation region only the ions of the desired species will materially improve the selectivity of ion detection as compared with that attainable with a single-pulse ionization. With this method, the selectivity of ion detection can be increased by three to four orders of magnitude.

The above method was used for trace analysis of boron in high-purity germanium. The boron atoms were excited by laser radiation to the Rydberg state in the following two steps (Fig. 6):

$$B(2^2P_{1/2}) \xrightarrow{\lambda_1 = 249.68\ \text{nm}} B(3^2S_{1/2}) \xrightarrow{\lambda_2 = 378.35\ \text{nm}} B(17p) \xrightarrow{\text{electric pulse}} B^+ .$$

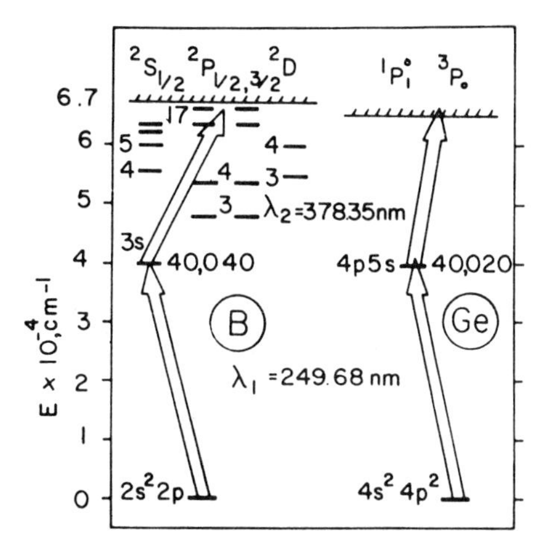


Fig. 6. Schematic energy-level diagram for resonance ionization of B atoms to the Rydberg state and nonresonance ionization of Ge atoms

The first-stage UV radiation pulses with an energy of about 1 μJ were obtained by frequency-doubling the output of a tunable dye (Coumarin-307 solution in ethanol) laser with a lithium formate crystal. The second-stage dye laser used a PBD solution in dioxane. The ionization scheme and laser radiation parameters used provided for about 10 % efficiency of ionization of boron atoms. Comparison between the energy level diagrams of the B and Ge atoms shows that germanium has a resonance line close to $\lambda_1$. The absorption of the first-stage laser radiation in the wing of this line results in the excitation of the Ge atoms into the $4s^24p5s\,^1P_1^0$ state, and the photon energy of the second-stage laser radiation ( $\lambda_2$ = 378.35 nm) is sufficient to ionize the germanium atoms from the $^1P_1^\circ$ level. Estimation of the selectivity of excitation of B atoms among Ge atoms, made according to the formula $S = 2(\Delta\omega)^2/\Delta\omega_{osc}\Gamma$[4] taking into account the transition oscillator forces, yields a value of about $10^6$ which is inadequate for nonresonance photoionization analyis of high-purity germanium containing from $10^{-4}$ to $10^{-7}$% B. The use of the double-pulse ionization method (pulse parameters $\mathcal{E}_- = 5$ kV/cm, $\tau_- = 30$ ns, $\mathcal{E}_+ = 7$ kV/cm, $\tau_+ = 10$ ns) made such a high-selectivity analysis possible. The detection method and experimental setup components remained basically the same as in [13].

A 10-mg germanium sample was placed in a graphite crucible annealed at t = 2500°C beforehand. The sample was then vaporized in a vacuum ($2 \times 10^{-6}$ Torr) at a temperature around 1700°C. By virtue of the different thermodynamic properties of germanium and boron, it was mainly germanium that evaporated at first, causing the concentration of boron in the remaining melt to rise gradually. Twenty minutes later, the temperature of the crucible was increased to 2200°C to vaporize effectively the germanium residue rich in boron. Figure 7 shows the relationships between the ion detector (secondary electron multiplier) current and the evaporation time at t = 2200°C for (a) an empty crucible, (b) a germanium sample (9.5 mg) containing $2 \times 10^{-8}$% B, and (c) a germanium sample (10 mg) containing $2\times 10^{-7}$% B. It is clear from comparison between the curves (b) and (c) that the ratio between the boron yields in these two cases is close to 10. Thus, the recorded signals reflect mainly the content of boron in the bulk of the sample and not in crucible surface contaminations. The absolute calibration of the entire detection system [12] against a reference boron beam showed that the integrated signal for the case (b) corresponded to almost complete escape of boron from the sample. All this supports the conclusion that the above analysis was correct. The factor limiting the sensitivity of the analysis in this experiment were traces of boron remaining in the crucible after annealing. Improving the effectiveness of ionization of B atoms by increasing the energy of the second-stage laser pulse, as well as improving the preliminary annealing of the crucible to free it from boron impurities, will enable one to realize the sensitivity of detection of boron in germanium at a level of $10^{-9}$%.

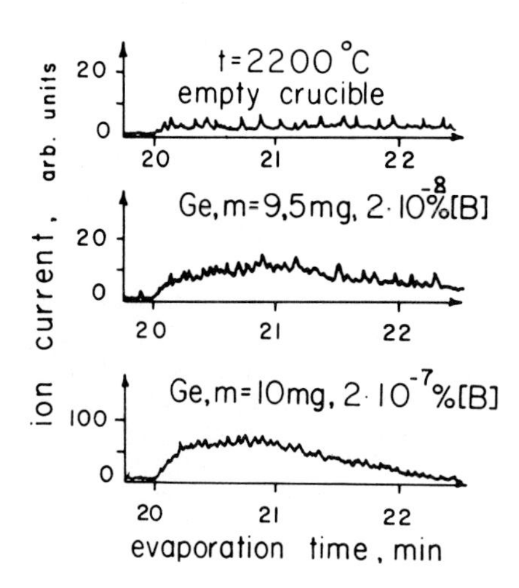


Fig. 7. Boron ion current as a function of evaporation time

Acknowledgements

The authors wish to thank M. A. Muchnik, E. Ya. Chernyak, and V. N. Radaev for their active participation in the experiments.

References

1. J. Amano: Thin Solid Films 92, 115 (1982)
2. V. S. Letokhov: Spectroscopy Lett. 8, 697 (1975)
3. V. S. Letochov and C. B. Moore: "Laser Isotope Separation", in Chemical and Biochemical Applications of Lasers, Vol. 3, ed. C. B. Moore (Academic, 1977) pp. 1-177
4. V. S. Letokhov, V. I. Mishin, and A. A. Puretsky: in "Progress in Quantum Electronics", Vol. 5 (Pergamon Press, Oxford, New York 1977) p. 139
5. J. I. Devis and E. B. Rockower: IEEE J. of Quantum Electronics QE-18, 233 (1982)
6. A. A. Isaev, G. Yu. Limerman: Sov. Kvantovaja Electron. 4, 1413 (1977)
7. V. A. Burmakin, A. P. Evtyunin, and M. A. Lesnoy: Sov. Kvantovaja Electron. 6, 1589 (1979)
8. M. L. Muchnik, Yu. V. Orlov, G. D. Parshin, E. Ya. Chernyak, V. S. Letokhov, and V. I. Mishin: Sov. Kvantovaja Electron. 10, 2331 (1983)
9. A. N. Zherikhin, V. S. Letokhov, V. I. Mishin, M. L. Muchnik, and V. N. Fedoseev: Appl. Phys. B30, 47 (1983)
10. V. S. Letokhov, V. I. Mishin, M. L. Muchnik, Yu. V. Orlov, and E. Ya. Chernyak: Sov. Kvantovaja Electron. 10, 1963 (1983)
11. G. I. Bekov and V. S. Letokhov: Appl. Phys. 30, 161 (1983)
12. R. Akelov and G. I. Bekov: Sov. Pis'ma JETP 13, 305 (1971)
13. R. Akelov, G. I. Bekov, V. S. Letokhov, G. A. Maximov, V. I. Mishin, V. N. Radaev, and V. N. Shishov: Sov. Kvantovaja Electron. 9, 1859 (1982)

# Optical Microanalysis of Device Materials and Structures[1]

S.R.J. Brueck

Lincoln Laboratory, Massachusetts Institute of Technology
Lexington, MA 02173-0073, USA

## I. Introduction

A vast array of optical techniques has been applied to diagnostics of semiconductor materials. A partial list of techniques includes absorption, photoluminescence, Raman scattering, ellipsometry, and nonlinear optical measurements. These measurements all depend on detecting optical signals generated through the interaction of light with the semiconductor material. Therefore, they are generally nondestructive and do not require special fabrication steps such as are required for electrical characterization. Often, optical diagnostics can be used at various stages during device fabrication and can probe the material changes induced during the processing. These techniques are also sensitive to the local environment within the sample and provide state specific information in contrast to ion and electron spectroscopies which are sensitive to atomic concentrations but often do not provide detailed information on internal energy levels and lattice structures. Additional information can be obtained from photoconductivity or photoacoustic techniques where the excitation is optical but the detection is through the electrical or acoustic properties of the material. These techniques are often more sensitive than all-optical measurements, but require additional contact with the material.

In this contribution, results for Raman measurements of stress in silicon-on-insulator and silicon-on-sapphire structures and for Raman measurements of thin crystalline Si films are discussed. Recent developments in surface photoacoustic spectroscopy which lead to a sensitivity to an absorbance of less than $2 \times 10^{-8}$ are also discussed.

Additional effects arise when these techniques are applied to samples with surface structures on the scale of the optical wavelength. The modifications of the electromagnetic boundary conditions associated with these microstructures can dramatically affect the results of the optical experiments. Results for both isolated structures (islands) and periodic surface structures (gratings) are presented.

In photoluminescence measurements, electron hole pairs are excited by radiation above the band gap and recombine via both band-to-band transitions which give information on the energy levels and carrier concentrations and via bound-free and bound-bound transitions which give information on impurity concentrations. Spatial resolutions are limited by both

---

[1]This work was sponsored by the Department of the Air Force, in part under a specific program sponsored by the Air Force Office of Scientific Research.

the wavelength of the exciting laser and carrier diffusion prior to recombination. In high mobility materials this is usually the dominant limitation and varies from ~ 10 μm for n-type GaAs to ~ 1 mm in high-purity Si. Quantitative analysis of impurity concentrations by photoluminescence is complicated by the competition between radiative and nonradiative recombination processes. A recent review of photoluminescence measurements is given by VOOS et al. [1]. Photoluminescence measurements of low-level impurity concentrations in Si [2] and of deep defects in III-V compounds [3] have been reviewed, as have the extensive measurements of luminescence from excitons in quantum-well heterostructures [4].

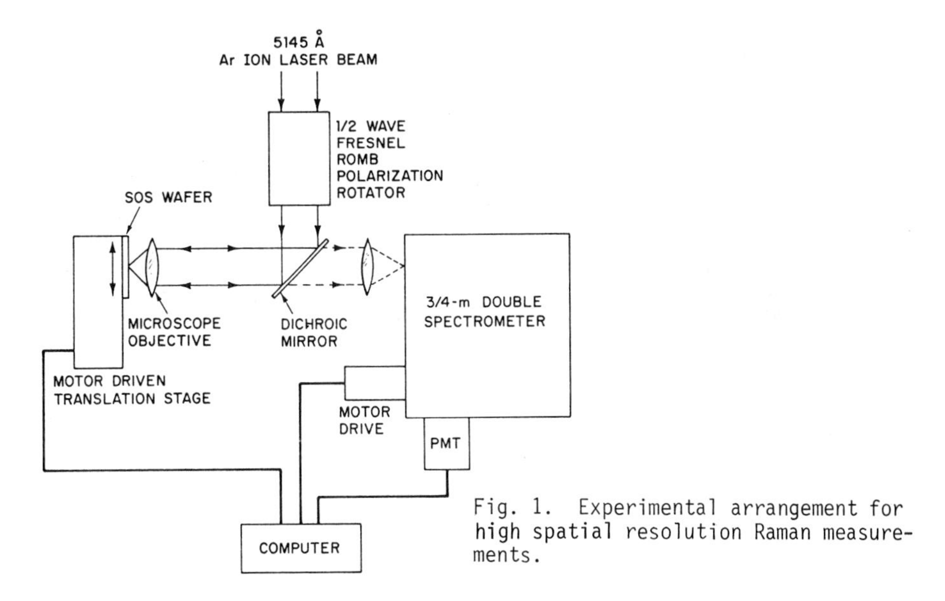


Fig. 1. Experimental arrangement for high spatial resolution Raman measurements.

Figure 1 shows a typical Raman scattering arrangement. A backscattering configuration, which provides a spatial resolution of the order of the laser wavelength, is shown. Raman scattering from optical phonons provides a probe for a number of important material parameters [5-7], including:

1) crystallinity - there are large differences between the Raman intensities and lineshapes of amorphous and single crystal materials. Intermediate lineshapes have been reported and attributed to very fine grain crystal structures. Some results on Raman scattering from very thin films of Si, as thin as 3 nm, will be presented below.

2) defect density - increased phonon scattering from lattice defects results in a shorter phonon lifetime and a broadened Raman linewidth;

3) strain - lattice strains affect the phonon energy and shift the Raman line. An example of spatially resolved analysis of strain variations at the edges of silicon-on-sapphire materials will be given later. Strain variations also affect electronic energy levels and occupations and hence carrier mobilities.

4) composition - for ternary and quaternary compounds the lattice frequencies and linewidths probe the composition and disorder.

For III-V compounds there is a coupling between the longitudinal optical phonon and the electron plasmon which provides information on the electronic properties. Measurements of the electron concentrations, mobility scattering times and surface depletion widths are possible. Raman measurements of the electronic properties in III-V bulk and heterostructure materials have recently been reviewed [8].

Raman cross sections are more readily quantified than luminescence intensities. However, care must be taken with the surface quality of the semiconductor. Damage layers can drastically affect the optical penetration and hence the signal strengths. Sensitivities in very small spatial regions are limited by local heating and carrier injection effects; low powers (~ 1-10 mW) must be used. The sensitivity of the Raman process can be enhanced by exploiting resonance effects between the incident laser energy and energy levels of the semiconductor material [9].

Ellipsometry relies on the measurement of changes in polarization of an incident optical beam upon interaction with the medium. Numerous configurations have been developed and recently reviewed [10,11]. Extensive studies of the wavelength dependent dielectric functions of thin metal and dielectric films as well as of bulk semiconductors have been reported [12,13]. Sensitivity to submonolayer adsorbed molecular films and to changes in the surface contamination of semiconductor surfaces following various surface cleaning treatments have been reported [14]. Ellipsometric measurements are routinely used for monitoring the thickness and dielectric constants of the thin oxide and nitride films used in semiconductor processing. Measurements with a spatial resolution approaching the laser wavelength have recently been reported [15].

Nonlinear optical probes of semiconductor properties are comparatively recent and have not yet been as fully developed as the more traditional probes. The most studied effect is second harmonic generation at surfaces and interfaces. Sensitivity to submonolayer molecular adsorbates and to the underlying material symmetry have been demonstrated [16]. Nearly degenerate four-wave mixing experiments which probe fast electron dynamics such as intraband energy relaxation and intervalley scattering have been reported [17]. Because of the weak signals and high laser intensities required for these measurements, they have not been applied to small spatial regions.

Photoacoustic measurements, in which acoustic waves generated by the conversion of absorbed energy in the electronic system to thermal energy and hence to acoustic waves, provide a very sensitive probe of weak absorptions at surfaces [18-20]. Some recent improvements in the measurements sensitivity using surface acoustic wave detection are presented below; submonolayer coverages of highly absorbing molecules such as dyes are readily detected. Techniques for temporarily bonding semiconductor substrates to SAW transducers have been developed so that elaborate sample preparation is not required. The spatial resolution is now limited by the acoustic wavelength which is typically 10-20 μm.

## 2. Raman Measurements

The experimental arrangement shown in Fig. 1 has been used for the measurement of stress profiles in silicon-on-insulator device structures. The 514.5-nm argon-ion pump laser was reflected from a dichroic mirror and focused onto the substrate with a 60X-microscope objective. A spot size of less than 1-μm diameter was inferred from the measured scattering intensity profiles. Typically, laser powers of less than 2 mW, corresponding to power densities of 500 $kW/cm^2$, were used. The backscattered Raman light was collected with the same objective, transmitted through the dichroic filter, analyzed with a 3/4-m computer-controlled double monochromator and detected with a small-area, S-20 surface, photomultiplier using photon-counting electronics. The computer also controlled a stepper-motor driven stage which was used to translate the sample across the laser focal plane with steps as small as 0.25 μm; Raman spectra were obtained at each position. These spectra were then analyzed to obtain the intensity, phonon frequency, and linewidth as a function of position. Raman spectra of (100) bulk Si were taken following each spatial scan and served as a calibration standard.

The devices were fabricated on silicon-on-sapphire and silicon-on-insulator wafers,with regions defined by both complete island etch (CIE) and coplanar techniques being investigated [21]. Figure 2 shows the Raman parameters measured in a scan across a 6-μm wide Si stripe on a fused quartz substrate fabricated by the CIE technique [22]. The penetration depth of the laser radiation is comparable to the Si thickness so the measurement probes the entire Si film. The integrated intensity of the Raman scattering signal is shown in the top trace; the rapid changes in intensity at the edges of the stripe indicate that a spatial resolution of $< 1$ μm has been achieved. The corresponding Raman frequencies are shown in the middle curve. As a result of the tensile stress of the silicon/quartz system the Raman frequencies are shifted to a lower frequency than that of bulk Si. A significant reduction in the stress is found near the edges of the stripe. The bottom trace shows the measured Raman linewidths. The increased linewidth at the edges of the stripe is due to inhomogeneities in the Raman frequency and does not appear to be due to increased scattering. Raman measurements of stress in silicon-on-insulator structures have also been reported by LYON _et al._ [23].

Raman parameters obtained for scans across 2-μm-wide SOS stripes fabricated by the CIE technique are displayed in Fig. 3. The noteworthy feature of these measurements is that the phonon frequency was nearly constant across the stripe and was strongly shifted from the large area SOS frequency of 524.6 $cm^{-1}$ toward that of bulk Si at 522.1 $cm^{-1}$. This corresponds to a 65% relaxation of the compressive stress across the entire width of the structure.

The observation of local stress variations extending as far as 1.5 μm from the edges of Si stripes in silicon-on-insulator and silicon-on-sapphire device structures clearly demonstrates the changes in materials parameters accompanying submicrometer fabrication and the sensitivity of these changes to the processing techniques used. Raman scattering has been shown to be a useful diagnostic tool for nondestructively probing these changes with micrometer resolution.

Raman spectra have frequently been employed to characterize the crystal quality of annealed Si films [22,23]. Typically, material exhibiting spectra that are broadened and asymmetrically shifted to lower frequencies than bulk Si are ascribed to small crystallite size, to inhomogeneous stress distributions, and to increased phonon scattering at grain boundaries. Unfortunately, a clear relationship between these parameters and the observed Raman spectra has not been theoretically or experimentally established. In an effort to assess the relative importance of purely dimensional effects on the Raman spectrum, we have made a study of the

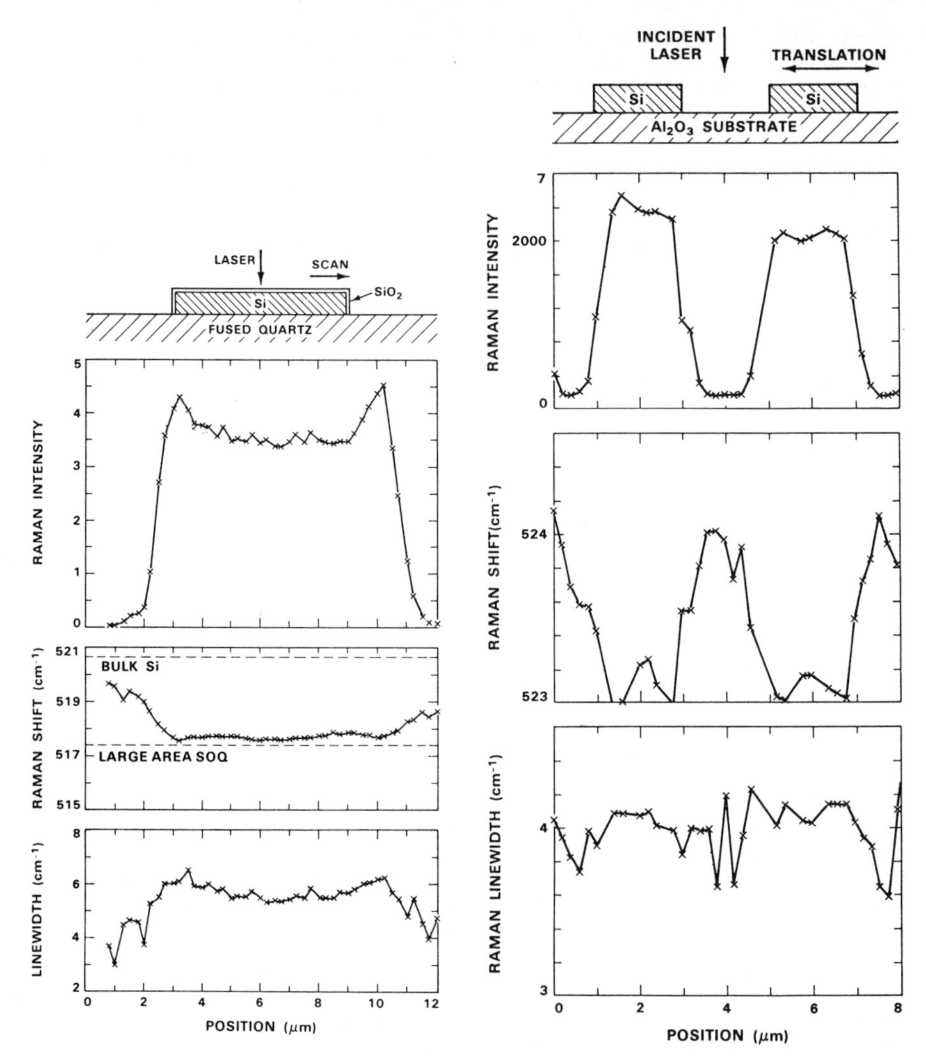


Fig. 2. Raman parameters measured for a Si-on-fused quartz stripe. Each data point corresponds to a 0.25-μm translation of the sample.

Fig. 3. Raman measurements for 2-μm wide SOS stripes.

effect of finite sample size on the Raman spectrum for films which have macroscopic transverse dimensions but are very thin, down to 3 nm, in the beam propagation direction. Films were prepared by oxidizing commercially grown SOS wafers until a very thin Si layer remained under a $SiO_2$ cap. Film thicknesses were determined by fitting the interference fringes apparent for the oxide-Si-sapphire structure.

As the film thickness decreases the Raman spectra broaden asymmetrically and shift to lower frequencies. Experimental results for the film thickness variation of the Si Raman linewidth are shown in Fig. 4. Dramatic broadening occurs only for thicknesses less than approximately 10 nm. Similar results are obtained both with and after removing the oxide cap layer. Qualitatively, these changes in the Raman spectra can be accounted for by the increasing contribution to the Raman signal of the lower-frequency phonon modes away from the zone-center as the wavevector selection rule is relaxed due to the small dimensions. Quantitative calculations of this effect, however, do not lead to good agreement with the experimental results. This suggests that changes in the phonon dispersion curves and damping coefficients are also important for these thin films.

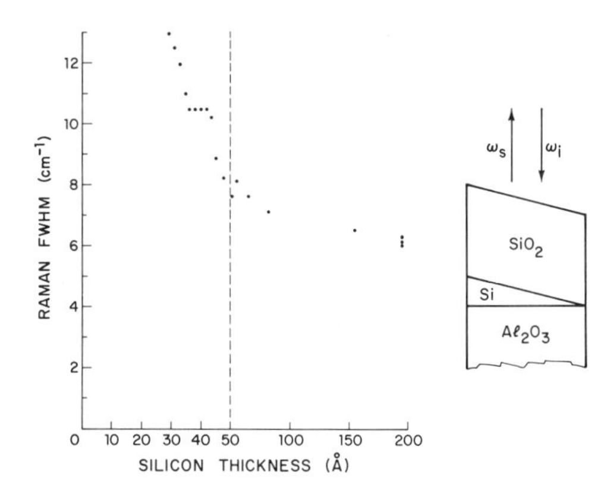


Fig. 4. Variation of the Raman linewidth with thickness for very thin SOS films.

## 3. Surface Photo-Acoustic Spectroscopy

Recently, a number of authors have reported on the detection of surface acoustic waves (SAW) generated on relaxation of energy optically absorbed in thin surface films [18,26]. We have recently extended this technique to the measurement of monolayer and submonolayer coverage surface adsorbates and to the detection of weak absorptions in thin films [20,27]. Both edge-bonded transducers (EBT) and interdigitated transducers (IDT) have been used to detect the SAW signals generated by absorption of the incident laser pulse. For most of the experiments, an EBT was used because its large bandwidth (~ 50 MHz) matched the frequency content of the very short (~ 10 ns) SAW pulses. Using a single line focus, a sensitivity to absorbances of as low as $1 \times 10^{-5}$ of the laser energy was demonstrated in these initial experiments and spectra of monolayer coverage R-590 dye molecules on quartz and $LiNbO_3$ were obtained.

Substantially more laser energy is available, but is not usable in this configuration because of laser damage to the film and substrate. To increase the detection sensitivity we have employed the multiple line image technique illustrated in Fig. 5. A 5-mm diameter collimated laser beam was used to illuminate the absorber which was a thin Au film in this case. The beam was passed through a mask with a 3 x 4 mm shaping aperture and a grating of 25-μm lines and spaces; the illumination pattern on the sample is a series of light and dark lines. This pattern acts like an interdigital transducer to produce a pulse of SAW energy over the entire illuminated area. The time duration of the SAW output shown in the figure simply corresponds to the SAW transit time across the spatial extent of the laser spot. With the grating removed, but still with the shaping aperture, very little high frequency SAW signal is generated. Straightforward signal-to-noise considerations show that this multiple spot technique improves the sensitivity by the square root of the number of cycles in the pattern. This is a factor of 25 for the present parameters. An additional factor of 10 improvement in the signal at constant laser fluence was observed for this multiple line technique. This is probably due to a better coupling to the SAW waves of the present sharply defined 25-μm lines than of the 30-μm Gaussian profile in the single line experiment. These improvements bring the minimum detectable absorbance to $2 \times 10^{-8}$ of the laser energy.

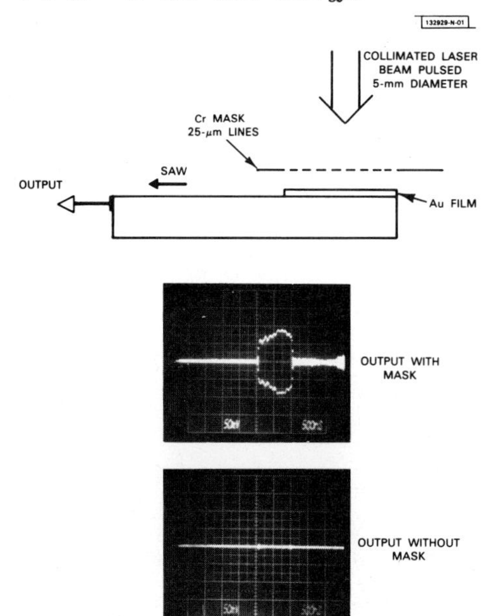


Fig. 5. Multiple line image technique used to improve the sensitivity of surface photoacoustic spectroscopy.

An additional advantage of the multiple pulse technique is the discrimination against the background absorption of the substrate illustrated in the bottom portion of the figure. If the absorber is patterned either lithographically or by laser processing, any unpatterned absorption in the substrate is automatically rejected; discrimination of over four orders of magnitude has been demonstrated. This will allow the investigation of many interesting systems such as adsorbates on metal films in which the substrate adsorption would otherwise mask the desired signals.

## 4. Surface Morphology Effects

The wavelength-scale surface morphology of materials which are being investigated with optical techniques can dramatically affect the local field intensity distribution and the consequent results of optical diagnostics. As optical probes are applied to smaller structures, these effects, which arise as a result of modifications in the electromagnetic boundary conditions due to the surface microstructures, become more important and must be understood in order to interpret the optical measurements properly. Various effects have been demonstrated depending on the material dielectric properties and the spatial frequency scale of the microstructure.

For planar interfaces between dielectric and metallic materials, the relevant surface mode is a surface plasma wave. Most efficient coupling into the radiation field is through a periodic surface structure or grating. This surface plasma wave coupling has been demonstrated to give enhanced Raman scattering from molecular adsorbates on Ag grating surfaces in a manner related to the surface-enhanced Raman scattering (SERS) from rough Ag surfaces [28]. Additionally, in many laser-surface interactions where the laser is actually being used for processing the material, a periodic structure has been found to form due to stimulated scattering of the incident laser radiation into these surface modes. We have previously modeled this process in analogy with stimulated Raman scattering and have calculated small-signal gain coefficients to describe the ripple growth rate for the cases of photodeposition of metal films and of laser-annealing of semiconductors [29,30]. Other workers [31-33] have also carried out detailed measurements and calculations on a number of interesting systems including laser annealing of semiconductors and laser vaporization of both solid and liquid metals. These calculations have shown that there can be significant scattering processes even for dielectric interfaces where there is no surface plasma wave. It is important in modeling these processes to consider the dynamical response of the material system to the laser radiation and to solve the boundary condition problem for the material parameters that exist during the interaction with the laser.

This is illustrated in Fig. 6 which shows the wavevector dispersion for ripples formed during laser irradiation of Ag films. Laser intensities were adjusted to produce a small but visible damage spot on the Ag film with a single laser spot. Typical intensities were 10 J/cm$^2$, sufficient to cause substantial heating and oxidation of the Ag film. The surface plasma wave dispersion curve calculated from the Ag optical constants is also shown in the figure. The ripple wavevector was determined by measuring the Littrow angle for diffraction of a cw-argon laser beam. Experimental points are shown for both single laser shot damage (circles) and multiple (50-100) exposure damage (x's). The experimental points for the single shot ripple formation are in good agreement with the calculated dispersion curve while the experimental points for multiple exposures are

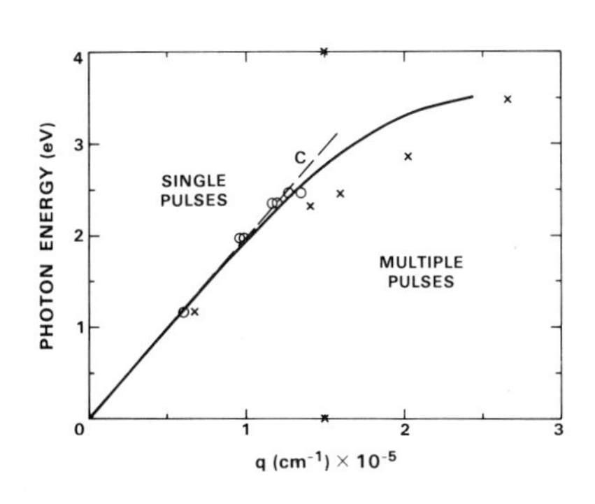


Fig. 6. Wavevector dispersion of the ripples formed during laser irradiation of Ag films. The results of both single (o) and multiple (x) pulse irradiation are shown.

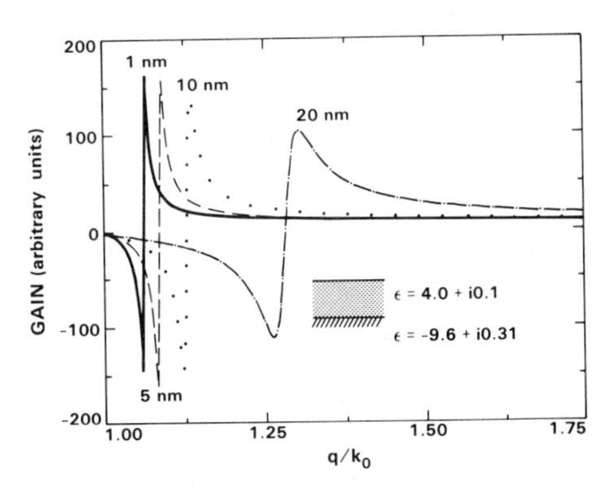


Fig. 7. Calculated gain for stimulated surface plasma wave scattering during irradiation of Ag films. Results are shown with the thickness of an oxide overlayer as a parameter.

systematically at higher spatial frequencies. We interpret this result as being due to the laser-induced formation of an AgO film on the surface. Auger measurements confirm the presence of an oxide overlayer of approximately 20-nm thickness. The effect of this overlayer is to shift the surface plasma wave dispersion curve as is shown in Fig. 7 which displays the calculated small signal gain for ripple formation as a function of the ripple wavevector for several values of the overlayer thickness. Even oxide coatings much less than a wavelength thick have a dramatic effect on the wavevector dependence of the ripple gain and shift the peak in the proper direction to be consistent with the experimental results.

There are also large changes in the local field distributions associated with small dielectric particles where the electromagnetic eigenmodes are related to cavity resonances. The light scattering properties of small dielectric particles show strong resonance effects when the frequency of the incident field approaches one of these eigenfrequencies. Such resonant excitation results in large internal fields and corresponds to sharp features in the absorption [34], scattering [35] and radiation pressure spectra [36] as well as in the luminescence and Raman scattering spectra [37]. Typically, these observations have been restricted to particles with low optical losses and large sizes relative to the optical wavelength. In contrast, laser diagnostic techniques are increasingly being used to probe micrometer and submicrometer sized particles in spectral regions where the materials are highly absorbing. There can also be large enhancements in this case; we have reported recently on enhancements of as much as 100 in the apparent Raman scattering cross section from a variety of Si structures having submicrometer dimensions [38].

For ~ 0.1-μm diameter Si spheroids on a silica substrate formed by strip heater annealing a 50-nm thick Si film deposited by chemical vapor deposition, both one- and two-phonon Raman spectra, taken using 488-nm Ar-ion laser excitation, were essentially identical to the Raman spectra of bulk Si with the significant exception of a factor of 15 greater intensity than that of the bulk Si. Factoring in the greater volume of Si contributing to the bulk signal (penetration depth ~ 750 nm) gives an enhancement per unit volume of ~ 110.

Some insight into this result can be obtained by performing a Mie calculation for the elastic scattering from Si spheres as a function of the particle size parameter. This calculation shows sharp features for small diameter particles which are the result of low order resonances of the first few terms of the Mie expansion and correspond to particle sizes which are resonant with the wavelength. These resonances are washed out at larger sizes due to the large absorption coefficient of Si at visible laser wavelengths. It is straightforward to show that the first peak corresponds to a particle diameter equal to the laser wavelength in the Si and the linewidth scales as $1/n^4$ where n is the Si index of refraction. Thus, these low order resonances are substantially sharper for high index media such as semiconductors than they are for lower index media such as glasses.

In order to calculate the Raman cross section for these spheroids it is necessary to carry out the Mie calculation to evaluate the intensity distribution within the sphere and then to add incoherently the contributions to the Raman scattering from all of the regions within the sphere. Within the approximation that only the first resonance of the magnetic dipole term in the Mie scattering series is important in resonantly enhancing the electromagnetic field strengths, this calculation can be carried out analytically [34]. Just as has been shown for surface-enhanced Raman scattering from rough metal surfaces, there are enhancements in the Raman cross section related to both the incident and scattered fields coupling to the cavity mode of the sphere. The maximum calculated enhancement is ~ 300 for a particle diameter of 110 nm, in good qualitative agreement with the observed value of 110 for a range of particle sizes.

Finally, it is also interesting to consider the effects of microstructure dimensionality on the enhancement. Figure 8 shows the calculated peak electromagnetic intensity enhancements for structures with one dimension comparable to a wavelength (slab), two small dimensions (cylinder), and three small dimensions (a sphere). In agreement with our experimental results, the enhancement is more pronounced for the three-dimensional structure.

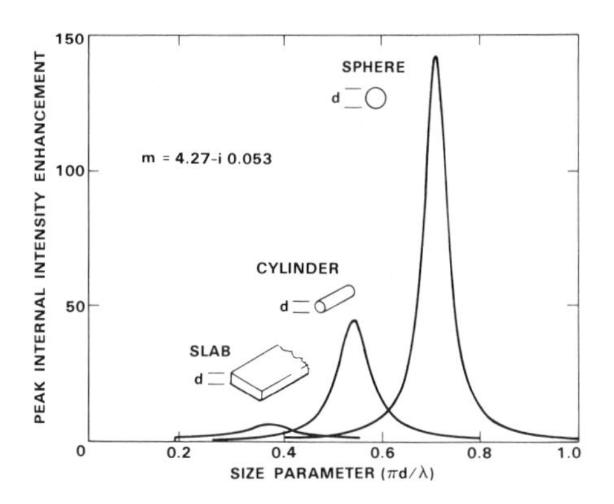


Fig. 8. Calculated internal intensity enhancement for one-, two-, and three-dimensional microstructures.

Substantially greater enhancements should be attained for measurements at wavelengths below the semiconductor bandgap where the attenuation is much lower. In addition, coherent optical processes such as four-wave mixing and second harmonic generation will show larger enhancements than this incoherent Raman process. This suggests that these microstructure enhancements will be very useful for optical device applications. They also clearly affect the results of optical measurements and must be understood in order to interpret properly the results of optical measurements on device structures using wavelengths on the order of the periodicity.

In summary, a very brief overview of a number of the optical techniques used for gaining information about semiconductor materials and devices has been presented. For each technique, the dominant types of information that can be provided and some of the advantages and disadvantages of the measurement were discussed. More detailed examples of two of the techniques, Raman measurements of stress and of the Si film thickness dependence of the Raman lineshape, and surface photoacoustic measurements of weak absorptions in semiconductors and adsorbed films, were presented. Finally, the effects of optical wavelength scale surface morphologies on the interpretation of the optical measurements were discussed.


## Acknowledgment

The work reported here was carried out in collaboration with T. F. Deutsch, D. J. Ehrlich, J. C. C. Fan, D. V. Murphy, D. E. Oates, D. J. Silversmith, J. Y. Tsao and B-Y. Tsaur. Expert technical assistance was provided by L. J. Belanger and R. C. Hancock.

References:


1. M. Voos, R. F. Leheny and J. Shah in Optical Properties of Semiconductors, M. Balkanski, Ed. Volume 2 of Semiconductor Handbook, T. S. Moss, Series Ed. (North-Holland, 1980).
2. M. Tajima, T. Masui, T. Abe and T. Iizuka in Semiconductor Silicon, 1981, H. R. Huff, R. J. Kriegler and Y. Takeishi, Eds. (The Electrochemical Society, 1981), p. 72.
3. U. Kaufman and J. Schneider in Festkorperprobleme XX - Advances in Solid State Physics (Vieweg, 1981), p. 87.
4. C. Weisbuch, J. Luminescence 24/25, 373 (1981).
5. E. M. Anastassakis in Dynamical Properties of Solids Vol. 4, G. K. Horton and A. A. Maradudin, Eds. (North-Holland, 1980), p. 157.
6. R. Tsu in Optical Characterization Techniques for Semiconductor Technology, D. E. Aspnes, S. So and R. F. Potter, Eds. (SPIE, 1981), p. 78.
7. D. V. Murphy and S. R. J. Brueck in Laser Diagnostics and Photochemical Processing for Semiconductor Devices, R. M. Osgood, S. R. J. Brueck and H. R. Schlossberg, Eds. (North-Holland, 1983), p. 81.
8. G. Abstreiter, M. Cardona and A. Pinczuk in Light Scattering in Solids IV, M. Cardona and G. Guntherodt, Eds. (Springer-Verlag, 1984).
9. M. Cardona in Light Scattering in Solids II, M. Cardona and G. Guntherodt, Eds. (Springer-Verlag, 1982).
10. D. E. Aspnes in Optical Properties of Solids: New Developments, B. O. Seraphin, Ed. (North-Holland, 1976), p. 801.
11. P. S. Hauge, Surf. Sci. 96, 108 (1980).
12. D. E. Aspnes, E. Kinsbron and D. D. Bacon, Phys. Rev. B 21, 3290 (1980).
13. D. E. Aspnes and A. A. Studna, Phys. Rev. B 27, 985 (1983).
14. D. E. Aspnes and A. A. Studna in Optical Characterization Techniques for Semiconductor Technology, D. E. Aspnes, S. So and R. F. Potter, Eds. (SPIE, 1981), p. 227.
15. T. Mishima and K. C. Kao, Optical Engineering 21, 1074 (1982).
16. H. W. K. Tom, T. F. Heinz, P. Ye and Y. R. Shen in Laser Spectroscopy VI, H. P. Weber and W. Luthy, Eds. (Springer-Verlag, 1983), p. 289.
17. K. Kash, P. A. Wolff and W. A. Bonner, Appl. Phys. Lett. 42, 173 (1983).
18. A. C. Tam in Ultrasensitive Spectroscopic Techniques, D. Kliger, Ed. (Academic Press, 1983).
19. F. Trager, H. Coufal and T. J. Chuang, Phys. Rev. Lett. 49, 1720 (1982).
20. S. R. J. Brueck, T. F. Deutsch and D. E. Oates, Appl. Phys. Lett. 43, 157 (1983).
21. S. R. J. Brueck, B-Y. Tsaur, J. C. C. Fan, D. V. Murphy, T. F. Deutsch and D. J. Silversmith, Appl. Phys. Lett. 40, 895 (1982).
22. This structure was provided by B-Y. Tsaur.
23. S. A. Lyon, R. J. Nemanich, N. M. Johnson and D. K. Biegelson, Appl. Phys. Lett. 40, 316 (1982).
24. Z. Iqbal, A. P. Webb and S. Veprek, Appl. Phys. Lett. 36, 163 (1980).
25. T. Kamiya, M. Kishi, A. Ushirokawa and T. Katoda, Appl. Phys. Lett. 38, 377 (1981).
26. A. C. Tam and H. Coufal, Appl. Phys. Lett. 42, 33 (1983).
27. D. E. Oates, S. R. J. Brueck and T. F. Deutsch in Ultrasonics Symposium Proceedings 1983, to be published.
28. S. S. Jha, J. R. Kirtley and J. C. Tsang, Phys. Rev. B 22, 3973 (1982).
29. S. R. J. Brueck and D. J. Ehrlich, Phys. Rev. Lett. 48, 1678 (1982).

30. D. J. Ehrlich, S. R. J. Brueck and J. Y. Tsao, Appl. Phys. Lett. 41, 630 (1982).
31. Z. Guosheng, P. M. Fauchet and A. E. Siegman, Phys. Rev. B 26, 5366 (1982).
32. J. E. Sipe, J. F. Young, J. S. Preston and H. M. van Driel, Phys. Rev. B 29, 184 (1983).
33. F. Keilman, Phys. Rev. Lett. 51, 2097 (1983).
34. G. J. Rosasco and H. S. Bennett, J. Opt. Soc. Am. 68, 1242 (1978).
35. P. Chylek, J. T. Kiehl and M. K. W. Ko, Appl. Opt. 17, 3019 (1978).
36. A. Ashkin and J. M. Dziedzic, Phys. Rev. Lett. 38, 1351 (1977).
37. H. Chew and D. S. Wang, Phys. Rev. Lett. 49, 490 (1982).
38. D. V. Murphy and S. R. J. Brueck, Opt. Lett. 8, 494 (1983).

# Laser Diagnostics of Submicron VLSI-Structures

J. Bille, T. Karte, M. Frieben, and A. Plesch

Institute of Applied Physics I, University of Heidelberg
D-6900 Heidelberg, Fed. Rep. of Germany

R.W. Wijnaendts and R. Kaplan

European Molecular Biology Laboratory
D-6900 Heidelberg, Fed. Rep. of Germany

## 1. Introduction.

In spite of the dramatic changes in feature size, die size and defect density, wafer inspection continues to be done manually. However, fast automatic wafer inspection will be a key element for efficient submicron VLSI-process technologies. A new two-step laser scanning procedure is described, resulting in processing speeds of up to 40 million pixels per second and spatial resolution down to 0.1 μm.

## 2. Experimental Arrangement.

The experimental arrangement is described in Fig. 1. In the fast scanning mode (40 MHz), a high speed polygon spinner is applied. The system performs linear and area dimensional as well as registration measurements. By evaluating reflected light of different wavelengths (green, UV) simultaneously, artefacts due to incidental interference effects can be avoided. The polarization-sensitive detection mode allows for calculation of surface dependent parameters. In addition, electrical parameters are obtained by exploiting the OBIC (optical beam induced current) method, where the laser beam induced photo-current is correlated to the laser-scan procedure.

In the second scanning mode of moderate speed (600 kHz) a high resolution confocal imaging technique is used. Confocal scanning microscopy consists of a coherent point source focused with an objective onto the scanned sample and viewed through an identical system with a point detector. This results in superresolution in image plane and in the depth of focus.

The principle of the scanning microscope is shown in Fig. 2. The laser beam illuminates a pinhole which is imaged to a diffraction limited spot by a high numerical aperture, quartz objective (Zeiss, Axiomat ultrafluor 125 x 1,25). The optical path is at rest while the sample is moved in x, y and z through the focus of the objective. Due to the pinhole in the image frame (confocal arrangement) virtually no light from the out of focus object planes is able to reach the reflection detector.

Magnification can be varied continuously by changing the mechanical scan amplitude and ranges between a field of a few microns to a maximum size of 1 mm. Vertically, the maximum scan is 0.2 mm. The electromechanical scanning part is based on a system originally constructed by Brakenhoff et al. [1] and has been described in

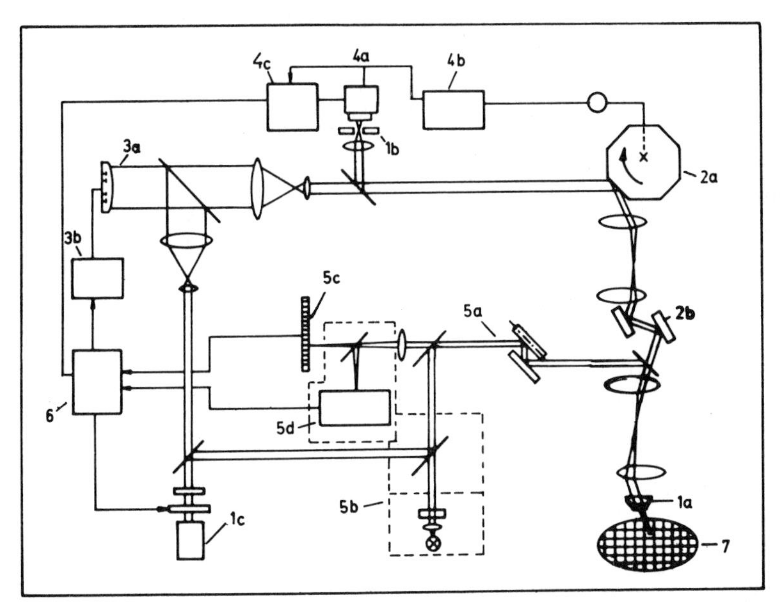


Fig. 1. Laser Scanning Microscope-Fast Scanning Mode
1) Confocal Laser Scan Microscope (1a) Objective Lens, 1b) Confocal Pinhole, 1c) UV Source)
2) X-Y Scanner (2a) X Deflection: Polygon Scanner, 2b) Y Deflection: Galvanometer Scanner or Mechanical Movement
3) Active Focus Control (3a) Active Mirror, 3b) Control Unit)
4) Detection Unit (4a) Photomultiplier, 4b) Synchronisation Logic, 4c) Image Buffer)
5) X-Y Sub-Scanner System (5a) Galvanometer Scanner, 5b) White Light Source, 5c) Diode Array, 5d) Spectrometer)
6) POLYP Multiprocessor System
7) Wafer Stage

detail [ 2 ] . The final image is collected in a frame memory and can be transferred to a large computer system. Two-dimensional images either x, y or x, z can be taken at a speed up to 1 image per second. The laser sources are a synchronously pumped dye laser (frequency doubled and modelocked), an argon ion laser and a helium-neon laser. At an excitation wavelength of 280 nm the system resolution is 0.097 µm in x and y and approximately 0.2 µm in the z direction. The z resolution is useful for the depth profiling of critical structures within integrated circuits.

## 3. Active Focusing of the Scanning Laser Microscope.

The scanning laser microscope (fast scanning mode) is equipped with an adaptive-optical focussing device. In Fig. 3 the four basic elements of an adaptive optical system are shown schematically; e.g. an optical set-up and receiver, a phase error sensor, a servo-control system and an optical phase-shifting element [ 3 ].

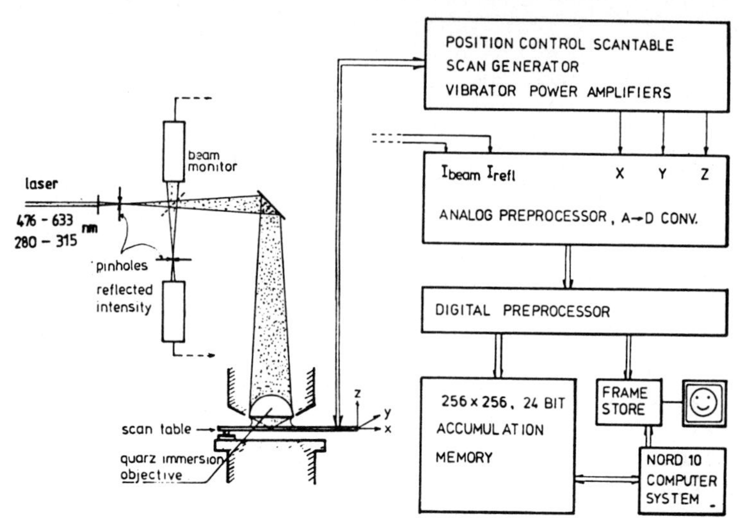


Fig. 2. Principle Diagram of Confocal Scanning Microscope

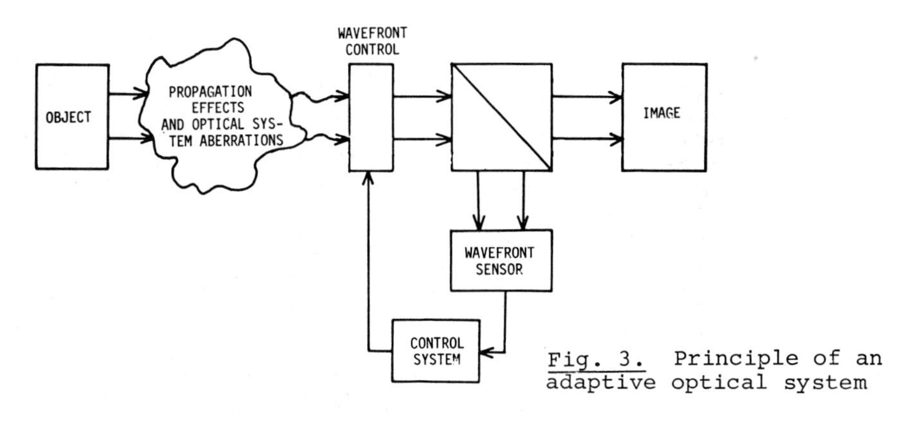


Fig. 3. Principle of an adaptive optical system

The distortion of the received wavefront is compensated by reflecting the laser beam from a deformable membrane mirror, which is electrostatically actuated [ 4 ] . The mirror surface is adjusted in real time to compensate the optical pathlength aberrations. The information required to deform the membrane mirror is obtained by analyzing the point spread function (PSF) of the combined system of the scanning laser microscope and the layer structure of the wafer. For wavefront reconstruction maximum likelihood methods and the Gerchberg-Saxton algorithm are applied [ 5 ] .

In Fig. 4, the iterative procedure for calculation the phase distribution in pupil plane based on the point spread function (PSF) measured in focal plane is shown.

With the wavefront reconstruction a map of wavefront errors at each instant of time is derived. Using this error map, the control system determines the signals required to drive the deformable mirror to null the wavefront errors [6].

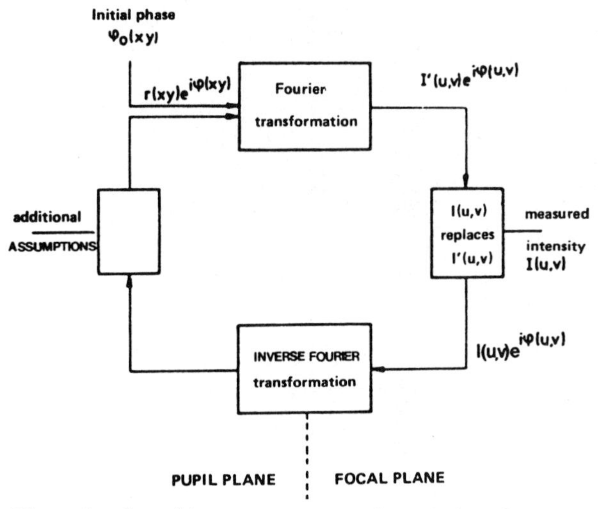


Fig. 4. Gerchberg-Saxton algorithm for wavefront reconstruction

The system essentially provides an elimination of optical aberrations due to refractive index inhomogeneities in the optical path of the focused laser beam. On the other hand, by active focus control layer structures of the wafer can be reconstructed due to their differences in refractive indices.

## 4. Experimental results.

In Fig. 5, the optical reflection (a) and the OBIC (b) images of a section of a 4 kbit-memory chip are shown. The images are recorded in the fast scanning mode (40 MHz).

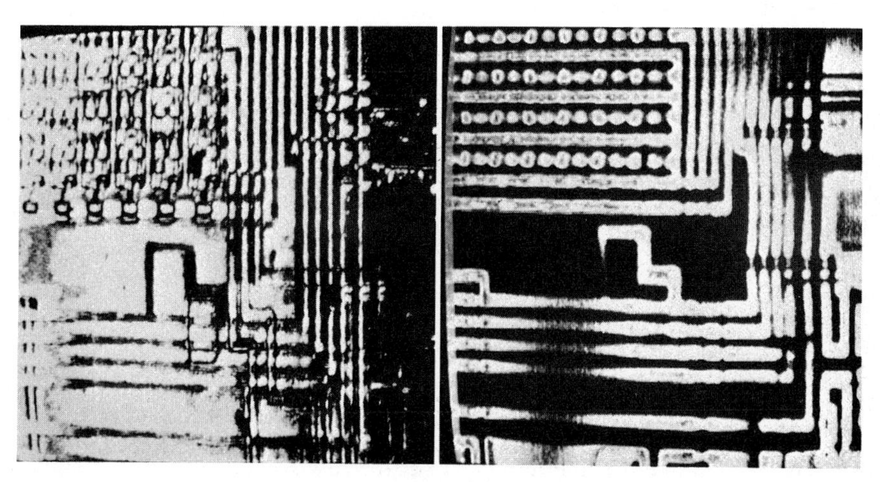

Fig. 5. Optical reflection (a) and OBIC (b) image of 4 kbit chip. Scanning rate: 40 Million pixels/second

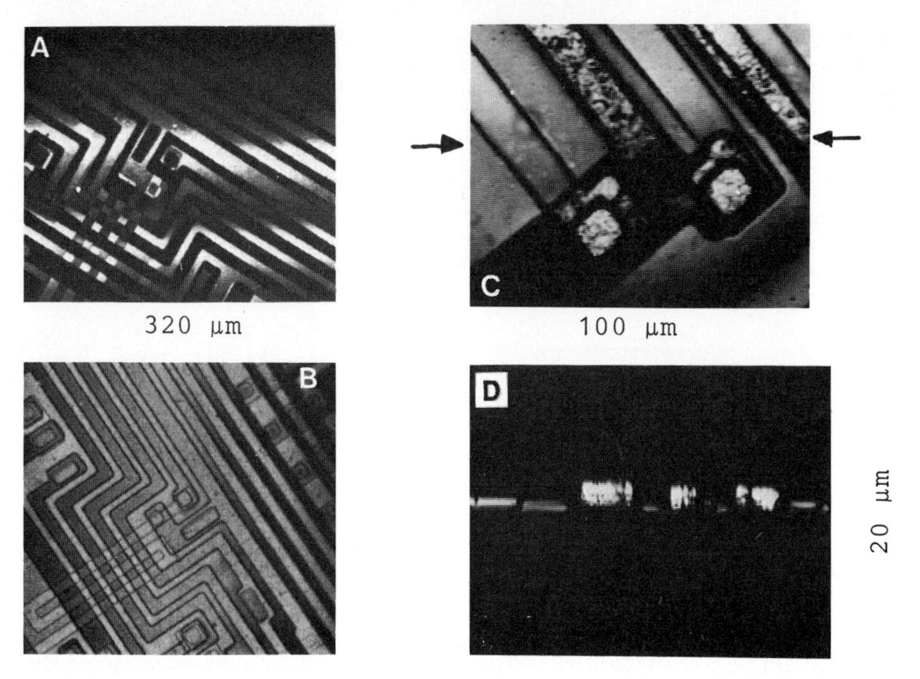


Fig. 6. Images of video IC taken with confocal scanning laser microscope

Figs. 6a and 6b illustrate the confocal effect of the scanning laser microscope. In Fig. 6a virtually no light which reflects from out of focus planes is able to reach the detector. The depth of focus is seen in Fig. 6a where submicron variations in wafer thickness show up in the form of bright and dark areas. In Fig. 6b the detector pinhole is removed and defocussed information is added to the image in Fig. 6a. These images were taken with UV light of 280 nm and a lateral resolution of 0.097 µm. The images shown in Figs. 6c and 6d were taken with an argon-ion laser set at 514 nm and have a somewhat lower resolution of 0.2 µm. Fig. 6d shows the vertical section of the integrated circuit at the positions indicated in Fig. 6c. Note that the vertical scale is not the same as the horizontal in order to show the height differences of the various layers more clearly.

## 5. Concluding Remarks.

In comparison to state of the art wafer inspection systems which usually apply vidicon image processing technology, the confocal laser scanning method combined with fast data processing allows for a factor of ten improvements in data acquisition rates and optical depth resolution.

Especially for linewidth measurements, the evaluation of active optically generated focal series of images in the confocal mode combined with digital 3D-reconstruction procedures [7] provide completely new experimental results.

Contact-free measurements can be made of optical and electronic characteristics of VLSI circuits during different stages of the production process. By mode-locking the laser beam, a sensitive lock-in measuring technique can yield even time resolved data characterizing the properties of electrons and holes as well as the semiconductor material.

## References


[1] G.J. Brakenhoff, P. Blom, and P. Barends, J. Micros. 117, 219-232 (1979)

[2] H.J.B. Marsman, G.J. Brakenhoff, P. Blom, R. Shricker, and R.W. Wijnaendts van Resandt: Rev. Sci. Instruments 54, 1047-1052 (1983)

[3] Hardy, J.W., Proc. IEEE 66, 651 (1978)

[4] Merkle, F., Freischlad, K., Bille, J., Proc. ESO Conference "Scientific Importance of High Angular Resolution at Infrared and Optical Wavelengths", Garching, March 1981, p. 41-52

[5] J. Bille, G. Jahn, A. Dreher Proceedings of the SPIE, Vol. 498 (SPIE's 28th Annual International Technical Symposium, 19-24 August 1984, San Diego, California)

[6] J. Bille, G. Jahn, M. Frieben Proceedings of the SPIE, Vol. 332, 269-275 (1982)

[7] G. Zinser, D. Komitowski, J. Bille Proceedings of the VIth International Congress for Pattern Recognition (ICPR), München (1982), p. 1173-1175

# Determination of the Mechanical Amplitude Distribution of Quartz Crystal Resonators by Use of a New Noninterferometric Laser Speckle Vibration Measurement System

S. Hertl, L. Wimmer, and E. Benes

Institut für Allgemeine Physik, Technische Universität Wien,
Karlsplatz 13/134, A-1040 Wien, Austria

## 1. Introduction

Using quartz crystals as sensors in thickness monitors the knowledge of the distribution of the mechanical vibration amplitude is of particular importance [1]. Basically, the crystals are used to determine the mass load caused by the deposited material for calculating the thickness of the thin film. This measurement is based on the change of the resonance frequency of the quartz crystal due to the mass load. For small mass loads the frequency shift during coating of the crystal is approximately proportional to the change in mass [2].

The ratio of frequency change and mass load $\Delta f/\Delta m$ depends on the type of the quartz crystal used as well as on the area of the deposited film. Unfortunately, the locally varying vibration amplitude influences the contribution of the local mass sensitivity of the crystal. To increase the accuracy in determining film thickness and evaporation rate, it is advisable to beware of the area of non-vanishing vibration amplitude in relation to the diameter of the deposited film which depends on the geometry of the crystal holder.

Looking for a method to measure the in-plane vibration amplitudes of quartz crystals oscillating in thickness-shear mode, which are commonly used as thickness monitors, we have developed a new technique [3] for this purpose. The benefits of this method are a simple mechanical setup being insensitive to environmental disturbances, a high spatial resolution as well as a sensitivity down to the order of some nanometers.

## 2. Principle of Operation

Illuminating a rough surface with laser light results in a granular appearance of the diffusely scattered light. The basic idea of our method is to use this speckle effect to investigate in-plane movements of a surface without using interferometric or holographic techniques. By positioning a photodiode anywhere in the speckle field, the photocurrent is proportional to the intensity of the detected light. An in-plane vibration of the reflecting surface causes an analogous movement of the speckle pattern and thus an amplitude modulation of the photocurrent.

Assuming that the displacement $u(x,y,t)$ of the illuminated spot $(x,y)$ is given by

$$u(x,y,t) = \hat{u}(x,y).\sin(\omega t) \quad (1)$$

where $\omega$ denotes the angular frequency of oscillation, the photocurrent $i(x,y,t)$ can be expressed by

$$i(x,y,t) = I_o(C_1(x,y) + C_2(x,y)\sin(\omega t)) \quad (2)$$

where $I_o$ is the intensity of the laser light. The coefficients $C_1(x,y)$ and $C_2(x,y)$ depend on the illuminated spot $(x,y)$. By averaging the signal of the photodiode at some adjacent points $(x,y)_i$, the following relationship between the averaged signal component $i_\omega(x,y)$ at frequency $\omega$ and the vibration amplitude $\hat{u}(x,y)$ via the constant K can be established [3]:

$$i_\omega(x,y) = \langle I_o C_2(x,y)\rangle = I_o K\hat{u}(x,y). \quad (3)$$

## 3. Experimental Results and Discussion

The principal arrangement of the amplitude measurement device is shown in Fig. 1. The photocurrent is the input signal of a spectrum analyzer, which is locked at the oscillation frequency of the quartz crystal and operates with a bandwidth of about 3 Hz. The data measured by the analyzer are read into the random access memory of a microcomputer via an IEEE-488 interface bus and stored on magnetic disk. The computer also controls two stepper motors to enable a scan across the entire surface of the vibrating object. The spatial resolution of the measurements is limited by the minimum step width of the stepper motors, which is one micrometer.

The vibration amplitude distribution of a plano-convex AT-cut quartz crystal oscillating in fundamental mode, which

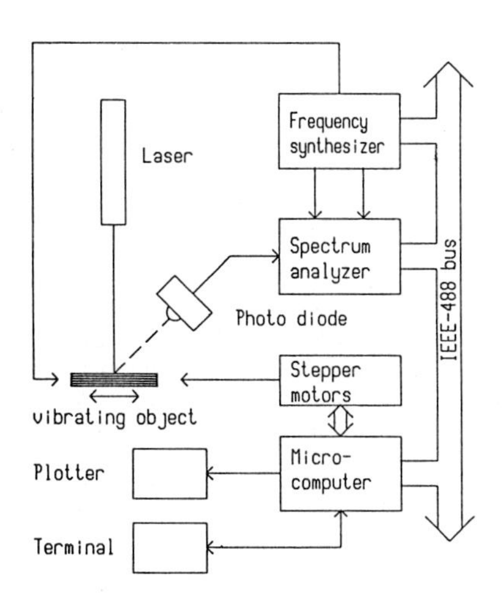


Fig.1: Block diagram of experimental setup

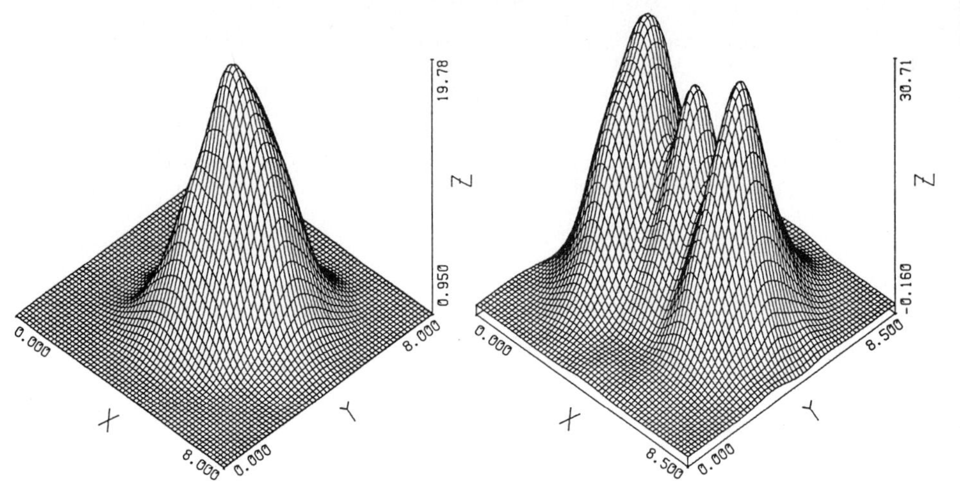


Fig.2: Vibration amplitude distribution of mode (1,1,1)

Fig.3: Vibration amplitude distribution of mode (1,1,3)

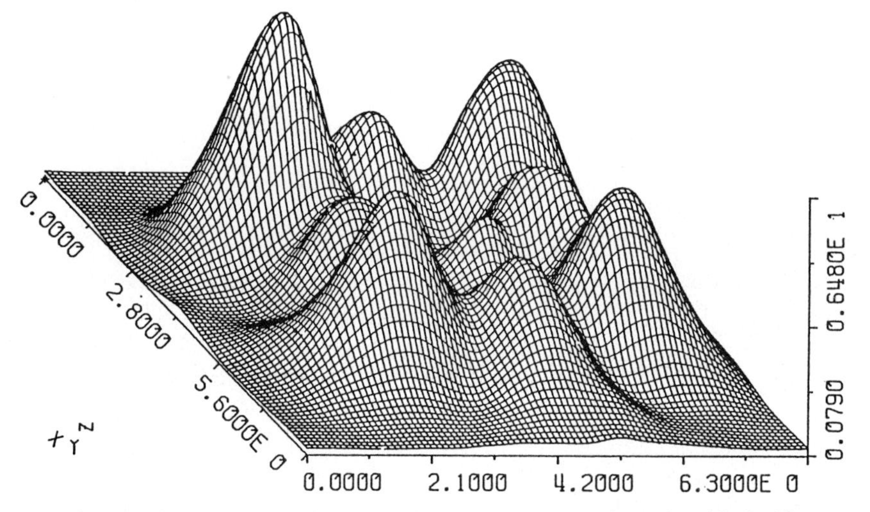


Fig.4: Vibration amplitude distribution of mode (1,3,3)

is identified as (1,1,1) mode according to WILSON [4], is shown in Fig. 2. Figures 3 and 4 present the amplitude distribution of modes (1,1,3) and (1,3,3), respectively.

To compare our measurements of amplitude distributions with theoretical functions derived by WILSON [4] or TIERSTEN [5], we calculated the vibration amplitude distribution of a plano-convex AT-cut quartz crystal as a function of the surface coordinates (x,y). For the thickness-shear mode the only large displacement is parallel to the x axis of the crystal. Neglecting other components the vibration amplitude in the x direction $\hat{u}_x(x,y)$ is given by WILSON [4] (and similarly by TIERSTEN [5]) as

$$\hat{u}_x(x,y) = H_{p-1}(\sqrt{\alpha_n}x)\exp(-\alpha_n x^2/2).$$
$$.H_{q-1}(\sqrt{\beta_n}y)\exp(-\beta_n y^2/2) \quad (4)$$

where $H_r$ denotes the Hermite polynomial of order r, r=0,1,2,3...; (n,p,q) is the mode number; and

$$\alpha_n = (n\pi)\sqrt{c_{66}/(Rl_Q{}^3 c_{11})} \quad (5)$$

$$\beta_n = (n\pi)\sqrt{c_{66}/(Rl_Q{}^3 c_{55})}. \quad (6)$$

The elastic stiffness constants effective for the AT cut are according to MINDLIN [6]:

$c_{11} = 86{,}74 \cdot 10^9$ Pa $\quad c_{55} = 68{,}81 \cdot 10^9$ Pa $\quad c_{66} = 29{,}01 \cdot 10^9$ Pa.

R denotes the radius of curvature of the crystal's convex side; $l_Q$ is the maximum thickness of the quartz crystal.

The results obtained by our calculations are in very good agreement with the experimental data. Figure 5 shows the measured vibration amplitude distribution of mode (1,1,3) using lines of equal amplitude. Figure 6 shows the calculated distribution of the same mode.

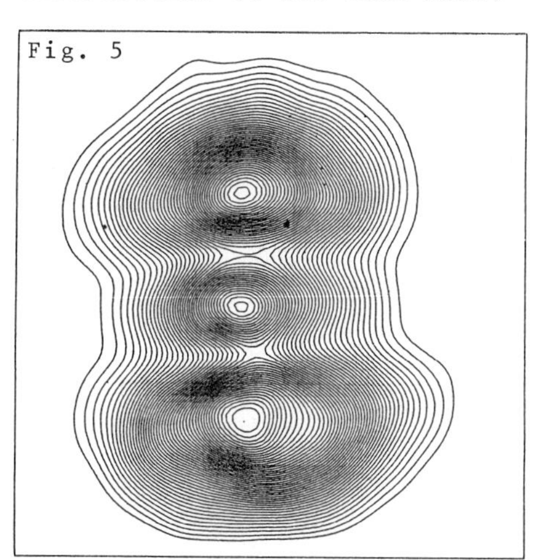


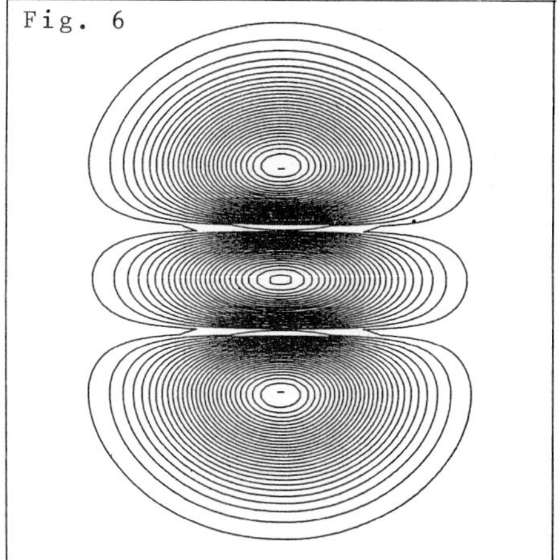


Fig.5: Measured vibration amplitude distribution of mode (1,1,3)

Fig.6: Calculated vibration amplitude distribution of mode (1,1,3)

## 4. Acknowledgements

This work has been sponsored by the Austrian Science Foundation (Österreichischer Fonds zur Förderung der wissenschaftlichen Forschung) under Project No. P4610. The crystal probes were supplied by Leybold-Heraeus/Inficon Inc.

## 5. Literature


1 H.K.Pulker et al. : Thin Solid Films 32 , 27 (1976)

2 C.Lu, O.Lewis: J. Appl. Phys. 43 , 4385 (1972)

3 L.Wimmer et al. : Rev. Sci. Instrum. 55 , 605 (1984)

4 C.J.Wilson: J. Phys. D 7 , 2449 (1974)

5 H.F.Tiersten, R.C.Smythe: Proc. of the 31st Annual Symp. on Frequency Contr. 1977, pp. 44-47

6 R.D.Mindlin: Quart. Appl. Math. 19 , 51 (1961)

# Characterization of Laser Induced Defects in (Al,Ga)As by Photoetching and TEM Measurements

B. Zysset and R.P. Salathé
Institute of Applied Physics, Sidlerstr. 5, CH-3012 Bern, Switzerland

J.L. Martin and R. Gotthardt
Institut de Gênie Atomique, Ecole Polytechnique Fédérale de Lausanne, PHB-Ecublens, CH-1015 Lausanne, Switzerland

F.K. Reinhart
Institut de Physique Appliquée, Ecole Polytechnique Fédérale de Lausanne, PHB-Ecublens, CH-1015 Lausanne, Switzerland

Laser generated defects in (Al,Ga)As have been investigated by photochemical wet etching and TEM measurements. Photoetching reveals a 500 nm wide zone in the center of the processed area where according to laser power either a luminescent or a nonradiative defect is present. In the adjacent regions (~10 μm wide) where the native luminescence is reduced, a third nonradiative defect is probably present. The luminescent defect has an etch rate similar to unprocessed material, the other two an enhanced one.

TEM measurements do not reveal any macroscopic defects (dislocations, microcracks, precipitates,etc.) but 0.5 μm wide lines are detected which show weak strain contrast. The visibility of the lines depends on the sample thinning process. From TEM it is concluded that the three defects are point defects or point defect complexes.

## 1. Introduction

In recent years laser light generated defects have been extensively investigated in III-V compound semiconductor structures [1-3]. Luminescence and electrical properties of the devices are strongly affected by the presence of these defects. Different types of defects can be introduced into semiconductor heterostructures. At very high laser power, these defects normally consist of dark line defects (DLD),i.e., the luminescence efficiency is strongly reduced. It was found that DLD's are mainly formed by extended dislocation networks and a large number of point defects [1]. Recently it was shown that highly efficient luminescence centers can be introduced by strongly focussing cw Kr-ion laser radiation into (Al,Ga)As three-layer structures [4]. Generation of these centers occurs at a critical irradiation density of ~ 0.49 MW/cm$^2$. At a slightly higher intensity of ~ 0.53 MW/cm$^2$ nonradiative defects are produced which strongly reduce the native luminescence efficiency of the material. Generation and properties of these centers are quite different from DLD's and therefore substantial differences in the internal structure have to be expected. In this work we report on photoetching and TEM measurements. The photoetching experiments show that at least two different defects, possibly even three, are generated through the laser processing. TEM measurements show evidence of weak strain contrast in the laser processed zone. No dislocations or microcracks (proposed by [5]) could be found. The TEM measurements indicate that the laser generated defects in our case should consist of point defects or point defect complexes.

## 2. Experimental Methods

The samples used in our experiment were three-layer structures, grown by liquid phase epitaxy onto a GaAs substrate [7]. The first and the third (top) layer consisted of 1 and 3 μm thick films of $(Al_{0.6}, Ga_{0.4})As$, respectively. They are transparent at the red Kr-ion laser wavelength. The second layer was 0.4 μm thick $(Al_{0.22}, Ga_{0.78})As$. The layers were p-type Sn doped at a level of $1\cdot10^{17}$ $cm^{-3}$. The defects were introduced into the second layer by focussing the beam of a krypton ion laser ($\lambda = 647$ nm) with a microscope-objective (40x; spot diameter 2.3 μm) into the second layer, where most of the light is absorbed. By moving the sample with a motor driven stage relative to the laser beam, lines of defects could be produced. At a power level of 0.49 $MW/cm^2$ a luminescent defect is induced in the center of the beam. The peak energy of this luminescence band is approximately 100 meV below the band gap energy [6]. At a slightly higher power level of 0.53 $MW/cm^2$ a nonradiative defect is produced. It was previously shown that the defect properties do not depend on conductivity or dopant type. Details of laser processing and luminescence properties can be found in refs. [4,6]. The two defects will subsequently be named B (bright) and D (dark) respectively. After laser processing, the samples were either photoetched or thinned for TEM measurements. Photoetching was performed in a solution of $H_3PO_4$, $H_2O_2$ and $CH_3OH$ at volume ratios of 1:1:13 and a temperature of 25°C. The etching cell was mounted on an optical microscope equipped with an infrared camera to monitor the luminescence. During etching the sample was illuminated with the unfocussed krypton laser at a power density of approximately 1 $W/cm^2$. The photoluminescence light of the 22 % layer was monitored and the etching stopped some seconds after the 22 % layer was reached. This time could be determined by a distinct drop in luminescence intensity due to a strong increase in surface recombination. The sample surface was then examined with optical and scanning electron microscopy.

For the thinning of the TEM samples the top layer was first removed by either concentrated HF or with the phosphoric acid etch described above. Etching was performed in the dark to avoid thickness variations due to the illumination. With both etchants, however, there is a faint contrast visible with Nomarski optical microscopy. The HF etch reveals only defect D while the phosphoric acid etches both B and D.

HF preferentially etches layers with a high Al content and it renders a smooth surface only when reaching the interface between top and second layer. Unfortunately, the interface which could contain important information is thereby removed. On the other hand the phosphoric acid etch gives a fairly smooth surface and can be used to etch close to the interface. In all cases the substrate of the sample was removed with a chemical jet and the first layer with HF. TEM investigations have been made with a 200 kV HITACHI microscope.

## 3. Results

### 3.1 Photochemical Etching

Figure 1 shows a luminescence micrograph of a laser processed sample. The lines B and D have been written at power densities of 0.49 and 0.53 $MW/cm^2$ respectively. At these power levels, the material is irreversibly changed. An interference filter of 752 nm placed before the vidicon has been used to accentuate the differences between the two lines. This filter transmits a part of the band-to-band luminescence (peak wavelength $\lambda = 730$ nm) and a part of the

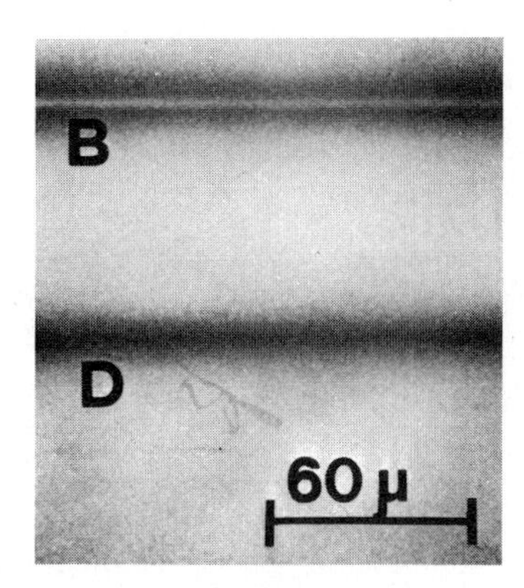


Fig. 1. Luminescence micrograph of laser processed $(Al_{0.22}Ga_{0.78})As$ layer with luminescent defect B and nonradiative defect D.

laser induced defect luminescence (peak wavelength λ= 790 nm) created in line B. The luminescent defect B is present only in the central zone. This zone is surrounded by ~10-15 µm wide adjacent regions where the luminescence efficiency is reduced. In the center of line D there is a strong decrease of the band-to-band luminescence. No defect luminescence is associated with this defect. In the adjacent region the luminescence is also decreased.

Two possible mechanisms could cause the decrease of the luminescence in the adjacent regions of lines B and D: First, diffusion of carriers toward the center of the lines and recombination there; second, recombination in the zone itself at defects induced through the laser processing.

Figure 2a shows a Nomarski micrograph of a photoetched sample and Figure 2b a SEM picture of a cleavage plane intersecting line B.

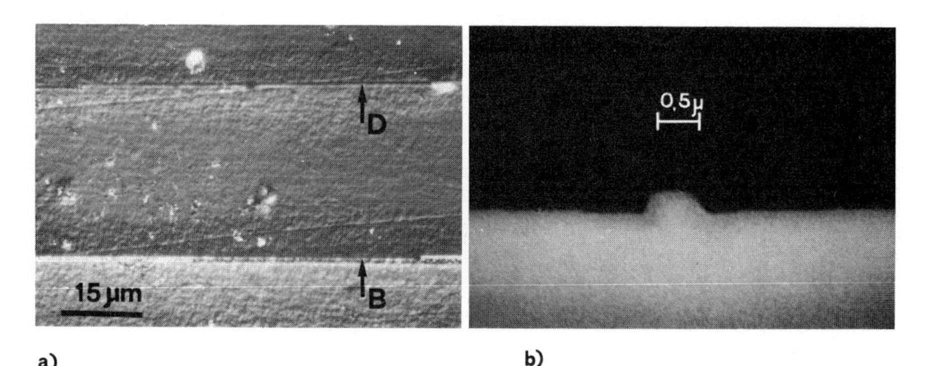


Fig. 2. (a) Nomarski micrograph of photoetched sample showing defect lines B and D (500 nm wide central zones) surrounded by 10 µm wide regions corresponding to dark shaded regions in Fig. 1, (b) SEM micrograph showing the profile of line B.

The shape of this line is the following. In the center, where defect B was present there is a mesa structure 500 nm wide and 260 nm high. This mesa is formed because the zones to the left and right etch faster than the center. The width of this zone is approximately 10 µm and corresponds to the dark shaded region of line B in Fig. 1. From optical interferometric measurements it was determined that the mesa has the same height as the parts of the sample which had not been affected by the laser processing,i.e., the etch velocity at the place of the luminescent defect B is the same as in untreated material. The etch profile at line D is different: it can be seen in Fig. 2a that the central zone ( ~ 0.5 µm) which appears black in the photoluminescence picture is slightly deepened, i.e.,the center etches faster than the adjacent regions. The depth of this trace was estimated from optical interferometric measurements to ~ 70 nm. To the left and right of the central zone, one finds a zone (~10 μm wide) etched equally as in the case of line B. Because no etch profiles develop by etching in the dark, the defect delineation is due to photoetching, which is a well-known process to reveal structural defects and inhomogeneities in semiconductors [8]. In p-type material the photoproduced carriers decrease the etch rate. At a defect site with a high recombination velocity and hence a lower minority carrier concentration, this decrease is less pronounced and a groove is formed [8]. This agrees well for defect D. In the adjacent regions to B and D the carrier concentration is obviously lowered, too. Defect B, however, is not active in photoetching of p-type material as seen above, i.e., it does not act as a fast recombination center. But in turn, this excludes the diffusion of carriers towards the center of line B from the outer region and a further defect C is needed to explain the etch feature. For line D this is not necessarily true. Neither carrier diffusion can be excluded nor the possibility that C and D are the same. However, carrier diffusion seems unlikely because the width of the zone is much larger than the carrier diffusion length (~1-2 μm). Former experimental work on luminescence decrease at dislocations done in [9] strongly supports this view.

It is concluded from photoetching that our laser processing introduces probably three different defects. The spatial extension is: defect D or defect B in a 500 nm wide central region of the beam, defect C in a ~10 μm wide region around the central zone of D and B. It can not be excluded, however, that D and C are the same.

### 3.2 TEM Measurements

Figures 3a and 3b show two TEM pictures of a line D made under two different imaging conditions. In the case of Fig. 3a the specimen was strongly inclined

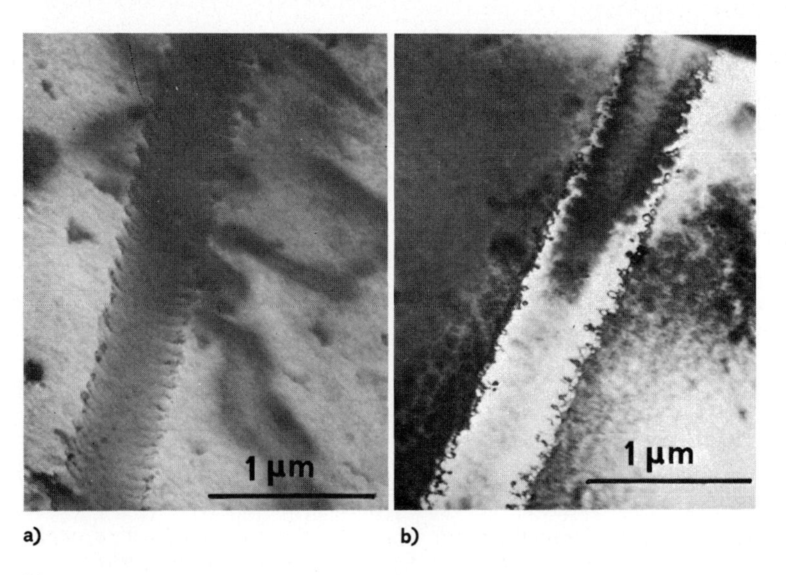


Fig. 3. TEM bright field image of defect line D. The contrast of the line depends on the imaging conditions (see text).

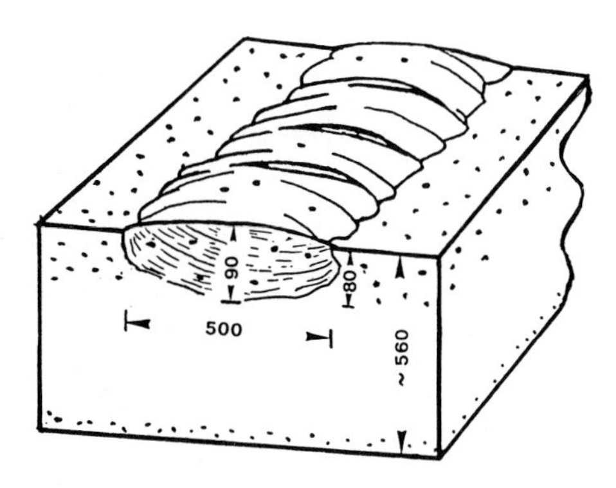


Fig. 4. Schematical representation of the active layer with a defect line D as seen by stereo microscopy (all dimensions in nm).

whereas it was nearly horizontal in Fig. 3b. The width of the line is 480 nm which corresponds well with the width of the central zone seen by the photoetch experiments. In Fig. 3a the line appears dark. Under the imaging condition of Fig. 3b contrast is partially reversed due to a bending contour crossing the line. The line appears segmented which is clearly seen in Fig. 3a. These segments terminate in the very sharp tiny loop contrasts at the border of the line in 3b. The visibility of these loops is strongly dependent on the imaging condition, but they are not due to dislocations or microcracks. An analysis of the change of contrast leads to the assumption that they are due to strain fields which are built in between the line and the surroundings. However, on the basis of the available information it can not be decided whether the segments are due to stress fields present in a geometrical homogeneous line or to real geometric segments introduced through etching. Stereoscopic observations show a cross section of the line as sketched in Fig. 4, with the segment structure appearing at the surface and extending inside the material. The height of the line is 600-800 Å. This does not mean that the laser modified zone corresponds to this value, but the latter could be due to etch effects. The HF etch with which this sample was thinned obviously attacks slower at the place of defect D. On both surfaces numerous grey contrasts, indicated as black dots in Fig. 4, down to 80 nm could be observed which are probably due to etch residues. Defects B and C are not detectable in HF-etched samples neither by Nomarski nor by TEM. It could be, however, that the laser modification is located at the interface and is removed through the thinning. To check this point, samples have been thinned with the phosphoric acid etch in the dark. Due to initial thickness variations in the top layer the etch time could be chosen so that in some areas a thin part remained. This could be checked with luminescence mapping. The results of these TEM experiments are summarized:

1) A very faint bright contrast is associated with line B and D. This contrast rapidly decreases with increasing top layer thickness.
2) No internal structure of the lines was detectable.
3) Strain contrasts associated with the lines are also observed.
4) Observations in regions with remaining parts of the top layer did not reveal dislocations or any other kind of defect detectable under our TEM conditions.
5) No defect structure could be detected by TEM in regions where defect C is present.
6) It follows from point 1) that contrast in TEM depends strongly on etching conditions.

These experimental observations rule out that the etching removes important detectable defect structures at the interface. It shows, however, that the whole etching process is critical for defect delineation in TEM.

## 4. Conclusion

Photoluminescence mapping and photoetching of laser processed samples reveal at least two different defect centers. There is strong evidence for a third one found in regions extending 10 μm away from the focus of the processing laser. This can be explained by outdiffusion of point defects from the focal zone. A strong correspondence between photoetch profiles and defect distribution as seen in photoluminescence is observed.

In TEM ~500 nm wide zones show up where defect B or defect D are present. No sign of defect C was detectable in TEM. No dislocations or even DLD and microcracks were visible which can be associated with laser processing. Our kind of laser processing therefore introduces substantially different defects than observed before. Since the defects are not directly visible in TEM it is most likely that the structures observed are revealed by etching and etching residues of the defects and the latter are point defects or point defect complexes.

## References


1 C.H. Henry, P.M. Petroff, R.A. Logan, and F.R. Merritt: J. Appl. Phys. 50, 3721 (1979)

2 Hajime Imai, Takao Fujiwara, Katsuharu Segi, Masahito Takusagawa, and Hirobumi Takanashi: Jap. J. of Appl. Phys. 18, 589 (1979)

3 S. Mahajan, H. Temkin, and R.A. Logan: Appl. Phys. Lett. 44, 119 (1984)

4 H.H. Gilgen, R.P. Salathé, and Y. Rytz-Froidevaux: Appl. Phys. Lett. 38, 241 (1981)

5 J.A. van Vechten: Europhys. J. Physica B and C 116, 575 (1983)

6 R.P. Salathé, H.H. Gilgen, and Y. Rytz-Froidevaux: IEEE J. Quantum Electron. 17, 1989 (1981)



7 The authors are grateful to Dr. R.A. Logan, Bell Telephone Laboratories, Murrey Hill, New Jersey, for providing the (Al,Ga)As heterostructures



8 F. Kuhn-Kuhnenfeld: J. Electrochem. Soc. 119, 1063 (1972)

9 K. Böhm and B. Fischer: J. Appl. Phys. 50, 5453 (1979)

# Optical Characterization of Implantation Damage Recovery and Electrical Activation in GaAs by Raman Scattering

B. Prevot and C. Schwab

Laboratoire de Spectroscopie et d'Optique du Corps Solide, Unité Associée au CNRS n° 232, Université Louis Pasteur, 5, rue de l'Université F-67000 Strasbourg, France

## 1 INTRODUCTION

Ion implantation is known to be an attractive method for selectively doping semiconductors, which however has the inherent drawback to require a post implantation treatment in order to anneal the associated lattice damage and to activate the implants by inserting them on the proper lattice sites.

Due to the dual aspect of the interatomic forces which govern the lattice vibrations, i.e. short and long range order forces, Raman Scattering (R.S.) by phonons constitutes a suitable tool for probing the lattice perfection. On the other hand, light scattering by free carrier excitations - mainly plasmons - may give valuable information about the electrical properties in a non-destructive and contactless manner.

In a previous publication [1], we have established the conditions for evaluating the pertinent R.S. parameters of the first-order scattering. In particular, besides the peak position (mode energy) and linewidth (vibration life time) we have demonstrated that the intensity scattered by the transverse and longitudinal modes (TO and LO) is an intrinsic parameter directly related to the crystal perfection. On these bases, the implantation induced damages could be evaluated for semi-insulating GaAs substrates subjected to B and Se ions implantations [2] and recently to Be bombardments [3].

In this paper we present a R.S. investigation of the annealing behavior of Be implanted layers in GaAs when submitted to successive and isochronal thermal steps in the 200 to 900°[C] temperature range. By taking advantage of the fact that only the LO phonons couple to charge density oscillations in the first order R.S. signature, the principal aim of the present study lies in the use of each line of the Raman signal as an independent probe for the simultaneous characterization of the lattice perfection using the TO signal and of the electrical activity using the LO phonon-plasmon coupled mode.

## 2 EXPERIMENTAL

The samples were L.E.C. Cr doped semi-insulating GaAs substrates cut 6° off a (100) surface and capped with a 100 [nm] thick layer of pyrolitic $Si_3N_4$ in order to prevent As evaporation during annealing. Room temperature implantations with 70 [keV] Be ions were performed at doses between $10^{14}$ and $10^{15}$ [ions.cm$^{-2}$] and at a constant current density of 23.5 [nA.cm$^{-2}$]. Taking the $Si_3N_4$/GaAs interface as a reference, the corresponding projected range $R_p$ is 150 [nm] with a range straggling of 76 [nm]. Polarized Raman spectra have been taken at room temperature in a Brewster angle geometry using excitation lines from an $Ar^+$ laser. The spectra have been analyzed with a Jarrell-Ash double monochromator equipped with a cooled RCA Quantacon photomultiplier and photon counting electronics. Further detailed experimental conditions can be found elsewhere [1]. The annealing procedure consisted in 12 [min] isochronal steps made under a purified Ar flow ; the $Si_3N_4$ film being transparent in the visible part of the spectrum, the Raman spectra could be obtained through the protective layer.

## 3 RESULTS

Figure 1 compares the R.S. response of an unimplanted reference sample with that observed on a Be implanted one at a $10^{15}$ [ions $cm^{-2}$] dose. In the geometry used, the selection rules allow first order scattering by the TO and LO phonons with natural energies of respectively 268.5 and 291.5 [$cm^{-1}$]. Their experimental width (FWHM) is of the order of 5 [$cm^{-1}$], whereas their intensity ratio R(TO/LO) is 0.47 as established previously in the case of a perfect crystal excited with the 488 [nm] argon line [1]. In this Fig. the effects of the implantation damage on the R.S. signal are clearly observable. The first-order lines are down shifted and broadened : typical values for the higher dose case (i.e. $10^{15}$ [$cm^{-2}$]) being $\nu(LO)$ = 285.5 [$cm^{-1}$] and $\Gamma(LO)$ = 12 [$cm^{-1}$] for the longitudinal optical mode. Similar observations have been noted in our previous study on B and Se implantations in GaAs [2] in agreement with other data reported for Si and Be [4] and for As [5]. In the lower part of the Raman shift, other modifications are noticeable : they consist of three intense and broad structures located around 70, 170 and 260 [$cm^{-1}$] whose origin will not be discussed here.

The R.S. modifications observed as a function of the successive isochronal annealing steps are summarized in Fig. 2 in the

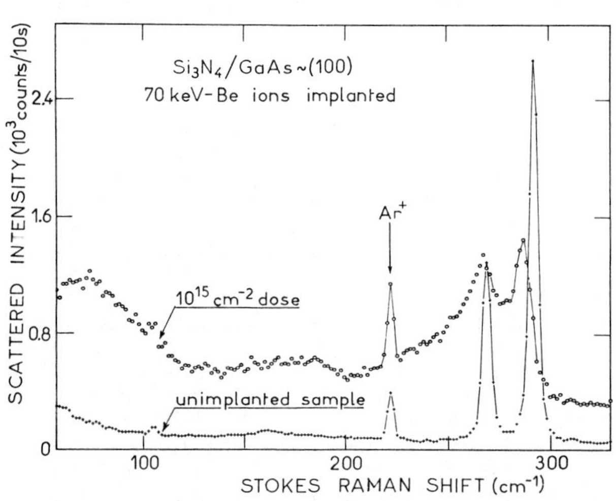


Fig. 1. The Raman spectrum of a Be implanted sample (open circles) compared with that of reference (crosses)

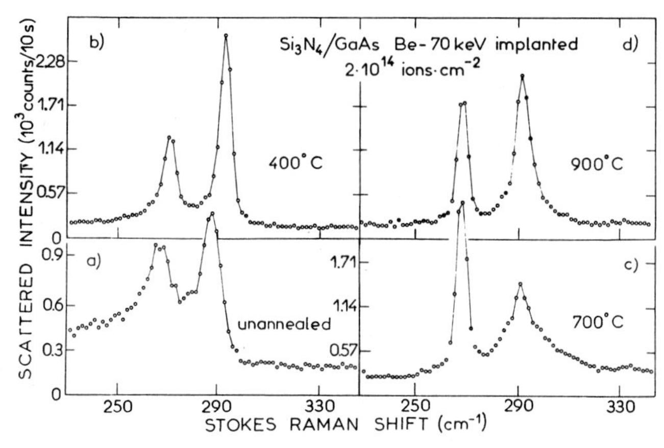


Fig. 2. Raman signatures of a Be implanted GaAs sample as function of the successive isochronal thermal steps performed till 400 (b), 700 (c) and 900°[C] (d). Note the change in the counting rate for the implanted but unannealed case (a)

case of the $2.10^{14}$ Be ions.[$cm^{-2}$] dose. Starting from the situation depicted in the part a) of the Fig., the R.S. first compares well with that of the reference sample (see Fig. 1) for a temperature step as low as 400°[C]. Both first-order TO and LO lines present peak energy and linewidth values which are characteristic of a nearly perfect substrate ; further the R(TO/LO) ratio has a value of 0.46 at T = 400°[C]. For the higher temperatures the signal in the LO part of the spectrum undergoes a sudden modification with a pronounced asymmetrical broadening and an apparent intensity reduction when compared with the TO line. At the ultimate annealing steps, the R.S. signal looks like the reference one although the LO linewidth remains rather broad (7.2 [$cm^{-1}$]) and R(TO/LO) has a value of 0.55 which is however higher than that of reference,i.e. 0.47 [1].

## 4 ANALYSIS

As pointed out briefly in the introduction, the lattice vibrational modes depend strongly on the actual long range order existing in the crystal. As a consequence any reduction of this long range order (or change in the electronic interactions) will affect the Raman signature. The same conclusions can be drawn about the basic mechanisms which are responsible for the scattered intensity [1]. Hence we interpret the spectrum shown in Fig. 1 as resulting from a partially amorphized medium subsequent to the implantation-induced damages. The situation is intermediate between that of a perfect crystalline sample where crystal momentum conservation is strictly obeyed and that reported for sputtered films where it does not apply anymore [6].

Light scattering by microcrystalline Si films presents similar behavior. The red shift of the zone center optical mode and its asymmetrical line shape broadening have been analyzed in terms of phonon wave vector reduction as due to the finite dimension of the crystallites [7]. We have analyzed our spectra within the same phenomenological model by introducing a Gaussian wave vector localization characterized by a width D. This allows the $q \neq 0$ optical phonons to participate in the Raman process, thus explaining the observed spectral modifications. A frequency shift and a broadening comparable to those reported in the previous section then correspond to a D value of the order of 3.5 [nm], which is only 6 times greater than the lattice unit parameter.

Conversely, the annealing procedure efficiency will be probed by a progressive recovery of the R.S. parameters towards their initial values. This trend is indeed observed for anneals performed till 400 - 500°[C] (cf. Fig. 2). Above this temperature only the LO line suffers modifications contrary to the TO one which remains unchanged till 900°[C]. Our interpretation is based on the fact that for $T \geqslant 500°$ [C], the implanted layer is electrically activated, giving rise to a charge carrier density wave which in turn modifies the involved scattering mechanisms. Indeed it is known that the longitudinal modes can interact with plasma oscillations due to their own electric field [8], thus giving rise to the coupled modes $L^+$ and $L^-$ whose frequencies are related to the carrier density.

The R.S. spectra for $T > 500°$[C] have been analyzed in the simplified hypothesis that the "longitudinal" intensity takes its origin from two different regions (or mechanisms) ; one where carriers are depleted through space charge effect, contributing with a pure unscreened LO signal and another one with active carriers, where the signal arises from the coupled LO phonon-plasmon mode. Lorentzian profiles have been introduced in the fitting procedure, the only fixed parameters being the position and width of the unscreened LO partner which have been constrained to their reference values. The results of this analysis are plotted in Fig. 3 in terms of a $L^+$ normalized mode intensity versus the temperature steps. From this Fig., it can be concluded that electrical activation occurs suddenly at T = 550°[C] in an almost fully recovered substrate. The $L^+$ intensity appears to increase slightly with temperature for the lower doses till a maximum around 700°[C], then decreases markedly for all doses. These observations are in good agreement with Hall differential measurements performed on similar samples[9].

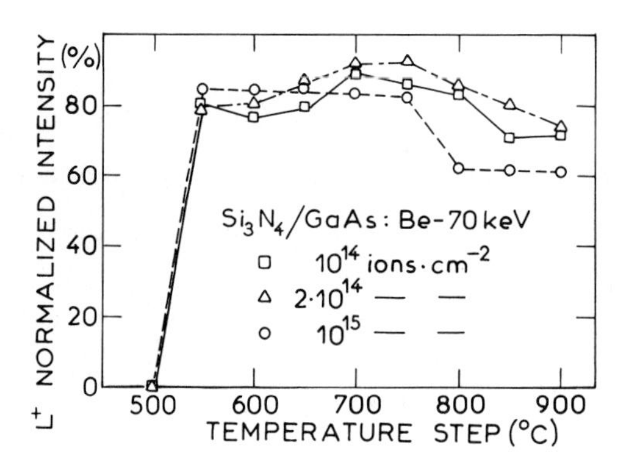


Fig. 3. Temperature variation of the $L^+$ normalized contribution in the "longitudinal" signal, for three implantation doses

However, for a proper treatment of the R.S. efficiency, one has to deal with the Raman cross-section as evaluated in the phonon-plasmon coupling case [8]. This involves the total dielectric function of the system in which the amount of plasmon damping (arising from the scattering of the carriers) plays an important role. Conversely, the analysis of the Raman signal in such a way gives valuable information about the electrical properties of the medium ; indeed the plasma frequency is related to the carrier density while its damping may be used to obtain their mobility, provided the carrier effective mass is known. Assuming that the electrically activated region gives now a complex coupled response, the results of a fit done on the spectrum shown in Fig. 2c lead to a mean hole density of 5.5 $10^{18}$[$cm^{-3}$] and a mobility of the order of 35 [$cm^2$/V.s].

To sum up, it has been demonstrated that the first-order R.S. signature can be very useful for assessing crystalline perfection and electrical activation of implanted layers. In the case of Be in GaAs, we have shown that the lattice recovery is almost complete for annealing temperatures in the 400 - 450°[C] range. Then the electrical activity suddenly occurs with a maximum of efficiency near 750°[C] ; for the higher temperatures, the observed decrease raises the problem of light dopant diffusion in GaAs in the case of high dose implantation rates [10].

We are greatly indebted to the Laboratoire d'Electronique et de Physique Appliquée, Limeil Brévannes, for providing us with the implanted samples and for stimulating discussions with Drs. J.B. Theeten, M. Erman and P. Chambon. This work has been supported by "Délégation Générale de la Recherche Scientifique et Technique".

1 J. Biellmann, B. Prévot, and C. Schwab, J. Phys.C : Solid State Phys. 16, 1135 (1983).
2 J. Biellmann, B. Prévot, C. Schwab, J.B. Theeten, and M. Erman, in Defects in Semiconductors II, edited by S. Mahajan and J.W. Corbett (North Holland, New York, 1983) p.517.
3 M. Erman, P. Chambon, B. Prévot, and C. Schwab, J. Phys. (Paris), Colloque C10, 44, 261 (1983).
4 L.L. Abels, S. Sundaram, R.L. Schmidt, and J. Comas, Appl. of Surface Science, 9, 2 (1981).
5 K.K. Tiong, P.M. Amirtharaj, F.H. Pollack, and D.E. Aspnes, Appl. Phys. Lett. 44, 122 (1984).
6 R. Shuker, and R.W. Gammon, Phys. Rev. Lett. 25, 222 (1970).
7 H. Richter, Z.P. Wang, and L. Ley, Solid State Commun. 39, 625 (1981).
8 W. Hayes, and R. Loudon : Scattering of Light by Crystals (Wiley, New York, 1978).
9 P. Chambon, B. Prévot, M. Erman, J.B. Theeten, and C. Schwab, Appl. Phys. Lett. (1984) in press.
10 J.P. Donnelly, Nucl. Inst. and Meth. 182/183, 553 (1981).

# Characterization of Gallium Arsenide Layers on Insulators with Germanium Interface Islands

M. Takai, T. Tanigawa, M. Miyauchi*, S. Nakashima*, K. Gamo, and S. Namba

Faculty of Engineering Science, *Faculty of Engineering, Osaka University
Toyonaka, Osaka 560, Japan

GaAs layers were grown by molecular beam epitaxy on single-crystal Ge-island layers, grown by zone melting recrystallization with $SiO_2$ capping layers, on the thermal oxide of Si wafers .

It was found, by microprobe laser Raman scattering, that local tensile stresses of 2.7 to 5.5 kbar remained in single-crystal Ge islands after zone melting recrystallization. The GaAs layers, grown on the single crystal Ge islands, show smooth surfaces without any grain boundaries, while those, grown on the $SiO_2$ layers, have grain boundaries. The GaAs layers on the single-crystal Ge islands emit photoluminescence (PL), the intensity of which was almost comparable to that of GaAs layers on bulk Ge crystals. The stress in the GaAs layers on the Ge islands was also estimated from the photoluminescence spectra and was found to range from 2.1 to 3.2 kbar, which was in good agreement with the value for the underlying Ge islands obtained from Raman scattering.

## 1. Introduction

Optical diagnostic techniques using laser beams such as Raman scattering and photoluminescence (PL) measurements have been widely used for probing semiconductor materials because they are nondestructive and contactless methods. Furthermore, spatial resolutions of less than 1 μm can be attained by focusing the laser beam. Laser Raman scattering methods, for example, provide information about stress, crystallinity, defect density, surface morphology, and temperature in materials [1].

Semiconductors-on-insulator (SOI) structures by laser or zone melting recrystallization have recently been studied extensively , especially for silicon, because of their features such as radiation hardness, higher speed, and three-dimensional integration. SOI structures with different semiconductor materials like III-V compound semiconductors on the same substrate, furthermore, provide hybrid integrated circuits including optical functions [2-6]. Although SOI structures with III-V compound semiconductors, such as GaAs or InP, are important, it is very difficult to prepare SOI structures with GaAs or InP because of the high vapor pressure of As or P and, hence, the difficulty in preserving the stoichiometry of constituents.

In this study, single crystal germanium islands were grown on the thermal oxide of Si wafers by zone melting with graphite strip heaters and $SiO_2$ capping layers,to provide interface layers for GaAs epitaxy. GaAs layers were grown by molecular beam epitaxy (MBE) on the single crystal Ge islands. Microprobe laser Raman scattering with a spatial resolution of 1 μm was used to detect local stresses in single-crystal Ge islands on insulators. Laser induced PL was used to qualify GaAs layers optically on insulators and to detect stresses in GaAs layers. The correlation between the stress obtained from the shift in Raman spectra and the peak shift in PL spectra is discussed.

## 2. Experimental Procedures

1 µm thick, (100)-oriented Ge islands with 100 µm x 80 µm sides connected with a narrow stripe (30 µm x 10 µm) were prepared on a 730 nm thick thermal oxide of a Si wafer by zone melting recrystallization with a 1 µm thick $SiO_2$ capping layer as described elsewhere [2,4]. The crystalline orientations of the islands were determined by TEM or etch pit pattern observation [2,4,6].

0.8 – 1.1 µm thick GaAs layers were grown on the Ge islands by MBE as shown in Fig. 1. A top surface of Ge island layers was lightly etched before MBE for 30 sec with Superoxol etchants ($HF:H_2O_2:H_2O$ = 1:1:10) [2]. GaAs layers were also grown on (100)- and (111)-oriented Ge wafers at the same time to prepare reference samples. Background and working pressures during MBE were less than $10^{-10}$ Torr and 2 x $10^{-8}$ Torr. The substrate temperature was maintained at 600°C, which was the optimum temperature in the range between 550 – 650°C. The growth rate of GaAs layers was about 1.1 µm/hr. GaAs layers were intentionally doped during MBE with Si at a dose of $10^{17}/cm^3$. Undoped GaAs layers were also grown for comparison.

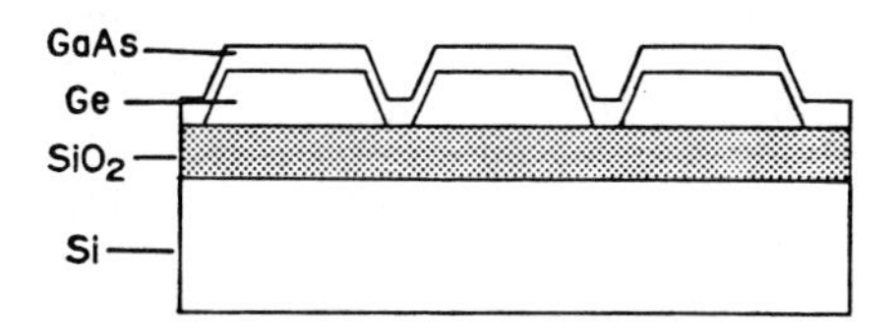


Fig. 1 A cross-sectional view of a sample

Raman spectra were obtained using a 514.5 nm line of an argon-ion laser. The scattered light was collected by an objective lens with a numerical aperture of 0.65 attached to a commercially available optical microscope as described elsewhere [5,7]. The measured diameter of the diffraction-limited focal-spot on the samples was about 1.0 µm. Samples were mounted on a rotatable X-Y stage with a precision of 1 µm. The sample temperature during measurements was maintained at room temperature. The Raman frequency shift was calibrated before and after runs using the argon laser lines. The accuracy of the frequency was better than 0.5 $cm^{-1}$. Sample heating was avoided by reducing an incident laser power on the sample to less than 10 mW and increasing the laser beam diameter to about 5 µm; no changes in the Raman spectra due to heat were observed [5,7].

PL was stimulated at 77 K by a focused 514.5 nm line of an Ar ion laser Special care was taken not to heat or damage GaAs layers during the measurements. The laser power during the measurements was maintained at less than 30 mW with a spot diameter of 200 µm. The luminescence spectrum was measured using a grating monochromator and photon-counting system coupled with an S-1 response photomultiplier [3].

## 3. Results and Discussion

Figure 2 shows the micrographs of MBE-grown GaAs layers on Ge islands recrystallized by zone melting with 1.0 µm $SiO_2$ capping layers. The GaAs layers, grown directly on $SiO_2$ layers, have dark-line contrast, corresponding to grain boundaries or subboundaries [3], while those on the single crystal Ge islands have smooth surfaces without dark-line contrast. Square-shaped etch-pit patterns and the change in the edge shape observed in the Ge islands are due to Superoxol etching before MBE growth [2,3]. This result together with the recent channeling measurements on MBE grown GaAs layers on (100)- and (111)-oriented Ge crystals [3] suggests

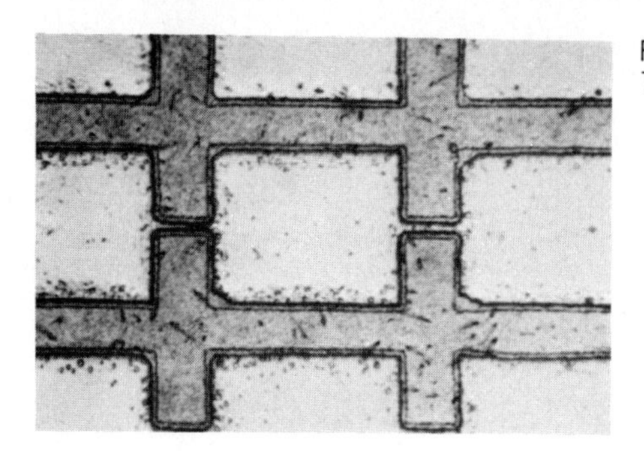

Fig. 2 Optical micrographs of MBE GaAs layers grown on Ge islands

that single-crystal GaAs layers can be grown only on the single crystal Ge islands, and the (100) orientation of the underlying Ge islands is superior for obtaining good crystallinity of MBE GaAs layers of (111) orientation.

GaAs layers with SOI structures, seeded by GaAs/Ge/Si [8] or GaAs [9], were reported to have film quality comparable to bulk GaAs materials, while GaAs layers grown on Ge/W/$SiO_2$ substrates were found to have grain boundaries in GaAs layers [10] presumably because underlying Ge layers did not have low-index orientation like (100). The GaAs layers grown on (100)-oriented Ge islands in this study were found to have smooth surfaces without grain boundaries (Fig. 2).

Figure 3 shows typical Raman scattering spectra obtained for (100)-oriented bulk Ge and a Ge island. The Raman scattering spectrum for the bulk Ge has a peak at 300.5 $cm^{-1}$, while the peak of the spectrum for the Ge island shifts to lower energy by 1.6 $cm^{-1}$. The frequency shift of the Raman band is reported to be due either to uniform strain in the sample [11,12] or to a size effect, i.e., small grain size [13]. The shift observed in this case is considered due to uniform strain in the Ge island by residual stresses, since the island is single crystal [2-6]. The observed shift to lower energy indicates that the stress in the Ge film is tensile [11,12]. The stress in the film can be calculated by solving the dynamical equations of the cubic lattice, following the analysis by ANASTASSAKIS et al.[11]. The shift of 1 $cm^{-1}$, corresponds to a stress of 3.4 kbar, provided that the deformation-potential constants (p.q) and the

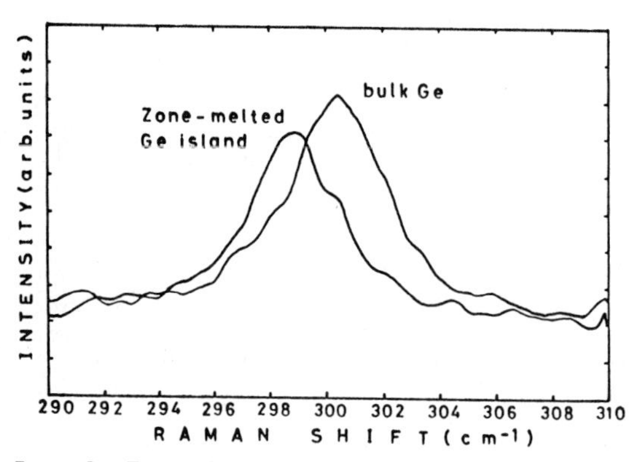


Fig. 3 Typical Raman scattering spectra for (100)-oriented bulk Ge and a Ge island

elastic compliance constants ($S_{11}, S_{12}$) for Ge are - 4.70 x $10^{27}$ $sec^{-2}$, - 6.17 x $10^{27}$ $sec^{-2}$, 0.9733 x $10^{-12}$ $dyne^{-1}cm^2$, - 0.2667 x $10^{-12}$ $dyne^{-1}cm^2$, respectively [12].

Table 1 compares the peak shifts of the Raman line measured at the three different positions, i.e., the middle (A) and the edge (B) of the island and the connecting stripe (C). Although the half width of the Raman lines for the three positions is almost the same, the energy shift of the Raman line for the island compared with that for the bulk Ge is slightly larger at the middle of the island (A) than that at the edge (B and C). The stress at three positions is 5.5 kbar, 3.4 kbar, and 2.7 kbar, indicating that the edge of an island suffers less stress than the middle. The stress at the edge may locally relax, presumably because of the presence of a lateral free surface.

Table 1 A summary of the Raman peak shifts and corresponding stresses

| Position | Peak shift [$cm^{-1}$] | Stress [kbar] |
|---|---|---|
| A | 1.6 | 5.5 |
| B | 1.0 | 3.4 |
| C | 0.8 | 2.7 |

These residual stresses in the Ge islands can be explained by the difference in thermal expansion coefficients between Ge (6.0 x $10^{-6}$/ °C) and underlying $SiO_2$/Si (5.5 x $10^{-7}$/ °C for $SiO_2$ and 4.0 x $10^{-6}$/ °C for Si) during zone melting recrystallization [5]. The stress in the Ge film is estimated to range from 1.4 to 3.9 kbar when the relation $s = \Delta\alpha \cdot \Delta T \cdot E_f$ is used, provided that the difference in thermal expansion coefficients ($\Delta\alpha$), the temperature difference ($\Delta T$) and the elastic modulus of Ge film ($E_f$) obtained from elastic compliance constants are 2.0 x $10^{-6}$/°C - 5.45 x $10^{-6}$ /°C, 917°C and 7.7 x $10^{10}$ N/$m^2$, respectively. The stress measured by Raman scattering is in good agreement with that estimated from the difference in thermal expansion coefficients, though the thermal expansion coefficient of $SiO_2$/Si substrates is ambiguous.

PL measurements on MBE GaAs layers grown simultaneously on the (100)-oriented Ge islands, (100)-oriented and (111)-oriented bulk Ge crystals were made to compare the optical quality of GaAs layers grown on different substrates. Figure 4 shows a comparison of PL spectra for GaAs layers grown simultaneously on three different substrates. The GaAs layers on the bulk Ge emit sharp PL signals located at 822 - 826 nm (1.51 - 1.50 eV), while a broad emission peak located at 840 nm (1.48 eV) is observed for the GaAs layer on the Ge island. The broad emission observed for the GaAs layer on the Ge island is thought to be due to a band-gap variation induced by the lattice strain in GaAs and/or impurity incorporation during MBE from Ge layers. Since stresses of 2.7 - 5.5 kbar due to the difference in thermal expansion coefficients between Ge islands and underlying $SiO_2$/Si substrates exist in the underlying Ge islands, and GaAs has almost the same thermal expansion coefficient as Ge (within 20 %), GaAs layers may also suffer such stress. The stress in GaAs layers can be estimated from the shift of PL emission lines from that of reference samples to be 2.1 - 3.2 kbar, provided that the peak shift of PL lines is due only to the band-gap variation induced by the lattice strain and the pressure coefficient of band gap is 11.3 x $10^{-6}$ eV/kg $cm^{-2}$. The stress estimated from the PL shift is in good agreement with that in the Ge islands obtained by Raman

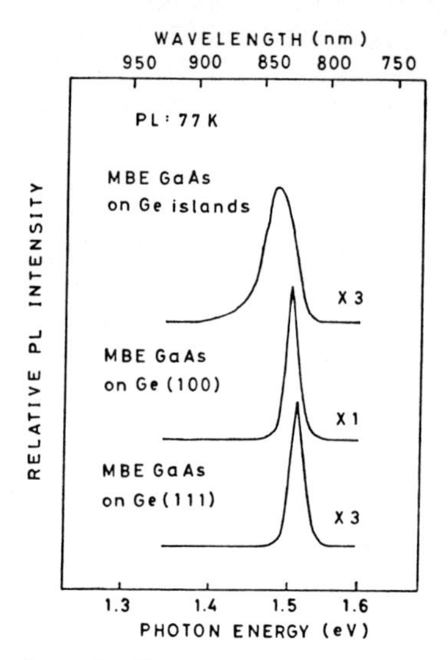


Fig. 4 PL spectra for MBE GaAs layers on the zone-melted Ge island, (100) and (111) bulk Ge. Multiplication factors stand for the values of the expanded scale.

scattering. The PL shift of the undoped MBE-GaAs layer on the Ge island was the same as that of the Si-doped MBE-GaAs layer on the Ge island. It should be noted that the integrated emission intensity for the GaAs layer on the Ge island , depending on the position of exciting laser beams because of the larger spot size than the island, is almost comparable to or about 30 % less than that for the GaAs layer on the (100)-oriented bulk Ge and is higher by a factor of 2.0 - 2.6 than that for the GaAs layer on the (111)-oriented bulk Ge. This result indicates that the GaAs layer on the Ge island has good quality applicable to device fabrication, though the GaAs-film thickness produced to date ranges from 0.8 to 1.1 μm. Further investigation, however, is necessary to characterize the GaAs layers on Ge islands, for example, using microprobe luminescence with good spatial resolution to obtain the local variation of GaAs-film quality, i.e., the quality of GaAs layers on the Ge island and on $SiO_2$.

## 4. Conclusion

Laser Raman scattering and photoluminescence measurements have been successfully applied to GaAs on $Ge/SiO_2$ structures. It was found that local tensile stresses of 2.7 - 5.5 kbar, which was induced by the difference in thermal expansion coefficients between Ge islands and underlying $SiO_2/Si$ substrates, exist in the Ge island recrystallized by zone melting with $SiO_2$ capping layers.

The GaAs layers, grown by MBE on single crystalline Ge islands, were also found by PL measurements to suffer stresses comparable to those remained in underlying Ge islands.

It was found that the GaAs layers, grown on the single-crystal Ge islands, have smooth surfaces without any grain boundaries, while those grown on the $SiO_2$ layers have grain boundaries. The GaAs layers on the single-crystal Ge islands were found to emit PL, the intensity of which was almost comparable to that of the GaAs layers on (100)-oriented bulk Ge crystals.

## Acknowledgements

The authors are indebted to Y. Yuba and H. Aritome for helpful discussions and to K. Kawasaki and K. Mino for their help in experiments.


## References


1. D.V. Murphy and S.R. Brueck: in Laser Diagnostics and Photochemical Processing for Semiconductor Devices, eds. R.M. Osgood, S.R.J. Brueck, and H.R. Schlossberg (North-Holland, New York, 1983) p.81
2. M. Takai, T. Tanigawa, K. Gamo, and S. Namba: Japan. J. Appl. Phys. 22, L626 (1983)
3. M. Takai, T. Tanigawa, T. Minamisono, K. Gamo, and S. Namba: Japan. J. Appl. Phys. 23, L308 (1984)
4. M. Takai, T. Tanigawa, K. Gamo, and S. Namba: Japan. J. Appl. Phys. 23, L357 (1984)
5. M. Takai, T. Tanigawa, M. Miyauchi, S. Nakashima, K. Gamo, and S. Namba: Japan. J. Appl. Phys. 23, L363 (1984)
6. M. Takai, T. Tanigawa, K. Gamo, and s. Namba: in Energy Beam-Solid Interactions and Transient Thermal Processing, eds. J.C.C. Fan and N.M. Johnson (North-Holland, New York, 1984) in press
7. S. Nakashima, Y. Inoue, M. Miyauchi, A. Mitsuishi, T. Nishimura, T. Fukumoto, and Y. Akasaka: Appl. Phys. Lett. 41, 524 (1982)
8. B.Y. Tsaur, R.W. McClelland, J.C.C. Fan, R.P. Gale, J.P. Salerno, B.A. Vojak and C.O. Bozler: Appl. Phys. Lett. 41, 347 (1982)
9. R.P. Gale, R.W. McClelland, J.C.C. Fan, and C.O. Bozler: Appl. Phys. Lett. 41, 545 (1982)
10. Y. Shinoda, T. Nishioka, and Y. Ohmachi: Japan. J. Appl. Phys. 22, L450 (1983)
11. E. Anastassakis, A. Pinczuk, E. Burstein, F.H. Pollak and M. Cardona: Solid State Commun. 8, 133 (1970)
12. F. Cerdira, C.J. Buchenauer, F.H. Pollak, and M. Cardona: Phys. Rev. 5, 580 (1972)
13. J.F. Morhange, G. Kanellis, and M. Balkanski: Solid State Commun. 31, 805 (1979)

# Surface-Enhanced Raman Scattering as a Diagnostic Method in Preparing Organic Semiconductor Films

E. Saad*, M.E. Lippitsch, A. Leitner, and F.R. Aussenegg

Institut für Experimentalphysik, Karl-Franzens-Universität Graz
A-8010 Graz, Austria

## 1. Introduction

Silicon is now the dominant semiconductor material in practical applications, accompanied by a few other compounds, all of inorganic nature. On the other hand, already some twenty years ago, strong interest has arisen in organic semiconductor materials, which in principle should be possible to be tailored according to purpose by organic chemistry. In reality, up to now we are far from this point, and most organic semiconductor materials are poorly characterized and of insufficient purity. Nevertheless, investigating this field seems promisable for the future. Up to now a few electronic devices, like diodes, thermistors, peltier elements, photoresistors, etc., have been built on the basis of organic semiconductors, and there are encouraging prospects even in the direction of more complex electronic functions. Prerequisite for this development is a reliable knowledge of the submicroscopic structure provided by suitable spectroscopic methods.

Among the organic semiconductors known up to now phtalocyanines belong to the most intensively studied /1/. This is due to the fact that phtalocyanines have the proven suitability for electronic applications and can be readily modified in their electric properties by controlling the crystal structure or "doping" the molecules with metal ions. The use of thin films of phtalocyanines seems promising for solid-state electronics as well as for a hypothetic "molecular" electronics, as recently discussed by several authors /3,4/.

Most structural information on phtalocyanines have been gathered by X-ray and infrared techniques. Both diagnostic methods can only be used in thin films of sufficient thickness ( >100 nm) on suitable substrates. In situ measurements of phtalocyanine films in electronic devices are therefore precluded. For that reason there is an urgent need of a method capable of delivering structural information on very thin phtalocyanine films deposited on arbitrary substrates. Raman spectroscopy could have the desired abilities, provided the sensitivity were high enough. This is usually not the case. Raman spectra recorded with conventional techniques from phtalocyanines have been rarely reported /5/, and usually are of rather poor quality. No such spectra are available from very thin films. The recently developed technique of surface-enhanced Raman scattering (SERS, for recent reviews, see, e.g., /6,7/) has made it possible, however, to record very good Raman spectra of phtalocyanine films down to less than one monolayer. In the following SERS spectra of phtalocyanines will be reported, showing the suitability of this technique as a diagnostic method with high content of structural information, which could be useful in controlling phtalocyanine film preparation in electronic device manufacturing.

* Permanent address: Faculty of Engineering, Department of Physics, Ain-Shams-University, Cairo, Egypt

## 2. Experimental

Surface-enhanced Raman scattering (SERS) is observed when the scattering molecule is situated close to a (usually submicroscopically rough) well-conducting metal surface (usually silver, gold, copper). The Raman intensity per molecule is enhanced by several orders of magnitude ($10^4$ - $10^8$). The mechanism is not yet understood in the subtle details, but it is generally accepted that enhancement of the electromagnetic field by photon-driven surface plasmons as well as enhancement of Raman cross section by charge-transfer interaction play the dominant role /6,7,8/. Especially suited for providing the necessary surface conditions for SERS are silver-island films /9/, consisting of isolated, nearly hemispherical silver particles on a substrate. These silver-island films can be easily produced by slow thermal evaporation and may be deposited on clean substrates (glass, quarz) as well as on top of molecular layers previously applied to the substrate. In our experiments island films were used with an average island diameter of 15 nm and an average spacing of 20 nm between the islands (total mass thickness 5 nm). As substrates glass or fused-silica slides were used. Phtalocyanine was deposited on the substrates or on the islands films by sublimation (evaporation from solid phtalocyanine in a $10^{-8}$ bar vacuum). The phtalocyanines were used as commercially available, without further purification. The Raman spectra were recorded with a double monochromator and single photon counting, using the visible lines of an Argon ion laser as an excitation source. The power density at the sample was kept low enough to avoid damage of the thin films. The Raman light was collected in a forward-scattering geometry.

## 3. Results and Discussion

Fig. 1 gives the surface-enhanced Raman spectrum of phtalocyanine, compared to a conventionally measured spectrum. It is obvious that the quality of the surface-enhanced spectrum is by far superior, despite the fact that it is taken from a 20 nm thin film, while the reference spectrum is from a bulk sample. This demonstrates clearly the advantage of using surface enhancement. The sensitivity of surface-enhanced Raman scattering is high enough to measure spectra of even sub-monolayers of phtalocyanines, as was proven by our investigations in agreement with other work /10/.

To be useful as a diagnostic tool in preparing organic semiconductor films, surface-enhanced Raman scattering must be able to provide some structural information. On the molecular level, this ability is proven by the comparison of the spectra of metal-free phtalocyanine and phtalocyanines containing a central

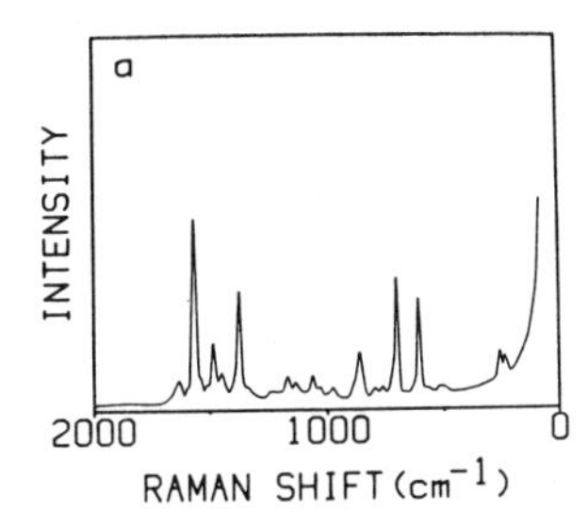


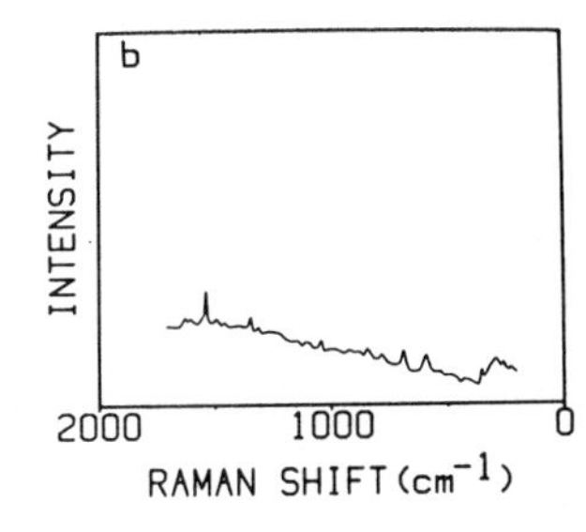


**Fig. 1:** Surface-enhanced spectrum of a Cu phtalocyanine thin film (a), compared to a Raman spectrum of solid CuPc recorded with usual Raman techniques (b). Exciting wavelength 514.5 nm, 1 W in both cases (also subsequent figs.), same intensity scale for both spectra

metal ion. The spectral change upon incorporating a metal ion is drastic, as shown in fig. 2 for Ni. It is quite interesting to see that the changes not only concern vibrations of the pyrrol rings, which directly interact with the metal, but also is reflected in vibrations ascribed to deformations of the benzene rings which have no direct connection to the ion /11/. The severe influence of the central ion on the total electronic structure of the molecule is thus well documented. Moreover, as shown in table 1, the position of certain bands is sensitive to the kind of metal ion incorporated, so that Raman spectroscopy could easily be used to detect areas of different "metal-doping" within a phtalocyanine film.

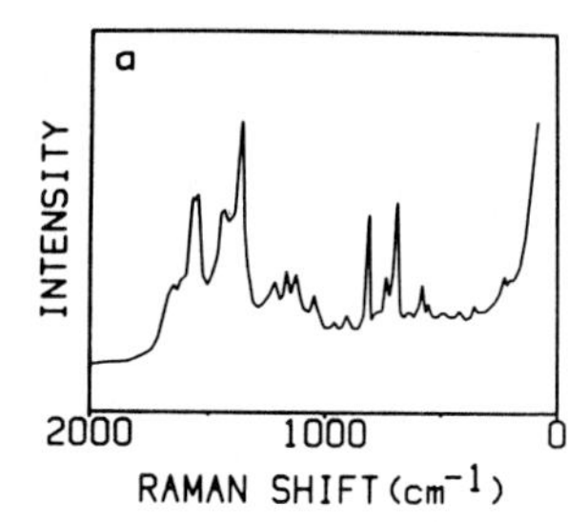


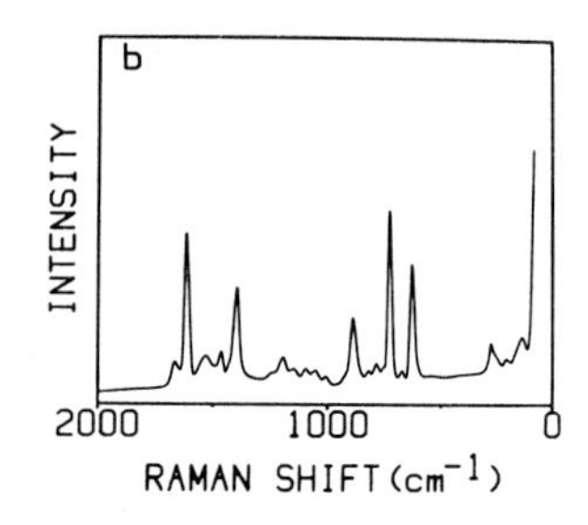


**Fig. 2:** SER spectra of metal-free phtalocyanine (a) and Ni phtalocyanine (b)

**Table 1:** Prominent SERS bands ($cm^{-1}$) of phtalocyanine (Pc) with different central metal ions (Ni, Co, Cu)

| NiPc | CoPc | CuPc |
|---|---|---|
| 256 | 255 | 244 |
| 273 | 273 | 266 |
| 607 | 607 | 603 |
| 700 | 696 | 692 |
| 856 | 846 | 848 |
| 1350 | 1350 | 1349 |
| 1487 | 1480 | 1465 |
| 1562 | 1552 | 1535 |

Also structural changes on the supra-molecular level show up in the surface-enhanced Raman spectra. Cu phtalocyanine can exist in at least two distinct modifications. The structure of these modifications is schematically shown in fig. 3. In the evaporation process, films of the $\alpha$ modification are formed. By the action of organic solvents or tempering for some hours this modification is transformed to the $\beta$ form. Usually these modifications in thin films can only be distinguished by X-ray techniques, which are difficult to apply in situ in an electronic device. In the Raman spectra significant reduction in intensity of about a factor of 2 is observed by going from $\alpha$ to $\beta$ accompanied by changes in the low-wavenumber region (ca. 250 $cm^{-1}$, fig. 4).

Another example for the detection of changes in crystalline structure by SERS is the following. From X-ray diffraction studies it had been concluded /2/ that in a thin film on a substrate the first few layers of phtalocyanine crystals have their long axis parallel to the surface, while subsequent layers have an upright position with the axis at about $20^{o}$ to the surface normal. This was investigated by SERS using silver islands below and atop the phtalocyanine film, respectively. Fig. 5 shows the wavenumber region from 1000 to 1150 $cm^{-1}$ for both cases. The first case (islands below) gives a single band at 1132 $cm^{-1}$, while the other case (islands atop) show an additional band at 1118 $cm^{-1}$. Comparative

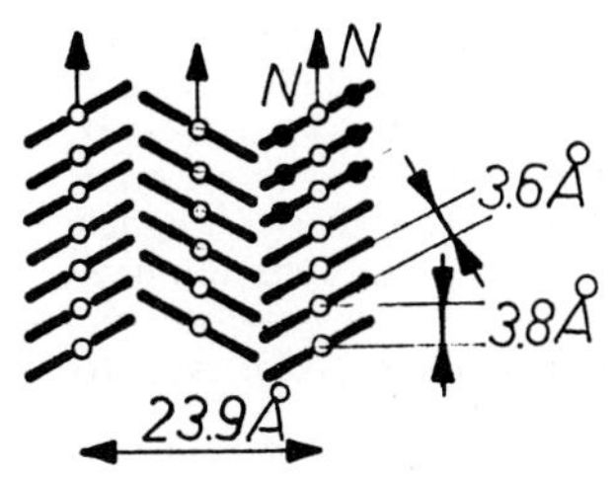

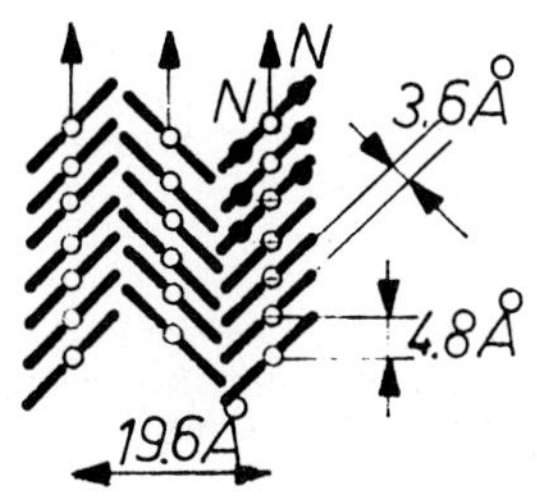


**Fig. 3:** Schematic structure of the two crystal modifications α and β of Cu phtalocyanine (from /2/)

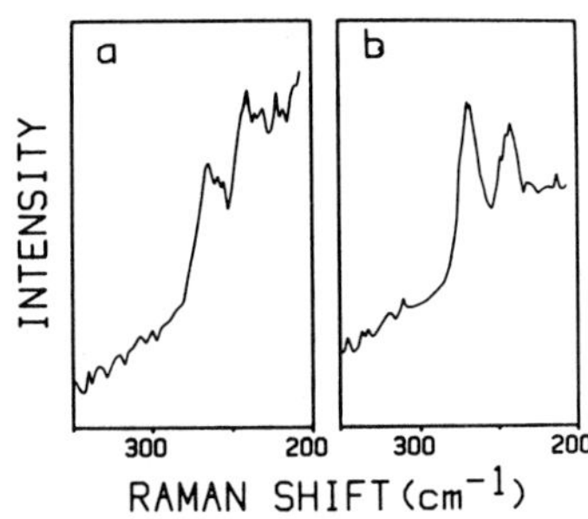


**Fig. 4:** Low-wavenumber region of the SER spectra of α (a) and β (b) phtalocyanine

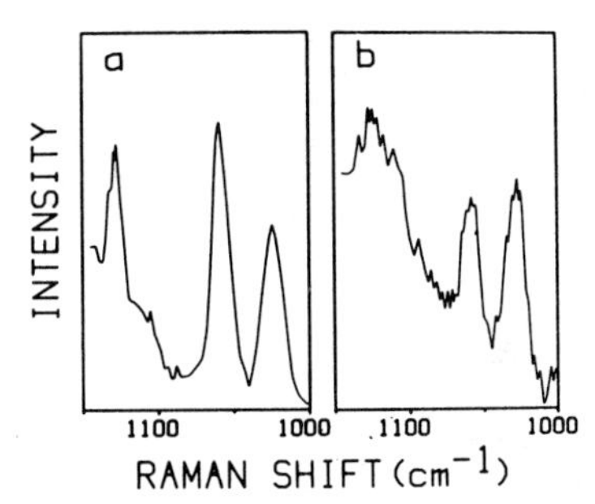


**Fig. 5:** SER spectra of Cu phtalocyanine with the Ag islands below (a) and on top (b) of a phtalocyanine film of ∿100 nm thickness. Spectral differences due to different crystal orientation

studies with other compounds, which have the same crystal orientation throughout the film, give the same Raman spectra with islands below and atop the film. Thus the conclusion seems justified that the 1132 $cm^{-1}$ band is characteristic for upright crystals.

## 4. Conclusion

The suitability of surface-enhanced Raman scattering as a diagnostic tool in preparing semiconductor films has been proven using phtalocyanine as an example. While conventional Raman spectra have a quality insufficient for diagnostic use, surface-enhanced spectra show excellent quality down to submonolayer films. Analytical information can be obtained on the molecular level (e.g. kind of central metal ion) as well as on the crystalline level (modification, direction of crystal axis with respect to the substrate). Surface-enhanced Raman scattering is superior to X-ray diffraction and infrared absorption in sensitivity and, due to its high spatial resolution, could also be used for direct measurements in future organic-semiconductor microcircuits.


## Acknowledgement

The authors are indebted to Miss Sonja Draxler for her help in performing the measurements.

## References


1 F. H. Moser and A. L. Thomas, The Phtalocyanines, Vols. I, II, CRC Press, Boca Raton 1983
2 C. Hamann, G. Lehmann, M. Starke, C. Tantzscher, and H. Wagner, in : C. Hamann, Organische Festkörper und dünne Schichten, Akademische Verlagsgesellschaft, Leipzig 1978
3 F. L. Carter, in: Second Ann. Report, R. B. Fox (ed.), NRL Memorandum, Report 4335, p. 35, Washington 1980
4 F. L. Carter (ed.), Molecular Electronic Devices, Marcel Dekker, New York 1982
5 I. V. Aleksandrov, Ya. S. Bobovich, V. G. Maslov, and A. N. Sidorov, Opt. i Spektroskopiya **37**, 467 (1974)
6 R. Chang and T. Furtak (eds.), Surface-enhanced Raman Scattering, Plenum, New York 1982
7 A. Otto, in: Light Scattering in Solids IV, M. Cardona and B. Güntherod (eds.), Topics in Applied Physics, Vol. 54, Springer, Berlin 1984
8 M. E. Lippitsch, Phys. Rev. **B29**, 3101 (1984)
9 S. Garoff, R. B. Stephens, C. D. Hanson, and G. K. Sorenson, Opt. Comm. **41**, 257 (1982)
10 C. A. Melendres, C. B. Rios, X. Feng, and R. Mc Mortes, J. Phys. Chem. **87**, 3526 (1983)
11 R. Aroca and R. O. Loutfy, J. Raman Spectr. **12**, 262 (1982)

# Raman-Microsampling Technique Applying Optical Levitation by Radiation Pressure

R. Thurn and W. Kiefer

Physikalisches Institut, Universität Bayreuth, Postfach 3008
D-8580 Bayreuth, Fed. Rep. of Germany

## 1. Introduction

Recently, there has been a rapid development in Raman microprobe spectroscopy [1]. It was shown that Raman spectra can be obtained from micrometer-size particles with reasonable signal-to-noise ratio. In these techniques specific precaution has to be taken into account to minimize spectral contributions arising from elastic and inelastic scattering from all possible sources other than the particle of interest. Particularly, inelastic scattering from the substrate which supports the particle for measurement must be avoided in order to keep spectral interference with the Raman spectrum of interest to a minimum.

A perfect sample arrangement for Raman microprobe studies would certainly be to have the particle free in space without any supporting element. This requirement can be fulfilled perfectly by the technique of optical levitation by radiation pressure which has been pioneered by ASHKIN and DZIEDZIC some years ago at the Bell Laboratories [2-6]. Here we report on results of the application of this technique to Raman spectroscopy.

## 2. Optical Levitation by Radiation Pressure

ASHKIN [2] showed that optical levitation is based on the ability of laser light to trap stably nonabsorbing particles by the force of radiation pressure. In this technique a continuous wave vertically directed focused $TEM_{00}$ Gaussian-mode laser beam supports the particle's weight and simultaneously pulls the particle transversely into the region of high light intensity on the beam axis. The radial inward force forms an optical potential, which is schematically shown in Fig. 1. Dependent on the laser

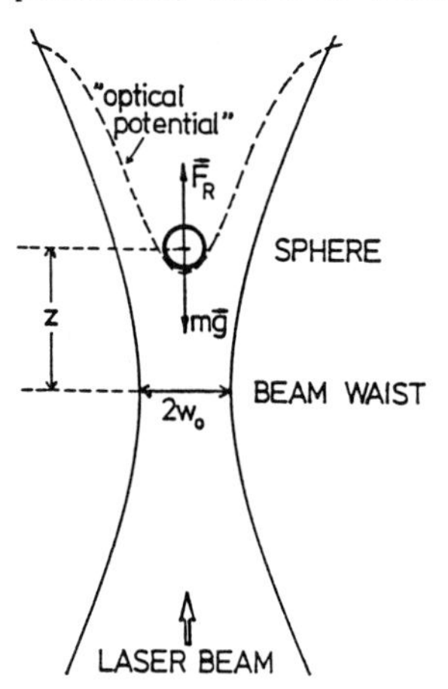


Fig. 1 A schematic diagram of a spherical particle sitting at the equilibrium position above the focus of a $TEM_{00}$-mode Gaussian beam, where gravity ($m\bar{g}$) and the axial light force in the upward direction ($F_R$) balance. Dashed line: schematically drawn optical potential due to the radial inward force.

intensity, the size of the particle and the focal length of the focusing lens, there is an equilibrium point some distance z above the beam waist of the focused $TEM_{oo}$-mode Gaussian beam, where gravity and the total axial light force acting in upward direction to the sphere balance. This equilibrium is stable since any vertical displacement from this point results in a restoring force due to the change in light intensity caused by the beam divergence, and any lateral displacement results in a restoring force due to the transverse gradient force. If spherical particles are brought in this optical potential well they will rest for hours stably at the equilibrium point. Thus, if this technique is applied such that at the sample position of a usual Raman spectrometer a vertically directed continuous wave laser beam stably traps and simultaneously excites a micronsized particle, microprobe Raman spectroscopy can ideally be performed. We have demonstrated experimentally that also non-spherical particles can be trapped long enough in order to take a Raman spectrum with reasonable signal-to-noise ratio.

## 3. Experimental

Several techniques can be employed to bring micron-sized particles to the stable minimum of the optical potential well, allowing then to take Raman spectra from the trapped particle. Fig. 2 describes schematically a technique where a single particle can be levitated and which we found to be a very efficient method [7]. A cw argon ion laser of about 500 mW operating at 514,5 nm in the $TEM_{oo}$ mode is focused by an f = 5 cm lens and directed vertically on a glass sphere of ~20 µm in diameter, initially at rest in position A on a glass plate (see Fig. 2). The power of the laser beam is such that the force of radiation pressure at the beam waist exceeds the gravity of the particle by several g and hence could levitate it. However, the van der Waals attraction of the 20 µm sphere is several orders of magnitude higher than the gravitational force of the particle [3] and, therefore, the particle could be levitated only if this strong van der Waals bond is broken. On the other hand, it is well known that the van der Waals force is proportional to $r^{-6}$ (r = distance of particle to supporting plate). Hence, it needs only a very short levitation distance to bring the particle in a region where the force of radiation pressure is higher than the gravitational plus van der Waals force of the particle. This is put into realization by setting up an eigenvibration of the centrally held

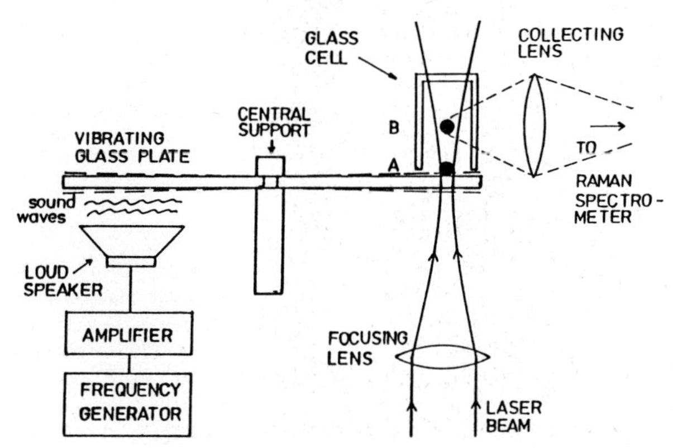


Fig. 2 Schematic diagram of an optical levitation technique by means of a vibrating glass plate which is resonantly driven by sound waves.

glass plate (see Fig. 2). With a closely mounted loud speaker, which is driven by an audio amplifier and a frequency generator (0.1 - 10 kHz), and by tuning the driving frequency rapidly through a mechanical resonance of the glass plate, one can momentarily shake the particle loose. The latter then begins to rise up into the diverging Gaussian beam. It comes to equilibrium where gravity and the axial light force in the upward direction balance, as mentioned above. By moving the focusing lens, the particle can easily be brought up to the right height for Raman excitation, which is the optical axis of the spectrometer (position B in Fig. 2).

In order to get experience in the optical levitation technique we first levitated spherical particles. The spheres used in our experiments were of glass. They were made commercially by Dragon Werk Wild, Bayreuth, F.R.G., for the purpose of manufacturing high reflectivity licence plates for automobiles. The glass spheres ranged in diameter between about 0.5 and 35 µm.

For demonstration of the applicability of the optical levitation technique to non-spherical particles we used microcrystals of quartz of size approximately 20 µm. The latter were obtained as $SiO_2$ p.a. from Merck. The particles were levitated and irradiated with a Spectra physics model 165 argon ion laser. We used mostly the green line at 514,5 nm with powers of the order of 500 mW at the sample. The beam was focused with lenses of focal lengths between 5 and 15 cm. The scattered light was collected with an 1:0.75 objective lense from KOWA, dispersed with a Spex triple monochromator (model 14018 plus model 1442) and photons were counted using an RCA C-31034-A-02 photomultiplier tube and a Photonic photon counter.

## 4. Raman Spectra of Optically Levitated Microcrystals

We have been successful in levitating spherical as well as non-spherical particles applying the method of eigenvibrations on the glass plate by means of sound waves as demonstrated in Fig. 2. However, it should be emphasized that the optical levitation of non-spherical particles with a Gaussian laser beam focused with a spherical lens is not as easy as for spheres. But after several trials we have also been successful to stably trap microcrystals in the focused laser beam. In the upper field of Fig. 3 we show for example the Raman spectrum of a microcrystal of quartz with size of about 20 µm. The lower field of Fig. 3 shows the same spectrum obtained from a pellet of pressed crystal powder of $SiO_2$. Because of the lower scattering signal from the microcrystal, the noise in the upper spectrum is slightly increased. Nevertheless all lines found in the crystal powder spectrum are also present in the one from the optically levitated particle. The spectrum shown of the microcrystal was obtained from one single scan.

## 5. Raman Spectra of Optically Levitated Microspheres

Fig. 4 shows the experimentally observed Raman spectrum (upper trace) from an optically levitated glass sphere with diameter of approx. 27 µm. In the lower part of Fig. 4 we display a Raman spectrum of a pellet pressed from spheres of the same glass material but with random diameters ranging between 0.5 and 35 µm. The relatively broad Raman lines in the spectrum of the pellet at about 500 and 1100 $cm^{-1}$ are well represented also in the spectrum of the levitated particle. Comparison of the upper and lower spectrum in Fig. 4 reveals that the general features in the Raman spectrum of the levitated microsphere are nicely reproduced. How-

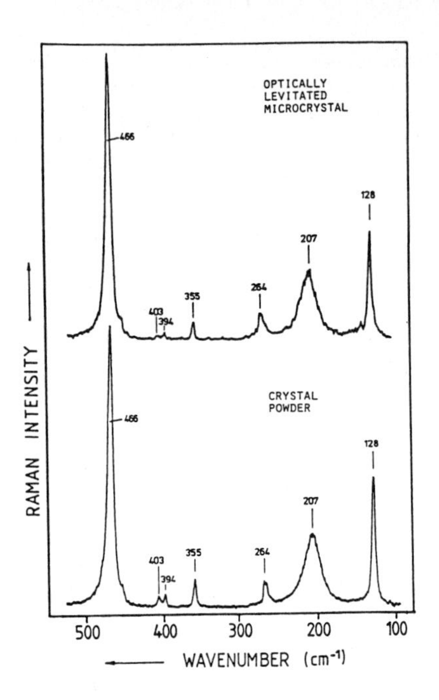


Fig. 3 Raman spectrum of an optically levitated microcrystal of quartz of size appr. 20 μm (upper spectrum). For comparison the low field shows the same spectrum from quartz crystal powder. Both spectra have been obtained under identical conditions. Excitation: 514,5 nm, 500 mW, slit width: 2 $cm^{-1}$, scan speed: 0,5 $cm^{-1}$/s, time constant: 2 s.

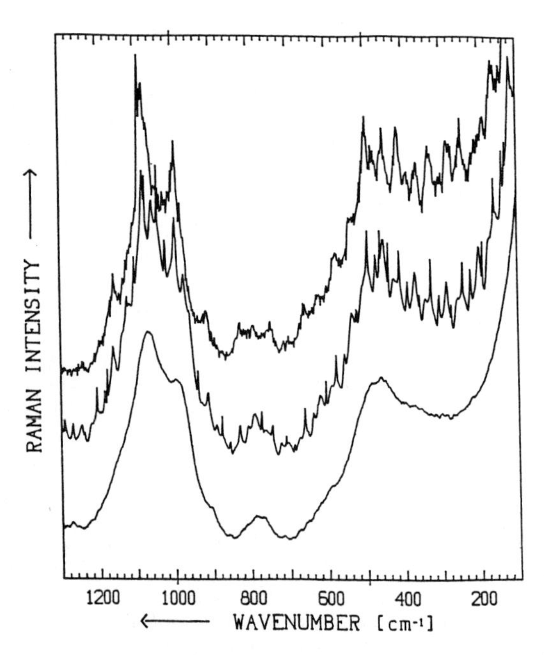


Fig. 4 Observed Raman spectrum of an optically levitated glass sphere of radius ~14 μm (upper spectrum). The middle spectrum shows a theoretically calculated spectrum (see text) and the lower spectrum is the Raman spectrum of the bulk glass material.

ever, in addition, we observe a regular structure of sharp peaks with spacing of about 40 $cm^{-1}$ in the spectrum of the micron-sized sphere. We interpret the observed ripple structure as structural resonances (MIE's [8] partial wave resonances) initiated by the Raman light scattered inside the glass sphere. Since the Raman spectrum of glass more or less is continuous in the region of interest, there are always frequencies which coincide with the frequencies of the structural resonances of the particular sphere. Based on the Mie theory we have calculated a synthetical Raman spectrum of a single glass sphere (radius 13.831 µm, refractive index n = 1.577) by modulating the Raman spectrum of the glass material with the extinction cross section of the sphere [8]. In Fig. 4 we display this synthetical Raman spectrum in the middle part. The observed and calculated Raman spectra of the microsphere show fairly good agreement.

## 6. Raman Spectra of Optically Levitated Liquid Drops

By means of the apparatus shown in Fig. 5 we have been able to trap liquid drops of sizes between appr. 20 and 40 µm diameter and simultaneously scan the Raman spectrum. Since liquid drops are perfect spheres one should expect the observation of the partial wave resonances also in the Raman spectrum of the droplets. Because water has a broad Raman spectrum which favors the observation of the resonances, but unfortunately has a high vapor pressure, we have made a mixture of water and glycerol. In Fig. 6 we compare part of the Raman spectrum of the liquid with the spectrum of a droplet of the same material. The latter nicely demonstrates the occurrence of electric and magnetic resonances of the dielectric sphere [10].

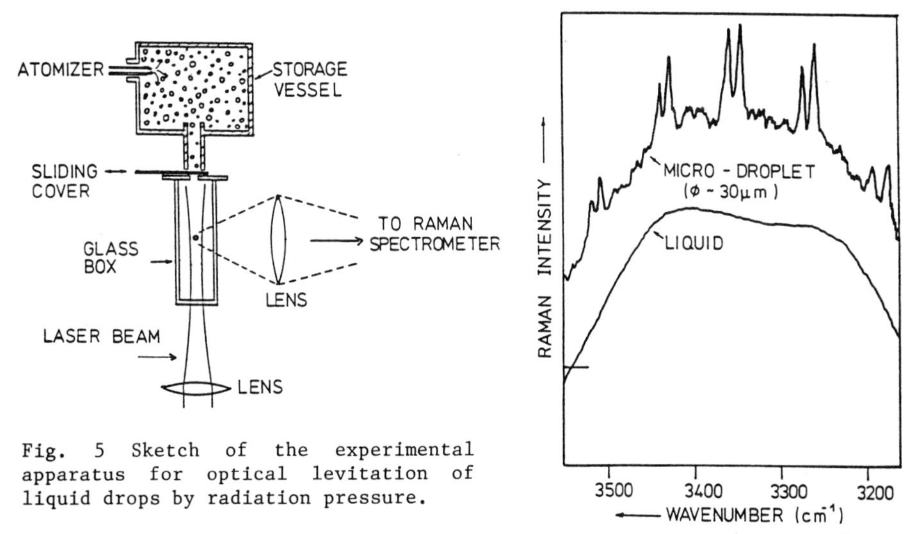


Fig. 5 Sketch of the experimental apparatus for optical levitation of liquid drops by radiation pressure.

Fig. 6 Part of the Raman spectrum of a 1:3 water-glycerol mixture. The lower spectrum shows the Raman spectrum of the liquid. The upper spectrum is a Raman spectrum of a droplet of size appr. 30 µm diameter. The doublet structure is due to electric and magnetic resonances of the dielectric sphere [10].

References


1 For a review see: G.J. Rosasco in: Advances in Infrared and Raman Spectroscopy, Vol. 7, R.J.H. Clark and R.E. Hester, editors, Heyden, London, 198, p. 223.
2 A. Ashkin, Phys. Rev. Letters 24, 156 (1970).
3 A. Ashkin and J.M. Dziedzic, Appl. Phys. Letters 19, 283 (1971).
4 A. Ashkin, Scientific American, February 1972, p. 63.
5 A. Ashkin and J.M. Dziedzic, Phys. Rev. Letters 30, 139 (1973), Appl. Phys. Letters 24, 586 (1974), Science 187, 1073 (1975), Appl. Phys. Letters 28, 333 (1976), Appl. Optics 19, 660 (1980), Phys. Rev. Letters 36, 267 (1976), Phys. Rev. Letters 38, 1351 (1977).
6 A. Ashkin, Science 210, 1081 (1980).
7 R. Thurn and W. Kiefer, Appl. Spectrosc. 38, 78 (1984).
8 G. Mie, Ann. d. Physik 25, 377 (1908).
9 R. Thurn and W. Kiefer, J. Raman Spectrosc., to be published.
10 R. Thurn and W. Kiefer, to be published.

# Photothermal Analysis of Thin Films

H. Coufal and P. Hefferle*

IBM Research Laboratory 5600 Cottle Road, K34/281
San Jose, California 95193 U.S.A.

## 1. Introduction

The photothermal effect can be observed whenever pulsed or modulated radiation is absorbed in a sample [1]. The sample under study is excited by the irradiation. Subsequent radiationless deexcitation causes local heating. If the lifetime of the excited states is short compared to the period of the excitation pulsed or modulated heat sources are generated giving rise to thermal waves. These thermal waves are critically damped, diffusive waves, *i.e*, within one wave length, the so-called thermal diffusion length $\mu$, the amplitude is attenuated by $e^{-2\pi}$. Therefore only heat generated within the diffusion length from the surface of a sample can contribute towards the temperature increase observed at this surface. These temperature waves can be readily detected at the surface using pyroelectric calorimeters [2] or other thermal or acoustic detectors [1]. At a modulation frequency f of 1 MHz thermal waves have typically a diffusion length of 1 $\mu$m. The thermal diffusion length is, however, frequency dependent $\mu \propto f^{-1/2}$. At very high modulation frequencies, therefore, only a very thin surface layer is seen in the photothermal signal. At slightly lower frequencies the same surface layer and heat from the adjacent layer reach the surface. The contribution by the additional layer can be determined if both layers are very thin by subtracting the signals at the two modulation frequencies. If the modulation frequencies differ substantially signals have to be corrected for the different amount of energy deposited during one excitation cycle. If the thickness of the individual layers is not negligible, a quantitative depth profile can not be readily reconstructed from frequency domain photothermal data, due to attenuation and dispersion of the thermal waves. Qualitative data, however, allow insight into the properties of samples. Two particularly interesting structures are discussed in the following paragraphs.

## 2. Phase Shifter

The interpretation of photothermal spectra is complicated due to the involvement of thermal and possibly also acoustic properties in the signal generation process. Considerable effort was, therefore, spent to compare optical features of otherwise identical samples [1] or to use reference samples with well defined and optimized optical and thermal properties [3]. Comparing two signals requires either a dual beam arrangement for real time recording of sample and reference spectra, which is crucial for compensation techniques, or the subsequent recording of these spectra with an off line normalization. For applications requiring utmost sensitivity such as weakly absorbing

*Permanent address: Institut für Physikalische und Theoretische Chemie der Technischen Universität München, Garching, Lichtenbergstr. 4, D-8046 Garching, Federal Republic of Germany.

samples [2,4] only the real time technique is suitable. For this type of sample there is, however, another alternative: weakly absorbing sample and well defined reference can be optically in series, the excitation being therefore simultaneous. If sample and reference are separated by a thermal delay line or a phaseshifter the detection can be sequential. Only one detector and subsequent electronics are required in this set up, thus eliminating noise sources and reducing cost considerably.

Assuming excitation of the composite sample from the front side and detection of the thermal wave at the back side of the reference sample, for example by a pyroelectric calorimeter, following modes of thermal wave propagation are of interest:

At low modulation frequencies the thermal wave from the sample reaches the detector unattenuated, but slightly later than the reference wave. By in-phase and out-of-phase detection the signal components could be separated and then the ratio of both signals determined. The same result can be conveniently obtained by recording the phase angle of the composite signal. Being a photothermal spectrum this spectrum is a convolution of the true absorption spectrum of the sample under study and the yield for radiationless deexcitation.

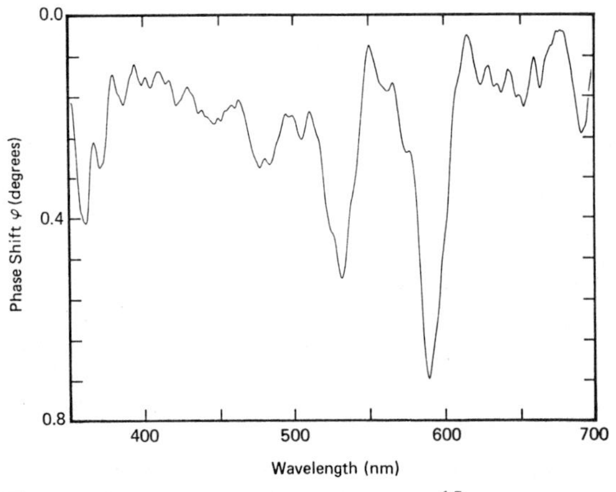


Fig. 1: Phase angle spectrum of $0.8 \times 10^{15}$ $Nd_2O_3$ molecules in a 1 μm thick PMMA film coated on top of a 0.1 mm thick undoped PMMA film on a silver substrate. Recorded at 2.2 Hz modulation frequency.

At high enough a modulation frequency the thermal wave from the sample does not at all reach the detector. The photothermal signal of the reference sample is then caused only by the light transmitted through the sample and allows the detection of the true transmission spectrum of the sample. The absorption spectrum of the sample can then be determined readily. By ratioing the above phase angle spectrum with the true absorption spectrum the quantum yield for radiationless deexcitation can be determined.

To demonstrate this concept a pyroelectric calorimeter with a silver electrode was coated with a 0.1 mm thick transparent PMMA film. The silver film serves as reference sample, the PMMA film as phase shifter. On top of this phase shifter a 1 μm thick PMMA film doped with $0.8 \times 10^{15}$ $Nd_2O_3$ was deposited as sample. The phase angle spectrum recorded at 2 Hz modulation frequency is shown in Fig. 1. It is in excellent agreement with spectra of identical samples obtained with much more sophisticated instrumentation [2]. By comparison with an absorption spectrum recorded with the same sample at 88 Hz modulation frequency the quantum yield for radiationless deexcitation was determined to be $90 \pm 5\%$ throughout the entire spectrum.

## 3. Multiplex Excitation

In the above example each modulation frequency had been excited and recorded separately. It would be convenient in this case and absolutely necessary for full depth profiling, which requires a complete modulation frequency spectrum to modulate and detect at many frequencies simultaneously. This has been done in photothermal spectroscopy in the wave length domain [6,7] and in photothermal imaging in the spatial domain [8,9]. This concept can be extended to the frequency domain, using Fourier transformations to obtain the information of interest. To generate as much intensity at high Fourier components as possible the otherwise stable output of a 6 mW HeNe laser was modulated with white noise. Figure 2 shows the light intensity incident on the sample in the time domain. A thin film of homogeneously carbon doped PMMA generates the response of Fig. 3. By ratioing response and excitation the frequency dependence of

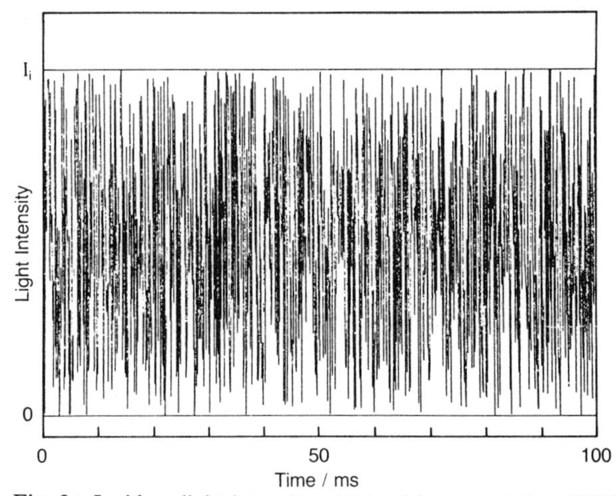


Fig. 2: Incident light intensity obtained by modulating CW laser with white noise.

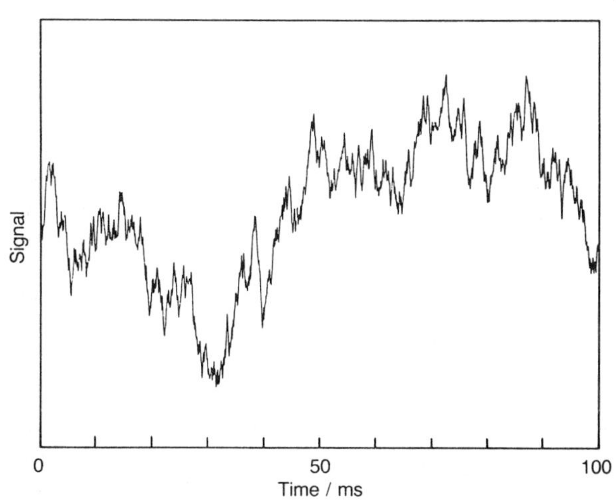


Fig. 3: Photothermal signal observed from a sample excited with the light intensity of Fig. 2.

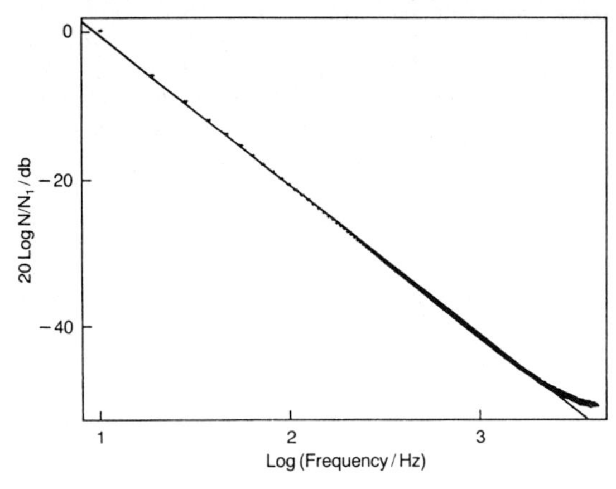


Fig. 4: Frequency dependence of the photothermal signal of a homogeneous, thin sample obtained by ratioing the Fourier transforms of Figs. 2 and 3.

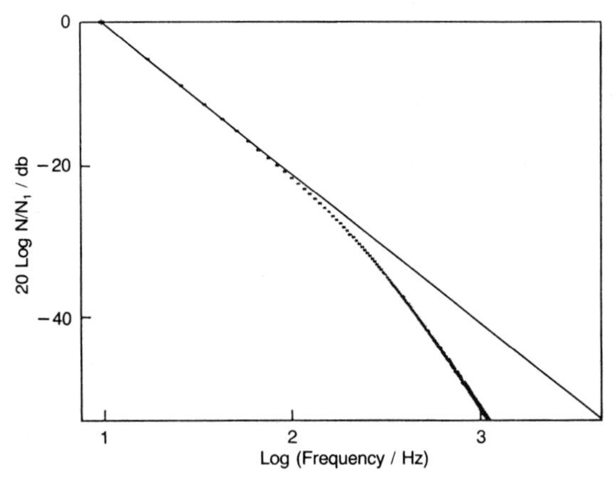


Fig. 5: Frequency dependence of the photothermal signal of a homogeneous, thick sample obtained by Fourier transform techniques.

the photothermal signal can be determined over the complete modulation frequency spectrum (Fig. 4). Data acquisition and Fourier transformation of the data required only 2.6 seconds. The frequency dependence determined with this technique is identical to the one determined conventionally one frequency at a time in more than 200 seconds. Both show clearly by their $f^{-1}$-frequency dependence that the sample was homogeneously doped [1]. Figure 5 shows clearly the frequency dependence of a thick sample obtained with the same technique.

## 4. Conclusion

It has been demonstrated that the photothermal analysis of thin films has a unique potential. Even without being able to construct an actual depth profile from photothermal data, mainly due to mathematical problems, valuable insight into the properties of the sample can be gained. In one example the known structure and thermal properties of a composite sample were used to obtain a spectrum of a thin surface layer with an amount of $Nd^{3+}$ ions corresponding to one monolayer. Furthermore the quantum yield for radiationless decay was obtained. In a second example with well defined optical and overall thermal properties the homogeneity of the doping was proven taking advantage of multiplex excitation.

## 5. Acknowledgments

The authors would like to thank R. Grygier, L. Kelley, and L. W. Welsh, Jr. for technical assistance. This work was supported in part by the Office of Naval Research.

## 6. References

[1] A. Rosencwaig, *Photoacoustics and Photoacoustic Spectroscopy*, (Wiley, New York, 1980).
[2] H. Coufal, *Appl. Phys. Lett.* **44**, 59 (1984).
[3] H. Coufal, *Appl. Optics* **21**, 104 (1982).
[4] H. Coufal, T. J. Chuang, and F. Träger, *Surf. Sci.*, in print.
[5] H. Coufal, *Appl. Phys. Lett.*, to be published.
[6] M. G. Rockley, *Chem. Phys. Lett.* **68**, 455 (1979).
[7] M. M. Farrow, R. K. Burnham, and E. M. Eyring, *Appl. Phys. Lett.* **33**, 735 (1978).
[8] H. Coufal, U. Möller, and S. Schneider, *Appl. Optics* **21** 116 (1982).
[9] H. Coufal, U. Möller, and S. Schneider, *Appl. Optics* **21** 2343 (1982).

# Part 5

# Laser Diagnostics in Reactive Gaseous Systems

# Raman Diagnostics of Heterogeneous Chemical Processes

G. Leyendecker[+], J. Doppelbauer, and D. Bäuerle
Angewandte Physik, Johannes Kepler Universität, A-4040 Linz, Austria

## 1. Introduction

A great many technical processes are based on heterogeneous chemical reactions at gas-solid interfaces. Among these are petrol refining or the production of electronic devices by means of chemical vapor deposition (CVD). Hydrodynamic transport mechanisms in the gas phase strongly influence the kinetics of such processes; furthermore, very little is known about the nature and role of intermediate species. A clarification of these questions requires precise knowledge of the fundamental parameters, namely the flow, temperature and concentration fields in the gas phase. In most cases the systems are too complex for satisfactory theoretical approaches. Conventional experimental methods such as thermocouple measurements or sampling techniques have many limitations resulting from perturbation of the system under study by the solid probe or from perturbation of the probe by the system. Optical techniques, in particular laser spectroscopy, however, besides being measurements of a non-intrusive character, meet the further requirements of in situ observation and high spatial resolution. While laser-induced fluorescence is suitable for qualitative detection of gas phase species with high sensitivity, laser Raman spectroscopy provides the possibility of simultaneous determination of local values of the temperature and the molecular concentrations.

Following the pioneering work of LAPP and PENNEY [1], in the past decade Raman scattering techniques have been applied in a number of investigations to the study of practical systems such as flames, combustion chambers or CVD reactors (for reviews see [2, 3]). Sophisticated techniques such as CARS have been developed to overcome the interferences inherent in these hostile environments [4]. As we have shown [5, 6], the accuracy and speed of temperature and concentration measurements may be improved by suitable selection of the Raman bands of the gases under consideration and by appropriate calibration techniques. Because many important technical processes are stationary, we have concentrated our interest on the investigation of stationary systems by means of spontaneous CW Raman spectroscopy, although Raman spectroscopy may be applied to time resolved studies [2]. In this paper we summarize our results obtained for the $CH_4/H_2$ CVD system and for catalytic hydrogenation of acetylene. After discussing theory, calibration and accuracy of measurement in general, we briefly comment on instrumentation aspects. Then we present experimental temperature and concentration profiles, and, finally, the Raman scattering technique is compared with other non-intrusive optical methods.

---

[+]Present address: Siemens AG, D-8000 München, Fed. Rep. of Germany

## 2. Theory

Raman scattering is inelastic light scattering in which the gas molecule changes its rotational or vibrational state. The intensity (in photons/s) of the scattered radiation is given by

$$I(i,f) = P_L \cdot N \cdot c \cdot f(i) \cdot l \cdot \sigma(i,f) \qquad (1)$$

$P_L$: power of the exciting radiation, N: Avogadro's number, c: molar concentration of the molecules, f(i): fraction of the molecules in the state $|i\rangle$, l: length of the scattering volume from which light is collected, $\sigma(i,f) = \int d\Omega\, d\sigma(i,f)/d\Omega$: scattering cross section for the solid angle over which light is collected. For non-resonant Raman scattering the differential scattering cross section can be written as

$$d\sigma(i,f)/d\Omega = K \cdot \nu(i,f)^3 \cdot P(i,f) \qquad (2)$$

K: collection of physical constants and molecular parameters independent of $|i\rangle$ and $|f\rangle$, $\nu(i,f)$: frequency of the scattered radiation, P(i,f): normalized Raman transition probability between states $|i\rangle$ and $|f\rangle$. The differential scattering cross section is of the order of $10^{-31}$ $cm^2$ $sr^{-1}$ (Rayleigh scattering: $10^{-27}$ $cm^2$ $sr^{-1}$) [7]. Resonant enhancement of the Raman scattering cross section by several orders of magnitude is possible when the incident frequency matches an electronic transition in the scattering molecule [8]. The angular and polarization properties of the scattered radiation depend on the symmetry of the states $|i\rangle$ and $|f\rangle$ [9]. For measuring temperatures or molecular concentrations, light collection at $90^0$ to the irradiating beam with its polarization perpendicular to the scattering plane is widely used because this arrangement measures the highest intensities. The differently polarized fractions of the scattered radiation are not separated for this purpose.

### 2.1. Determination of Local Temperatures

In equilibrium systems or when the concept of local equilibrium is valid - which is certainly the case for stationary systems with only thermal excitation - f(i) from (1) is given by the Boltzmann distribution function. Therefore, from the relative intensities of two or more Raman lines of a molecular species the relative population of the corresponding initial states, and thereby the local temperature, can be derived. Since only relative intensities are required, most of the factors determining the measured intensities cancel, for example, the optical collection efficiency. Only the frequency-dependent response of the detection system has to be considered. The lines used for temperature determination should be carefully selected to obtain high accuracy of measurement with short measuring times. One frequently used procedure is to take the intensity ratio of the corresponding Stokes and anti-Stokes transitions between the same two states [2]. However, in most cases there are other pairs of lines whose intensity ratios yield smaller errors in the temperature. Local temperatures are often derived from the pure rotational Raman spectra. For diatomic and linear molecules, the level populations are according to the Boltzmann distribution function

$$f(J) = g(J) \cdot (2J + 1) \cdot \exp(-E(J)/k_B T) \;/\; Q_{rot}(T) \qquad (3)$$

g(J): nuclear spin degeneracy factor, E(J): energy of the level J, $Q_{rot}$: rotational partition function, which is the sum of all f(J). For determination of a single temperature value, earlier workers (for a review see [2]) have plotted ln $(I(J,J')/k_J)$ against $E(J)$ ($k_J$ is a J dependent factor) for the entire measured Stokes or anti-Stokes branch. The temperature was then derived from the slope of the resulting straight line. The advantage of such a procedure is that deviations from the equilibrium population can be detected. On the other hand, recording a complete rotational spectrum is very time consuming and the necessary correction for the response of the detection system has to be determined for a wide spectral range. However, the local temperature can readily be obtained by taking the ratio of any two different rotational lines. For diatomic and linear molecules, the temperature derived from the intensity ratio of the Raman lines corresponding to the transitions $J = i \to j$ and $J = k \to l$, respectively, is given by

$$T = \frac{(E(k) - E(i))/k_B}{\ln\left(\frac{I(i,j)}{I(k,l)}\cdot r\cdot n\right) + 3\ln\frac{\nu(k,l)}{\nu(i,j)} + \ln\frac{(2k+1)\cdot g(k)\cdot P(k,l)}{(2i+1)\cdot g(i)\cdot P(i,j)}} \tag{4}$$

r: detection system response correction coefficient, n: intensity correction coefficient due to nonrigidity [3] for the lines under consideration. Because values for n taken from the literature (for $H_2$ [10]) seem to be quite uncertain, and both n and r are independent of temperature, it is appropriate to evaluate the product $n\cdot r$, using (4) and the corresponding molecular constants, by measuring the intensity ratio at a known temperature, e.g. room temperature. Thereby one also avoids trouble with the determination of the detection system response function. According to the law of error propagation, the random error of the temperatures derived according to (4) is given by

$$\Delta T = \frac{T^2\cdot k_B}{E(k) - E(i)}\cdot\frac{\Delta R}{R} \tag{5}$$

$R = I(i,j)/I(k,l)$: intensity ratio of the two lines. Compromising between a good signal-to-noise ratio in the intensity ratio and a large energy separation $(E(k) - E(i))$ one can always select an optimal pair of lines which minimizes the random error of the derived temperatures. The optimum choice depends on the collection efficiency of the apparatus and on the concentration of the molecules; it may change with temperature. $H_2$ is the ideal specimen for the determination of temperatures in this way. Because of its large rotational constant only a few rotational levels are appreciably populated even at temperatures of 1500 K. For our apparatus, random errors according to (5) are shown in Fig. 1 for 1000 mbar $H_2$. Below about 600 K, the pair of lines $J = 1 \to 3$ and $J = 3 \to 5$ yields the smallest error in the derived temperatures. Between about 600 and 1500 K, the most suitable Raman lines of $H_2$ are due to the transitions $J = 1 \to 3$ and $J = 5 \to 3$. For other molecules, e.g. $N_2$, the optimum choice changes more often with temperature [11]. Nevertheless, we believe that the method described above has even in this case several advantages in comparison to those methods which make use of a great number of rotational lines for the determination of a single temperature value: the attention is directed only to a limited number of lines chosen to give a minimum error and for which the intensity corrections can be determined with high accuracy. Furthermore, in gas mixtures the pair of lines can be selected to avoid spectral interferences from Raman scattering of other molecules than those of interest.

The spectra of rotational vibrational bands contain information on both the relative populations of the rotational levels and of the vibrational

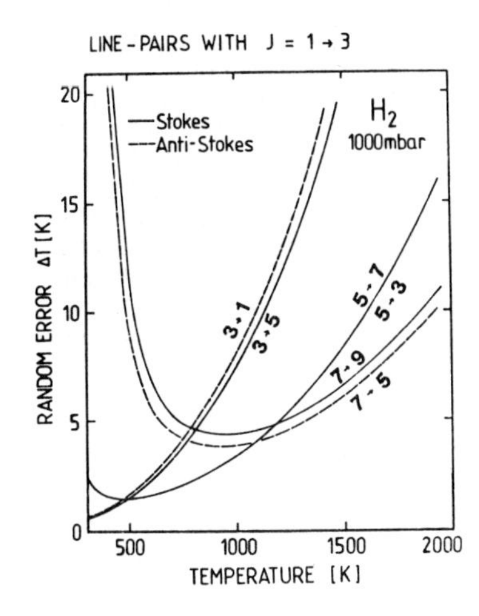


Fig. 1. Calculated random error of temperatures derived from the intensity ratio of two rotational lines of hydrogen for several line pairs with J = 1 → 3

states. However, because of their higher intensities, temperature determination from the pure rotational lines - if possible - will be more accurate than evaluation of the intensity distribution of the single lines of the rovibrational branches. Due to anharmonic coupling, the vibrational bands may include "hot bands" [9]. From the relative intensities of the hot bands to the fundamental the relative populations of the vibrational states can be determined; this kind of temperature measurement was first applied to $N_2$ [7]. If a quantitative interpretation of the hot bands is not possible (e.g. because of missing data for the anharmonicity constants), the temperature dependence of the relative intensities of the hot bands and the fundamental may be calibrated. We have successfully applied such a procedure to $CH_4$ (Sect. 4).

## 2.2. Determination of Local Concentrations

The Raman scattered intensity is directly proportional to the number of scattering molecules. At known temperature, the concentration may be determined by normalization of the scattered intensity to that at a reference temperature and known concentration, but optical misalignment and changes of window transmission may cause serious errors. In gas mixtures, relative concentrations can be derived from relative intensities of the Raman bands of the constituents. In this way one avoids the problems mentioned above. Generally, for the determination of local concentrations the most intense Raman bands of the molecules under consideration are employed. Except for the case of $H_2$, these are the Q branches of the totally symmetric vibrational bands. To measure the intensity with high accuracy, instead of scanning through the bands it is appropriate to use a spectral bandpass such that almost the whole contour of a Q branch can be detected at once. The measured count rate of a Raman band j of the molecular species A can then be written as

$$I(j) = P_L \cdot N \cdot c_A \cdot \sigma_A(j) \cdot l \cdot \Delta_{A,j}(T) \cdot R(\nu_j) \tag{6}$$

$\sigma_A(j)$: part of the scattering cross section independent of the individual lines, $\Delta_{A,j}(T)$: correction factor explained below, (7), $R(\nu_j)$: response of the entire optical detection system at the frequency of the scattered radiation. The correction $\Delta_{A,j}(T)$ originates from the temperature dependence of the band contour: as the temperature is raised, increasing proportions of the contour fall outside the bandpass which in our experiments is positioned to transmit most of the contour at room temperature. (The question of optimal setting of the bandpass was discussed in detail in [2]). Thus, $\Delta_{A,j}$ (T) may be written as

$$\Delta_{A,j}(T) = \sum_i f_j(i) \cdot P(i,f) \cdot S(\nu(i,f)) \tag{7}$$

where the sum is over all initial states $|i\rangle$ of the band. $S(\nu(i,f))$ is the spectral transmission at the Raman shifted frequency. While for the vibrational bands of diatomic molecules such as $N_2$ this correction may be ignored at moderate temperatures if sufficiently wide bandpasses are used, it is significant for the vibrational bands of diatomic molecules even at temperatures between room temperature and 500 K [6]. In principle, $\Delta_{A,j}$ (T) may be calculated; for complicated molecules for which no simple relations exist for the contour of their rovibrational bands and for which the relevant molecular constants are not known, $\Delta_{A,j}$ (T) can be determined experimentally only.

In mixtures containing sufficient amounts of hydrogen, the rotational Raman line $J = 1 \rightarrow 3$ is particularly suitable as a reference for the determination of local concentrations. We define

$$\Sigma_A(j) = \frac{\sigma_A(j) \cdot R(\nu_j)}{\sigma_{H_2}(1,3) \cdot R(\nu(1,3))} \tag{8}$$

as a measure of the relative scattering cross sections. For quantitative concentration measurements it is necessary to determine only the calibration factors $[\Delta_{A,j}(T)/\Delta_{A,j}(T_{ref})]$ and $[\Sigma_A(j) \cdot \Delta_{A,j}(T_{ref})]$. The ratio of the molar fractions is then determined from

$$\frac{x_A}{x_{H_2}} = \frac{I_A(j)}{I_{H_2}(1,3)} \; \frac{f_{H_2,J=1}(T)}{f_{H_2,J=1}(T_{ref})} \; \frac{[\Delta_{A,j}(T_{ref})/\Delta_{A,j}(T)]}{[\Sigma_A(j) \cdot \Delta_{A,j}(T_{ref})]} \tag{9}$$

$x_A$, $x_{H_2}$: molar fractions, $f_{H_2,J=1}$: population of the $H_2$ rotational level. (The functions $\Delta_{A,j}$ (T) can be included in the calculations only if the local temperature is known. The local temperature can be derived simultaneously from the intensity ratio of two rotational lines of $H_2$). The molar fractions can then be calculated using the fact that the sum of the molar fractions is 1; neglecting trace amounts of minor species has little effect on the accuracy of major species concentrations. The procedure described above can be transferred to any multicomponent mixture.

## 2.3. Accuracy of Measurement and Limits

The accuracy of both the temperature and the concentration measurements are determined by the signal-to-noise ratios of the measured count rates of the Raman bands. Because the Raman scattering cross sections are very small, in many practical applications of Raman techniques interference from other sources of radiation such as thermal radiation or fluorescence strongly affects the accuracy of measurements. Usually, pulsed lasers together with gated detection are employed for background suppression when necessary. In some systems, however, there is a strong laser-induced background which limits the applicability even of pulsed Raman techniques [12]. Some authors use multipass or intracavity configurations. With such arrangements, the available laser power is multiplied; on the other hand, fluctuations will be strongly amplified. We believe that in stationary systems with limited background single pass operation of CW lasers will be the best choice for Raman investigations. With our experimental arrangement [5, 6], for example, with 10 mbar $H_2$ we obtain at room temperature count rates higher than $10^3$ cps from the rotational line $J = 1 \rightarrow 3$. Consequently, with 30 s integration time, the statistical fluctuations are averaged so that the signal-to-noise ratio is limited just by the low frequency output fluctuations of the laser ($\leq$ 0.3 %). The standard deviation of the temperature derived from the $H_2$ rotational spectrum is then less than 0.5 K; the detection limit is about $10^{-2}$ mbar. However, spectral interferences from Raman scattering of other molecules than those of interest are a serious problem in the determination of minor species concentrations in multicomponent mixtures. This problem can be solved partially by suitable choice of the Raman bands.

## 3. Instrumentation Aspects

The instrumentation of laser Raman temperature and concentration measurements is well established [2]. The major components are the laser source, the light collecting and frequency selection optics, and the detection and signal processing unit. The availability of low cost microcomputers now offers the possibility of on-line signal processing of the digital information from the photon counting system together with control of the monochromator setting. Apart from the convenience of direct readout of temperatures and concentrations, time-optimization routines may be implemented on such systems. These routines integrate the counts from a band until the desired signal-to-noise ratio is reached. A practical set-up, used for the experiments presented in the next sections, is shown in Fig. 2.

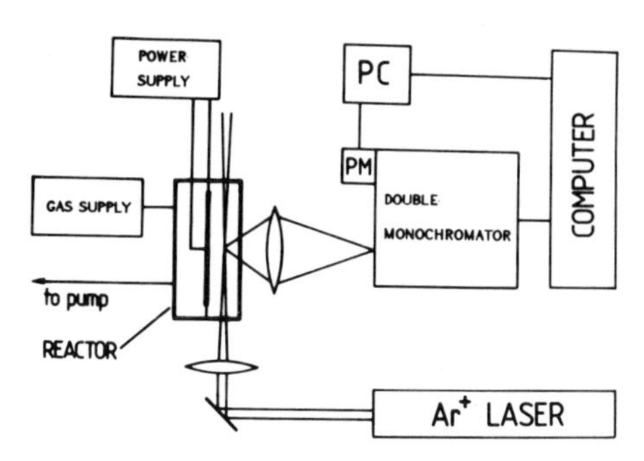


Fig. 2: Experimental set-up for Raman temperature and concentration measurements in a model reactor (PM: photomultiplier tube, PC: photon counting system)

## 4. The $CH_4/H_2$ CVD System

Chemical vapor deposition (CVD) is widely used for the production of electronic devices, glass-fiber optics, and coatings [13]. The lack of understanding of the basic mechanisms of the CVD process makes Raman scattering techniques highly interesting for the investigation of CVD systems [14 - 16]. Our intention was to test the suitability of the method for hydrocarbon CVD used for the deposition of carbon. Because $H_2$ is in any case a reaction product in the decomposition of hydrocarbons such as methane, we investigated temperature profiles in a model reactor (50 mm square by 300 mm height) filled with $CH_4$, $H_2$, and mixtures of both. A resistance heated platinum wire centered on the vertical axis of the reactor served as the substrate material (for details see [5]). Raman temperature measurements were performed in a plane perpendicular to the wire in the center of the reactor for wire temperatures of 773 K and of 1473 K and various gas pressures between 30 and 1000 mbar. Temperatures were

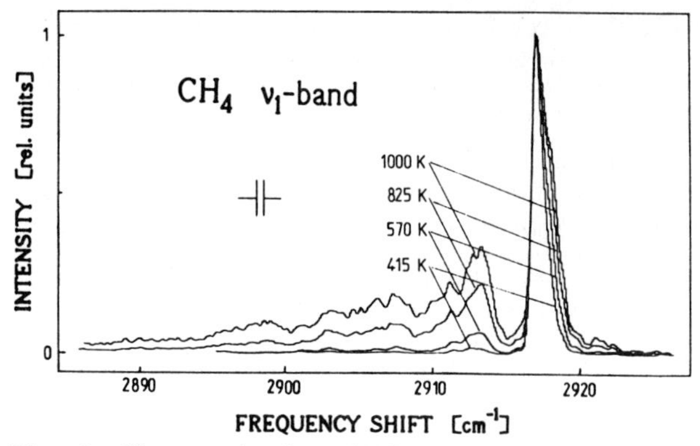

Fig. 3. $CH_4$ $\nu_1$ - band at different temperatures

derived from the pure rotational spectrum of $H_2$ and from the $\nu_1$ band of $CH_4$ of which typical spectra are shown in Fig. 3. It was not possible to interpret quantitatively the distinct hot band structure near the fundamental. These lines were used for temperature measurements, in spite of the difficulties in quantitative interpretation, by calibrating the temperature dependence of the relative peak heights of the fundamental and the hot band near 2913 $cm^{-1}$, which can probably be assigned as $\nu_1 + \nu_4 - \nu_4$. The calibration was performed in mixtures of $CH_4$ and $H_2$ via the temperature derived from the $H_2$ rotational spectrum.

Typical temperature profiles are shown in Fig. 4. Error bars indicate standard deviations derived from a large number of single data points. For

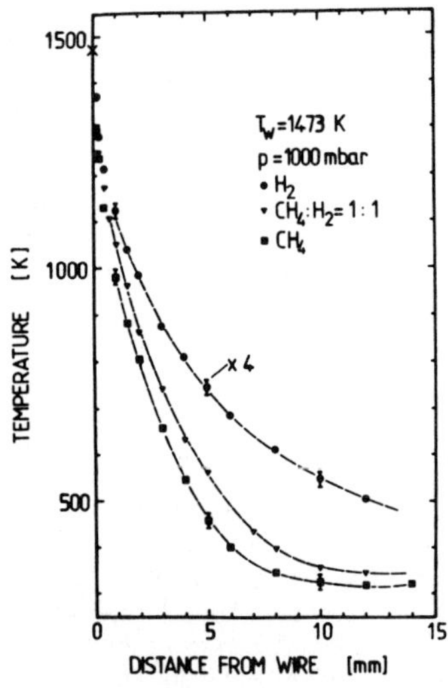

Fig. 4. Temperature profiles in the model reactor at a wire temperature of 1473 K and a gas pressure of 1000 mbar. The bars indicate standard deviations and are expanded four times for clarity. The dashed lines are guides for the eye

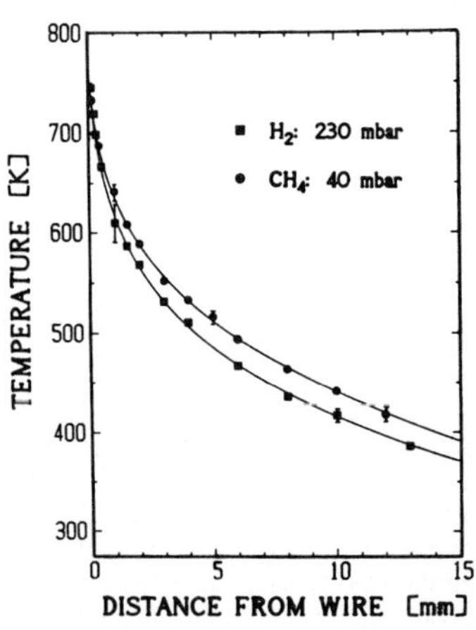

Fig. 5. Temperature profiles in the model reactor at a wire temperature of 773 K. The bars indicate standard deviations and are expanded two times for clarity. The solid curves are theoretical solutions for the temperature distribution

example, with $CH_4$ at 1 mm distance from the wire we found standard deviations of 3 K (wire temperature 773 K, 1000 mbar), 4 K (773 K, 40 mbar), and 4 K (1473 K, 1000 mbar). Our results show a significant improvement of the accuracy of measurement compared with results of other authors obtained under similar conditions [17, 18]. This is especially remarkable in view of the short recording times of less than 3 min for a single data point. To confirm the validity of our experimental findings, we have obtained independent theoretical solutions for the temperature distribution in our model reactor using the model of free convection in a vertical concentric annular cavity. The hydrodynamic characteristics of the system are determined by the dimensionless Rayleigh number which is proportional to the square of the average gas density [5]. At atmospheric pressure, the steep temperature gradient near the inner cylinder is much more pronounced in the case of $CH_4$ - due to much higher Rayleigh numbers than with $H_2$ (Fig. 4). At reduced pressures, the temperature profile in the center of the reactor is due to only heat conduction perpendicular to the wire. When the minor effects of temperature jump at the wire (Knudsen effect) and the actual square cross section are considered, quantitative agreement between the experimental data and the theoretical results is obtained (Fig. 5). Disregarding the temperature jump effect would yield a shift of the theoretical curves towards higher temperatures which is clearly more than the error of the measurement.

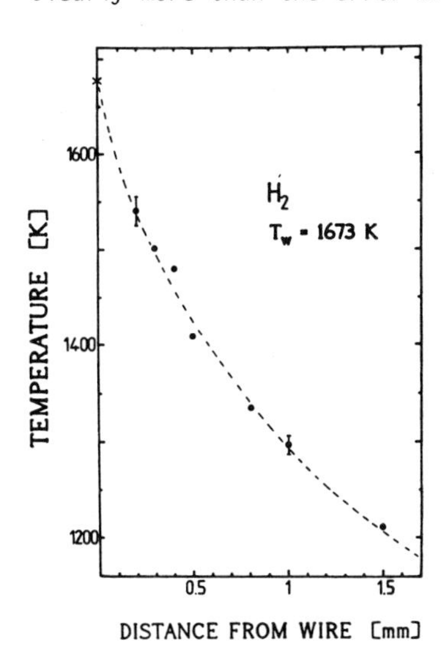


Fig. 6. Temperature profile with 1000 mbar $H_2$ at a wire temperature of 1673 K

The present method can be used to make measurements with sufficient accuracy close to the thermally radiating substrate even at substrate temperatures above 1500 K (Fig. 6). However, with $CH_4$, the onset of particle nucleation within the gas phase at even higher temperatures (in our system this would be about 1600 K at 1000 mbar) leads to a strong laser-induced background which may be due to particulate incandescence [12] or fluorescence. This limits the applicability of the Raman scattering technique.

## 5. Catalytic Hydrogenation of Acetylene

To demonstrate the power of CW Raman scattering for the investigation of mass transport phenomena, we have studied as a model system the catalytic hydrogenation of acetylene ($C_2H_2$) to ethylene ($C_2H_4$) over Pt. Metal catalyzed hydrogenation of acetylene has been the subject of numerous experimental studies (for a recent review see [19]). We chose this reaction because of the simple molecules involved and because of the high reaction rates at temperatures of about 500 K. Temperature and concentration profiles were measured in the same model reactor as used for the investigation of the $CH_4$ CVD system; the polycrystalline platinum wire here served as the catalyst.

The factors $[\Delta_{A,j}(T)/\Delta_{A,j}(T_{ref})]$ from (9) have been calibrated for the most intense Raman bands of $C_2H_2$ and $C_2H_4$, respectively. The trapezoidal spectral slit function of our monochromator had a flat top of about 10 $cm^{-1}$. These experiments were performed in a homogeneously heated cell with the pure gases and with mixtures with $H_2$. In the latter case, the intensities were compared to those of the $H_2$ rotational line $J = 1 \rightarrow 3$ to eliminate possible errors due to optical misalignment. The standard deviations of the data were less than 1 % in the temperature range between room temperature and 500 K. The calculated values for $C_2H_2$ agree with the experimental results within 1 %. The other relevant quantities for Raman concentration measurements $[\Sigma_A(j)\cdot\Delta_{A,j}(T_{ref})]$ were measured for each gas ($C_2H_2$, $C_2H_4$) from several different concentrations of the gas in $H_2$. With a suitable arrangement the systematic error in this calibration factor was reduced to less than 1 %; the systematic error of the derived concentration values is thus less than 2 %.

Metal catalysts can be readily poisoned by impurities. In our system, we could not observe any reaction when using commercial acetylene without further purification. Using purified gas, we observed the highest rates at wire temperatures between about 450 K and 550 K and at a molar fraction of about 2 % $C_2H_2$ in $H_2$. After an increased transient activity in the early stages of the reaction, the rate became constant. Representative concentration profiles, measured after any initial transients, with continuous flow, are shown in Fig. 7a. Because the wire acts as a sink of $C_2H_2$, this species is depleted with decreasing distance from the wire. On the other hand, $C_2H_4$ is produced at the surface of the wire. If only ordinary diffusion occurred, the sum of the molar fractions of $C_2H_2$ and $C_2H_4$ should be roughly constant for any distance from the wire, since one molecule of $C_2H_4$ is built from one molecule of $C_2H_2$. The additional effect of temperature gradients on the spatial variations of the gas concentrations is demonstrated in Fig. 7b. Here, we show concentration profiles measured under similar conditions but with a deactivated catalyst. Thermal diffusion contributes significantly to the mass transport in systems with large temperature gradients. This fact is of great importance when hydrogen is either used as the carrier gas or produced during the chemical reaction, for example, the widely used CVD reactions for the deposition of Si from $SiH_4$ and of C from $CH_4$. In contrast to Sect. 4, here, theoretical calculations cannot be used to check the experimental results. Firstly, in multicomponent mixtures the equations of change which describe the transport phenomena are more complicated; secondly, the relevant transport coefficients are rarely known. So, in this case determination of local temperatures and concentrations by Raman spectroscopy would allow to verify new theoretical models. However, our principal result is that Raman methods are accurate enough that different contributions to the mass transport can be distinguished clearly. The systematic errors and the recording times of the method are suitable for useful application to technological problems.

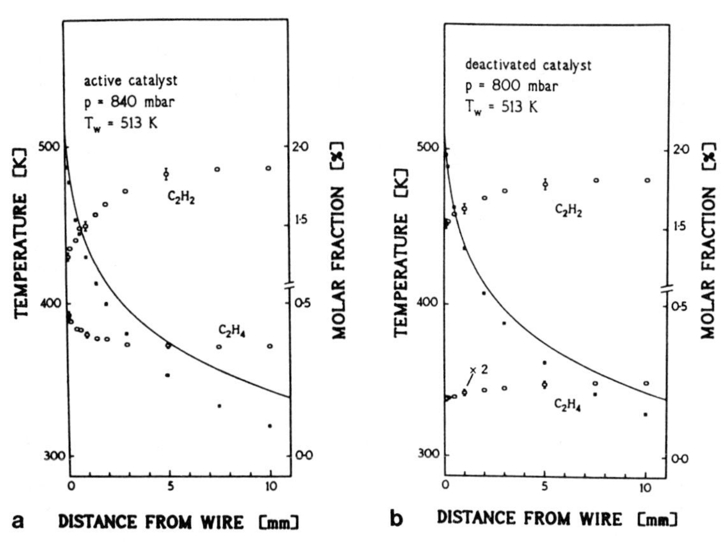


Fig. 7. Temperature (▪) and concentration (**o**) profiles of $C_2H_2$ and of $C_2H_4$; (a) with an active catalyst and continuous flow, and (b) with a deactivated catalyst. The full lines are theoretical temperature profiles calculated for pure $H_2$. The bars indicate the total error and in (b) (for $C_2H_4$) are expanded two times for clarity

## 6. Alternative Optical Techniques

A number of other optical techniques have been used for non-intrusive investigation of technological systems. Optical emission and absorption techniques can provide very sensitive measurements of species concentrations but are limited in spatial resolution. Laser excited fluorescence which uses the same general type of instrumentation as Raman spectroscopy is also very sensitive. It suffers from the influence of quenching so that quantitative measurements are barely possible. Applications to the study of CVD systems are described by HO et al. [20] and by HARGIS [21]. The methods described above are suitable for the detection of minor species and of reaction intermediates. The nonlinear process CARS (Coherent Antistokes Raman Scattering) has been looked upon as a promising tool for temperature and concentration measurements. There are a number of recent papers concerning the application of CARS in combustion probing and in other highly luminous and particle laden systems (for example [22, 23]). With CARS, the data reduction process is much more complicated than with spontaneous Raman scattering. Many molecular parameters such as Raman linewidths which are rarely known enter the calculations and can give rise to serious errors [24]. Despite the fact that with typical instrumentation CARS signals are many orders of magnitude stronger than spontaneous Raman scattering, the CARS sensitivity for minor constituents of a gas mixture is limited to about 0.1 % by the occurrence of a nonresonant background [4, 24]. Therefore, in clean environments spontaneous Raman scattering offers distinct advantages over CARS.

## 7. Conclusion

CW laser Raman spectroscopy is a diagnostic tool particularly suitable for the investigation of heterogeneous chemical processes. It allows nonperturbing simultaneous determination of temperature and concentration fields in the gas phase and thereby characterization of transport phenomena. At present there are no alternative experimental techniques which would yield similar information.

## Acknowledgements

The authors are indepted to Dr D.J. Dunstan for valuable discussions and for critical reading of the manuscript. Financial support by the Austrian Fonds zur Förderung der wissenschaftlichen Forschung is gratefully acknowledged.

## References

1. M. Lapp, L.M. Goldman, C.M. Penney: Science 174, 112 (1972)
2. M. Lapp, C.M. Penney: In Advances in Infrared and Raman Spectroscopy, Vol. 3, ed. by R.J.H. Clark, R.E. Hester (Heyden, London 1977) pp. 204-261
3. M.C. Drake, G.M. Rosenblatt: In Characterization of High Temperature Vapors and Gases, ed. by J.W. Hastie, NBS Special Publication 561 (US Govt. Printing Office, Washington, DC 1979) pp. 609-646
4. B. Attal, M. Pealat, J.P. Taran: J. de Physique 44, Colloque C7, 287 (1983)
5. G. Leyendecker, J. Doppelbauer, D. Bäuerle, P. Geittner, H. Lydtin: Appl. Phys. A30, 237 (1983)
6. J. Doppelbauer, G. Leyendecker, D. Bäuerle: Appl. Phys. B33, 141 (1984)
7. M. Lapp: In Laser Raman Gas Diagnostics, ed. by M. Lapp, C.M. Penney (Plenum, New York 1974) p. 108
8. D.L. Rousseau, J.M. Friedman, P.F. Williams: In Raman Spectroscopy of Gases and Liquids, ed. by A. Weber (Topics in Current Physics 11, Springer, Berlin, Heidelberg, New York 1979) pp. 203-252
9. G. Herzberg: Molecular Spectra and Molecular Structure, Vol. 2: Infrared and Raman Spectra of Polyatomic Molecules (Van Nostrand, New York 1945)
10. L.M. Cheung, D.M. Bishop, D.C. Drapcho, G.M. Rosenblatt: Chem. Phys. Lett. 80, 445 (1981)
11. J.A. Salzman, W.J. Masica, T.A. Coney: NASA TN D-6336 (1971)
12. A.C. Eckbreth: J. Appl. Phys. 48, 4473 (1977)
13. J. Bloem, L.J. Giling: In Current Topics in Materials Science, Vol. 1, ed. by E. Kaldis (North Holland, Amsterdam 1978) p.147
14. T.O. Sedgwick, J.E. Smith, Jr.: J. Electrochem. Soc. 123, 254 (1976)
15. W.G. Breiland, M.J. Kushner: Appl. Phys. Lett. 42, 395 (1983)
16. M. Koppitz, R. Bahnen, M. Heyen, W. Richter: this volume
17. J. Bouix, M.P. Berthet, M. Boubehira, J. Dazord, H. Vincent: J. Electrochem. Soc. 129, 2338 (1982)
18. G.H. Miller, A.J. Mulac, P.J. Hargis, Jr.: In Characterization of High Temperature Vapors and Gases, ed. by J.W. Hastie, NBS Special Publication 561 (US Govt. Printing Office, Washington 1979) p. 1135
19. G. Webb: In Comprehensive Chemical Kinetics, ed. by C.H. Bamford, C.F.M. Tipper (Elsevier, Amsterdam 1978) p. 50
20. P. Ho, M.E. Coltrin, W.G. Breiland: this volume
21. P.J. Hargis, Jr.: this volume
22. R.J. Hall, J.A. Shirley: Appl. Spectr. 37, 196 (1983)
23. M. Hanabusa, H. Kikuchi: Jap. J. Appl. Phys. 22, L712 (1983)
24. W.M. Tolles, R.D. Turner: Appl. Spectr. 31, 96 (1977)

# Laser Spectroscopy and Gas-Phase Chemistry in CVD

Pauline Ho, Michael E. Coltrin, and William G. Breiland

Sandia National Laboratories, Division 1126, P.O. Box 5800
Albuquerque, NM 87185, USA

Experimental studies of CVD utilizing laser-diagnostic techniques are closely coordinated with theoretical modelling. Laser Raman spectroscopy, laser velocimetry and laser-excited fluorescence techniques are used to probe the gas phase. The model carefully treats the coupled fluid dynamics and gas-phase chemistry of silane CVD. Deposition rates predicted by the model agree with data from the literature. The presence of $Si_2$ was predicted by the model and observed with laser-excited fluorescence. The results indicate that gas-phase chemical kinetics and reactive intermediate species are important in silane CVD.

## I. Introduction

We are pursuing a closely coordinated experimental [1-3] and theoretical [4] program to investigate the fundamentals of chemical vapor deposition (CVD). The experimental work involves the use of laser spectroscopic techniques for measurements in a CVD reactor. The theoretical work consists of a computer model for CVD that carefully treats the coupled fluid dynamics and gas-phase chemical kinetics of the CVD process. We use the deposition of silicon from silane as a relatively simple, yet representative, system for these studies. The use of laser techniques for measuring species concentration profiles and local gas temperatures and velocities allows us to make rigorous tests of the predictions of the model.

## II. Laser Diagnostic Techniques

Analytical measurements in a CVD reactor during deposition pose a difficult challenge to the experimentalist. The ideal probe for such measurements must be non-intrusive, selective, sensitive, general, and capable of high spatial resolution in the presence of rapidly changing chemical and temperature fields. Laser techniques come close to meeting all these requirements.

### A. Laser Raman Spectroscopy

Laser Raman spectroscopy can be used during deposition to measure local species concentrations and gas temperatures [1,5-11]. The primary advantages of Raman techniques are high spatial resolution, selectivity, and generality--virtually all species exhibit Raman spectra. The disadvantage of spontaneous Raman spectroscopy is its insensitivity, which limits it to the study of stable reactant or product species. In the presence of large continuous background signals, such as susceptor blackbody radiation in CVD, the use of pulsed lasers and gated detection greatly improves signal-to-noise and detection limits.

We have used rotational Raman spectroscopy to measure gas-phase temperatures as a function of height above the susceptor in a CVD cell. Fig. 1 shows temperature profiles obtained for identical flow conditions in nitrogen and helium carrier gases. A small amount of hydrogen was added to the helium as a "thermometer" to provide temperature measurements. Two features relevant to CVD are illustrated in Fig. 1. First, inert carrier gases such as nitrogen and helium are not equivalent; their fluid dynamic properties differ sufficiently to produce drastically different temperature profiles, which in turn could affect the deposition chemistry. Second, fairly high temperatures are achieved in the gas phase for distances up to 1 cm above the susceptor when helium carrier gas is used. Similar profiles occur in hydrogen. Because the chemical reactants typically used in CVD are chosen to be unstable at high temperatures, this strongly suggests that substantial gas-phase chemistry occurs under such circumstances.

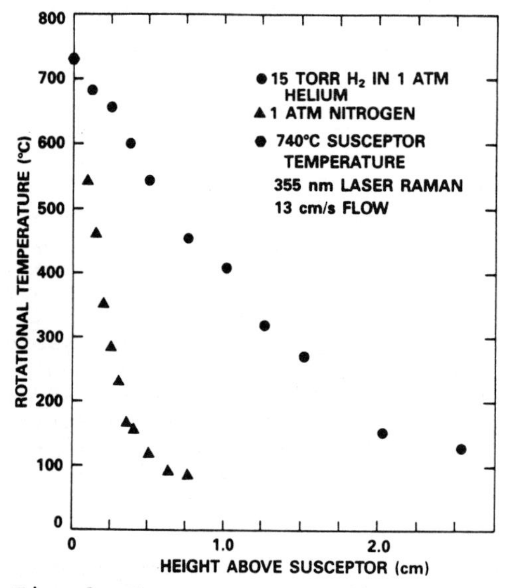


Fig. 1 Temperature profiles obtained from rotational Raman spectra in a CVD cell for nitrogen and helium carrier gases under identical flow conditions.

We have also used vibrational Raman spectra for the measurement of silane densitites as a function of position in the CVD reactor (Fig. 2). The Raman technique yields absolute measurements of gas densities, allowing quantitative comparisons. Partial pressures can be obtained from density measurements and local temperature measurements. We have also used laser Raman spectroscopy to monitor species such as $WF_6$, $SiCl_2H_2$ and $TiCl_4$.

B. Laser Velocimetry

Laser velocimetry provides measurements of gas-flow velocities [12, 13] as a function of position, which allows the flow proper-

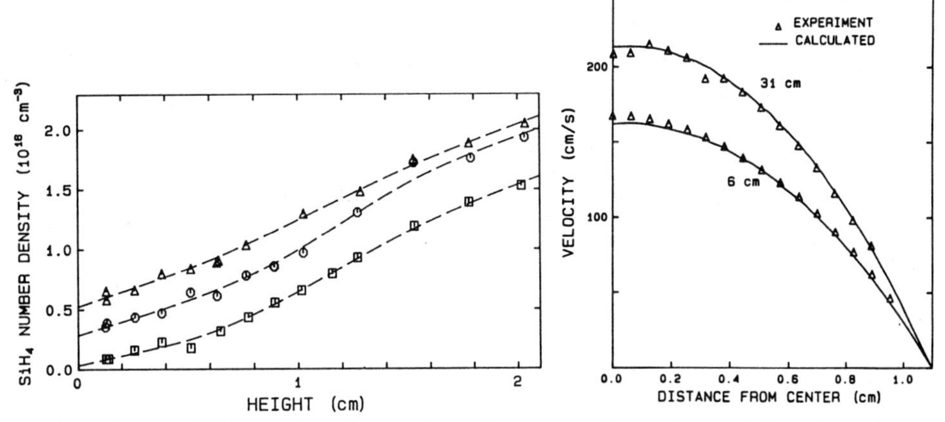


Fig. 2 Profiles of silane density as a function of height above the susceptor for three susceptor temperatures obtained using laser Raman spectroscopy. Susceptor temperatures: triangles = 550°C, circles = 650°C, squares = 750°C

Fig. 3 Comparison of experimental gas velocity measurements made using laser velocimetry with calculated velocity profiles. Velocities were measured 6 cm and 31 cm from the beginning of a 150°C heated section of the tube. Room-temperature maximum velocity of the helium gas was 162 cm/s. As the gas heats up, it expands and the velocity increases.

ties of a given CVD reactor to be characterized. Since the theory of fluid mechanics is well understood for laminar flow, it is possible to construct specialized research CVD reactors whose geometries are simple enough to be accurately described by theoretical fluid-dynamic models. We have used laser velocimetry measurements to verify calculations of gas velocities within a reactor. By using special cell geometries, it should be easier to separate the effects of fluid dynamics, gas-phase chemistry and surface processes in CVD.

The results from laser velocimetry measurement on a heated, vertical, cylindrical cell are shown in Fig. 3. The fluid dynamics of this geometry are well understood, and the agreement between experiment and theory confirms that this cell can be modeled successfully. The data in Fig. 3 also show the precision and the accuracy of the experimental technique, demonstrating that laser velocimetry could also be used as a diagnostic tool to characterize the flow patterns in conventional CVD reactors.

C. Laser-excited Fluorescence

Laser-excited fluorescence (LEF) is a very sensitive technique that can be used to detect chemical species that are present in extremely low concentrations. LEF is routinely used to detect species present at the level of $10^{10}$ molecules cm$^{-3}$ ($10^{-6}$ Torr), which makes the technique especially useful for monitoring highly-reactive chemical intermediates in the gas phase. The LEF method can also provide a means for unequivocal identification of a given species. The extremely high sensitivity and selectivity of LEF is somewhat offset by its lack of generality. For the technique to be successful, the molecule of interest must have a reasonable number of absorption and emission lines. In addition, very few molecules exist for which quantitative determinations of absolute concentration are possible, although relative concentrations can usually be obtained. Despite these shortcomings, LEF is one of the most powerful tools for identifying highly unstable chemical intermediates in the gas phase.

Using laser-excited fluorescence, we have observed the reactive intermediate species HSiCl during dichlorosilane CVD [2]. HSiCl was detected above a 750°C susceptor both in pure dichlorosilane (4 Torr) and in a mixture of dichlorosilane (4 Torr) and an atmosphere of helium carrier gas. Fig. 4 shows the observed fluorescence excitation spectrum of HSiCl, where each lettered band contains several vibronic transitions. Fig. 5 is an expanded plot of the band labeled "B" in Fig. 4 and shows the calculated line positions [14] for the rotational substructure of the band. The observed spectral features in Fig. 5 can all be assigned to HSiCl subbands. The main progression in the observed spectrum is the 'r' rotational K-subband of the 000-000 vibronic transition. The HSiCl dispersed fluorescence spectrum is shown in Fig. 6, which also shows the calculated line positions for three HSiCl vibronic progressions. The excellent agreement between the experimental and calculated line positions clearly identifies the emitting species as HSiCl.

The emission shown in Fig. 6 was previously observed in CVD by Sedgwick et al.[7, 15], but they misassigned it to $SiCl_2$. Figure 7 shows profiles of HSiCl fluorescence intensity, which is proportional to the HSiCl density, as a function of height above the susceptor for both low and atmospheric total pressure. The fact that the profiles exhibit maxima above the surface indicate that these species are products of gas-phase reactions rather than products of surface reactions diffusing into gas.

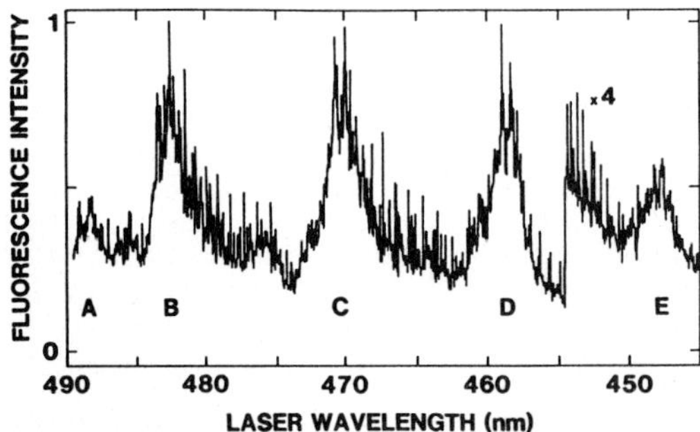


Fig. 4 Fluorescence-excitation spectrum of HSiCl observed during dichlorosilane CVD. The bands labeled A-E contain the following vibronic band origins ($v_1'$, $v_2'$, $v_3'$, $-v_1''$, $v_2''$, $v_3''$) as calculated from the constants of Herzberg and Verma [14]: A = (010-000), (001-010); B = (000-000), (001-001), (010,001), C = (010-000), (001-000), (011-001), (020-001); D = (020-000), (011-000), (021-001), (030-001; E = (030-001), (021-000), (031-001), (040-001).

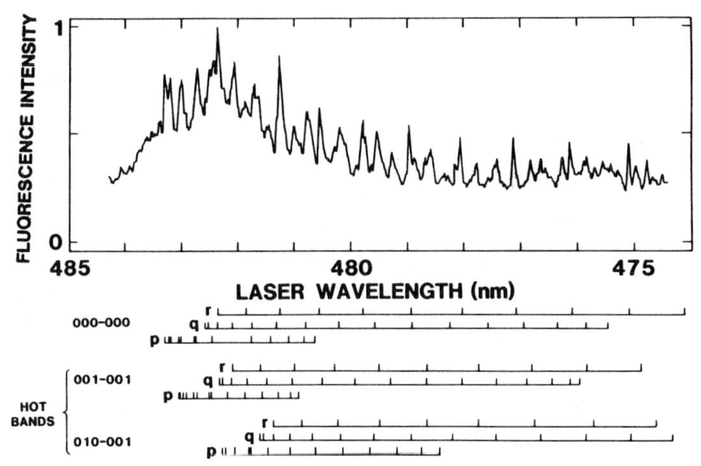


Fig.5 Rotational K-Subband assignments near the origin, labeled as band B in Fig.4. Calculated line positions are plotted below the spectrum.

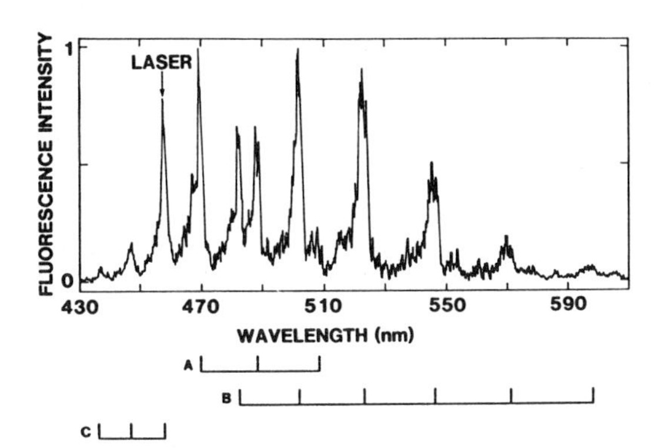


Fig.6. Spectrum of HSiCl fluorescence observed during dichlorosilane CVD. The emission is a result of excitation by a dye laser at 457.5 nm as indicated in the figure. The calculated vibronic progressions are A=(010-000) to (010-020), B=(000-000) to (000-050), C=(040-000) to (020-000).

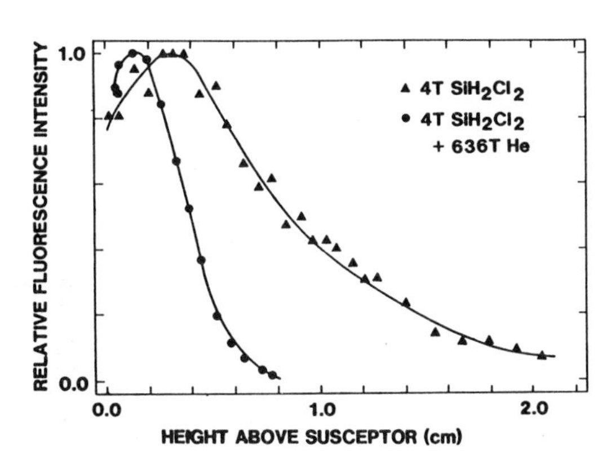


Fig.7 Profiles of the relative HSiCl density as a function of height above the susceptor at atmospheric and low total pressures. HSiCl fluorescence intensities have been normalized to a maximum of 1.0; the HSiCl was excited at 482.4 nm.

## III. Theoretical Model for Silane CVD

Our model [4] contains a detailed treatment of the coupled gas-phase chemistry and fluid mechanics in a CVD reactor. This treatment of the gas phase is unique among CVD models, which have often concentrated on surface reactions and treated the gas-phase very simply. The chemical reaction mechanism is comprised of 20 sets of forward and backward elementary reactions (see Table). This was derived from an initial 120-reaction mechanism using a sensitivity analysis. Kinetic parameters for gas-phase reactions were taken from the literature or estimated using standard techniques. Our model has a very simple treatment of surface reactions. Silane is assumed to react on the surface with the small probability measured by Farrow [16]. In the absence of experimental measurements, unstable intermediate species such as $SiH_2$, $Si_2H_2$, etc., are assumed to form Si(s) with unit probability upon collision with the silicon surface.

TABLE: REACTION MECHANISM

| Reaction | Reaction | A[(a)] | $E_a$[(a)] |
|---|---|---|---|
| R1 | $SiH_4 \rightarrow SiH_2 + H_2$ | 5.00E12 | 52.2 |
| R2 | $SiH_4 \rightarrow SiH_3 + H$ | 3.69E15 | 93.0 |
| R3 | $SiH_4 + SiH_2 \rightarrow Si_2H_6$ | 5.01E12 | 1.29 |
| R4 | $Si_2H_4 + H_2 \rightarrow SiH_4 + SiH_2$ | 6.22E16 | 2.0 |
| R5 | $SiH_4 + H \rightarrow SiH_3 + H_2$ | 1.04E14 | 2.5 |
| R6 | $SiH_4 + SiH_3 \rightarrow Si_2H_5 + H_2$ | 1.77E12 | 4.4 |
| R7 | $SiH_4 + SiH \rightarrow SiH_3 + SiH_2$ | 1.38E12 | 11.2 |
| R8 | $SiH_4 + SiH \rightarrow Si_2H_5$ | 2.93E12 | 2.0 |
| R9 | $SiH_4 + Si \rightarrow 2SiH_2$ | 9.31E12 | 2.0 |
| R10 | $Si + H_2 \rightarrow SiH_2$ | 1.15E14 | 2.0 |
| R11 | $SiH_2 + SiH \rightarrow Si_2H_3$ | 1.26E13 | 2.0 |
| R12 | $SiH_2 + Si \rightarrow Si_2H_2$ | 7.24E12 | 2.0 |
| R13 | $SiH_2 + Si_3 \rightarrow Si_2H_2 + Si_2$ | 1.43E11 | 18.8 |
| R14 | $H_2 + Si_2H_2 \rightarrow Si_2H_4$ | 2.45E14 | 2.0 |
| R15 | $H_2 + Si_2H_4 \rightarrow Si_2H_6$ | 9.31E12 | 2.0 |
| R16 | $H_2 + SiH \rightarrow SiH_3$ | 3.45E13 | 2.0 |
| R17 | $H_2 + Si_2 \rightarrow Si_2H_2$ | 1.54E13 | 2.0 |
| R18 | $H_2 + Si_2H_3 \rightarrow Si_2H_5$ | 2.96E13 | 2.0 |
| R19 | $Si_2H_2 + H \rightarrow Si_2H_3$ | 8.63E14 | 2.0 |
| R20 | $Si + Si_3 \rightarrow 2Si_2$ | 2.06E12 | 24.1 |

(a) Arrhenius parameters in the form $K_i = A_i \exp(-E_a/RT)$. The units of $A_i$ depend on the reaction order, but are given in terms of moles, cubic centimeters, and seconds. $E_a$ is in kcal/mole. For details, see Ref. [4].

The model predicts gas-phase temperature and velocity profiles, concentration profiles for 14 chemical species, deposition rates and deposition uniformity as a function of the various operating parameters. Deposition rates predicted by our model as a function of temperature, carrier gas, and total pressure are plotted in Fig. 9. This figure represents a wide range of conditions of interest to test the model. Experimental deposition rates for a simple cell geometry that can be well described by our two-dimensional model are available only for the case of $H_2$ carrier gas [17]. These data are plotted in Fig. 8 as the solid triangles.

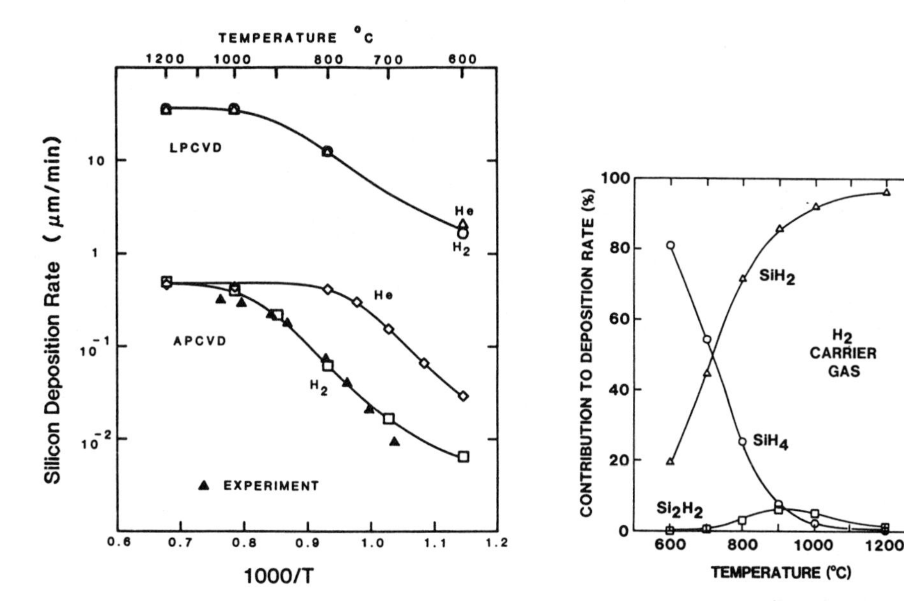


Fig. 8 Deposition rates predicted by the model (open symbols) as a function of temperature, total pressure and carrier gas. Conditions for all calculations: average gas velocity = 60 cm/s, 0.76 torr $SiH_4$ in either 760 Torr of carrier gas (APCVD) or 7.6 Torr of carrier gas (LPCVD). Experimental data from Ref. [17] are given by the solid triangles. The solid curves have been drawn to distinguish between sets of calculated results.

Fig. 9 Percent contribution made to the deposition rate by various chemical species as a function of temperature in $H_2$ carrier gas. The chemical species and symbols are: $SiH_4$ (open circle), $SiH_2$ (open triangle), $Si_2H_2$ (open square).

Agreement between experimental and theoretical deposition rates is excellent over the temperature range 700-1000°C. The model quantitatively predicts the deposition rates, as well as the transition between the high-temperature behavior (weak temperature dependence) and low-temperature behavior (much higher apparent activation energy). The correct prediction of the low-temperature behavior is important because our model includes only a simple surface reaction mechanism. In our model, the activated character of the deposition rate at low temperature is principally due to the temperature dependence of the gas-phase reactions. The remaining carrier-gas and total pressure dependences of the deposition rate shown in Fig. 8 are also in qualitative agreement with experimental deposition rate behavior.

The model predicts that the chemical species that are primary contributors to the deposition process change with the experimental conditions. Fig. 9 gives the percent contribution to the deposition rate of the various silicon-containing chemical species in $H_2$ carrier gas over the temperature range 600-1200°C. At low temperature the surface decomposition of silane itself contributes most to deposition. Below about 700°C, the gas-phase reactions are very slow in $H_2$ carrier gas because the excess $H_2$ inhibits the decomposition rate by shifting the equilibrium toward the reactants. At higher temperatures, $SiH_2$ becomes the most important species contributing to deposition.

Figure 10 is a similar plot for He carrier gas. Gas-phase chemistry is much faster in He than in $H_2$, so the surface decomposition of $SiH_4$ is a minor contribution to the solid, even at 600°C. At temperatures below about 1000°C, $Si_2H_2$ contributes most to the deposition rate. At higher temperatures, $Si_2$ and $Si_3$ make the largest contribution to the deposition rate. Formation of these species is also suppressed in $H_2$.

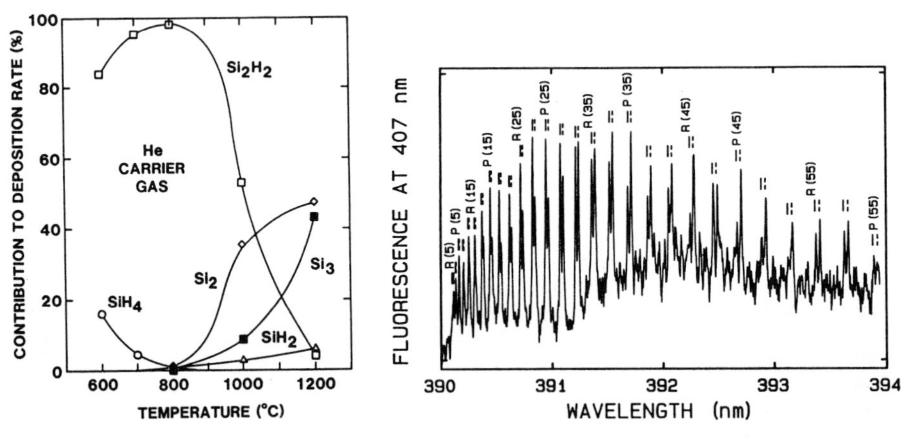


Fig. 10 Percent contribution made to the deposition rate by various chemical species as a function of temperature in He carrier gas. The chemical species and symbols are: $SiH_4$ (open circle), $SiH_2$ (open triangle), $Si_2H_2$ (open square), $Si_2$ (open diamond), $Si_3$ (closed square).

Fig. 11 Fluorescence-excitation spectrum of $Si_2$ during silane CVD, obtained by monitoring total fluorescence while tuning the laser frequency. Dashed and solid lines indicate calculated line positions for the P and R branches, respectively, of the 5-0 vibronic band of the H-X transition of $Si_2$.

## IV $Si_2$

Our model for silane CVD predicts that large concentrations of $Si_2$ and $Si_3$ should be present in the gas phase, close to the susceptor. Based on this prediction, we used laser-excited fluorescence to detect the intermediate species $Si_2$ (Figs. 11, 12) during silane CVD [3]. Figure 11 shows the fluorescence excitation spectrum of $Si_2$ we observed using 0.3 Torr silane in an atmosphere of helium carrier gas about a 740°C susceptor. Fig. 11 also shows line positions calculated from the known spectroscopic constants for $Si_2$ [18, 19]. The dashed and solid lines indicate the calculated positions for the P and R branches, respectively. The dispersed fluorescence spectrum for $Si_2$ is shown in Fig. 12. The labels (v' - v") indicate the calculated

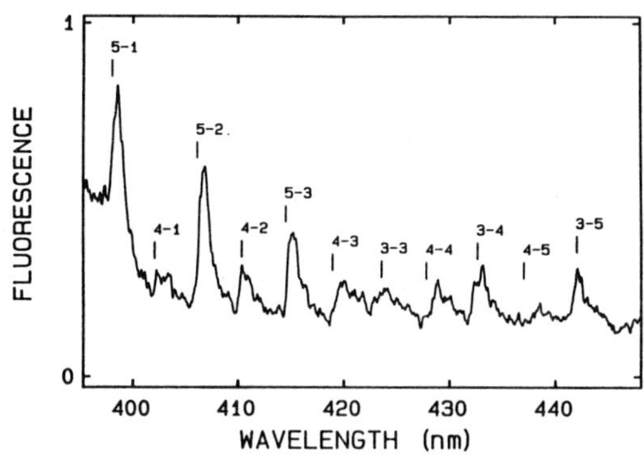


Fig. 12 Spectrum of the $Si_2$ fluorescence observed during silane CVD. Labels (v' - v") mark the calculated positions of the vibronic origins for the $Si_2$ H-X electronic transition.

positions of the vibronic origins for the $Si_2$ H - X transition. The excellent agreement between the observed and calculated line positions in both spectra shows that the emitting species is indeed $Si_2$.

Our LEF experiments on $Si_2$ constitute the first observation of a reactive intermediate species in the silane CVD system. This observation is also a dramatic confirmation that the gas is far from thermodynamic equilibrium. At equilibrium, the $Si_2$ concentration would be roughly $2 \times 10^{-18}$ Torr under the conditions of our experiments which is far below the detection limit of our LEF experiments.

Our model predicts that the $Si_2$ concentration should increase rapidly with increasing temperature, and be suppressed by the addition of hydrogen. As shown in Fig. 13, the $Si_2$ fluorescence is indeed strongly dependent on the amount of added hydrogen,

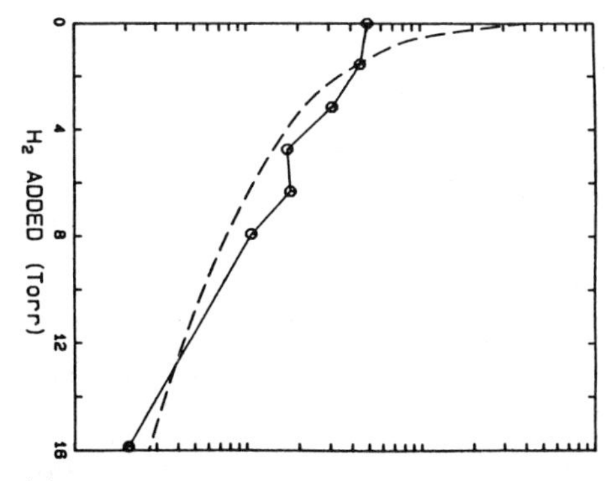


Fig. 13 Dependence of $Si_2$ density on added hydrogen. Points represent measurements of relative $Si_2$ fluorescence. Dashed curve represents $Si_2$ densities predicted by the computer model for silane CVD. Relative scaling arbitrary.

but the experimentally observed suppression is not as strong as that predicted by the model. It is also interesting that the behavior of the $Si_2$ and $Si_3$ concentrations correlate with experimental observations of gas-phase nucleation of particles. Particulates are observed to form very rapidly above a threshold temperature and are suppressed in a hydrogen carrier gas. Thus, $Si_2$ and $Si_3$ may be precursors to gas-phase nucleation of particles.

## V. Conclusion

We have developed a detailed mathematical model of the coupled fluid dynamics and gas-phase chemical kinetics in the CVD of silicon from silane. The model predicts gas temperatures, velocities, deposition rates and chemical species concentrations as a function of position in the cell, susceptor temperature, initial gas composition, pressure and flow velocity. Deposition rates predicted by the model quantitatively agree with data taken from the literature, without use of adjustable parameters. We have used laser diagnostic techniques to measure gas temperatures and velocities, and to monitor reactant species and unstable intermediate species profiles. The presence of $Si_2$ was predicted by the model and confirmed by laser-excited fluorescence experiments. This is the first direct observation of a gas-phase intermediate species in the silane CVD system. In contrast to previous work in the CVD field, our work thus far shows that gas-phase chemical kinetics are very important in chemical vapor deposition.

## References:


1. W. G. Breiland and M. J. Kushner: Appl. Phys. Lett. 42, 395 (1983)
2. P. Ho and W. G. Breiland: Appl. Phys. Lett. 43, 125 (1983)
3. P. Ho and W. G. Breiland: Appl. Phys. Lett. 44, 51 (1984)
4. M. E. Coltrin, R. J. Kee and J. A. Miller: J. Electrochem. Soc. 131, 425 (1984)
5. T. O. Sedgwick, J. E. Smith, Jr., R. Ghez and J. E. Cowher: J. Cryst. Growth 31, 264 (1975)
6. T. O. Sedgwick and J. E. Smith, Jr.: J. Electrochem. Soc. 123, 254 (1976)
7. J. E. Smith, Jr. and T. O. Sedgwick: Thin Solid Films 40, 1 (1977)
8. J. Bouix, M. P. Berthet, M. Boubehira, J. Dazord and H. Vincent: J. Electrochem. Soc. 129, 2339 (1982)
9. J. E. Smith, Jr., and T. O. Sedgwick: Lett. In Heat and Mass Transfer 2, 329 (1975)
10. G. Leyendecker, J. Doppelbauer, D. Bäuerle, P. Geittner and H. Lydtin: Appl. Phys. A30, 237 (1983)
11. J. Doppelbauer, G. Leyendecker and D. Bäuerle: Appl. Phys. B33, 141 (1984) see also: G. Leyendecker, J. Doppelbauer, D. Bäuerle: this volume
12. L. E. Drain: "The Laser Doppler Technique" (John Wiley and Sons, New York, 1980)

13. W. G. Breiland and P. Ho: "In Situ Measurements of Silicon CVD", Proceedings of the Ninth International Conference on CVD, Electrochemical Society, 1984
14. G. Herzberg and R. D. Verma: Can. J. Phys. 42, 395 (1964)
15. T. Sedgwick and G. V. Arbach: Proc. 10th Mat. Res. Symp. on Characterization of High Temp. Vapors and Gases (NBS Special Publication 561, Gaithersburg, Maryland, 1979) p. 885
16. R. F. C. Farrow: J. Electrochem. Soc. 121, 899 (1974)
17. C. H. J. van den Brekel: Thesis, University of Nijmegen, p. 66, 1978
18. R. D. Verma and P. A. Warsop: Can. J. Phys. 41, 152 (1963)
19. I. Dubois and H. Leclercq: Can. J. Phys. 49, 3053 (1971)

# Laser Diagnostic Studies of Plasma Etching and Deposition*

P.J. Hargis,Jr., R.W. Light, and J.M. Gee

Sandia National Laboratories, Albuquerque, NM 87185, USA

Laser excited fluorescence spectroscopy was used to determine that $CF_2$ radicals control the silicon dioxide to silicon etch ratio in fluorocarbon discharges used to etch silicon and silicon dioxide. $CF_2$ was found to control the etch ratio through polymer formation which selectively inhibits the silicon etch rate.

## 2 Introduction

Even though laser spectroscopy was first used for plasma diagnostics as early as 1972 [1-2], it is only in the last two years that this versatile technique has been applied to the study of glow discharges used in plasma etching and deposition [3-7]. Laser spectroscopic measurements are of increasing interest because they are generally non-perturbing, provide an unambiguous identification of atomic and molecular species, directly measure the concentration of ground state species, and can be used to achieve high spatial and temporal resolution. In this paper we discuss the application of laser spectroscopy to the study of the fluorocarbon plasma etching of silicon and silicon dioxide. Emphasis will be placed on the use of laser-excited fluorescence spectroscopy and pulsed-ultraviolet laser Raman spectroscopy to measure the concentration of gas-phase molecular species. Correlations between the concentration of molecular species and measured deposition and etch rates provide new insights into the mechanisms occurring in plasma etching processes.

## 3 Fluorocarbon Plasma Etching

The krypton-fluoride excimer laser is a convenient fluorescence excitation source for detecting ground-state $CF_2$ radicals in fluorocarbon discharges used to etch silicon and silicon dioxide [3]. Since ground-state concentrations are directly measured, etch rates can be correlated with the ground-state density of $CF_2$ to provide new insights into etching mechanisms.

Experiments to measure the correlation between the ground state concentration of $CF_2$ and silicon dioxide and silion etch rates were carried out in a Plasma-Therm model PK-2440 plasma etching reactor. All measurements were carried out with $CHF_3$ as the etchant gas. Typical measurements of the silicon dioxide to silicon etch ratio in this reactor are shown in Fig. 1 for wafers

*This work was performed at Sandia National Laboratories supported by the U.S. Department of Energy under contract number DE-AC04-76DP00789.

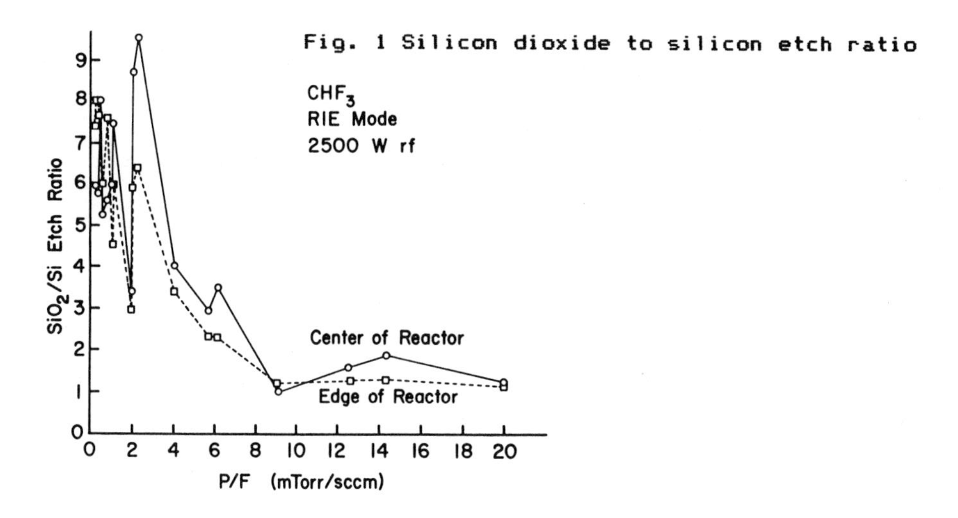


Fig. 1 Silicon dioxide to silicon etch ratio

placed in the center of the reactor and near the edge of the reactor.

Fluorescence measurements were carried out with a Lambda-Physics Model EMG-500 Krypton-fluoride excimer laser operating at a pulse repetition rate of 10 Hz and an energy of about 10 mJ/pulse. For all measurements the krypton-fluoride excimer laser was used to excite the X(0,0,0) to A(0,6,0) transition. A small 0.125 meter monochromator with an RCA C31034A photomultiplier tube was used to detect a single vibronic fluorescence line. A Princeton Applied Research Model 162 Boxcar integrator was used to read out the fluorescence signal. Absolute $CF_2$ number densities were determined from our flourescence measurements by calibrating the $CF_2$ fluorescence signal with respect to the Raman signal from a known density of nitrogen. This calibration was carried out in situ without disturbing the fluorescence instrumentation by backfilling the plasma etching reactor with a known density of nitrogen. The measured $CF_2$ ground state number density in the center of the reactor is shown in Fig. 2 for the same experimental conditions given in Fig.1.

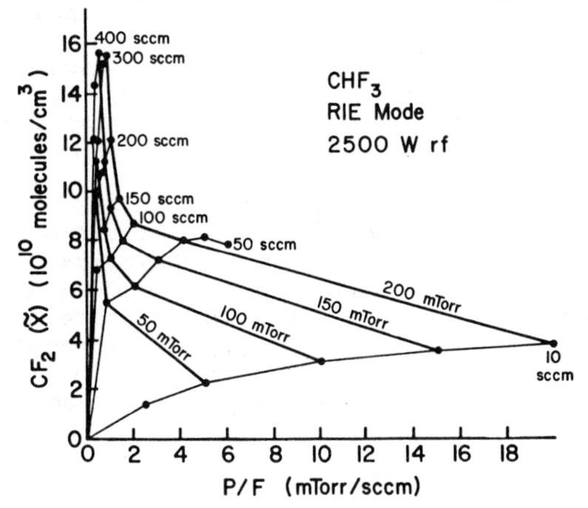


Fig. 2. $CF_2$ number density in plasma etching reactor

Figures 1 and 2 demonstrate that $CF_2$ is intimately related to the silicon dioxide to silicon etch ratio. This correlation is more evident when the silicon dioxide and silicon etch rates and ratio are plotted as a function of $CF_2$ number density in Fig. 3. Figure 3 shows that the oxide etch rate is independent of the $CF_2$ number density, whereas the silicon etch rate drops dramatically for $CF_2$ number densities between 4 and 8 X $10^{10}$ molecules/$cm^3$. This is more apparent from the etch ratio which also plotted in Fig. 3.

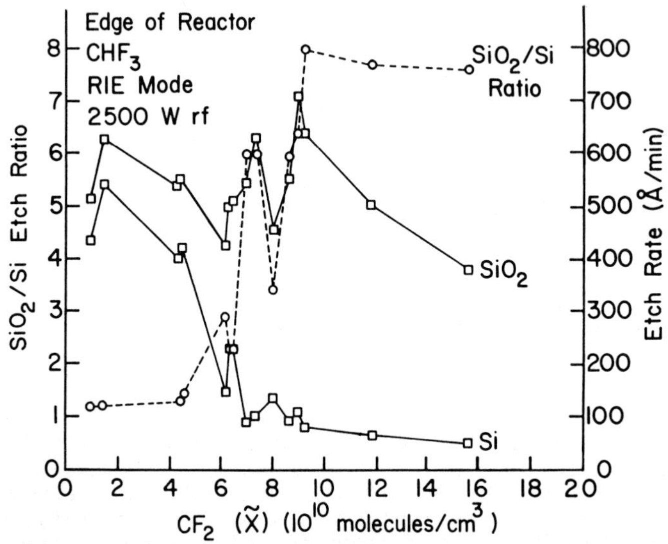


Fig. 3 Silicon dioxide and silicon etch rates and ratio as a function of $CF_2$ number density

Mass spectrometer measurements of the relative abundance of high mass fluorocarbon species in our reactor have shown that these species increase in abundance for $CF_2$ number densities greater than about 6 X $10^{10}$ molecules/$cm^3$. Since high mass fluorocarbons are the precursors for polymerization, it appears that $CF_2$ is intimately related to polymerization. This is even more apparent from our visual observation of polymer formation on the reactor sidewalls under conditions corresponding to high $CF_2$ number densities.

The precipitous increase in the oxide to silicon etch ratio for $CF_2$ number densities between 4 and 8 X $10^{10}$/$cm^3$ can thus be interpreted in terms of a polymerization model which results in the selective decrease of the silicon etch rate. Additional evidence for this interpretation comes by performing the same measurements in an $O_2$ - $CHF_3$ discharge. Oxygen addition to fluorocarbon discharges is known to result in a dramatic increase in the oxide and silicon etch rates. However, despite the differences in absolute etch rates, the oxide to silicon etch ratio shows an identical dependence on the $CF_2$ number density. Figure 4 shows the dependence of the oxide to silicon etch ratio on $CF_2$ number density for both the $CHF_3$ and $O_2$ - $CHF_3$ discharges.

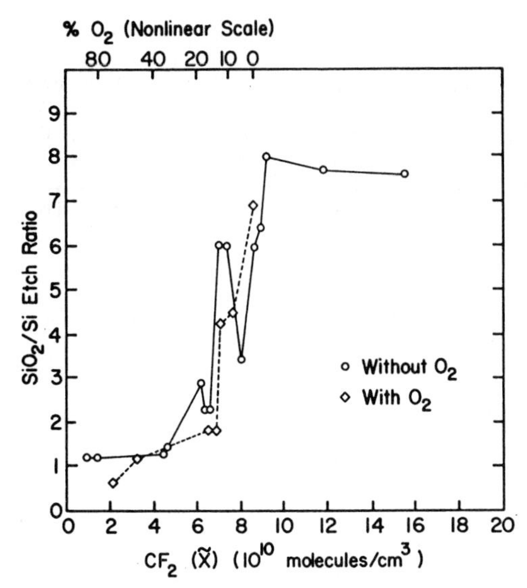


Fig. 4 Oxide to silicon etch ratio dependence on $CF_2$ number density

## 4 Conclusion

$CF_2$ radicals control the oxide to silicon etch ratio in fluorocarbon plasma etching reactors through polymer formation which selectively inhibits silicon etching. The oxide to silicon etch ratio is thus a unique function of the $CF_2$ number density in the reactor. This means that the performance of a given plasma etching reactor con be optimized by measuring the $CF_2$ number density in the reactor.

Acknowledgments
The authors would like to acknowledge the expert technical assistance of William Curtis in all aspects of this experiment.

## References

1. C.F. Burrell and H.-J. Kunze: Phys. Rev. Lett. 28, 1 (1972)
2. R.M. Measures and R.B. Rodrigo: Appl. Phys. Lett. 20, 102 (1972)
3. P.J. Hargis, Jr. and M.J. Kushner: Appl. Phys. Lett. 40, 779 (1982)
4. J.C. Knights, J.P.M. Schmitt, J. Perrin, and G. Guelachvili: J. Chem. Phys. 76, 3414 (1982)
5. R.A. Gottscho, G. Smolinsky, and R.H. Burton: J. Appl. Phys. 53, 5908 (1982)
6. V.M. Donnelly, D.L. Flamm, and G. Collins: J. Vac. Sci. Technol. 21, 817 (1982)
7. S. Pang and S.R.J. Brueck: In Laser Diagnostics and Photochemical Processing for Semiconductor Devices. ed. by R.M. Osgood, S.R.J. Brueck, and H.R. Schlossberg (North-Holland, New York, 1983) p. 161

# Light Scattering Diagnostics of Gas-Phase Epitaxial Growth (MOCVD-GaAs)

**M. Koppitz and W. Richter**
1. Physikalisches Institut and SFB 202, RWTH Aachen, Templergraben 55
D-5100 Aachen, Fed. Rep. of Germany

**R. Bahnen**
Technische Thermodynamik, RWTH Aachen, Templergraben 55
D-5100 Aachen, Fed. Rep. of Germany

**M. Heyen**
Institute of Semiconductor Electronics and SFB 202, RWTH Aachen,
Templergraben 55, D-5100 Aachen, Fed. Rep. of Germany

## 1. Introduction

In gas phase epitaxial processes the species forming the crystal lattice are transported in a carrier gas as gaseous compounds into a reactor. The compounds decompose in a high temperature region and are deposited on the substrate (see Fig. 1). Two main processes control the growth rate of the layer: (i) the transport of the reacting species to the substrate and (ii) kinetic processes at the surface, like adsorption and chemical reactions. In most cases during growth of GaAs from metalorganic compounds and $AsH_3$ (MOCVD) it appears that the transport to the surface is the growth rate limiting and controlling step. In this situation the hydrodynamics in the epitaxial reactor determine the growth process. Thus, at stationary conditions, the process is determined by the flow velocity $\underline{v}(\underline{r})$, the temperature $T(\underline{r})$ and the partial pressure of the reactants $p_i(\underline{r})$, where $\underline{r}$ gives the position in the reactor. The current density of reactants in the gas phase can be described by [1]

$$\underline{j}_i = p_i \cdot \underline{v} / (k \cdot T) - D_i (\nabla p_i + \alpha \cdot p_i \cdot \nabla \ln T) / (k \cdot T) \quad (1)$$

where $D_i$ is the diffusion coefficient of reactant i and $\alpha$ the thermodiffusion coefficient. The latter contribution may be especially important in cold wall reactors because of the considerable temperature gradients (only the substrate is heated). Since the partial pressures $p_i$ ( usually $10^{-3}$ to $10^{-2}$ bar) are much smaller than the carrier gas pressure (0.1 to 1 bar), the velocity

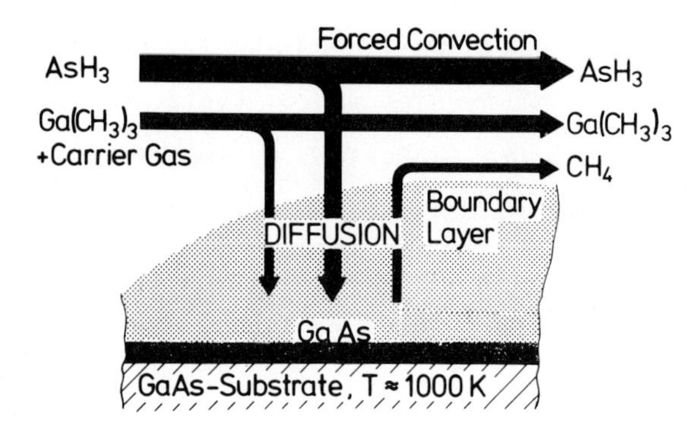


Fig. 1. Schematic diagram of the GaAs-MOCVD (Metal Organic Chemical Vapour Deposition) process. Typical conditions:
$p(AsH_3) = 10^{-3}$ bar
$p(Ga(CH_3)_3) = 10^{-4}$ bar
p (carrier gas, $N_2, H_2$) = 0.1 ... 1 bar

profiles $\underline{v}(\underline{r})$ and the $T(\underline{r})$ are essentially determined by the carrier gas properties. Even under this simplifying assumption a complete theoretical analysis, which must include the simultaneous solution of the partial differential equations of motion and thermal conductivity, is impossible. Only some numerical results for a two-dimensional system using the finite element method have been published [2].

Therefore, most discussions up to now are of a qualitative nature based on the assumption of a stagnant boundary layer above the substrate surface [3]. However, the experimental data for verification of this assumption are very limited. It is thus the purpose of this paper to demonstrate that light scattering is an ideal experimental method to analyze the hydrodynamic situation in an epitaxial reactor.

## 2. MOCVD Process and Reactor

Our interest here is focused on the growth of III-V compounds from metalorganic compounds and $AsH_3$ (MOCVD) [4]. A schematic diagram of the process has been shown in Fig. 1 for the case of GaAs. Although this method is well established for the growth of GaAs and GaAlAs films, the understanding of the mechanism of transport and reactions taking place in the gas phase or the growing surface is very limited. In addition the growth of InP based compounds along similar lines has been confronted with several difficulties [5], and makes a detailed investigation of the MOCVD process very desirable. As an example we have taken the GaAs growth which follows the overall reaction :

$$Ga(CH_3)_3 + AsH_3 \longrightarrow GaAs + 3CH_4 \qquad (2)$$

as shown in Fig. 1. The reactants are transported at room temperature in a carrier gas ($N_2$, $H_2$ at atmospheric pressure) into the reactor and react at the hot substrate surface. Since the forced flow is essentially parallel to the surface the main contribution for transport to the surface is caused by diffusion (second term in (1)). The experimental reactor designed specifically for light scattering investigations is shown in Fig. 2. Laser beams can enter the reactor through several windows as indicated in the diagram. The scattering volume from which information is sampled and which determines the spatial resolution can be as small as 50 μm in diameter.

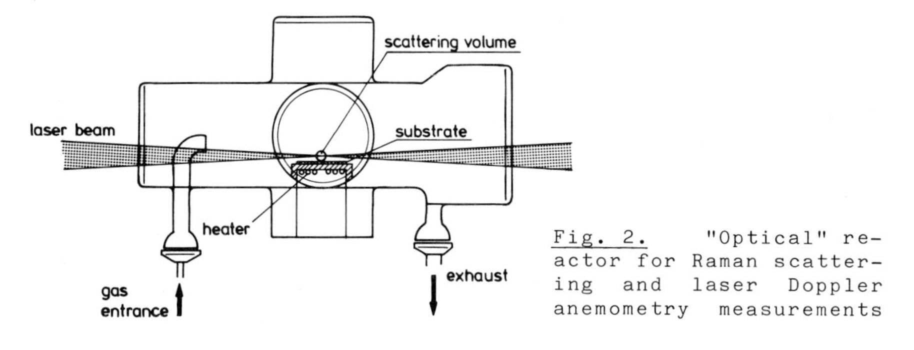


Fig. 2. "Optical" reactor for Raman scattering and laser Doppler anemometry measurements

Three different methods have been applied for the characterisation of the reactor: (i) velocity measurements by using laser Doppler anemometry, (ii) temperature measurements with the aid of rotational Raman scattering and (iii) concentration measurements of reactants by using vibrational Raman scattering. Since growth experiments have shown that the carrier gas can affect the growth process (rate, morphology), experiments were carried out in $H_2$ as well as in $N_2$.

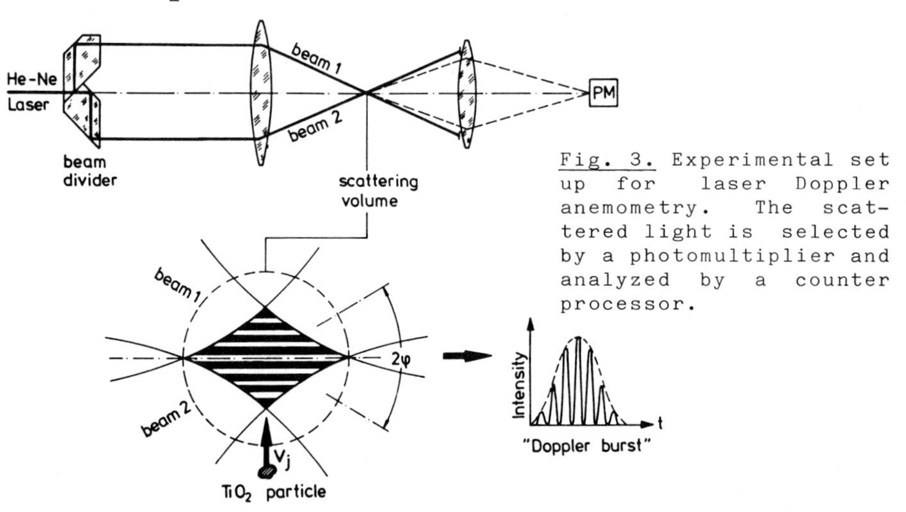


Fig. 3. Experimental set up for laser Doppler anemometry. The scattered light is selected by a photomultiplier and analyzed by a counter processor.

## 3. Velocity Measurements

For velocity determination two-beam laser anemometry has been used (Fig. 3). $TiO_2$ particles (approx. size 1 μm) were introduced into the gas stream and the two beams obtained from a He-Ne laser were guided perpendicular to the flow direction through the reactor. The scattered light measures the velocity component $v_j$ normal to the interference fringes as displayed in Fig. 3. This velocity is obtained by

$$v_j = \lambda \cdot \nu / (2 \sin \rho) \tag{3}$$

where $2\rho$ is the angle between the two beams and $\nu$ the measured frequency. By rotating the two beams into a different plane a second velocity component $v_k$ is obtained. Both $v_j$ and $v_k$ give the components of $\underline{v}$ in a plane perpendicular to the substrate. The results for the carrier gases $H_2$ and $N_2$ are shown in Fig. 4. For each point approximately 50 $TiO_2$ particles were sampled. The halfwidth ($2\,\Delta v$) of the Gaussian distribution within the 50 samples is a measure for the degree of turbulence ($\Delta v/v$) accompanying the laminar flow. The turbulence was 20% for $N_2$ and 2% for $H_2$. At large distances from the substrate the form of the velocity profiles in Fig. 4 is governed by entrance effects. Boundary layer effects show up close to the substrate (distance approx. 7 mm for hydrogen and 3 mm for nitrogen).

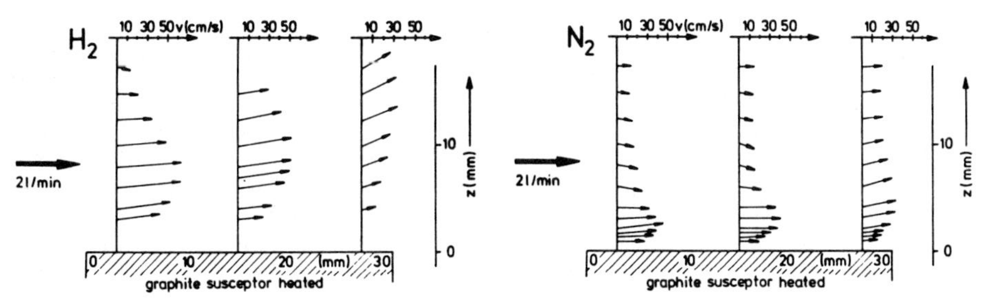


Fig. 4. Velocity profiles for $H_2$ and $N_2$

## 4. Temperature Measurements

For the determination of the local temperature the rotational Raman spectra of the diatomic carrier gas molecules have been utilized. By making the safe assumption of thermal equilibrium for all excitations within the scattering volume, the Maxwell-Boltzmann distribution governs the scattering intensity for high rotational quantum numbers and allows a very accurate determination of temperature [5,6]. The results in Fig. 5 again for $H_2$ and $N_2$ are plotted in the same plane as the velocity profiles in Fig. 4.

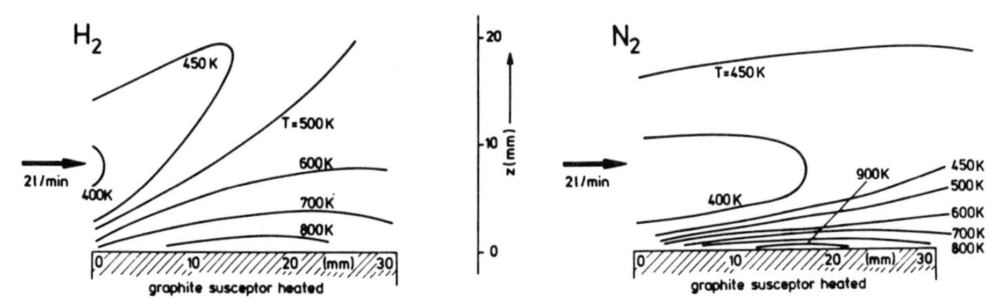


Fig. 5. Temperature profiles (isotherms) for $H_2$ and $N_2$

## 5. Discussion of v,T Profiles

For each carrier gas the velocity and temperature profiles are consistent. The boundary layer [3] has approximately the same size in the v and in the T plot. This is indeed expected for gases with Prandtl numbers close to one. The fact that the boundary region in $N_2$ is smaller than in $H_2$ is caused by the larger viscosity and larger thermal conductivity of the former. This causes a much steeper temperature gradient normal to the surface in $N_2$ (Fig. 5). Buoyancy driven convection effects are visible in both velocity profiles (Fig. 4) at the downstream edge of the susceptor as indicated by the direction of the velocity. They are pronounced in the case of $H_2$. Since no velocity measurements have been made perpendicular to the plane of the plot in Fig. 4, we cannot exclude that lateral vortex formation also takes place as has been observed by interference experiments in $N_2$ or Ar [7] since the Rayleigh numbers for nitrogen flow in the present reactor are in the order of 10000 (critical value: 1700).

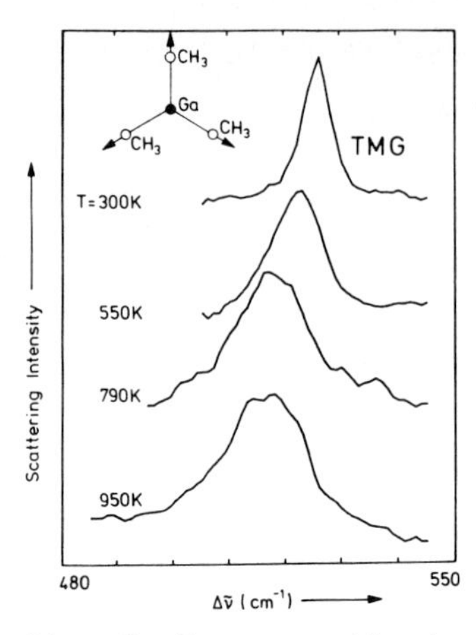


Fig. 6. Raman scattering spectra of $Ga(CH_3)_3$ (TMG) at different temperatures ($p_i = 10^{-2}$ bar)

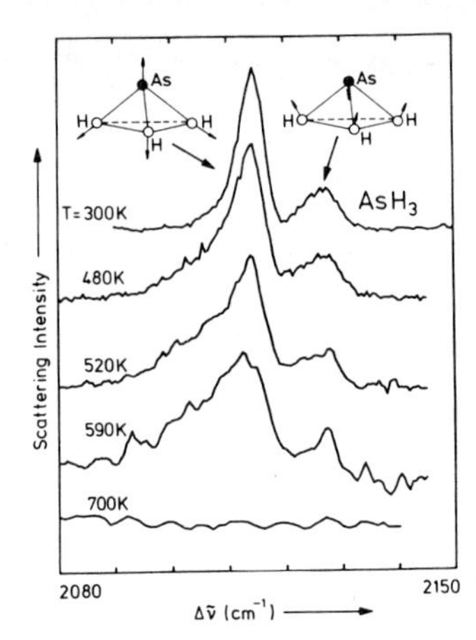


Fig. 7. Raman scattering spectra of $AsH_3$ at different temperatures ($p_i = 10^{-2}$ bar)

In the temperature profiles (Fig. 5) the bending of the isotherms at 400 and 450 K is also noteworthy. It is caused by heating (radiation, thermal convection) of the upper reactor wall. It could be avoided by the use of a water-cooled reactor [8].

## 6. Concentration Measurements

Concentrations of reactants were obtained from vibrational Raman scattering. Figures 6 and 7 show data for TMG (without $AsH_3$) and $AsH_3$ (without TMG) at different temperatures, which correspond to certain distances from the substrate. The normal modes measured are indicated in the top. The data describe the thermal decomposition of the two kinds of molecules. In contrast to what is known from plug flow measurements [9] TMG appears to be more stable than $AsH_3$. From such measurements the concentration (inte-

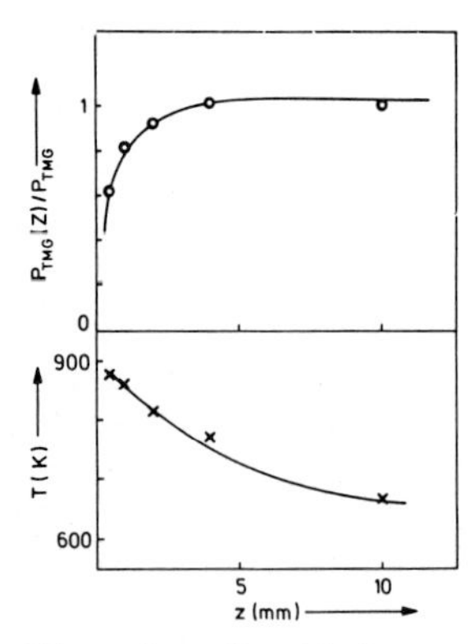


Fig. 8. Partial pressure of TMG normalized to the reactor input pressure at different heights and corresponding temperatures above the substrate

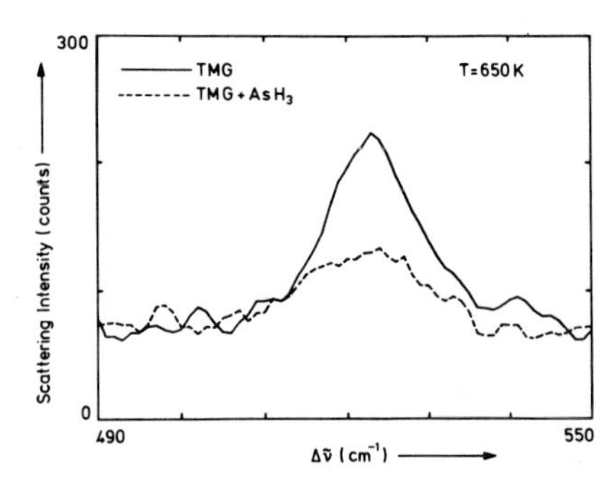


Fig. 9. Raman spectrum of TMG alone and in the presence of $AsH_3$

grated peak area) can be determined. Figure 8 gives the partial pressure as a function of height above the substrate for TMG. The depletion of TMG obviously occurs then in a very narrow region below 3 mm. The figure also shows that without $AsH_3$ being present, Ga is transported essentially in the form of TMG to the surface. This changes drastically when $AsH_3$ is added. Figure 9 shows two spectra of TMG with and without $AsH_3$. Clearly in the presence of $AsH_3$ the TMG structure becomes much weaker. This observation is in agreement with ref. [9]. However, a first search for new spectroscopic features was not successful.

## 7. Conclusions

It has been proven that light scattering is an ideal method for the in situ characterisation of CVD reactors. From the experimental data velocity, temperature and pressure gradients can be obtained. They allow for an estimate of the diffusion current of TMG with the help of (1). Assuming $D_i = 2\ cm^2/s$ and $\alpha = 1$ [2] (experimental values for TMG seem to be not available in the literature) we obtain j (TMG, normal to surface) = $4 \cdot 10^{20}\ m^{-2}s^{-1}$. Since TMG is the growth rate determining reactant in the MOCVD process a transport limited growth rate for a GaAs (100) surface of 60 µm/h can be calculated. This is in the same order of magnitude as experimental values (30 µm/h [4]).

## References


1. R.B. Bird, W.E. Stewart, E.N. Lightfoot: Transport Phenomena (Wiley, New York 1962)
2. V. Lewe, PhD. Diss. 1982, RWTH Aachen; C.W. Manke and L.F. Donaghey, in: Proc. 6th Int. Conf. CVD, Electrochem. Soc. Inc. 1977, p. 151
3. J .Bloem and L.J. Giling, in: Current Topics in Materials Science 1, p. 147 (North-Holland, Amsterdam 1978)
4. L. Hollan, J.P. Hallais and J.C. Brice, in: Current Topics in Materials Science 5, p. 5 (North-Holland, Amsterdam 1980)
5. M. Koppitz, O. Vestavik, W. Pletschen, A.Mircea, M.Heyen and W.Richter: J. Crystal Growth 68, 6 (1984)
6. G. Leyendecker, J. Doppelbauer, D. Bäuerle, P. Geittner and H. Lydtin: Appl. Phys. A39, 237 (1983)
7. L.J. Giling: J. Electrochem. Soc. 129, 634 (1982)
8. S.J. Bass, C. Pickering and M.L. Young: J. Crystal Growth 64, 68 (1983)
9. M.R. Leys: private communication and to be published

# On the Generation of $C_2$-Radicals by IR-Multiple-Photon Dissociation

H. Albrecht, H. Hohmann, and R. Grunwald

Central Institute of Optics and Spectroscopy of the Academy of Sciences of the GDR, Rudower Chaussee 6, DDR-1199 Berlin - Adlershof

## 1 INTRODUCTION

In most cases of laser assisted photolytic reactions, for example deposition, etching and doping of electronic materials, the laser was used to dissociate the parent molecules, i.e. to generate free radicals [1]. Among these laser assisted photolytic reactions the IR multiple photon dissociation (IR-MPD) is a powerful technique for the generation of free radicals [2]. In the present paper we give some results concerning the investigation of the production of $C_2$ radicals by IR-MPD of molecules, such as $C_2H_4$ and $C_2H_5Cl$, with TEA-$CO_2$-laser pulses. The spontaneous and laser induced fluorescence were used to detect the carbon radicals. We have investigated the pressure, excitation wavelength and time dependences of the (relative) concentration of the $C_2$ radicals in the $d^3\Pi_g$ and $a^3\Pi_u$ states of the well-known Swan band.

Dissociation of ethylene molecules in the intense IR field of a pulsed $CO_2$ laser and $C_2$ radicals as a fragment of this process were first observed in [3]. Furthermore the $C_2$ fragment had been detected in the $d^3\Pi_g$ and $a^3\Pi_u$ states, following the IR-MPD of a number of organic molecules [2]. Nevertheless, up to now the mechanism of the formation of $C_2$ radicals via IR-MPD is under discussion and an open question [4].

We observed in the tail of the laser pulses a remarkable production rate for $C_2$ radicals in either the ground or first excited triplet states. These results suggest the formation of highly excited primary radicals, which can be further dissociated to $C_2$ by relatively low laser intensities.

## 2 THE EXPERIMENTAL SETUP

We used an experimental setup typical for such investigations. The $CO_2$-laser radiation is focused into a stainless steel gas cell through a NaCl window by a NaCl lens (f = 6 cm ). Dissociation of the molecules occurs in the focal region of the lens. The ordinary and laser induced fluorescence from this region were directed by means of a two-lens condenser onto a photomultiplier FEU-106. The signal from the photomultiplier was amplified and monitored on a recorder after boxcar integration (BCl-280, 40 nsec gate and in most cases 16 samples) or on an oscillograph C-8-12. An interference filter ($\Delta\lambda$=10 nm ) was placed inside the condenser, which has a transparency maximum at 516 nm (ordinary fluorescence measurements). For LIF measurements the filter was turned to obtain the transparency maximum at 512,9 nm. These values coincide with the (0,0) and (1,1) lines of the $d^3\Pi_g \rightarrow a^3\Pi_u$ transition of the $C_2$ radical, respectively. To probe the laser induced fluorescence a 5.5 nsec dye laser pulse from an oscillator-amplifier system (Coumarin 102) pumped by a XeCl laser was directed into the gas cell perpendicular to both the excitation and observation directions. In all experiments the probing laser was tuned to 473.6 nm, i.e. to the (0,1) vibrational transition of the Swan band $d^3\Pi_g \leftarrow a^3\Pi_u$ of the $C_2$ radical. We always worked under saturation conditions. Pulses of the $CO_2$ laser and the probing laser were synchronized by means of an electronic circuit with 10 ns jitter.

We worked with two different TEA-$CO_2$-laser pulse shapes, i.e. a laser pulse with a "high" intensity tail containing about 50% of the total pulse energy ( 0.55 J ) and pulses with a "low" intensity tail containing about 25% of the total energy (0.36 J ). The gain-switch part of the laser pulses has the same shape in both cases and contains nearly the same amount of energy. The pulse shapes were controlled during the experiments by means of a photon drag detector and were held constant for all excitation wavelengths under investigation. Also for the pulses with "low" intensity tail the fluence in the focal region of the NaCl lens is always higher than 500 J/cm$^2$ and therefore has a value which is about one order of magnitude higher than the threshold value for IR-MPD of $C_2H_4$ [5].

## 3 EXPERIMENTAL RESULTS and DISCUSSIONS

Figure 1 shows the dependence of the normalized LIF signal on time for different excitation wavelengths and pulses with high

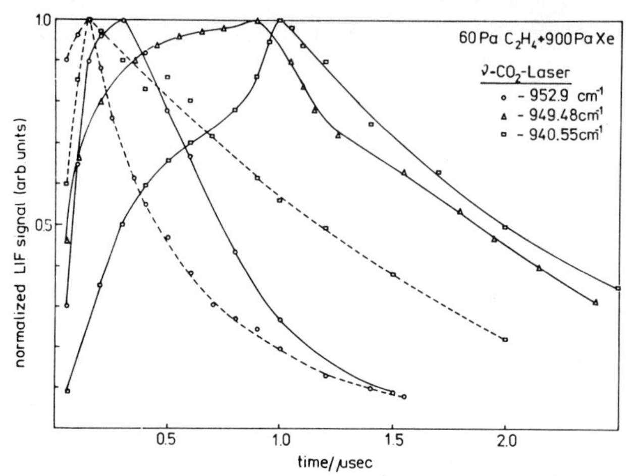


Fig. 1. Dependence of the normalized LIF signal on time for excitation pulses with high ( —— ) and low ( - - - )intensity tail

and low intensity tail exciting $C_2H_4$ molecules. Here t = 0 is the onset of the fluorescence signal. Under our experimental conditions we obtain a delay of ~40 nsec between the onsets of the fluorescence pulses. Because the LIF signal is proportional to the concentration of $C_2$ radicals in the $a^3\Pi_u$ state, we can compare the decays of the curves shown in Fig. 1 with the reaction rate constant for the reaction

$$C_2\ (a^3\Pi_u) + C_2H_4 \longrightarrow 2C_2H_2$$

measured in [6]. From the data in 6 for this reaction we calculate a lifetime of ~ 200 nsec $torr^{-1}$ for $C_2$ radicals in the $a^3\Pi_u$ state. Only for the 10P(10) $CO_2$-laser line ( $\nu$ = 952.9 $cm^{-1}$) and especially for excitation pulses with a low intensity tail we observed a fluorescence decay, which corresponds to this value. In all other cases, especially for longer laser wavelengths, the decays are considerably slower than expected from this lifetime.

Quantitatively the same behaviour was observed for ordinary fluorescence measurements, i.e. only for excitation pulses with a low intensity tail we obtained a fluorescence decay, which is comparable with the fluorescence lifetime of $C_2$ radicals in the $d^3\Pi_g$ state (~120 nsec [7]), whereas for high intensity tail pulses the fluorescence decay is considerably slower.

The observed slow decay of the radical concentration in both the ground and first excited triplet states and especially the increase of the radical concentration during the tail of the laser pulse ( see Fig. 1) result at least from two processes: from (probably internal) relaxation processes and from multiphoton excitation caused by the IR-laser field of the pulse tail, which has durations of up to 3 $\mu$sec or 2 $\mu$sec for high and low intensity tails, respectively. Because from the energetic point of view the consecutive detachment of two $H_2$ molecules is the more probable dissociation process for $C_2H_4$ in an intense IR-laser field[5], these results suggest the formation of probable highly excited primary radicals, which can be further dissociated to $C_2$ by relatively low laser intensities.

As for LIF measurements [5] we observed also for the ordinary fluorescence signal by IR-MPD of $C_2H_4$ a linear pressure dependence at pressures below 20 Pa, indicating the possibility of the $C_2$-radical production in the $d^3\Pi_g$ state under collisionless conditions. The quadratic pressure dependence above 20 Pa suggests the onset of rotational relaxation at that pressure value, which increases the number of molecules which can be excited by the IR-laser field. Adding a buffer gas, the rotational relaxation and therefore the yield of $C_2$ radicals can be **considerably** increased. As an example Fig. 2 shows the Xe pressure dependence of the LIF signal. Similar results were obtained for the ordinary fluorescence signal.

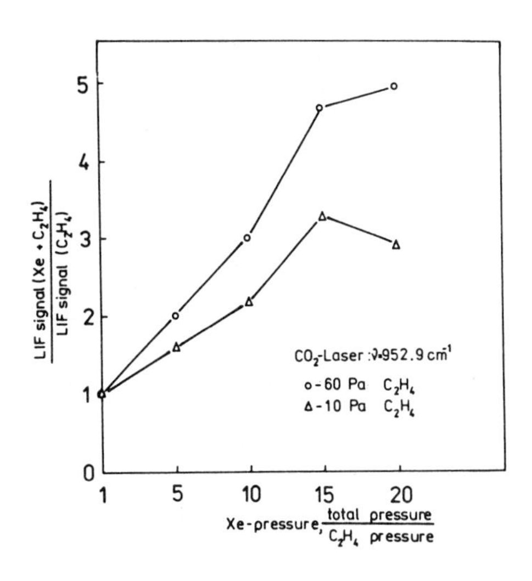


Fig. 2. The influence of Xe buffer gas on the peak LIF signal by the IR-MPD of $C_2H_4$

Investigations of the infrared multiphoton decomposition of $C_2H_5Cl$ [8] show that the following reaction takes place

$$C_2H_5Cl \xrightarrow{nh\nu} C_2H_4 + HCl,$$

i.e. the $C_2H_4$ molecule is a primary product, which can be further dissociated by IR-MPD. We have carried out experiments on IR-MPD of $C_2H_5Cl$ to obtain $C_2$ radicals. We observed qualitatively the same pressure dependence of the ordinary fluorescence signal by the excitation of $C_2H_5Cl$ as for $C_2H_4$ (see Fig. 3). This result suggests that below 30 Pa (linear pressure dependence) the excited $C_2$ radicals can be produced under collisionless conditions. For $C_2H_5Cl$ pressures below 30 Pa we observed two different decay processes, which dominate the time dependence of the ordinary fluorescence. Immediately after the peak, the fluorescence falls down with a time constant, which is comparable with the radiation lifetime of $C_2$ radicals in the $d^3\Pi_g$ state and - after that - starting at a time which is approximately equal to the rotational relaxation time ( $\tau_{RR}$~34 nsec $torr^{-1}$ , calculated from Fig. 3) it changes to a considerably slower decay regime.

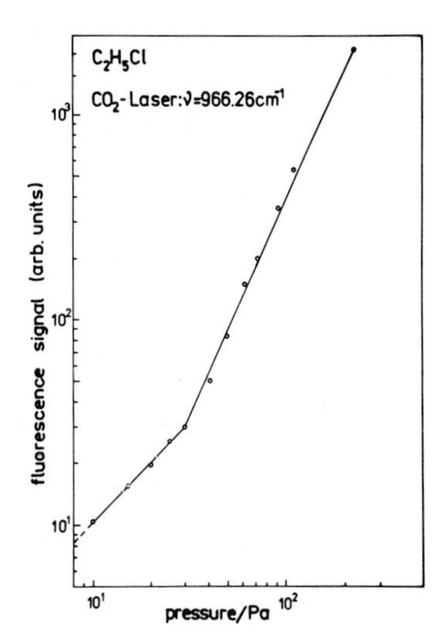


Fig. 3. The pressure dependence of the peak ordinary fluorescence signal exciting $C_2H_5Cl$ by $CO_2$-laser pulses with high intensity tail. The peak follows 150 nsec after the onset of the fluorescence signal

Figure 4 shows the IR multiple photon excitation wavelength dependence of the peak ordinary fluorescence signal for $C_2H_5Cl$ together with results concerning the decomposition of $C_2H_5Cl$ taken from [8]. In contrast to the decomposition rate measure-

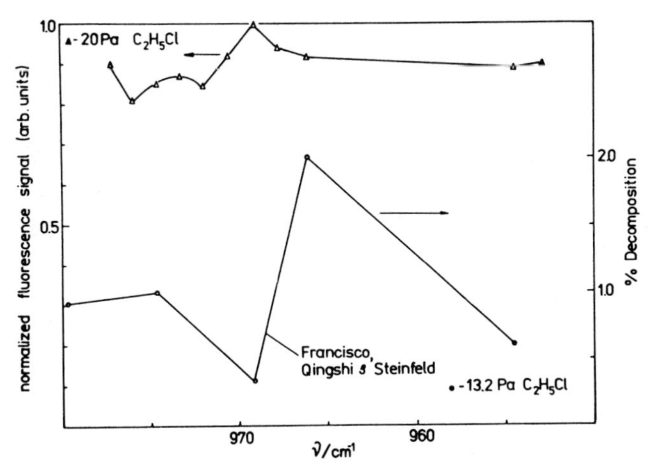


Fig. 4. The IR-MP excitation wavelength dependence of the peak ordinary fluorescence signal for $C_2H_5Cl$. The peaks follow 100-150 nsec after the onset of the fluorescence signal. Results from 9, concerning the decomposition of $C_2H_5Cl$, are also shown

ments we observed no significant excitation wavelength dependence of the fluorescence signal. Probably the further excitation of primary products (may be highly excited $C_2H_4$) to produce $C_2$ $(d^3\Pi_g)$ radicals **smears out this dependence.**

Further detailed investigations of the IR-MPD of $C_2H_5Cl$ **and $C_2H_4$ are in progress.**


1 "Surface Studies with Lasers" (Ed.: F.R. Aussenegg, A. Leitner, M.E. Lippitsch) Springer-Verlag Berlin, Heidelberg, New York, Tokyo (1983).

2 M.R. Levy, H. Reisler, M.S. Mangir, C. Wittig, Optical Engineering 19, 29 (1980).

3 R.V. Ambartzumian, N.V. Chekalin, V.S. Letokhov, E.A. Ryabov, Chem. Phys. Lett. 36, 301 (1975).

4 J.F. Caballero, C. Wittig, J. Chem. Phys. 78, 7169 (1983).

5 N.V. Chekalin, V.S. Letokhov, V.N. Lokhman, A.N. Shibanov, Chem. Physics 36, 415 (1979).

6 V.M. Donelly, L. Pasternack, Chem. Physics 39, 427 (1979).

7 N.V. Chekalin, V.S. Dolzhikov, V.S. Letokhov, V.N. Lokhman, A.N. Shibanov, Appl. Phys. 12, 191 (1977).

8 J.S. Fransisco, Zhu Qingshi, J.I. Steinfeld, J. Chem. Phys. 78, 5339 (1983).

# Index of Contributors

# Subject Index

# Springer Series in Chemical Physics

Editors: **V. I. Goldanskii, R. Gomer, F. P. Schäfer, J. P. Toennies**

Volume 1
**I. I. Sobelman**
## Atomic Spectra and Radiative Transitions
1979. 21 figures, 46 tables. XII, 306 pages.
ISBN 3-540-09082-7

Volume 2
**M. A. Van Hove, S. Y. Tong**
## Surface Crystallography by LEED
**Theory, Computation and Structural Results**
1979. 19 figures, 2 tables. IX, 286 pages.
ISBN 3-540-09194-7

Volume 3
## Advances in Laser Chemistry
Proceedings of the Conference on Advances in Laser Chemistry, California Institute of Technology, Pasadena, USA, March 20–22, 1978
Editor: **A. H. Zewail**
1978. 242 figures, 2 tables. X, 463 pages.
ISBN 3-540-08997-7

Volume 5
**W. Demtröder**
## Laser Spectroscopy
**Basic Concepts and Instrumentation**
2nd corrected printing. 1982. 431 figures.
XIII, 696 pages. ISBN 3-540-10343-0

Volume 6
## Laser-Induced Processes in Molecules
**Physics and Chemistry**
Proceedings of the European Physical Society, Divisonal Conference at Heriot-Watt University, Edinburgh, Scotland, September 20–22, 1978
Editors: **K. L. Kompa, S. D. Smith**
1979. 196 figures, 31 tables. XIV, 367 pages.
ISBN 3-540-09299-4

Volume 7
**I. I. Sobelman, L. A. Vainshtein, E. A. Yukov**
## Excitation of Atoms and Broadening of Spectral Lines
1981. 34 figures, 40 tables. X, 315 pages.
ISBN 3-540-09890-9

Volume 8
**Y. N. Molin, K. M. Salikhov, K. I. Zamaraev**
## Spin Exchange
**Principles and Applications in Chemistry and Biology**
1980. 68 figures, 41 tables. XI, 242 pages.
ISBN 3-540-10095-4

Volume 9
## Secondary Ion Mass Spectrometry SIMS-II
Proceedings of the Second International Conference on Secondary Ion Mass Spectrometry (SIMS II) Stanford University, Stanford, California, USA, August 27–31, 1979
Editors: **A. Benninghoven, C. A. Evans, Jr., R. A. Powell, R. Shimizu, H. A. Storms**
1979. 234 figures, 21 tables. XIII, 298 pages.
ISBN 3-540-09843-7

Volume 10
## Lasers and Chemical Change
By **A. Ben-Shaul, Y. Haas, K. L. Kompa, R. D. Levine**
1981. 245 figures. XII, 497 pages.
ISBN 3-540-10379-1

Volume 11
## Liquid Crystals of One- and Two-Dimensional Order
Proceedings of the Conference in Liquid Crystals of One- and Two-Dimensional Order and Their Applications, Garmisch-Partenkirchen, Federal Republic of Germany, January 21–25, 1980
Editors: **W. Helfrich, G. Heppke**
1980. 218 figures (some in color), 19 tables. XII, 416 pages. ISBN 3-540-10399-6

Volume 12
**S. A. Losev**
## Gasdynamic Laser
1981. 100 figures. X, 297 pages. ISBN 3-540-10503-4

Volume 13
**I. Lindgren, J. Morrison**
## Atomic Many-Body Theory
1982. 96 figures. XIII, 469 pages.
ISBN 3-540-10504-2

Volume 14
## Picosecond Phenomena II
Proceedings of the Second International Conference on Picosecond Phenomena, Cape Cod, Massachusetts, USA, June 18–20, 1980
Editors: **R. Hochstrasser, W. Kaiser, C. V. Shank**
1980. 252 figures, 17 tables. XII, 382 pages.
ISBN 3-540-10403-8

Volume 15
## Vibrational Spectroscopy of Adsorbates
Editor: **R. F. Willis**
With contributions by numerous experts
1980. 97 figures, 8 tables. XII, 184 pages.
ISBN 3-540-10429-1

Volume 17

**Inelastic Particle-Surface Collisions**

Proceedings of the Third International Workshop on Inelastic Ion-Surface Collisions
Feldkirchen-Westerham, Federal Republic of Germany, September 17–19, 1980
Editors: **E. Taglauer, W. Heiland**
1981. 194 figures. VIII, 329 pages. ISBN 3-540-10898-X

Volume 18

**Modelling of Chemical Reaction Systems**

Proceedings of an International Workshop, Heidelberg, Federal Republic of Germany,
September 1–5, 1980
Editors: **K. H. Ebert, P. Deuflhard, W. Jäger**
1981. 163 figures. X, 389 pages. ISBN 3-540-10983-8

Volume 19

**Secondary Ion Mass Spectrometry SIMS III**

Proceedings of the Third International Conference, Technical University, Budapest, Hungary,
August 30 – September 5, 1981
Editors: **A. Benninghoven, J. Giber, J. László, M. Riedel, H. W. Werner**
1982. 289 figures. XI, 444 pages. ISBN 3-540-11372-X

Volume 20

**Chemistry and Physics of Solid Surfaces IV**

Editors: **R. Vanselow, R. Howe**
1982. 247 figures. XIII, 496 pages
ISBN 3-540-11397-5

Volume 21

**Dynamics of Gas-Surface Interaction**

Proceedings of the International School on Material Science and Technology, Erice, Italy, July 1–15, 1981
Editors: **G. Benedek, U. Valbusa**
1982. 132 figures. XI, 282 pages. ISBN 3-540-11693-1

Volume 22
**V. S. Letokhov**

**Nonlinear Laser Chemistry**
**Multiple-Photon Excitation**
1983. 152 figures. XIV, 417 pages. ISBN 3-540-11705-9

Volume 23

**Picosecond Phenomena III**

Proceedings of the Third International Conference on Picosecond Phenomena Garmisch-Partenkirchen, Federal Republic of Germany,
June 16–18, 1982
Editors: **K. B. Eisenthal, R. M. Hochstrasser, W. Kaiser, A. Laubereau**
1982. 288 figures. XIII, 401 pages. ISBN 3-540-11912-4

Volume 24

**Desorption Induced by Electronic Transitions, DIET I**

Proceedings of the First International Workshop, Williamsburg, Virginia, USA, May 12–14, 1982
Editors: **N. H. Tolk, M. M. Traum, J. C. Tully, T. E. Madley**
1983. 112 figures. XI, 269 pages. ISBN 3-540-12127-7

Volume 25

**Ion Formation from Organic Solids**

Proceedings of the Second International Conference, Münster, Federal Republic of Germany,
September 7–9, 1982
Editor: **A. Benninghoven**
1983. 170 figures. IX, 269 pages. ISBN 3-540-12244-3

Volume 26
**B. C. Eu**

**Semiclassical Theories of Molecular Scattering**

1984. 17 figures. XII, 229 pages. ISBN 3-540-12410-1

Volume 27

**EXAFS and Near Edge Structures**

Proceedings of the International Conference, Frascati, Italy, September 13–17, 1982
Editors: **A. Bianconi, L. Incoccia, S. Stipcich**
1983. 316 figures. XII, 420 pages. ISBN 3-540-12411-X

Volume 33

**Surface Studies with Lasers**

Proceedings of the International Conference, Mauterndorf, Austria, March 9–11, 1983
Editors: **F. R. Aussenegg, A. Leitner, M. E. Lippitsch**
1983. 146 figures. IX, 241 pages. ISBN 3-540-12598-1

Volume 34

**Inert Gases**
**Potentials, Dynamics, and Energy Transfer in Doped Crystals**
Editor: **M. L. Klein**
With contributions by R. A. Aziz, S. S. Cohen, H. Dubost, M. L. Klein
1984. 89 figures. XI, 266 pages. ISBN 3-540-13128-0

Volume 35

**Chemistry and Physics of Solid Surfaces V**

Editors: **R. Vanselow, R. Howe**
1984. 303 figures. XXI, 554 pages. ISBN 3-540-13315-1

Volume 36

**Secondary Ion Mass Spectrometry SIMS IV**

Proceedings of the Fourth International Conference, Osaka, Japan, November 13–19, 1983
Editors: **A. Benninghoven, J. Okano, R. Shimizu, H. W. Werner**
1984. 415 figures. XV, 503 pages. ISBN 3-540-13316-X

Springer-Verlag
Berlin
Heidelberg
New York
Tokyo

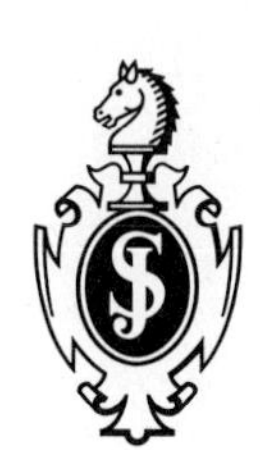